Nutrition, Weight, and Digestive Health

Carolyn Newberry • Janese Laster
Octavia Pickett-Blakely
Editors

Nutrition, Weight, and Digestive Health

The Clinician's Desk Reference

Springer

Editors
Carolyn Newberry
Division of Gastroenterology
Weill Cornell Medical Center
New York, NY, USA

Octavia Pickett-Blakely
GI Nutrition, Celiac Disease
and Obesity Program
University of Pennsylvania, Perelman
School of Medicine
Philadelphia, PA, USA

Janese Laster
Gastroenterology, Obesity Medicine
Nutrition and Bariatric Endoscopist
Gut Theory Total Digestive Care
George Washington University Hospital
Washington, DC, USA

ISBN 978-3-030-94952-5 ISBN 978-3-030-94953-2 (eBook)
https://doi.org/10.1007/978-3-030-94953-2

This Springer imprint is published by the registered company Springer Nature Switzerland AG
The registered company address is: Gewerbestrasse 11, 6330 Cham, Switzerland

Preface

In the last couple of decades, a deeper understanding of the link between nutrition, weight, and digestive health has come to the forefront of both patient and provider interest. Despite a growing body of literature and increased awareness, lack of medical practitioner knowledge and comfort level in the nutrition space often limits practical application. The aim of this book is to serve as a definitive nutritional reference for medical providers who care for patients with digestive diseases.

The book is divided into four sections, serving as a comprehensive reference tool as follows:

- The first section discusses basic nutritional concepts that lay a foundation for future chapters. This includes discussion of the gastrointestinal tract's role in digestion and metabolism, an outline of dietary composition and associated deficiencies, and a review of nutritional assessment and general therapeutic principles.
- The second section outlines dietary and nutritional implications of specific digestive diseases organized by affected gastrointestinal organ. It additionally discusses the use of prebiotics, probiotics, and herbal supplements and reviews food allergies and intolerances.
- The third section reviews appetite regulation, weight management, and obesity's association with gastrointestinal diseases. It also discusses the importance of comprehensive, multi-disciplinary obesity care including a review of dietary, pharmacological, endoscopic, and surgical options that promote weight loss.
- The fourth section discusses foundational nutritional support concepts. It additionally details management of both parenteral and enteral nutrition for use when oral diets are insufficient, not tolerated, or contraindicated in care.

Overall, our hope is this book empowers practitioners to incorporate nutrition and weight management principles into their care for patients with digestive diseases.

New York, NY, USA — Carolyn Newberry
Washington, DC, USA — Janese Laster
Philadelphia, PA, USA — Octavia Pickett-Blakely

Acknowledgments

The editors would like to acknowledge the work of all their talented authors, who helped bring this important desk reference to press. Additionally, they would like to thank the publisher, dedicated staff, and supportive family and friends for helping them recognize their goal of building a comprehensive textbook highlighting the intersection between nutrition and digestive diseases.

Contents

Contributors

Sarah Barenbaum, MD Department of Internal Medicine, Division of Endocrinology, Comprehensive Weight Control Center, NewYork-Presbyterian Hospital, Weill Cornell Medicine, New York, NY, USA

Sara Bonnes, MD Department of General Internal Medicine, Mayo Clinic, Rochester, MN, USA

Christian Brown, MD University of Florida, UF Health, Department of Surgery, Gainesville, FL, USA

Nicholas Caminiti, MD University of Louisville, Department of Surgery, Louisville, KY, USA

Perica Davitkov, MD Department of Gastroenterology and Hepatology, Digestive Health Institute, VA Northeast Ohio Healthcare System, Case Western Reserve University School of Medicine, Cleveland, OH, USA

Pratima Dibba, MD Department of Gastroenterology and Liver Disease, New York Presbyterian Brooklyn Methodist Hospital, Brooklyn, NY, USA

Russ Dolan, MD Brigham and Women's Hospital and Harvard Medical School, Boston, MA, USA

Andrew Eidelberg, BS Weill Cornell Medical College, New York, NY, USA

Ryan Fecteau, MD, PhD Department of Radiation Oncology, NewYork-Presbyterian Hospital, New York City, NY, USA

Anita Ganti, MD Department of Medicine, The Donald and Barbara Zucker School of Medicine at Hofstra-Northwell, Manhasset, NY, USA

Irwin Grosman, MD Department of Gastroenterology and Liver Disease, New York Presbyterian Brooklyn Methodist Hospital, Brooklyn, NY, USA

Ryan T. Hurt, MD, PhD Department of General Internal Medicine, Mayo Clinic, Rochester, MN, USA

Pichamol Jirapinyo, MD, MPH Brigham and Women's Hospital and Harvard Medical School, Boston, MA, USA

Jeanette N. Keith, MD Department of Medicine, Section of Gastroenterology, Decatur Morgan Hospital, Decatur Morgan GI and Nutrition, Decatur, AL, USA

Keerthana Kesavarapu, MD Robert Wood Johnson, Department of Gastroenterology, New Brunswick, NJ, USA

AnnMarie Kieber-Emmons, MD Department of Medicine, Division of Gastroenterology and Hepatology, Weill Cornell Medical College, New York City, NY, USA

Sindhura Kolli, MD Department of Internal Medicine, NYU Langone Comprehensive Program on Obesity, NYU School of Medicine, New York, NY, USA

Megha Kothari, MD Department of Gastroenterology and Liver Disease, New York Presbyterian Brooklyn Methodist Hospital, Brooklyn, NY, USA

Janese Laster, MD Gastroenterology, Obesity Medicine, Nutrition and Bariatric Endoscopist, Gut Theory Total Digestive Care, George Washington University Hospital, Washington, DC, USA

Elissa Lin, MD Department of Medicine, NYU Langone Health, New York, NY, USA

W. Aaron Marshall, MD University of Louisville, Department of Surgery, Louisville, KY, USA

Arnon Matan, MD Robert Wood Johnson, Department of Gastroenterology, New Brunswick, NJ, USA

Amit Mehta, MD Divison of Gastroenterology, The Johns Hopkins Hospital, Baltimore, MD, USA

Robin Mendelsohn, MD Division of Gastroenterology, Memorial Sloan Kettering Cancer Center, New York, NY, USA

Dejan Micic, MD Department of Internal Medicine, Section of Gastroenterology, Hepatology and Nutrition, University of Chicago, Chicago, IL, USA

Danny Mou, MD Department of Surgery, Brigham and Women's Hospital, Boston, MA, USA

Neil Nadpara, MD Temple University Hospital, Department of Internal Medicine, Philadelphia, PA, USA

Carolyn Newberry, MD Division of Gastroenterology, Weill Cornell Medical Center, New York, NY, USA

Lena B. Palmer, MD, MSCR Medicine, Gastroenterology, Southeast Louisiana Veterans Health Care System, New Orleans, LA, USA

Henry P. Parkman, MD Gastroenterology Section, Department of Medicine, Temple University School of Medicine, Philadelphia, PA, USA

Parita Patel, MD Department of Internal Medicine, Section of Gastroenterology, Hepatology and Nutrition, University of Chicago, Chicago, IL, USA

Violeta Popov, MD, PhD Department of Medicine, NYU Langone Health, New York, NY, USA

New York VA Harbor Healthcare System (Manhattan), New York, NY, USA

Ilana P. Redmond, MD Department of Internal Medicine, Division of Endocrinology, Comprehensive Weight Control Center, NewYork-Presbyterian Hospital, Weill Cornell Medicine, New York, NY, USA

Martin Rosenthal, MD University of Louisville, Department of Surgery, Louisville, KY, USA

Ennaliza Salazar, MD Department of Gastroenterology and Hepatology, Singapore General Hospital, Singapore, Singapore

Sagarika Satyavada, MD Department of Gastroenterology and Hepatology, Digestive Health Institute, University Hospitals Cleveland Medical Center, Case Western Reserve University School of Medicine, Cleveland, OH, USA

Katherine H. Saunders, MD Division of Endocrinology, Diabetes and Metabolism, New York-Presbyterian Hospital and Weill Cornell Medical Center, New York, NY, USA

Jessica Schucht, MD University of Louisville, Department of Surgery, Louisville, KY, USA

Shawn L. Shah, MD Division of Digestive and Liver Diseases, UT Southwestern Medical Center, Dallas, TX, USA

Raj Shah, MD Department of Gastroenterology and Hepatology, Digestive Health Institute, University Hospitals Cleveland Medical Center, Case Western Reserve University School of Medicine, Cleveland, OH, USA

Dariush Shahsavari, MD, FACP Gastroenterology Section, Department of Medicine, Temple University School of Medicine, Philadelphia, PA, USA

GI Motility Fellow, Gastroenterology Section, Department of Medicine, Lewis Katz School of Medicine at Temple University, Philadelphia, PA, USA

Reem Z. Sharaiha, MD, MS Division of Gastroenterology and Hepatology, New York-Presbyterian Hospital and Weill Cornell Medical Center, New York, NY, USA

Konika Sharma, MD Division of Gastroenterology, Memorial Sloan Kettering Cancer Center, New York, NY, USA

Nicha Somlaw, MD Department of Medicine, King Chulalongkorn Memorial Hospital and Chulalongkorn University, Bangkok, Thailand

Ali Tavakkoli, MD Division of General and GI Surgery, Brigham and Women's Hospital, Boston, MA, USA

Beverly G. Tchang, MD Department of Internal Medicine, Division of Endocrinology, Comprehensive Weight Control Center, NewYork-Presbyterian Hospital, Weill Cornell Medicine, New York, NY, USA

Matthew J. Whitson, MD, MSEd Division of Gastroenterology, The Donald and Barbara Zucker School of Medicine at Hofstra-Northwell, Manhasset, NY, USA

Aaron Justin Yeoh, MD Department of Medicine, NYU Langone Health, New York, NY, USA

Part I

Basic Nutrition Principles

1 Normal Gastrointestinal Tract Physiology

Dariush Shahsavari and Henry P. Parkman

Introduction

The gastrointestinal (GI) tract plays several important roles in body homeostasis including regulating the transit of ingested food down the GI tract for efficient digestion and absorption of essential nutrients. The GI tract is responsible for providing the body with supply of water, electrolytes, essential nutrients, and vitamins [1]. The main functions of the gastrointestinal tract include (1) movement of food through GI tract (motility), (2) digestion of food by mechanical and chemical (secretion of digestive enzymes) mechanisms, (3) absorption, (4) barrier and immune defense, (5) and interactions with microbiota. In this chapter, each of these areas is discussed, starting out with a brief overview of the topic, followed by a discussion of that area, and ending with a summary of the important aspects of the topic.

D. Shahsavari (✉)
Gastroenterology Section, Department of Medicine, Temple University School of Medicine, Philadelphia, PA, USA

GI Motility Fellow, Gastroenterology Section, Department of Medicine, Lewis Katz School of Medicine at Temple University, Philadelphia, PA, USA
e-mail: dariush.shahsavari@tuhs.temple.edu

H. P. Parkman
Gastroenterology Section, Department of Medicine, Temple University School of Medicine, Philadelphia, PA, USA
e-mail: henry.parkman@temple.edu

GI Motility

Overview of GI Motility There are two main purposes of GI motility: (1) propulsion of food bolus along the alimentary tract and (2) grinding and mixing of the content with digestive enzymes. This is achieved by a series of phasic and tonic contractions which are under local and neuroendocrine regulations and reflexes leading to movement of the ingested/digested food.

Contractions

The intestinal wall consists of several layers including (1) the serosa, (2) a longitudinal smooth muscle layer, (3) a circular smooth muscle layer, (4) the submucosa, and (5) the mucosa. The longitudinal and circular muscle layers are closely connected through numerous gap junctions and bundles of muscle fibers which are interconnected with connective tissue forming essentially a matrix of smooth muscle bundles [1].

1. *Phasic contractions*. The smooth muscle in the alimentary tract shows a continuous electrical activity which has two types: (1) slow waves and (2) spikes [1, 2]. Slow waves are

C. Newberry et al. (eds.), *Nutrition, Weight, and Digestive Health*,
https://doi.org/10.1007/978-3-030-94953-2_1

slow changes in the resting cell membrane potential with a varying frequency depending on the location in the GI tract, ranging from 3/min in the body of stomach, to 8/min in the terminal ileum, to 12/min in duodenum [3]. Slow waves set the rhythm of contractions in different parts of GI tract [4, 5]. The mechanism of slow wave generation is complex but seems to start in the interstitial cells of Cajal (ICCs), the GI pacemaker cells [6]. The slow waves are not able to generate muscle contraction by themselves, but by bringing the membrane potential closer to threshold, they facilitate the generation of "spike potentials" which are true action potentials and can lead to muscle contraction [1, 2]. Unlike action potential in nerve fibers which is caused by influx of sodium, GI muscle fibers rely mostly on calcium ion entry through calcium-sodium channels, which are much slower compared to sodium channels, which aids longer duration of action potentials [2]. Acetylcholine release (parasympathetic) facilitates action potential, whereas norepinephrine (sympathetic) and epinephrine (adrenal medullary stimulation) can inhibit action potential [7].

2. *Tonic contractions*. In addition to the phasic contractions, some muscles in the GI tract exhibit continuous tonic contractions. The gastrointestinal sphincters, such as the lower esophageal sphincter, rely on this mechanism to maintain their tone. Phasic contractions may be superimposed on tonic activity and, therefore, tone can increase the efficiency of phasic contractions by diminishing the diameter of the lumen [8]. On the other hand, tone partly determines the wall tension and contributes to the perception of distention [9].

Gastrointestinal Movements

There are two types of movements in GI tract: (1) peristalsis to move contents forward and (2) mixing movements which facilitate the mixing of GI tract contents.

1. Peristalsis

These propulsive movements cause forward movement of food in an aboral direction (away from mouth). A ring-like contraction begins in a part of GI tract and then moves forward. It usually is trigged by gut wall distention which then causes contraction [1, 4]. Table 1.1 shows the reflexes associated with GI tract. Other factors that increase peristalsis are chemical or physical irritants, as well as parasympathetic stimulation. This mechanism relies on the presence and proper function of the myenteric plexus. The congenital absence of this structure (such as in Hirschsprung's disease) leads to weak or non-existent peristalsis [4].

When a segment of GI tract is stimulated usually by distention, a contraction several centimeters behind the bolus begins which moves in the anal direction for 5–10 centimeter before fading out. Simultaneously, the gut wall downstream relaxes for several centimeters ("receptive relaxation") [1, 2]. This allows food to be propelled forward. This "peristaltic reflex" depends on the myenteric plexus. Together with forward propulsion of food, this is called "law of gut" (also known as Bayliss and Starling's law of the intestines) [1, 10].

2. Mixing Movements

Peristaltic contractions can also participate in mixing if the forward contractions are blocked by a closed sphincter, such as in the stomach with the pyloric sphincter. In addition, there are specific mixing movement patterns which are specific to each part of the GI tract. The purpose of these movements is to facilitate food contact with digestive enzymes and absorptive surfaces. They also help with temporary storage in certain regions of the gut, prevent retrograde movement of the content, and promote disposition of the residues [8].

Mastication (Chewing)

Chewing is an important part of digestion of food, especially for fruits and raw vegetables as they

Table 1.1 Gastrointestinal Reflexes

Reflex	Mechanism
Receptive relaxation (myenteric or peristaltic reflex)	A vasovagal reflex that relaxes the muscles of the proximal stomach to accommodate incoming food
Chewing reflex	A reflex involving cranial nerves and brain stem to organize rhythmic chewing movements
Gastroenteric reflex	Stomach wall distention increases peristalsis in small intestine via local myenteric and vagal nerves
Gastroileal reflex	Stomach wall distention increases motility in terminal ileum and release of chyme into cecum
Gastrocolic and duodenocolic reflexes	Distention of gastric and duodenal walls leads to increased colonic motility
Intestino-intestinal reflex	Overdistention of a portion of small intestine results in inhibition of motility of the rest of the small bowel
Enterogastric reflexes	Distention of small bowel wall inhibits gastric motility and increases pyloric tone via myenteric and sympathetic nerves
Rectosphincter reflex (rectoanal inhibitory reflex)	Distention of rectal wall leads to relaxation of internal anal sphincter and urge to defecate
Defecation reflexes	A series of reflexes involved in the defecation process
Peritoneoinstetinal reflex	Irritation of peritoneum (peritonitis) can inhibit excitatory enteric nervous system which leads to ileus
Renointestinal and vesicointestinal reflex	Irritation of kidney or bladder can inhibit excitatory enteric nervous system which leads to ileus

have indigestible cellulose membranes that need to be broken down. Teeth play an initial vital role. The front teeth (incisors) help with cutting and the posterior teeth (molars) are involved with grinding [10]. Digestive enzymes act on the surface of food particles and chewing helps break down the bolus into smaller pieces with larger total surface to be digested. Furthermore, this facilitates easier passage of food through GI tract [1].

Mastication is a well-orchestrated process which involves a series of voluntary and involuntary movements. Muscles of mastication include the masseter, the temporalis, and the medial and lateral pterygoids which are innervated by the mandibular division of the trigeminal nerve (cranial nerve V). The chewing process is controlled by the nuclei in the brain stem which control the rhythmic chewing movements [11]. Although the initiation is voluntary, much of the process happens as a part of "chewing reflex" [1]. Initially, when bolus enters the oral cavity, muscles of mastication are inhibited via a reflex mechanism. This allows the lower jaw to drop and trigger a "stretch reflex" of the mastication muscles to contract, which raises the jaw, pushing the bolus against the oral mucosa which leads to jaw drop and this repetitive cycle continues.

Deglutition (Swallowing)

Swallowing is a complex process which involves safe passage of bolus into the alimentary tract while protecting airway. There are three phases of deglutition: (1) voluntary stage, (2) pharyngeal stage, and (3) esophageal stage [1, 12].

1. *Voluntary phase*: When the mastication process is complete, food is pushed to the pharynx with the help of tongue. The movement is upward against soft palate and especially on the tonsillar pillars which have swallowing receptors, and this triggers the automatic part of swallowing [1].
2. *Pharyngeal phase*: This phase is involuntary and begins after epithelial swallowing receptors start sending afferent signals to the brainstem deglutition centers in medulla oblongata [13]. Initially, the soft palate is pulled upward to protect the nasopharynx, so food does not enter the nasal cavities. The palatopharyngeal folds are pulled medially to provide a slit through which food can pass to the posterior pharynx. It also acts as a filter to allow smaller food particles to pass and the larger parts are pushed to the front for more mastication [1].

The vocal cords are closed and larynx is pulled up and anteriorly by the neck muscles while epiglottis swings backward to cover the opening of larynx due to the presence of ligaments. This prevents food from getting into trachea [14]. Upward movement of trachea also pulls up the upper opening of esophagus, and the upper esophageal sphincter (UES) relaxes which allows food to be passed to esophagus. Once the passageway is open, pharyngeal wall muscles contract starting from the superior part going downward which pushes food into esophagus. During the swallowing process, which lasts less than 2 seconds, the swallow center inhibits the respiratory center in medulla [14]. Cranial nerves V, IX, X, XII, and nucleus ambiguous are involved in the motor function of swallowing [13, 15].

3. *Esophageal phase*: There are two types of peristaltic movements which propel food to the stomach. *Primary peristalsis* is continuation of the pharyngeal contraction wave. The wave propagates down the entire length of esophagus which lasts about 8–10 seconds [1, 8]. In upright position, gravity also facilitates the food passage. These waves in the upper one-third of the esophagus, which contains striated muscles, happen mostly through a brainstem reflex [13, 15]. *Secondary peristalsis* of esophagus is a result of local distention by residual food if bolus does not pass completely [8, 10]. These waves continue until the bolus is cleared. In the lower two-thirds of the esophagus, which contains smooth muscle, the myenteric plexus plays a major role. Vagus nerve through its connections with myenteric plexus also facilitates the process. Before these peristaltic waves reach the lower esophageal sphincter (LES), a "receptive relaxation" of LES (via release of vasoactive intestinal peptide [VIP] and nitric oxide) and also the stomach (through inhibitory myenteric fibers) facilitate passage and storage of food in the stomach (accommodation) [1, 8, 16]. Synchrony between longitudinal and circular muscle layers is important for effective esophageal contractility which leads to shortening of esophagus and opening of LES [17]. Lack of proper LES relaxation during swallowing occurs in achalasia, and weak baseline LES tone, can lead to gastroesophageal reflux (GERD). Crural diaphragm, which is superimposed on the LES, plays an important role in the EGJ function. These striated muscle bundles which contract during inspiration exert effective boosting of EGJ pressure [18]. Other factors increasing LES tone include acetylcholine (parasympathetic system), gastrin, motilin, and protein-rich food. Factors decreasing LES tone include sympathetic system, VIP, nitric oxide, cholecystokinin (CCK), gastric inhibitory peptide (GIP), secretin, progesterone, prostaglandin E, and fat-rich food [10].

Stomach

The stomach has various functions which include temporary storage of food after ingestion, digestive enzymes secretion, and mixing food with gastric secretions. This process results in the production of a semifluid mixture termed chyme which is slowly emptied through the pylorus into the small intestine [1]. Anatomically, stomach consists of cardia, fundus, body (corpus), antrum, and pylorus. The orad portion of the stomach (fundus and body) is responsible for storage. As food enters the stomach, it stretches stomach walls causing a vasovagal reflex to reduce the tone of wall muscles to allow for more compliance (increase in volume without increase in pressure). This is known as "accommodation" and is mediated by nitric oxide and VIP [1, 8, 16]. A completely relaxed stomach can accommodate 0.8–1.5 liters [1]. Gastric secretory glands, which are present in the entire stomach lining except for lesser curvature, secret digestive enzymes which act on the ingested food's surface. A set of peristaltic waves called *mixing waves* begin in the upper and mid portion of stomach and progress toward the antrum every 15–20 seconds [2]. They are generated by the background slow waves discussed earlier. As they move toward the antrum, they become stronger and form constrictor rings which are action potential-driven that push the content toward pylorus [10]. Since the pyloric sphincter is contracted, only a small amount of content can pass through pylorus (less than 0.25 mm in diameter). This results in upstream movement of food back toward the body ("retropulsion"), which essentially leads to mixing and pulverization of food and this cycle continues [1, 10]. About 20% of these peristaltic waves are more intense and begin in the mid portion of the body and progress toward pylorus in a ring-like formation, which facilitate stomach emptying. When food has been exposed to gastric secretions and acid thoroughly, the soft fluid/semifluid mixture chyme is formed which can be pushed through pylorus to duodenum. This action is called "pyloric pump" [19]. As the stomach becomes empty, these constriction rings move proximally and this helps push the remaining food distally. Higher food volume in the stomach enhances emptying from stomach by activating local myenteric reflexes that inhibit pylorus constriction and intensify the pyloric pump. Another factor that promotes pylorus pump and gastric emptying is gastrin secretion by antral G cells. The rate of emptying is generally faster for liquids, small solids, and carbohydrates. Proteins, fats, acidic food, and food with higher osmolarity have slower emptying [10].

As food enters the small bowel, several regulatory mechanisms control the rate of gastric emptying. As the volume of chyme increases in the small intestine (causing wall distention), several local and systemic reflexes are activated which act mostly through enteric and sympathetic nervous systems, and this decreases gastric emptying and increases pyloric tone [2]. These "enterogastric reflexes" ensure enough time for digestion. Other factors that can trigger these reflexes in duodenum are acidity and osmolality of chime, and presence of irritants, proteins, and possibly fat breakdown products. There are small intestinal inhibitory feedback hormones which also regulate gastric emptying. Cholecystokinin (CCK) is released from jejunum in response to fatty content which decreases gastric motility. Secretin, triggered by acidic chyme and gastric inhibitory peptide (GIP) secretion in response to fat and probably carbohydrates, can also reduce stomach motility and emptying [10, 20].

The stomach movements do not exclusively happen in the presence of food. The stomach exhibits regular contractions every 90–120 minutes called "migrating motor complex (MMC)" [1, 8, 10], which start when stomach has been empty for several hours. The hormones motilin (secreted by M cells in the upper small intestine) and ghrelin (secreted by P-/D1-cells in the gastric fundus and epsilon cells in the pancreas) play a role in generating these rhythmical movements in the body of the stomach which gradually increase in intensity, culminate in strong peristaltic contractions [21]. There are four phases of a normal MMC. Phase I is a quiescent period with no contractions. During phase II, irregular and intermittent low-amplitude contractions occur. Phase III (main phase) consists of regular and high-amplitude contractions, and finally phase IV is a short transition period back to phase I. During the phase III portion of the MMC, the pyloric sphincter remains open to evacuate large non-digestible food left in the stomach and small intestine as well as mucus, sloughed cells, and bacteria from the small intestine [10]. This process functions as a housekeeping process and also prevents bacterial overgrowth. When meal ingestion occurs, these complexes are converted to the fed motor activit state and this conversion relies on an intact vagal nerve function [8].

Ghrelin, an endogenous ligand of growth hormone receptor, is a gastric peptide hormone which exerts various physiological actions in the body including growth hormone secretion, appetite stimulation, long-term body weight regulation, and glucose homeostasis [22]. In addition, ghrelin increases gastric acid secretion by stimulating vagal signal and histamine release and promotes gastric motility and migration motor complexes (MMC) via vagal stimulation as mentioned above [23, 24]. Ghrelin is secreted in a pulsatile manner and its levels increase before the onset of meal and during fasting and decrease with feeding [25]. This may suggest that ghrelin may act as a hunger signal for meal initiation [22].

Small Intestine

Small intestine also has two types of movements: segmentation (mixing) and peristalsis (propulsion) [1].

When any segment of small intestine is distended (e.g., due to the presence of chyme), transient concentric contractions occur which are called "segmentation" [26]. It creates a sausage-like chain of segments which alternate between contraction and relaxation of different parts generating mixing motions of food with digestive secretions. The maximum frequency of these contractions is based on the frequency of slow waves in different parts of small intestine from 12/min in duodenum to 8/min in terminal ileum [3].

Peristaltic waves happen in any part of the small intestine. They are usually faster in the proximal intestine. Each wave can travel about 3–5 centimeters before dying down. The net result is usually a velocity of 1 cm/min forward movement which translates into 3–5 hours of time required for chyme to pass from pylorus to ileocecal valve [1]. These waves increase after meal consumption. This results from stomach distention (gastroenteric reflex) as well as duodenal distention which leads to activation of myenteric plexus [1, 2]. Hormones such as gastrin, CCK, insulin, motilin, and serotonin can enhance these movements. Conversely, secretin, epinephrine, and glucagon decrease small bowel motility. Overdistention of a portion of small intestine results in inhibition of motility of the rest of the small bowel (intestino-intestinal reflex). When chyme reaches the terminal ileum, it stops behind the ileocecal sphincter for several hours until the next meal when gastric distention leads to "gastroileal reflex" which increase the peristaltic waves and pushes chyme into cecum. This ensures ample time for digestion and absorption in small intestine. While stomach empties 7–10 liter of chyme into small intestine every day, only 1.5–2 liter of chyme is emptied into the cecum [10]. Although these waves are relatively weak, local irritation of mucosa (e.g., inflammation or infection) can cause stronger and more frequent waves called "peristaltic rush" which facilitate expulsion of toxins and irritants into colon causing diarrhea. On the other hand, distention of cecum or presence of irritation in the cecal area (e.g., acute appendicitis) intensifies ileocecal sphincter tone and inhibit ileal peristalsis sometimes to the point of total paralysis (i.e., ileus) [10]. Local myenteric plexus and sympathetic nervous system are involved in the process [2].

Colon

Large intestine also has mixing (haustrations) and peristaltic movements (mass movements) [1, 27]. The purpose of these movements is absorption of water and electrolytes and formation of solid feces. The proximal part of colon is mostly involved in absorption and stool formation and the distal part is mainly for storage of fecal matter until defecation.

Haustrations in colon happen similar to segmentation in the small bowel. Large circular rings form constricting segments of colon along with longitudinal taeniae coli. The result is balloon-like sacculation of other segments (haustra). These movements peak in about 30 seconds and then gradually disappear which result in mixing and rolling of the fecal matter, thereby exposing more surfaces to mucosa for water and electrolyte absorption. These movements show a diurnal variation, i.e., they are less pronounced during sleep and increase dramatically with waking [28, 29].

Haustrations do have some slow forward movement toward the anus, but the main propulsive action is causes by the so-called "mass movements" which can happen 1–3 times a day, especially in the morning after breakfast [30, 31]. These peristaltic waves begin with a constrictive ring which rapidly move and stimulate a large segment of colon to contract, often forming a block of more than 20 centimeters, pushing the fecal matter forward. The contraction peaks at about 30 seconds and then dissipates within the next 2–3 minutes. Similar series of movements repeat for 10–30 minutes and then stop [1]. Meal ingestion (distention of stomach and duodenum) triggers mass movements (gastrocolic and duodenocolic reflexes). Composition of the meal seems to influence these reflexes [8]. Fat and carbohydrate stimulate colonic activity, while amino acid and protein inhibit it. Local irritation of colon (e.g., inflammatory bowel disease) also can cause persistent mass movements.

There is a cyclic motor activity, especially in the rectum, called "rectal motor complex" which is not synchronized with the small intestinal MMC, and its regulation and purpose are not fully understood; perhaps this generates the urge to defecate [8].

Defecation

Defecation is the process of expelling feces when it reaches the rectum. Rectal vault is usually empty most of the time due to a sharp angle between the sigmoid colon and rectum [1, 32]. When a series of mass movements propel fecal matter into rectum, the sensation to defecate is triggered. It initiates "rectosphincter reflex" (also known as the rectoanal inhibitory reflex [RAID]) resulting in contraction of the rectum and relaxation of the internal anal sphincter which is the involuntary smooth muscle sphincter of anus [2]. The external sphincter, which is composed of voluntary striated muscles, prevents leakage of stool until willful evacuation [32]. If defecation is prevented, the rectum slowly pushes the material back into the sigmoid colon and the urge to defecate disappears until the next mass movement [10]. There are a number of "defecation reflexes" involved in the process of defecation [2, 32]. The "intrinsic reflex" (through myenteric plexus) is a result of rectal wall distention which leads to intensification of peristaltic movements in the descending colon, sigma, and rectum to push feces toward anus, which in turn relaxes the internal anal sphincter as described above. Rectal distention also triggers a parasympathetic defecation reflex (through S2-S4 spinal segments) which leads to much stronger peristaltic waves and even more relaxation of the internal sphincter. When defecation is started, other processes are triggered via spinal cord including taking a deep breath and downward movement of the diaphragm, closure of the glottis, abdominal muscle contraction, and pelvic floor relaxation. These activities together help push more feces down and distend the rectal wall, which in turn trigger new set of reflexes [1].

Summary of Important Aspects of GI Motility

- GI motility involves propulsion and mixing of the nutrients along the digestive tract. This is achieved by a series of phasic and active movements which are under local and neuroendocrine regulations and reflexes.
- Chewing is an important part of food breakdown, especially indigestible fibers. This is followed by swallowing, which through a series of voluntary and involuntary movements involving higher brain centers leads to the safe passage of food to the stomach.
- The stomach cavity relaxes in response to incoming food to receive, store, and expose food to acid and digestive enzymes.
- The stomach movements are well coordinated and under many local and system reflexes and hormones. They ultimately bring about mixing of food with enzymes and formation of chyme which passes to the small intestine.
- The small intestine continues to mix (segmentation) and propel chyme while further digestion and absorption happens.
- Mixing movements in the colon (haustrations) ensure the maximal absorption of water and electrolytes, and together with peristalsis (mass movements), condensed fecal matter is formed and expelled through a complex process involving coordinated movements called defecation.

Gastrointestinal Secretions

Overview of GI Secretions There are numerous secretory glands distributed throughout the alimentary tract. These have mainly two purposes: mucous production and digestion. The secretion process is regulated by local and autonomic nervous systems as well as various hormones. Gastrointestinal secretions from different areas of the GI tract are listed in Table 1.2.

Mucous Production

"Mucus" is a thick secretion which mainly consists of water, electrolytes, and certain glycopeptides [33]. The composition slightly varies based on the anatomical location, but the function is the same, namely, lubrication and protection of the gut wall. Due to its viscous quality, it can adhere to the food tightly and fully cover food particles with a thin and slimy film which facilitates movement along the GI tract (lubrication) [1]. In the colon, it helps fecal particles to adhere to one another to form stool. It forms an effective coating of the GI lumens to prevent direct contact of food or digestive enzymes with the mucosa. It is very resistant to digestion by digestive enzymes. Mucus also contains a moderate amount of bicarbonate ions which helps to neutralize acidic products. It is secreted by billions of "mucous glands" (also known as goblet cells) [34]. Epithelial stimulation from coming in contact with food leads to increase in mucous production. Other factors promoting mucous section include enteric nervous system activation, local distention, and chemical irritation [1].

In general, parasympathetic stimulation increases most GI glandular secretions via muscarinic (M3) receptors on acinar cells. Sympathetic nervous system has a dual effect on secretion [10]. Norepinephrine binds to β-2 adrenergic receptors on acinar cells which stimulates secretion modestly. If secretion is already high due to parasympathetic or hormonal factors, sympathetic stimulations lead to reduction of the secretions by causing local vasoconstriction.

Saliva

Saliva contains two types of secretions: serous and mucus. Parotid gland produces serous secretions, buccal glands produce mucus, and submandibular and sublingual glands are mixed

Table 1.2 Gastrointestinal secretions

Location	GI secretion	Stimulated by	Inhibited by	Function
Oral cavity	Saliva (mucus and serous)	ACh (M3 receptors), NE (β2 receptor)	Antimuscarinic medications, dehydration, stress	Lubrication, digestion of complex carbohydrates and lipids
Alimentary tract from esophagus to rectum	Mucus	ACh (M3 receptors)		Lubrication, mucosal protection
Stomach	Hydrochloric acid	ACh (M3 receptors), histamine (H2 receptors), gastrin (CCK_B receptor, histamine)	Secretin, somatostatin, GIP, prostaglandins, PPIs, H2 blockers	Food digestion, pepsinogen activation, bactericidal effect
	Intrinsic factor (IF)	ACh (M3 receptors)		Vitamin B12 absorption
	Pepsin	ACh (M3 receptors)	High gastric pH	Protein digestion
	Mucus	ACh (M3 receptors)		Lubrication, stomach mucosa protection
Pancreas	Bicarbonate	Secretin, ACh		Neutralization of acidic chyme
	Digestive enzymes (protease, amylase, lipase)	CCK, ACh, enterokinase	Trypsin inhibitor	Digestion
Liver	Bile	CCK, ACh, more bile return in the enterohepatic circulation		Fat digestion, and cholesterol and toxin excretion

glands. Serous secretions have "ptyalin" (a form of α-amylase) which aids in digestion of complex carbohydrates and "lingual lipase" which starts the digestion of triglycerides [1, 34].

Saliva also plays a vital role in maintaining healthy oral hygiene. As saliva flows (0.5 cc/min while awake), it washes the harmful bacteria constantly [1]. There are various bactericidal factors in saliva including proteolytic enzymes (e.g., lysozyme), lactoferrin, and thiocyanate ions. In addition, IgA immunoglobulin content in saliva also activates immune system to reduce the pathogen burden in the oral cavity. The importance of this function is manifested in patients with Sjogren's disease, in whom salivation is absent, and this leads to oral ulceration and tooth decay [10].

Average daily saliva production is around 1 liter with a pH of 6.0–7.0 [1, 34]. The saliva is secreted in stages. In the first stage, acini secretes the "primary saliva" which contains ptyalin and mucin. Electrolyte composition is similar to extracellular component. As the "primary saliva" passes through the ductal system, the electrolyte content changes [1, 10]. Sodium ions are actively reabsorbed in exchange for potassium secretion. Chloride is passively reabsorbed to keep the electrical balance. Bicarbonate is absorbed partly passively in exchange for chloride and partly by active secretion. This is called the "secondary saliva" which is rich in potassium and bicarbonate but has lower concentration of sodium and chloride compared to plasma. When there is copious salivation, this composition may be different as there may not be enough time for primary saliva produced in acini to undergo these changes as it passes through ducts.

Salivation centers in the brain stem which include superior and inferior salivatory nuclei regulate secretion of the saliva by parasympathetic fibers in facial and glossopharyngeal nerves which increase saliva production and secretion in response to both taste and tongue tactile stimuli. These nerve endings release acetylcholine (ACh) which acts on the acinar cells to increase the volume of saliva. ACh also releases kallikrein which activates bradykinin (a vasodilator) and promotes blood flow to the glandular cells [10].

Higher cortical areas, hypothalamus and amygdale, also influence salivary secretion. Smelling or eating the food that is desirable generates more salivation than otherwise. Even seeing or thinking about food stimulates saliva production (conditioned reflexes) [2, 10].

The sympathetic supply of the salivary glands comes from superior cervical ganglia. As discussed before, it has a dual effect and its stimulatory effect is weaker than parasympathetic system [10]. Finally, any irritation in the stomach or small bowel also promotes saliva secretion to help remove the irritating factor [2].

Esophagus

The esophageal tract is almost entirely mucus-producing to facilitate lubrication and protection [35]. In the upper part, there are mainly simple mucous glands, but in the area closer to the esophagogastric junction (EGJ), there are numerous compound mucous glands to protect the esophageal mucosa against the acidic gastric pH [1].

Stomach

In addition to simple mucous cells that are present in the entire stomach lining, there are two distinct types of glands in the stomach: gastric (oxyntic) glands and pyloric glands [36, 37].

Gastric Glands Oxyntic (acid-forming) glands, which are mostly located in the body and fundus, mostly secrete stomach acid, pepsinogen, intrinsic factor, and mucus. They are composed of three types of cells: (1) peptic (chief) cells that secrete pepsinogen, (2) parietal (oxyntic) cells that secrete hydrochloric acid and intrinsic factor, and (3) mucous (neck) cells that produce mucus [37].

Hydrochloric acid secreted by parietal cells is isotonic but extremely acidic (pH ~ 0.8) [1, 36]. Basal acid output (BAO) is the amount of hydrochloric acid produced in the absence of any stimulation (usually less than 10 mmol/hour). Maximal acid output (MAO) is the amount of acid produced when stimulated, which is usually around 50 mmol/hour [10].

In parietal cells, when stimulated, water is dissociated into H^+ and OH^- in the cytoplasm and the hydrogen ion is actively transported to the apical branching canaliculi by hydrogen-potassium pump (H-K-ATPase pump, also known as "proton pump"). This is the pump that is the target for proton pump inhibitors (PPIs) [10, 37]. Sodium is reabsorbed from the lumen by Na^+-K^+-ATPase pump on the basolateral side. Potassium accumulated in the cells leaks back into the gastric lumen which is exchanged for more hydrogen ions. OH^- by-product combines with CO_2 to form bicarbonate which is transported to blood in exchange for chloride ions which enters the cells toward the gastric lumen. Finally, water follows the ions secreted into the lumen via osmosis [36]. The net result is the secretion of hydrochloric acid, water, potassium chloride, and small amount of sodium chloride. It is important that this acidic juice does not come into direct contact with stomach mucosa. This is achieved by generous secretion of alkaline mucus as well as tight junctions between epithelial cells [33]. Any compromise of either or both factors leads to gastric mucosal injury which can lead to gastritis or gastric ulcer formation. This process makes the venous gastric blood alkaline during active acid secretion leading to "alkaline tide" which is partly neutralized by the acidic blood coming from pancreas when producing sodium bicarbonate as explained later [38].

Intrinsic factor secreted by parietal cells is vital for vitamin B12 absorption in terminal ileum. As a result, destruction of parietal cells leads to achlorhydria and pernicious anemia (a consequence of vitamin B12 deficiency) [10].

Pepsinogen produced by chief cells breaks down into its active form "pepsin" as soon as it enters the acidic stomach environment. This is the active enzyme form which helps with protein digestion (proteolysis). This enzyme is only active in acidic medium and becomes inactive as it enters more alkaline environment (i.e., duodenum) [1, 36].

Parasympathetic or enteric nervous system (ACh secretion) stimulate all three types of secretions (hydrochloric acid, pepsinogen, and mucus), whereas gastrin and histamine only stimulate acid secretion. Acid secretion can cause additional enteric nervous reflexes which promotes pepsinogen secretion as well. Enterochromaffin-like (ECL) cells are in the deep recesses of the gastric glands and release histamine which promotes acid secretions when it comes into direct contact with parietal cells (paracrine) [1, 10]. These cells are in turn activated by the hormone gastrin which reaches them through blood (endocrine).

Vagal stimulation leads to muscarinic (M3) receptors activation which stimulates H+-K+-ATPase pump. On the other hand, gastrin stimulates parietal cells to secrete H+ by interacting with cholecystokinin B (CCK-B) receptors. Histamine acts on H_2 receptors on parietal cells and activates the proton pump. These stimuli can potentiate each other [10].

Pyloric Glands These glands consist mostly of mucous cells, few chief cells, and G cells that produce gastrin. There are no parietal cells in this region [36]. Gastrin is secreted by "gastrin cells" ("G cells") located mostly in the antrum [39]. When they come into contact with meat or other protein-rich food, they release the hormone into the bloodstream which stimulates the ECL cells to secrete histamine as described above.

Phases of Gastric Secretion

1. *Cephalic phase*: gastric secretion begins with the sight, smell, taste, or even thought of food and when it is being chewed. These signals originate from the appetite centers in amygdala and hypothalamus as well as cortical areas. Emotional stress can also provoke gastric juice secretion which in the long run can lead to peptic ulcer disease. This phase leads to 30 percent of total gastric secretion (total daily volume is about 1.5 liter) [1, 2, 36].
2. *Gastric phase*: 60 percent of secretion occurs when food enters the stomach. It involves

local enteric reflexes, vasovagal reflexes, and gastrin secretion.

3. *Intestinal phase*: Presence of food in the duodenum initially also stimulates gastric secretion (10 percent), but as more chyme enters the small intestine, due to enterogastric reflex, stomach secretion is inhibited. After gastric emptying, if gastric pH remains low, "somatostatin" secreted from D cells surpasses acid secretion by inhibiting gastrin and histamine secretion [40]. Abnormally high gastrin secretion (e.g., in Zollinger-Ellison syndrome) leads to unchecked increase in gastric acid production which can lead to multiple drug-resistant gastric and duodenal ulcers [10].

Other factors inhibiting gastric secretions include the hormone secretin (secreted as the acidic chyme enters duodenum), gastric inhibitory peptide (GIP), vasoactive intestinal peptide (VIP), and prostaglandins [1, 37]. During fasting, gastric secretions continue which contain mostly mucus and some pepsin and almost no acid [36].

Small Intestine

There are numerous mucous glands called "Brunner's glands" in the proximal duodenum which secrete a large amount of alkaline mucus [33]. This secretion along with pancreatic and hepatic alkaline secretions protects the duodenal mucosa when the acidic chyme enters the small intestine. Local distention, vagal stimulation, and secretin increase mucous secretion by these cells. Sympathetic stimulation inhibits mucous secretion which possibly explains the higher risk of duodenal ulcers in people who are under stress [41].

In addition, the entire surface of the small intestine is covered with villi and microvilli which facilitate nutrient absorption. Between these villi, there are crypts of Lieberkühn which contain numerous goblet cells that secrete mucus [1]. There are also enterocytes which secrete large quantities of water and electrolytes. Subsequently, these alkaline secretions along with the nutrients in the chyme are quickly reabsorbed by intestinal villi [1, 42]. As with other parts of GI tract, enteric nervous system in response to the small intestine's wall distention or irritation plays a major role in regulation of these secretions [2].

Large Intestine

Alkaline mucus production in the large intestine is similar to that in the small intestine [43]. There are crypts of Lieberkühn but no villi and digestive enzymes in the large intestine [1]. This is important to lubricate the colon and form solid stool which can slide and be expelled. Mucous production also protects the colonic wall against excoriation by fecal material as well as billions of bacteria in feces.

Local enteric nervous system also regulates mucous production and secretion in the colon. Local irritation such as infection can increase water and electrolyte secretion tremendously in order to dilute and expel toxins, i.e., diarrhea [10]. Parasympathetic stimulation via pelvic nerves also can increase mucous secretion in the distal half of colon. This may lead to copious mucoid diarrhea during emotional stress.

Pancreas

Pancreatic exocrine glands are structurally very similar to salivary glands [34]. The pancreatic acini produce the digestive enzymes, and sodium bicarbonate solution is added to the secretion by the ductal epithelial cells which is emptied through the pancreatic ducts and papilla of Vater into the duodenum. The total daily amount secreted is about 1 liter [1].

Digestive enzymes Enzymes secreted by pancreas are involved in the digestion of all three types of food components: proteins, fats, and carbohydrates [43].

Enzymes involved in protein digestion are "trypsin' (the most common one) and "chymotrypsin," which digest polypeptides into smaller peptides (but not single amino acids), and "carboxypolypeptidase," which can split some peptides into amino acids. These enzymes are initially synthesized in their inactive precursor forms which are called trypsinogen, chymotrypsinogen, and procarboxypolypeptidase respectively [1, 43]. They are activated once they enter the duodenum. Trypsinogen is activated by enterokinase (also called enteropeptidase), an enzyme secreted by the intestinal mucosa. Trypsin itself can activate additional trypsinogen molecules, as well as chymotrypsin, and procarboxypolypeptidase. It is imperative that these activations do not happen inside the acini or in the pancreatic ducts. Otherwise, these enzymes "autodigest" the pancreas itself [1]. The same cells that produce these enzymes also secrete a "trypsin inhibitor" into the acini to prevent this conversion inside the pancreas. If pancreatic tissue is damaged or in case of an obstruction (e.g., gallstone), the secretions build up quickly in the ductal system and overwhelm trypsin inhibitor, which leads to pancreatic injury i.e., acute pancreatitis [44].

"Amylase" is the enzyme involved in the digestion of starch, glycogen and polysaccharides (except cellulose). "Lipase" is responsible for breaking up triglycerides into fatty acids and monoglycerides, "cholesterol esterase" hydrolyzes cholesterol molecules, and "phospholipase" breaks up phospholipids [1, 43].

Bicarbonate Secretion Water and sodium bicarbonate are secreted by the epithelial cells in the ductules and ducts and are added to the digestive enzymes [43]. These cells have carbonic anhydrase which facilitates HCO_3- synthesis by combining water and carbon dioxide ($CO_2 + H_2O=HCO_3- + H^+$). Hydrogen ions are transferred into circulation in exchange with sodium ions at the basal surface. Bicarbonate ions together with sodium ions are actively transported to the luminal surface to form sodium bicarbonate [1]. Water follows the electrolytes into the lumen by osmosis.

Regulation Parasympathetic activation (ACh secretion) and cholecystokinin (CCK) stimulate the acinar cells to produce large amounts of digestive enzymes but small amount of bicarbonate or water [45]. Without these components, the digestive enzymes remain in the acinar cells and ducts. The hormone secretin, on the other hand, stimulates water and bicarbonate secretion, which carries the digestive enzymes into the small intestine. These stimuli have potentiating and additive effect.

Much like gastric secretions, the pancreatic secretions have similar phases [1]. Cephalic and gastric phases lead to 25–30% of secretion, mainly through ACh stimulation. The intestinal phase, when chyme, is associated with most of pancreatic secretions as CCK and secretin are activated (through blood stream). Secretin is a hormone that is secreted by "S cells" in the duodenum and jejunum. The precursor form is called "prosecretin" which is activated when acidic chyme enters the duodenum. Secretin promotes luminal chloride absorption in exchange for bicarbonate by acting on the cystic fibrosis transmembrane conduction regulator (CFTR) receptor [10]. This leads to copious secretion of water and sodium bicarbonate that neutralize the acidic chyme. The lower the pH, the more secretin is released which leads to more voluminous secretion. This is essential for protection of the duodenal epithelia as they cannot withstand such acidic environment. CCK is produced by "I cells" in the duodenal and upper jejunal mucosa after being exposed to protein by-products and long-chain fatty acids [1, 45].

Bile Production and Secretion

Bile production is one of the many liver functions [46]. Bile acids are important for fat digestion and absorption. Bile also is a carrier of various waste products including bilirubin (hemoglobin end-product) and cholesterol.

Bile is secreted from hepatocytes which consists of bile acids (most common substance), cholesterol, lecithin, and bilirubin. It is secreted in bile canaliculi and empties into the terminal bile ducts which eventually form the hepatic duct and common bile duct. Bile from here either is diverted to gallbladder through the cystic duct for storage or is secreted into the duodenum. As bile passes through the bile ducts, the epithelial cells secrete water and sodium bicarbonate similar to pancreatic secretions which add to the bile volume and facilitate its flow [46]. If bile ends up in the gallbladder, sodium is reabsorbed via active transport through gallbladder wall and chloride and water follow passively. This leads to more concentrated bile which allots more storage capacity in gallbladder [47].

Every day about 1 liter of bile is secreted which contains 6 grams of bile acids [1]. These bile acids are synthesized in liver from cholesterol precursors which are converted to cholic acid and chenodeoxycholic acid. These acids are then conjugated with glycine and taurine to form "primary bile salts" [10, 46]. These salts subsequently undergo alteration in the intestinal lumen by bacteria to form "secondary bile salt" which includes conjugated deoxycholate and lithocholate. They play an important role in fat digestion and absorption by emulsification of hydrophobic fat droplets (fatty acids, monoglycerides, cholesterols) into complexes called "micelles" which are semi-soluble in the chyme, and thence they carry small fat globules to intestinal mucosa to be absorbed [48]. In the absence of these bile salts, as much as 40% of ingested fat can be lost in stool [1].

Bile salts are also an important means of removing cholesterol from blood as cholesterol is completely insoluble in water and needs to be excreted in the form of a colloid (i.e., micelles) [48]. People who have a high cholesterol diet are at risk of cholesterol precipitation in the gallbladder and stone formation (most common type) [10].

As these bile salts go through the small intestine, about 94% are reabsorbed in the terminal ileum into blood by both active transport and diffusion which enter portal circulation and go back to liver and hepatocytes through "enterohepatic circulation" to be resecreted into the bile. These cycles continue on average for 17 times before these salts are excreted in feces [1, 48]. Bile acids also stimulate colonic motility and secretions. High exposure of colonic mucosa to bile acids in case of bile acid malabsorption has been shown in a subgroup of patients with diarrhea-predominant IBS [49]. On the other hand, bile acid synthesis defect may lead to constipation-predominant IBS [50].

The amount of bile secreted by liver depends on the presence of bile salts in enterohepatic circulation. The higher their concentration in the portal circulation, the higher the rate of bile secretion [1, 48].

Gallbladder contraction, sphincter of Oddi relaxation, and bile secretion are stimulated by CCK mostly as a result of fatty food reaching duodenum. Acetylcholine through enteric or parasympathetic nervous system also stimulates gallbladder contraction. Secretin stimulates the production of sodium bicarbonate and water here similar to pancreas [1, 46].

Summary of Important Points of GI Sections

- The main purposes of various secretions throughout the alimentary tract are mucous production and digestion. The secretion process is regulated by local and autonomic nervous systems as well as various hormones.
- Mucus, a thick alkaline secretion which is present throughout the GI tract, facilitates food movement by lubrication and forms an effective protective coating which protects the GI tract against digestive enzymes, bacteria, and other pathogens.
- Saliva consists of mucous and serous secretions that contain enzymes (amylase and lipase) which play some role in digestion.
- Gastric secretions include hydrochloric acid and pepsin which are important in protein breakdown. These secretions are under several neuronal and hormonal regulations.

- The small intestine, the principal place of digestion and absorption, is where many digestive enzymes and regulatory hormones are secreted. These include pancreatic secretions which contain neutralizing bicarbonate and digestive enzymes. Biliary secretions play a vital role in fat digestion and absorption.

Digestion and Absorption

Overview on Digestion and Absorption Digestion is the process of chemical and mechanical breakdown of food into absorbable components. Absorption is the movement of nutrient molecules from the GI lumen into enterocytes and then into bloodstream or lymph [10].

Digestion and Absorption

There are three types of main nutrients in food: carbohydrates, proteins, and fats which cannot be absorbed in their native forms and need to be digested. In addition, food contains water, minerals, and vitamins which are necessary for bodily functions.

Most major nutrients are absorbed in the small intestine. The colon (mostly the proximal half) is mainly involved in fluid and electrolyte absorption. It is able to absorb up to 8 liters of fluid and electrolytes each day [1].

The wall of the small intestine consists of millions of folds (folds of Kerckring), villi, and microvilli which increase the surface area available for absorption tremendously [1, 42]. The strategic location of the blood vessels and lymph lacteal in the center of villi facilitates this absorption. The absorptive capacity of a normal small intestine is thousands of grams of carbohydrates, 500 grams of fat, 500–700 grams of proteins, and more than 20 liters of water each day [1].

Carbohydrates

Most carbohydrates in food are either polysaccharides or disaccharides that are essentially monosaccharides bound together with glycosidic bonds, which means a hydrogen ion has been removed from one side and a hydroxyl ion has been removed from the other side forming water in the process of binding (see Fig. 1.1) [8, 51]. During digestion, this process is reversed through a process called "hydrolysis," which means adding a water molecule to break up the bond [1]:

$$R'' - R' + H_2O \rightarrow R''OH + R'H$$

Three major sources of carbohydrates in a normal diet include a large polysaccharide in plant-based foods called starch (the most common), sucrose (disaccharide), and lactose which is a disaccharide found in milk. Other carbohydrates which are in small quantities include amylose, glycogen, lactic acid, pyruvic acid, and dextrins.

In addition, there are often non-digestible carbohydrates e.g. cellulose in food which humans do not have the enzyme to digest its β-acetyl bond and therefore mostly stay in the GI tract and are ultimately exerted feces. These non-absorbable fibers have multiple benefits [10]. In the stomach, they bind water molecules. This leads to increase in bolus size which, after reaching the duodenum, can slow gastric emptying (by local distention) prevent overeating by inducing satiety. In the ileum and colon, more wall distention results in lowers transit time which leads to more voluminous and softer stool. These fibers also bind cholesterol and bile acids and facilitate their excretion. Glucose absorption is also hindered by a high-fiber diet. Finally, fibers bind ammonia which leads to increased nitrogen excretion in feces. This is especially important in people with liver or renal disease [10].

Digestion of carbohydrates begins when food enters mouth. Saliva contains ptyalin (an α-amylase) which mainly hydrolyzes α-1-4 glycosidic bonds in starch into maltose, maltotriose, and α-limit dextrins (disaccharides) [10]. The process continues in the stomach for a while but since the enzyme is blocked by stomach acid, this only accounts for about 30–40% of total starch digestion [1]. As chyme enters the duodenum, pancreatic amylase, which is more potent than the salivary enzyme, digests almost all carbohydrates within 15–30 minutes. Enterocytes in the small intestine have multiple disaccharidases (lactase, maltase, sucrase, α-dectrinase) on their

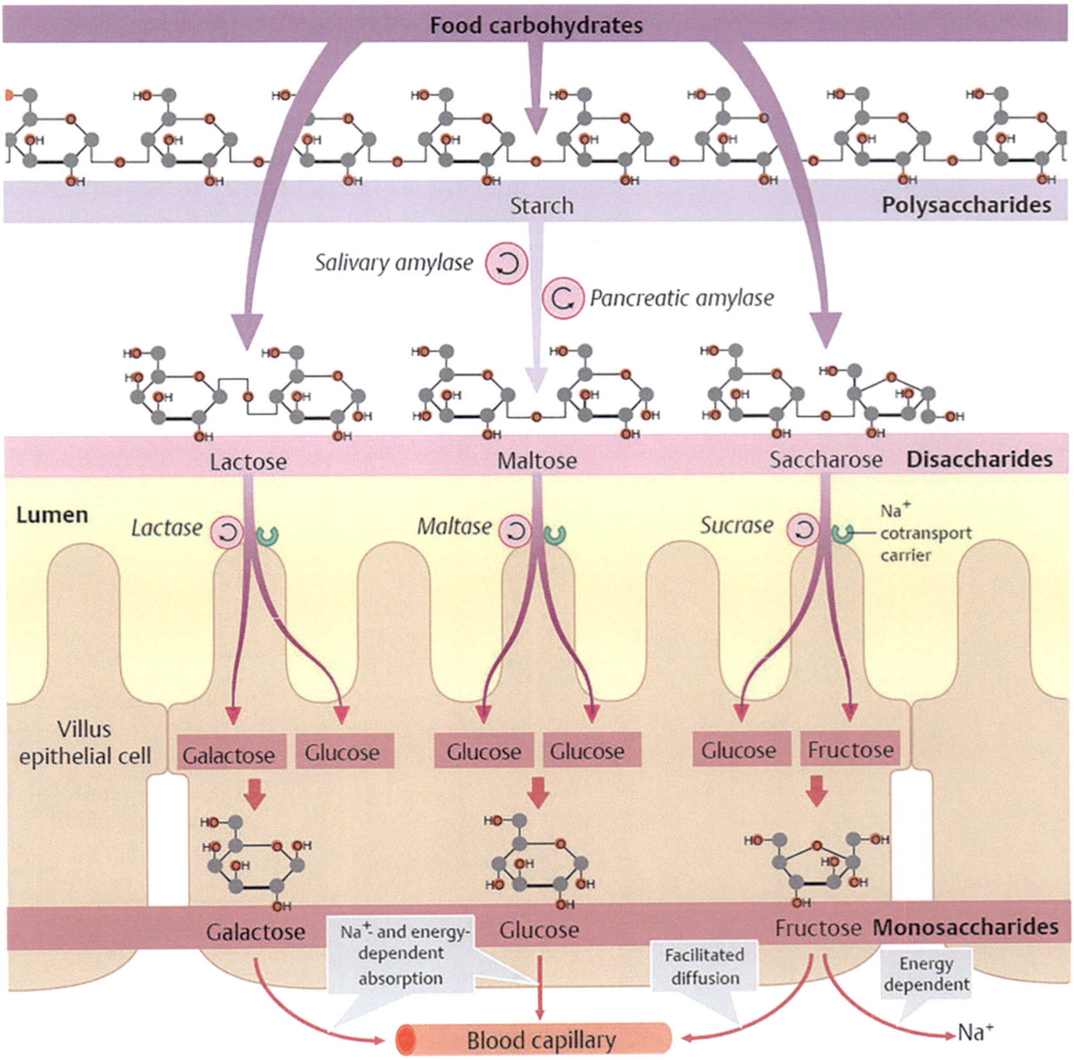

Fig. 1.1 Carbohydrate breakdown and metabolism in human body. Most carbohydrates in food are either polysaccharides or disaccharides that are essentially monosaccharides bound together with glycosidic bonds, which means a hydrogen ion has been removed from one side and a hydroxyl ion has been removed from the other side forming water in the process of binding. During digestion, this process is reversed through a process called "hydrolysis." (*Adopted from* TannerThies [102]. *Reprinted with permission from Thieme publishers.*)

surface, which split disaccharides into monosaccharides as shown in Fig. 1.1.

Monosaccharides are water soluble and easily absorbed, mostly via active sodium co-transporters. These transporters rely on active transportation of sodium through the basolateral membranes of the enterocytes by Na^+-K^+-ATPase pump [52]. This creates a gradient for sodium which drags more sodium along with the monosaccharides at the luminal brush border. This process is called "secondary active transport" which also relies on the presence of their other substrate, i.e., monosaccharides to be "co-transported" with sodium. Glucose and galactose then enter the portal circulation by facilitated diffusion (GLUT2) at the basolateral membrane. Fructose has different absorption mechanism which is facilitated diffusion on the apical side (GLUT5) [51, 53]. When fructose enters enterocytes, it is immediately phosphorylated and mostly converted to glucose which is transported to the bloodstream. This is a slower process compared to secondary active transport. In general, the rate of absorption of carbohydrates is greater in the proximal bowel and most carbohydrates are absorbed by the middle of jejunum [10].

Proteins

Proteins consist of arrays of amino acids which are linked by peptide bonds. Gastric acid denatures protein structures by unfolding them and exposes more bonds to pepsin (see Fig. 1.2) [8, 10]. Pepsin is an important stomach enzyme in digesting proteins [1, 53]. It is only active under acidic pH and splits larger proteins into smaller polypeptides, proteoses, and peptones. It is exceptionally able to break up collagen which is a major connective tissue protein in meat which allows other meat proteins to be digested and absorbed. Lack of pepsin leads to poor meat digestion [10]. Pepsin provides 10–20% of total protein digestion via hydrolysis mechanism similar to carbohydrates. When proteins enter the small bowel, pancreatic peptidases (trypsin, chymotrypsin, elastase, carboxypolypeptidase) break up more peptide bonds [1]. Trypsin, chymotrypsin, and elastase split proteins into smaller polypeptides and carboxypolypeptidase A and B are able to cleave single amino acids from

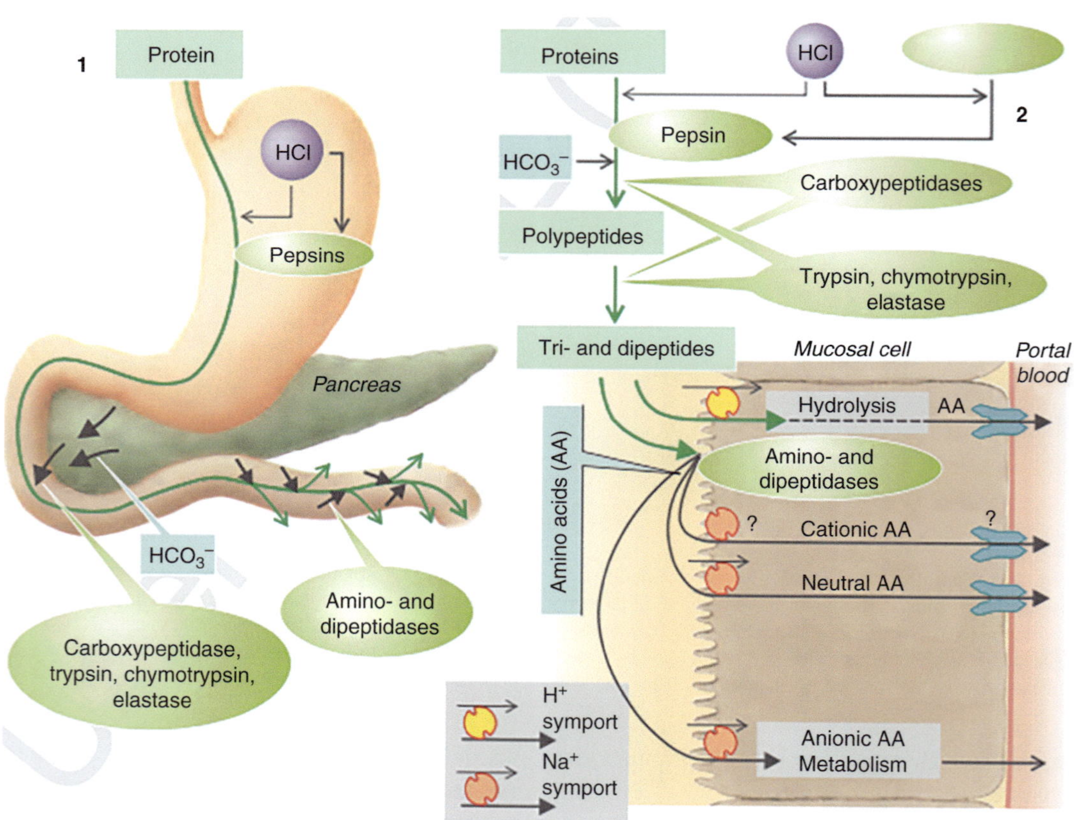

Fig. 1.2 Protein metabolism. Proteins consist of arrays of amino acids which are linked by peptide bonds. Gastric acid denatures protein structures by unfolding them and exposes more bonds to pepsin. Pepsin is an important stomach enzyme for digesting proteins. When proteins enter the small bowel, pancreatic peptidases (trypsin, chymotrypsin, elastase, carboxypolypeptidase) break up more peptide bonds. Trypsin, chymotrypsin, and elastase split proteins into smaller polypeptides, and carboxypolypeptidase A and B are able to cleave single amino acids from the carboxyl end of protein chains. Finally, in duodenum and jejunum, enterocytes at their brush border have various peptidases including aminopolypeptidase and dipeptidases which split the remaining polypeptides intro tripeptides, dipeptides which are absorbed by H^+-dependent active transporter (PepT1), and a few amino acids which are absorbed by sodium-dependent secondary active transport similar to carbohydrates mostly in jejunum. (*Adopted from* TannerThies [102]. *Reprinted with permission from Thieme publishers.*)

the carboxyl end of protein chains. Finally in duodenum and jejunum, enterocytes at their brush border have various peptidases including aminopolypeptidase and dipeptidases which split the remaining polypeptides intro tripeptides, dipeptides which are absorbed by H^+-dependent active transporter (PepT1), and a few amino acids which are absorbed by sodium-dependent secondary active transport similar to carbohydrates mostly in jejunum [10].

In the cytosol of enterocytes, there are more peptidases which break up the remaining peptide bonds and free amino acids enter into the blood through the basolateral side. This is imperative as if larger polypeptides are absorbed into blood stream, they can cause serious allergic or immune reactions [1].

Lipids

Fat in the food consists of triglycerides (mostly in animal-based meals), phospholipids, cholesterol, and cholesterol esters [1, 53]. Lingual lipase starts the digestion of triglycerides (mostly short-chained water-soluble lipids) which accounts for less than 10% of total digestion. The main step of fat digestion occurs in the small intestine (See Fig. 1.3) [8, 54]. As chyme

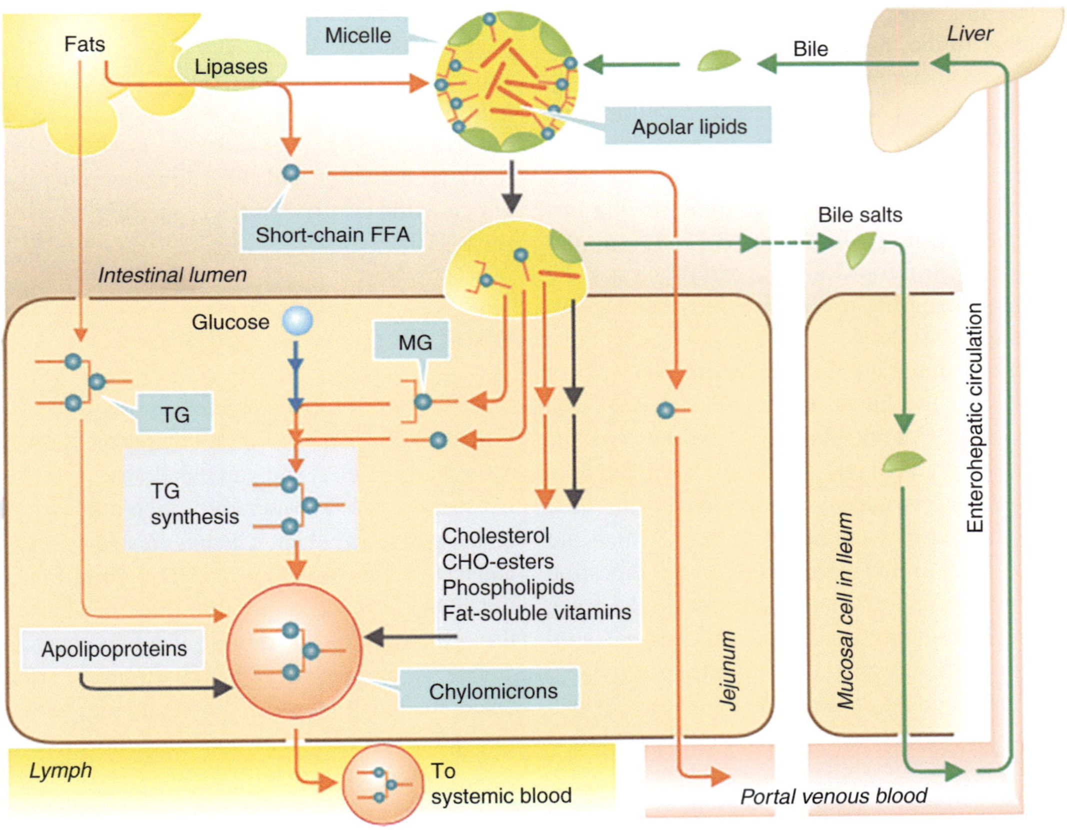

Fig. 1.3 Lipid metabolism. Fat in the food consists of triglycerides, phospholipids, cholesterol, and cholesterol esters. Lingual lipase starts the digestion of triglycerides (mostly short-chained water-soluble lipids) which accounts for less than 10% of total digestion. The main step of fat digestion occurs in the small intestine. As chyme enters duodenum, bile is secreted and "emulsifies" fat by binding to fat globules. Bile does not have any enzymatic activity but contains bile salts and lecithin which is a phospholipid with two ends. The fat-soluble portion binds to and engulfs the fat particles, while the polar (water soluble) end projects on the outer surface, which decreases interfacial tension of the fat, and breaks down fat into smaller particles. Pancreatic lipase can digest triglycerides very quickly in the small intestine by removing two fatty acids from positions 1 and 3 of triglycerides through hydrolysis similar to carbohydrates and proteins, resulting in two free fatty acids and a 2-monoglyceride. (*Adopted from* TannerThies [102]. *Reprinted with permission from Thieme publishers.*)

enters duodenum, bile is secreted and, as explained before, "emulsifies" fat by binding to fat globules. Bile does not have any enzymatic activity but contains bile salts and lecithin which is a phospholipid with two ends. The fat-soluble portion binds to and engulfs the fat particles while the polar (water soluble) end projects on the outer surface, which decreases interfacial tension of the fat, and breaks down fat into smaller particles with agitation in the small intestine, thereby increasing the total surface area of the fatty particles to almost 1000-fold [1]. This is important because lipases are water-soluble enzymes and can only act on the surface of fat particles. Even though bile salts help lipase this way, they also inhibit lipase from binding to the fat droplets. "Colipase" secreted from the pancreas alleviates this problem by binding to the C-terminal of lipase and forming a conformation that is more hydrophobic [55]. Pancreatic lipase can digest triglycerides very quickly in the small intestine by removing two fatty acids from position 1 and 3 of triglycerides through hydrolysis similar to carbohydrates and proteins, resulting in two free fatty acids and a 2-monoglyceride [1, 53]. This process leads to rapid accumulation of these end-products which can hinder the lipase activity. Fortunately, bile salts in the vicinity can absorb and remove free fatty acids and monoglycerides from the area around the enzymes by forming micelles. These are small (3–6 nanometer) spheres which are water soluble and carry triglyceride digestion products through the small intestine to the brush borders of enterocytes where they are released and immediately absorbed into the cells [54].

Small amount of short- and medium-chained fatty acids can be absorbed into the portal blood with passive diffusion without needing to form chylomicrons and going through the lymphatics, as they are relatively more water soluble. The long-chain fatty acids and lipids require transporters, namely the plasma membrane fatty acid-binding protein (FABPpm), the fatty acid transport protein 4 (FATP4), and the fatty acid translocase (FAT/CD36) [10].

Free fatty acids and monoglycerides enter the enterocyte's smooth endoplasmic reticulum, where they form triglycerides again (re-esterification) and are carried in the form of chylomicrons by exocytosis to the lymph ducts and then to the systemic circulation via thoracic duct (thereby bypassing portal circulation). Bile salts are released into the small intestine and remain in the chyme to participate in fat digestion again [1, 53].

Free fatty acids are also released from cholesterol esters and phospholipids by pancreatic enzymes (cholesterol ester hydrolase and phospholipase A2 respectively). Bile salt micelles carry cholesterol and phospholipids in a similar manner to triglyceride products. Without micelles, almost no cholesterol and only 40–50% of other fat particles are absorbed [10].

If pancreatic lipase is absent (e.g., chronic pancreatitis), or inactivated (e.g., in case of Zollinger-Ellison syndrome where stomach acid inhibits pancreatic lipase), or if bile acids are deficient (e.g., liver disease or ileal resection), fat digestion and absorption are impaired, which leads to oily and foul-smelling "steatorrhea" [10].

Water, Electrolytes, and Minerals

Water absorption is completely through passive diffusion by osmosis which happens through cells (transcellular) and gap junctions (paracellular) paths [56, 57]. Water absorption relies solely on the osmotic gradient which is created by active and passive transportation of electrolytes from GI lumen. As a result, water absorption depends on the osmolality of the chyme. If a hyperosmotic chyme is discharged from the stomach, water enters the small intestine, so the chyme remains isosmotic with plasma.

Sodium is absorbed by an active mechanism of Na^+-K^+-ATPase at the basolateral surface of intestinal epithelial cells which drags sodium from the GI lumen [58]. It can be co-transported with other nutrients through "secondary active transport" which was discussed earlier. It also can be exchanged with hydrogen ions (Na^+-H^+ exchanger) in ileum. Aldosterone (similarly to renal tubules) can enhance sodium absorption, and along with it chloride and water, greatly [1, 57]. This leads to increase in absorption especially in the colon if a person is dehydrated. The tight junctions in the large intestine are better sealed compared to the small intestine which prevents back-leak and makes sodium absorption much more effective [1].

The intestine must be able to absorb 25–35 grams of sodium each day as 20–30 grams of sodium are secreted in the GI secretions daily and the average diet consists of 5–8 grams of salt [1]. In case of intestinal epithelial damage or extreme secretion due to inflammation or infection, total body sodium reserves can be depleted rapidly.

In the upper GI tract, negatively charged chloride ions are dragged with positively charged sodium passively by diffusion. In some parts of ileum and the entire colon, chloride is absorbed by chloride-bicarbonate exchanger. This provides a protective alkaline environment in the colon. Cholera toxin can cause a widespread chloride channels via a cAMP pathway and lead to massive secretion of chloride ions and consequently sodium and water in the intestines, and this can lead to severe dehydration and death if left unchecked [10].

Since both bile and pancreatic secretions contain large amounts of bicarbonate ions, they need to be reabsorbed. Hydrogen ions coming from the stomach as well as those secreted by Na^+-H^+ exchanger combine with bicarbonate in the duodenum and jejunum to form water and carbon dioxide molecules, both of which are absorbed by diffusion [1, 57].

Potassium is absorbed passively mostly in a paracellular manner [10]. It can be secreted in the colon (via a mechanism similar to secretion in renal distal tubules) by aldosterone-sensitive stimulation of Na^+-K^+-ATPase pump [58].

Calcium ions are actively absorbed mostly in the duodenum via channel-like calcium transporter (CaT1), the Na+-Ca2+ exchanger (NCX1), and the plasma membrane Ca2+-ATPase (PMCA1) [10]. This process is vitamin D dependent, and parathyroid hormone (PTH) regulates calcium absorption through vitamin D activation. Calcium can also be passively absorbed through paracellular pathway in the rest of small intestine.

Iron is absorbed in the proximal small intestine [10]. When exposed to the stomach acid, ingested iron in the form of ferric ions (Fe3+) is reduced to ferrous ions (Fe2+). Ferric reductase on the brush border of proximal small intestine and also vitamin C (ascorbic acid) are able to reduce ferric ions. Ferrous form is transported into enterocytes by the heme carrier protein 1 (HCP1) [59] and the divalent metal ion transporter (DMT1, also involved in zinc absorption) [60]. Fe^{2+} is then transported by ferroprotein-1 at the basolateral membrane into blood where it binds to transferrin which acts as a vehicle for ferric ion delivery to various tissues such as the liver, spleen, and bone marrow.

Vitamins

Fat-soluble vitamins (vitamin A, D, E, and K) are absorbed in a similar way to fat, namely in micelles formed by bile salts and then are incorporated into chylomicrons. SR-B1 is involved in vitamin E uptake, and NPC1L1 and ABCA1 probably play a role in vitamin A absorption [10].

Water-soluble vitamin (except vitamin B12) are mostly absorbed by Na+-dependent mechanisms [10]. Vitamin B12 is a relatively large molecule and is present in dietary protein, which is released after acid exposure in the stomach [61]. It then binds to R proteins secreted in saliva. In the duodenum, trypsin digests the R protein that forms with intrinsic factor secreted by the gastric parietal cells. The complex is resistant to trypsin and carries vitamin B12 to terminal ileum where it is absorbed via a receptor-mediated endocytosis if pH is more than 5.6 and calcium ions are available [10].

Summary of Important Points on Digestion and Absorption

- Digestion is the process of chemical and mechanical breakdown of food into absorbable components. Absorption is the movement of nutrient molecules from the GI lumen into enterocytes and then into bloodstream or lymph.
- There are three main classes of nutrients in food: carbohydrates, proteins, and fats. These are mostly digested (through hydrolysis) and absorbed in the small intestine.

- The absorptive capacity of a normal small intestine is thousands of grams of carbohydrates, 500 gram of fat, 500–700 gram of proteins, and more than 20 liters of water each day.
- The colon (mostly the proximal half) is mainly involved in fluid and electrolyte absorption.

GI Mucosal Barrier Function

Overview of GI Mucosal Barrier Function The alimentary tract, as one of the largest body surfaces exposed to the outside world, has an important role in protecting against external environment through a tightly regulated intestinal barrier [8, 62, 63]. This is also where millions of microbes and environmental antigens come into close contact with the host immune system [64].

Normal Function

The gastrointestinal system has a very complex task of selectively allowing the absorption of essential nutrients, while limiting the transport of potentially harmful antigens. This delicate balance plays an important role in maintaining intestinal integrity and immune homeostasis [65]. There are several mechanisms by which gut protects the body against potentially harmful pathogens.

The GI secretions including saliva, gastric acid, and pancreatic juice degrade bacteria and other pathogens in the lumen [64]. Almost the entire alimentary tract is covered with a constantly supplied layer of alkaline mucus which provides a barrier between bacteria and the epithelial cells. The most abundant mucous protein secreted by the goblet cells in the small and large intestine is mucin 2 (Muc2). The gene expression for Muc2 is critical in gastrointestinal tract barrier function, as Muc2-knockout mice spontaneously develop colitis [66].

Furthermore, enterocytes in the small intestine also have an extra layer of glycocalyx on top of the mucous layer which is a matrix of mucopolysaccharides and glycoprotein which provides additional surface for absorption [8]. The colon also has two mucous layers: the outer layer harbors and allows colonization of crucial commensal bacteria and the inner layer provides a sterile barrier [64]. The secretion of antimicrobial protein (AMPs) such as defensins by Paneth cells and secretory immunoglobulin A (IgA) adds another layer of defense against bacteria.

At the epithelial level, cells are tightly sealed by three types of junctional structures: (1) tight junctions, (2) adherent junctions, and (3) desmosomes. Starting from the apical side, tight suctions consist of protein complexes formed by Claudius, occludin, and tricellulin. Actin fibers via zona occludens (ZO)-1 and ZO-2 strengthen these complexes [62]. Main function of these junctions is sealing of the paracellular space and regulating transportation. Many factors including intercellular signaling, cytokines, and post-translational modifications dynamically modulate the tight junction protein complexes to allow passage of essential molecules and restrict harmful substances. This is referred to as the "leak pathway" [67]. An imbalance in these regulations leads to weak barrier integrity which is associated with various diseases. Underneath tight junctions lie adherent junctions which consist of protein complexes such as E-cadherin and catenins which are also strengthened by actin cytoskeleton. Adherent junctions with desmosomes which are located on the basolateral aspect of cells form strong adhesive bonds which provides mechanical strength to the epithelial wall [8].

Finally, the innate and adaptive immune cells such as T cells, B cells, macrophages, and dendritic cells reside in the lamina propria which is underneath the mucosal layer, and this adds another layer of protection against pathogens [64, 68].

Factors Affecting Barrier Function

Many factors are involved in dysfunction of the gut barrier [8]. Certain genetic predispositions make gut wall barrier more vulnerable to failure. Patients who carry a polymorphism in the cadherin-1 gene (a part of adherent junctions) are more likely to develop post-infectious IBS [69].

Patients with diarrhea-predominant IBS have lower level of glutamine synthase, which is crucial in glutamine production, which is a major energy source for enterocytes [70]. Psychological stress, extreme temperatures, or pain results in the release of cytokines by mast cells which can increase the permeability of gut wall [71].

The role of a balanced diet for gut homeostasis and gut barrier integrity has become an increasingly important area of research as food plays an important role as a modulator of GI functions including intestinal barrier function [72, 73].

Flavonoids are present in fruits, green and black tea, coffee, red wine, and chocolate [74]. Flavonoids are able to modulate gut microbiota and improve the gut barrier integrity [75]. The average intakes seem to be lower than recommendations in most people.

The impact of high-sugar and high-fat diet commonly referred to as "Western diet" has been extensively studied on barrier function. In one study, feeding such diet to mice led to a decrease in mucous thickness and goblet cell expression, and an increase in gut permeability and inflammatory markers [76]. To make matters worse, common food additives such as carboxymethylcellulose and polysorbate-80, which are added to improve food taste, have been associated with similar effect on the mucosal function and resulted in colitis and metabolic syndrome in mice [77].

Heavy alcohol use has shown to increase intestinal permeability, mainly through its main metabolite, acetaldehyde. It activates the oxidative stress pathways and disrupts tight and adherent junctions [78]. Bacteria in the gut also play an important role in ethanol-induced injury as chronic alcohol use is associated with increase in gram-negative bacteria which interrupt normal microbiota and damage barrier function [79].

Non-steroidal-anti-inflammatory agents (NSAIDs) have demonstrated increased intestinal permeability as a result of cyclooxygenase inhibition, as well as direct damage to the epithelia [64, 80].

Psychological stress and its association with GI barrier function (gut-brain interaction) have been extensively studied [64]. In animal models, physical and psychological stress including noise, heat/cold, crowding, and maternal deprivation has shown deterioration of the intestinal barrier function [81]. This has been seen in human volunteers who showed concomitant increased small intestinal permeability and salivary cortisol after a public speech test [82].

Defects in the intestinal barrier have been implicated in a broad range of GI disorders including inflammatory bowel disease (IBD), celiac disease, colon cancer, and systemic diseases such as diabetes type 1, obesity, depression and chronic liver disease [64].

In IBD patients (both Crohn's disease and ulcerative colitis), alterations in intestinal permeability due to changes in expression of tight junction and mucous layer leading to bacterial penetration have been observed [83]. Furthermore, abnormal immune response to microbiota in the intestine in patients with genetic predisposition and release of inflammatory markers seems to threaten the integrity of the epithelia [84]. This impairment has been seen in asymptomatic Crohn's patients as far as one year before clinical symptoms appear [85].

Celiac disease induces increased permeability and tight junction defects, which allows gliadin to leak into the lamina propria and provoke the immune system [86]. In addition, gluten fractions in food alter the gut barrier function that causes tight junction disintegration with ensuing inflammatory response [87].

In non-alcoholic fatty liver disease (NAFLD), intestinal permeability and tight junction disruption correlate with the severity of liver disease [88]. Higher bacterial translocation and endotoxin levels are seen in these patients [89].

Microbiota

Overview of GI Microbiota The human colon hosts a large group of microorganisms [8]. Nondigestible meal residues serve as feeding substrate for the microbiota. The human microbiome is formed by bacteria, archaea, viruses, and other microbes [90].

Microbiota in Health

Two large databases characterizing human microbiota are the European Metagenomics of the Human Intestinal Tract (MetaHIT) and the Human Microbiome Project (HMP). These databases combined with 368 Chinese samples were converged into the most comprehensive database of 9.8 million unique gene sequences which is believed to contain nearly all the bacteria in most human guts [91]. Data analysis from HMP database has identified the community types of these microbiota [92]. It seems like each individual has a relatively stable group of residing organism in their intestine. One study found that in adults not taking antibiotics, 70% of the fecal species remained stable over 1 year and some up to 5 years [93]. Evidence of "shared" species within family members indicates that these species may be stably present perhaps more than decades if not for a lifetime [90].

The relationship between human host and these organisms is mutual. Human organism feeds and hosts these organisms, and in return, they play several crucial roles in our body including modulation of the immune system (e.g., development of immune tolerance), development of central nervous system, regulation of metabolic activity and growth, and regulation of digestive functions. Factors like prebiotics and probiotics modify the microbiome and facilitate intestinal transit. Microbiota are also involved in visceral sensitivity and pain perception [8]. Microbiota play a key role in normal digestive physiology. They can release short-chain fatty acids (SCFA) from indigestible fibers. These products are important nutrients for intestinal mucosa and are involved in modulating immune system and carcinogenesis [90].

Microbiota in Diseases

In recent years, there has been an increasing interest in finding the link between microbiota and diseases. Alterations of this delicate microbial balance by eating habits, medications, and other environmental factors have been seen in various conditions. It often is challenging to discern whether these alterations are the cause or the result of the disease [90].

Clostridium difficile infection (CDI) is a classic example of how alterations in microbiota conformation in the gut can lead to pathology. Different classes of antibiotics are associated with CDI. There have been promising results when a "healthy" conformation of species is added to these patients (fecal microbial transplant [FMT]). FMT in patients with recurrent CDI has shown significant superiority compared to treatment by oral vancomycin or vancomycin therapy followed by bowel lavage [94]. These patients had higher diversity of microbiota, higher population of Bacteroidetes, and lower number of Proteobacteria after FMT.

IBD is associated with changes in the microbiota [95]. Patients with Crohn's disease have less diversity of their microbiota [90]. In one study, certain microbial classes were strongly associated with disease phenotype in ileal and rectal samples [96].

Microbiota plays a crucial role in GI motility and functional gastrointestinal disorders (FGID) [97]. This effect is mediated by short chain fatty acids (SCFA) produced by these organisms as discussed earlier, modulation of GI hormone secretions, and inflammatory signaling by immune responses to microbiota. The receptors for SCFA and GI hormones are present in the neural, endocrine, and immune cells. It has been suggested that normalization of the gastric microbiota by probiotics may be an effective treatment in FGID [98].

The microbiota have been implicated in irritable bowel syndrome (IBS). Diets low in fermentable oligosaccharides, disaccharide, monosaccharides, and polyols (FODMAPs) have shown improvement of symptoms in patients with IBS by altering gut microbiota [99]. Furthermore, FMT, which is used in recurrent CDI, has shown promising results in IBS in some studies [100, 101].

Summary of Important Points on GI Microbiota

- The GI tract, as one of the largest body surfaces exposed to the outside world, plays an important role in protecting against external threats through a tightly regulated intestinal barrier, where millions of microbes and environmental antigens come into close contact with the host immune system.

- This system maintains a delicate balance of selectively allowing the absorption of essential nutrients, while limiting the transport of potentially harmful antigens via epithelial junctions (tight junction, adherent junction, and desmosomes).
- There are additional layers of protection which include mucous, saliva, gastric acid, and pancreatic secretions which neutralize bacteria and other pathogens.
- Factors that can damage the gut barrier include genetic predispositions, Western diet, alcohol use, stress, and certain medications including NSAIDS.
- Impairment of this barrier has been associated with many disorders including IBD, celiac disease, colon cancer, chronic liver disease, type 1 diabetes, obesity, and depression.
- Microbiota refers to the large group of microorganisms which reside in the GI tract. There have been remarkable advances in recognizing the role of these organisms and their interaction with the host (human body) in normal development, immune modulation, and metabolic activities. Certain diseases including *C. difficile* infection can occur as a result of disturbance of this delicate balance.

Conclusion

The GI tract plays important role in body homeostasis including regulating the transit of ingested food down the GI tract for efficient digestion and absorption of essential nutrients. The enteric nervous system, such as the "gut brain," plays an important role in generating and harmonizing these activities both directly and through a number of enteric reflexes. Furthermore, the intestinal tract has vast number of endocrine (and paracrine) activities which regulate bodily functions inside and outside the GI tract. Ingested food goes through series of steps including mastication (oral cavity), deglutition (pharynx and esophagus), mixing and digestion (stomach), further digestion and absorption (intestines), and finally storage and defecation (colon). Each organ has a unique structure, movement pattern, and secretion well suited to its task. The gut wall is a crucial barrier against external pathogens while maintaining a healthy and essential interaction with the millions of microorganism that reside inside the gut (microbiota).

References

1. Hall J. Guyton and Hall textbook of medical physiology. 13th ed. Elsevier Health Sciences; 2016.
2. Furness JB. The enteric nervous system and neurogastroenterology. Nat Rev Gastroenterol Hepatol. 2012;9:286.
3. Cheng LK, Du P, O'Grady G. Mapping and modeling gastrointestinal bioelectricity: from engineering bench to bedside. Physiology (Bethesda). 2013;28(5):310–7.
4. Huizinga JD, Lammers WJ. Gut peristalsis is governed by a multitude of cooperating mechanisms. Am J Physiol Gastrointest Liver Physiol. 2009;296:G1.
5. Lammers WJ, Slack JR. Of slow waves and spike patches. News Physiol Sci. 2001;16:138.
6. Sanders KM, Ward SM, Koh SD. Interstitial cells: regulators of smooth muscle function. Physiol Rev. 2014;94:859.
7. Mittal R, Debs LH, Patel AP, et al. Neurotransmitters: the critical modulators regulating gut-brain axis. J Cell Physiol. 2017;232(9):2359–72.
8. Boeckxstaens G, Camilleri M, Sifrim D, et al. Fundamentals of neurogastroenterology: physiology/motility - sensation. Gastroenterology. 2016;150:1292–304.
9. Distrutti E, Azpiroz F, Soldevilla A, et al. Gastric wall tension determines perception of gastric distention. Gastroenterology. 1999;116:1035–42.
10. TannerThies R. Physiology: an illustrated review. New York: Thieme Medical Pub; 2012.
11. Lund JP, Kolta A. Brainstem circuits that control mastication: do they have anything to say during speech? J Commun Disord. 2006;39(5):381–90.
12. Matsuo K, Palmer JB. Anatomy and physiology of feeding and swallowing: normal and abnormal. Phys Med Rehabil Clin N Am. 2008;19(4):691–707, vii.
13. Lang IM. Brain stem control of the phases of swallowing. Dysphagia. 2009;24(3):333–48.
14. Costa MM, Lemme EM. Coordination of respiration and swallowing: functional pattern and relevance of vocal folds closure. Arq Gastroenterol. 2010;47(1):42–8.
15. Bieger D. Neuropharmacologic correlates of deglutition: lessons from fictive swallowing. Dysphagia. 1991;6:147–64.

16. Tack J, Demedts I, Meulemans A, et al. Role of nitric oxide in the gastric accommodation reflex and in meal induced satiety in humans. Gut. 2002;51:219–24.
17. Mittal RK, Padda B, Bhalla V, et al. Synchrony between circular and longitudinal muscle contractions during peristalsis in normal subjects. Am J Physiol Gastrointest Liver Physiol. 2006;290:G431–8.
18. Mittal RK, Balaban DH. The esophagogastric junction. N Engl J Med. 1997;336:924–32.
19. Browning KN, Travagli RA. Central control of gastrointestinal motility. Curr Opin Endocrinol Diabetes Obes. 2019;26(1):11–6.
20. Côté CD, Zadeh-Tahmasebi M, Rasmussen BA, et al. Hormonal signaling in the gut. J Biol Chem. 2014;289:11642.
21. Takahashi T. Interdigestive migrating motor complex -its mechanism and clinical importance. J Smooth Muscle Res. 2013;49:99–111.
22. Delporte C. Structure and physiological actions of ghrelin. Scientifica (Cairo). 2013;2013:518909.
23. Asakawa A, Inui A, Kaga T, et al. Ghrelin is an appetite-stimulatory signal from stomach with structural resemblance to motilin. Gastroenterology. 2001;120(2):337–45.
24. Fujino K, Inui A, Asakawa A, Kihara N, Fujimura M, Fujimiya M. Ghrelin induces fasted motor activity of the gastrointestinal tract in conscious fed rats. J Physiol (Lond). 2003;550(Pt 1):227–40.
25. Tschöp M, Wawarta R, Riepl RL, et al. Post-prandial decrease of circulating human ghrelin levels. J Endocrinol Invest. 2001;24(6):RC19–21.
26. Huizinga JD, Chen JH, Zhu YF, et al. The origin of segmentation motor activity in the intestine. Nat Commun. 2014;5:3326.
27. Kumral D, Zfass AM. Gut movements: a review of the physiology of gastrointestinal transit. Dig Dis Sci. 2018;63(10):2500–6.
28. Steadman CJ, Phillips SF, Camilleri M, et al. Variation of muscle tone in the human colon. Gastroenterology. 1991;101:373–81.
29. Ford MJ, Camilleri M, Wiste JA, et al. Differences in colonic tone and phasic response to a meal in the transverse and sigmoid human colon. Gut. 1995;37:264–9.
30. Furukawa Y, Cook IJ, Panagopoulos V, et al. Relationship between sleep patterns and human colonic motor patterns. Gastroenterology. 1994;107:1372–81.
31. Bampton PA, Dinning PG, Kennedy ML, et al. Prolonged multi-point recording of colonic manometry in the un- prepared human colon: providing insight into potentially relevant pressure wave parameters. Am J Gastroenterol. 2001;96:1838–48.
32. Palit S, Lunniss PJ, Scott SM. The physiology of human defecation. Dig Dis Sci. 2012;57(6):1445–64.
33. Allen A, Flemström G. Gastroduodenal mucus bicarbonate barrier: protection against acid and pepsin. Am J Physiol Cell Physiol. 2005;288:C1.
34. Humphrey SP, Williamson RT. A review of saliva: normal composition, flow, and function. J Prosthet Dent. 2001;85(2):162–9.
35. Long JD, Orlando RC. Esophageal submucosal glands: structure and function. Am J Gastroenterol. 1999;94(10):2818–24.
36. Schubert ML. Gastric secretion. Curr Opin Gastroenterol. 2011;27(6):536–42.
37. Soybel DI. Anatomy and physiology of the stomach. Surg Clin North Am. 2005;85(5):875–94, v.
38. Johnson CD, Mole DR, Pestridge A. Postprandial alkaline tide: does it exist? Digestion. 1995;56(2):100–6.
39. Dimaline R, Varro A. Novel roles of gastrin. J Physiol. 2014;592:2951.
40. Makhlouf GM, Schubert ML. Gastric somatostatin: a paracrine regulator of acid secretion. Metab Clin Exp. 1990;39(9 Suppl 2):138–42.
41. Browning KN, Travagli RA. Central nervous system control of gastrointestinal motility and secretion and modulation of gastrointestinal functions. Compr Physiol. 2014;4(4):1339–68.
42. Johansson ME, Sjövall H, Hansson GC. The gastrointestinal mucus system in health and disease. Nat Rev Gastroenterol Hepatol. 2013;10(6):352–61.
43. Pallagi P, Hegyi P, Rakonczay Z. The physiology and pathophysiology of pancreatic ductal secretion: the background for clinicians. Pancreas. 2015;44(8):1211–33.
44. Manohar M, Verma AK, Venkateshaiah SU, Sanders NL, Mishra A. Pathogenic mechanisms of pancreatitis. World J Gastrointest Pharmacol Ther. 2017;8(1):10–25.
45. Chandra R, Liddle RA. Neural and hormonal regulation of pancreatic secretion. Curr Opin Gastroenterol. 2009;25(5):441–6.
46. Boyer JL. Bile formation and secretion. Compr Physiol. 2013;3:1035.
47. Shiffman ML, Sugerman HJ, Moore EW. Human gallbladder mucosal function. Effect of concentration and acidification of bile on cholesterol and calcium solubility. Gastroenterology. 1990;99(5):1452–9.
48. Staels B, Fonseca VA. Bile acids and metabolic regulation: mechanisms and clinical responses to bile acid sequestration. Diabetes Care. 2009;32 Suppl 2:S237–45.
49. Wong BS, Camilleri M, Carlson P, et al. Increased bile acid biosynthesis is associated with irritable bowel syndrome with diarrhea. Clin Gastroenterol Hepatol. 2012;10:1009–1015 e3.
50. Abrahamsson H, Ostlund-Lindqvist AM, Nilsson R, et al. Altered bile acid metabolism in patients with constipation-predominant irritable bowel syndrome and functional constipation. Scand J Gastroenterol. 2008;43:1483–8.
51. Wright EM, Martín MG, Turk E. Intestinal absorption in health and disease--sugars. Best Pract Res Clin Gastroenterol. 2003;17(6):943–56.
52. Wright EM, Loo DD, Hirayama BA. Biology of human sodium glucose transporters. Physiol Rev. 2011;291:733.
53. Goodman BE. Insights into digestion and absorption of major nutrients in humans. Adv Physiol Educ. 2010;34(2):44–53.

54. Black DD. Development and physiological regulation of intestinal lipid absorption. I. Development of intestinal lipid absorption: cellular events in chylomicron assembly and secretion. Am J Physiol Gastrointest Liver Physiol. 2007;293:G519.
55. Lowe ME. Structure and function of pancreatic lipase and colipase. Annu Rev Nutr. 1997;17:141–58. https://doi.org/10.1146/annurev.nutr.17.1.141.
56. Banks MR, Farthing MJ. Fluid and electrolyte transport in the small intestine. Curr Opin Gastroenterol. 2002;18(2):176–81.
57. Kunzelmann K, Mall M. Electrolyte transport in the mammalian colon: mechanisms and implications for disease. Physiol Rev. 2002;82:245.
58. Bachmann O, Juric M, Seidler U, et al. Basolateral ion transporters involved in colonic epithelial electrolyte absorption, anion secretion and cellular homeostasis. Acta Physiol (Oxf). 2011;201:33.
59. Przybyszewska J, Zekanowska E. The role of hepcidin, ferroprotein, HCP1, and DMT1 protein in iron absorption in the human digestive tract. Prz Gastroenterol. 2014;9(4):208–13.
60. Yamaji S, Tennant J, Tandy S, Williams M, Singh Srai SK, Sharp P. Zinc regulates the function and expression of the iron transporters DMT1 and IREG1 in human intestinal Caco-2 cells. FEBS Lett. 2001;507(2):137–41.
61. O'leary F, Samman S. Vitamin B12 in health and disease. Nutrients. 2010;2(3):299–316.
62. Camilleri M, Madsen K, Spiller R, et al. Intestinal barrier function in health and gastrointestinal disease. Neurogastroenterol Motil. 2012;24:503–12.
63. Neunlist M, Van Landeghem L, Mahe MM, et al. The digestive neuronal-glial-epithelial unit: a new actor in gut health and disease. Nat Rev Gastroenterol Hepatol. 2013;10:90–100.
64. Vancamelbeke M, Vermeire S. The intestinal barrier: a fundamental role in health and disease. Expert Rev Gastroenterol Hepatol. 2017;11(9):821–34.
65. Salvo Romero E, Alonso Cotoner C, Pardo Camacho C, Casado Bedmar M, Vicario M. The intestinal barrier function and its involvement in digestive disease. Rev Esp Enferm Dig. 2015;107(11):686–96.
66. Van der Sluis M, De Koning BA, De Bruijn AC, et al. Muc2-deficient mice spontaneously develop colitis, indicating that MUC2 is critical for colonic protection. Gastroenterology. 2006;131(1):117–29.
67. Chelakkot C, Ghim J, Ryu SH. Mechanisms regulating intestinal barrier integrity and its pathological implications. Exp Mol Med. 2018;50(8):103.
68. Turner JR. Intestinal mucosal barrier function in health and disease. Nat Rev Immunol. 2009;9(11):799–809.
69. Villani AC, Lemire M, Thabane M, et al. Genetic risk factors for post-infectious irritable bowel syndrome following a waterborne outbreak of gastroenteritis. Gastroenterology. 2010;138:1502–13.
70. Zhou Q, Souba WW, Croce CM, et al. MicroRNA-29a regulates intestinal membrane permeability in patients with irritable bowel syndrome. Gut. 2010;59:775–84.
71. Santos J, Saperas E, Nogueiras C, et al. Release of mast cell mediators into the jejunum by cold pain stress in humans. Gastroenterology. 1998;114:640–8.
72. Shimizu M. Interaction between food substances and the intestinal epithelium. Biosci Biotechnol Biochem. 2010;74(2):232–41.
73. De Santis S, Cavalcanti E, Mastronardi M, Jirillo E, Chieppa M. Nutritional keys for intestinal barrier modulation. Front Immunol. 2015;6:612.
74. Vogiatzoglou A, Mulligan AA, Lentjes MA, et al. Flavonoid intake in European adults (18 to 64 years). PLoS One. 2015;10(5):e0128132.
75. Anhê FF, Roy D, Pilon G, et al. A polyphenol-rich cranberry extract protects from diet-induced obesity, insulin resistance and intestinal inflammation in association with increased Akkermansia spp. population in the gut microbiota of mice. Gut. 2015;64(6):872–83.
76. Martinez-Medina M, Denizot J, Dreux N, et al. Western diet induces dysbiosis with increased E coli in CEABAC10 mice, alters host barrier function favoring AIEC colonization. Gut. 2014;63(1):116–24.
77. Chassaing B, Koren O, Goodrich JK, et al. Dietary emulsifiers impact the mouse gut microbiota promoting colitis and metabolic syndrome. Nature. 2015;519(7541):92–6.
78. Elamin EE, Masclee AA, Dekker J, Jonkers DM. Ethanol metabolism and its effects on the intestinal epithelial barrier. Nutr Rev. 2013;71(7):483–99.
79. Malaguarnera G, Giordano M, Nunnari G, Bertino G, Malaguarnera M. Gut microbiota in alcoholic liver disease: pathogenetic role and therapeutic perspectives. World J Gastroenterol. 2014;20(44):16639–48.
80. Bjarnason I, Takeuchi K. Intestinal permeability in the pathogenesis of NSAID-induced enteropathy. J Gastroenterol. 2009;44(Suppl 19):23–9.
81. Rodiño-Janeiro BK, Alonso-Cotoner C, Pigrau M, Lobo B, Vicario M, Santos J. Role of corticotropin-releasing factor in gastrointestinal permeability. J Neurogastroenterol Motil. 2015;21(1):33–50.
82. Vanuytsel T, van Wanrooy S, Vanheel H, et al. Psychological stress and corticotropin-releasing hormone increase intestinal permeability in humans by a mast cell-dependent mechanism. Gut. 2014;63(8):1293–9.
83. Johansson ME, Gustafsson JK, Holmén-Larsson J, et al. Bacteria penetrate the normally impenetrable inner colon mucus layer in both murine colitis models and patients with ulcerative colitis. Gut. 2014;63(2):281–91.
84. De Souza HS, Fiocchi C. Immunopathogenesis of IBD: current state of the art. Nat Rev Gastroenterol Hepatol. 2016;13(1):13–27.
85. Vogelsang H. Do changes in intestinal permeability predict disease relapse in Crohn's disease? Inflamm Bowel Dis. 2008;14(Suppl 2):S162–3.
86. Heyman M, Abed J, Lebreton C, Cerf-Bensussan N. Intestinal permeability in coeliac disease: insight

into mechanisms and relevance to pathogenesis. Gut. 2012;61(9):1355–64.
87. Fasano A. Zonulin and its regulation of intestinal barrier function: the biological door to inflammation, autoimmunity, and cancer. Physiol Rev. 2011;91(1):151–75.
88. Giorgio V, Miele L, Principessa L, et al. Intestinal permeability is increased in children with non-alcoholic fatty liver disease, and correlates with liver disease severity. Dig Liver Dis. 2014;46(6):556–60.
89. Harte AL, da Silva NF, Creely SJ, et al. Elevated endotoxin levels in non-alcoholic fatty liver disease. J Inflamm (Lond). 2010;7:15.
90. Shreiner AB, Kao JY, Young VB. The gut microbiome in health and in disease. Curr Opin Gastroenterol. 2015;31(1):69–75.
91. Li J, Jia H, Cai X, et al. An integrated catalog of reference genes in the human gut microbiome. Nat Biotechnol. 2014;32:834–41. PubMed PMID: 24997786.
92. Ding T, Schloss PD. Dynamics and associations of microbial community types across the human body. Nature. 2014;509(7500):357–60.
93. Faith JJ, Guruge JL, Charbonneau M, et al. The long-term stability of the human gut microbiota. Science. 2013;341(6141):1237439.
94. Van Nood E, Vrieze A, Nieuwdorp M, et al. Duodenal infusion of donor feces for recurrent Clostridium difficile. N Engl J Med. 2013;368(5):407–15.
95. Kostic AD, Xavier RJ, Gevers D. The microbiome in inflammatory bowel disease: current status and the future ahead. Gastroenterology. 2014;146(6):1489–99.
96. Gevers D, Kugathasan S, Denson LA, et al. The treatment-naive microbiome in new-onset Crohn's disease. Cell Host Microbe. 2014;15(3):382–92.
97. Fukui H, Xin X, Miwa H. Role of gut microbiota-gut hormone axis in the pathophysiology of functional gastrointestinal disorders. J Neurogastroenterol Motil. 2018;24:367.
98. Igarashi M, Nakae H, Matsuoka T, et al. Alteration in the gastric microbiota and its restoration by probiotics in patients with functional dyspepsia. BMJ Open Gastroenterol. 2017;4:e000144.
99. Halmos EP, Power VA, Shepherd SJ, et al. A diet low in FODMAPs reduces symptoms of irritable bowel syndrome. Gastroenterology. 2014;146(1):67–75. e5.
100. El-Salhy M, Mazzawi T. Fecal microbiota transplantation for managing irritable bowel syndrome. Expert Rev Gastroenterol Hepatol. 2018;12:439–45.
101. Johnsen PH, Hilpüsch F, Cavanagh JP, et al. Faecal microbiota transplantation versus placebo for moderate-to-severe irritable bowel syndrome: a double-blind, randomized, placebo-controlled, parallel-group, single-centre trial. Lancet Gastroenterol Hepatol. 2018;3:17–24.
102. TannerThies R. Physiology—an illustrated review. 1st ed; 2011.

Dietary Composition and Nutritional Deficiencies

2

Andrew Eidelberg and Carolyn Newberry

Introduction

Both macronutrients and micronutrients are essential for human health and nutrition. Macronutrients, such as carbohydrates, proteins, and fats, provide foundational energy to meet basic requirements of the body. Micronutrients, like vitamins and trace metals, are additional important components of metabolic processes and overall health, presenting with standard symptoms in times of deficiency (Table 2.1). This chapter will examine the basic structure and function of each type of nutrient, the recommended daily intake amounts as set forth by the US Food and Nutrition Board, and the causes and symptoms of specific nutrient deficiencies, including how they relate to the gastrointestinal tract.

A. Eidelberg
Weill Cornell Medical College, New York, NY, USA
e-mail: Ase2009@med.cornell.edu

C. Newberry (✉)
Division of Gastroenterology, Weill Cornell Medical Center, New York, NY, USA
e-mail: Can9054@med.cornell.edu

Macronutrients

Carbohydrates

Carbohydrates, in their most basic form, can be identified by the formula $C_x(H_2O)_y$, which describes the ratio between carbon, hydrogen, and oxygen in the compound [1]. Carbohydrates are formed from the transition of solar energy into chemical energy [2]. This chemical energy is then processed through glycolysis and respiration, yielding ATP, which stores energy in an easily accessible form for host use [2]. Carbohydrates are among the most common naturally occurring compounds and serve a wide variety of functions, both in the human body and in the diet. Some of these roles include providing energy, assisting with intercellular communication, and providing structure to cells and tissue [1].

Carbohydrates occur in countless different forms and can be derived from other compounds through oxidation/reduction or dehydration reactions [1]. This yields several notable forms, including monosaccharides (i.e., glucose, fructose, galactose), which cannot be further hydrolyzed, and disaccharides (i.e., sucrose, lactose, maltose), which are composed of two monosaccharide residues [3]. Oligosaccharides (i.e., maltodextrins, inulin) are characterized typically by three to nine monosaccharide polymers, whereas polysaccharides (i.e., amylose and other

C. Newberry et al. (eds.), *Nutrition, Weight, and Digestive Health*,
https://doi.org/10.1007/978-3-030-94953-2_2

starches, cellulose, glucomannans) are typically characterized by greater than ten [3].

Carbohydrates serve a crucial role in clinical nutrition. They can be separated into two main classes: those that are readily available for metabolism, such as glucose or starch, and those that must be metabolized before they can be utilized, such as cellulose and other types of fibers [1, 4]. Generally, carbohydrates are digested in the small intestine and fermented in the large intestine [5]. Because of the complex structure of some carbohydrates, there remains a difference in the net metabolizable energy that could be made available for energy [5]. The differences in carbohydrate digestion do not, however, alter the recommended dietary allowance (RDA) set forth by the Food and Nutrition Board, which recommends 130 grams of carbohydrates per day for healthy adults [6]. Thus, the Acceptable Macronutrient Distribution Range (AMDR) for carbohydrates should be 45–65% of the total energy consumed [6].

Proteins

Proteins are macronutrients that are composed of amino acids, of which there are twenty [7–9]. Of the twenty amino acids, twelve are produced in the body, whereas the other eight must be obtained through the diet (which are termed essential) [9]. When paired together by peptide bonds, these amino acids form different proteins containing a hydrocarbon backbone and nitrogenous residues [7, 8]. Ultimately, protein molecules are digested by specific enzymes secreted by glands in the oral cavity (salivary amylase) and pancreas (pancreatic amylase), which converts them to single peptide and dipeptides that can absorbed in the small intestine and incorporated into DNA, enzymes, or energy-providing structures for proper growth and development [7, 8].

Proteins can be obtained through the diet from both animal and plant sources. Animal proteins contain all essential amino acids and may provide more health benefits, especially in certain groups like pregnant patients and the elderly [8]. Animal proteins, however, are also associated with increased risk of cardiovascular disease and osteoporosis when consumed in excess [8, 10]. Plant proteins, in contrast, must be consumed in large amounts and varieties to ensure that all essential amino acids are consumed, but provide enhanced health benefits including decreased cardiovascular risk and enhanced bone density [8].

Overall, the RDA for proteins is 0.8 gram/kilogram of body weight/day in a healthy adult [11]. Consumption of less than this recommended amount can increase the risk for protein deficiency syndromes such as marasmus and kwashiorkor. Marasmus is classified as a total calorie deficit due to food insecurity, HIV infection, mal-

Table 2.1 Summary of micronutrients and associated deficiencies

	Micronutrient	Risk of deficiency	Deficiency symptoms
Fat-soluble vitamins	Vitamin A	Resource-poor settings Infants Cystic fibrosis patients	Xeropthalmia Low-light blindness Impaired immunity
	Vitamin D	Breastfed infants The elderly People with dark skin Malabsorptive disorders	Rickets, failure to thrive, cardiomyopathy in children Osteomalacia, osteoporosis, multiple sclerosis, cardiovascular disease in adults
	Vitamin E	Malabsorptive disorders	Impaired immunity/increased infection risk Neuropathy Myopathy Retinopathy
	Vitamin K	Infants Patients on anticoagulants Malabsorptive disorders	Hemorrhage in severe cases Osteoporosis

Table 2.1 (continued)

	Micronutrient	Risk of deficiency	Deficiency symptoms
Water-soluble vitamins	Vitamin C	Smokers Infants Individuals with restrictive diets	Fatigue Malaise Gingivitis Poor wound healing Hyperkeratosis Petechiae Corkscrew hair
	Vitamin B1	Alcoholism Elderly HIV/AIDS patients Diabetics	Beriberi: peripheral neuropathy, congestive heart failure, death Wernicke encephalopathy: nystagmus, ataxia, confusion Korsakoff syndrome: amnesia, confabulation, disorientation
	Vitamin B2	Vegans Pregnant women Infants IBD patients Alcoholism	Skin disorders Hyperemia Angular stomatitis Cheilosis Hair loss Degeneration of the liver and nervous system
	Vitamin B3	Limited diets Alcoholism HIV/AIDS patients IBD Carcinoid syndrome Hartnup disease	Pellagra: dermatitis, diarrhea, dementia Depression Hallucination Memory loss Psychosis
	Vitamin B5	Pantothenate kinase-associated neurodegeneration (PKAN)	Peripheral neuropathy Irritability Fatigue Anorexia
	Vitamin B6	Alcoholism Malabsorption disorders Homocystinuria Medications	Microcytic anemia Cheilosis Glossitis Depression Peripheral neuropathy Suppressed immunity
	Vitamin B7	Biotinidase deficiency Alcoholism	Thin hair Conjunctivitis Dermatitis Metabolic acidosis Depression Paresthesia
	Vitamin B12	Pernicious anemia Malabsorptive disorders Bariatric surgery Vegan diet	Peripheral neuropathy Paresthesia Depression Dementia Psychosis Ataxia Macrocytic anemia
	Folate	Alcoholism Pregnancy Malabsorptive disorders Medications	Macrocytic anemia Depression Dementia Fatigue Stomatitis

(continued)

Table 2.1 (continued)

	Micronutrient	Risk of deficiency	Deficiency symptoms
Trace metals	Zinc	Malabsorptive disorders Pregnancy Sickle cell disease Diabetics Acrodermatitis enteropathica	Growth restriction Diarrhea Appetite suppression Impaired immunity Hair loss Hypogonadism
	Chromium	Deficiency syndrome not well defined	Hyperglycemia Peripheral neuropathy Weight loss
	Selenium	Insufficient intake Dialysis HIV/AIDS patients	Impaired immunity and cognition Keshan disease
	Iodine	Pregnancy Vegan diet Low soil iodine or iodized salt intake	Growth restriction and cretinism in children Hypothyroidism in adults
	Copper	Celiac disease High zinc or protein intake Menke disease	Anemia Skin/hair hypopigmentation Osteoporosis Impaired immunity Hyperlipidemia
	Iron	Pregnancy Infants Women of reproductive age Cancer patients Chronic kidney disease Malabsorptive disorders Hookworm infections	Anemia Fatigue Decreased concentration Pica Restless leg syndrome Impaired immunity Plummer-Vinson syndrome

absorption, or anorexia of any etiology [12–14]. Marasmus is characterized by failure to thrive, dehydration and weight loss, hypotension, bradycardia, and signs and symptoms of other nutrient deficiencies [12, 15, 16]. Kwashiorkor, in contrast, is specifically caused by protein deficiency. Kwashiorkor is similar to marasmus in terms of causes and symptoms, with the added findings of edema, thin and hyperpigmented skin, hepatomegaly, dermatitis, and muscle wasting due to inadequate protein provision [16, 17].

Fats

Fats in the diet are usually found in the form of triglycerides, which consist of three fatty acids attached to a glycerol moiety [11, 18]. Fatty acids can be obtained both through the diet and endogenously through metabolic processes, although the amount acquired via these mechanisms is dependent on what is consumed and varies with age and geography [18]. Two fatty acids in particular, linoleic acid (n-6) and alpha-linolenic acid (n-3), must be obtained through the diet and are considered essential [19]. The main roles of fatty acids are to provide structure to cell membranes, provide energy to most tissues, and assist in cellular signaling [18].

Fatty acids can differ in their structure, which affects their utilization in the body. In general, fatty acids are typically 6–24 carbon units long and can vary in the number of double bonds they have [11, 18]. Saturated fatty acids contain no double bonds, are usually solid at room temperature (i.e., butter), and should be limited in the diet according to the Food and Nutrition Board [6, 11, 18, 20]. In contrast, monounsaturated fats have one double bond, whereas polyunsaturated fats have two or more [11]. These can be further broken down based on whether the double bonds are on the same side (*cis* configuration) or on opposite sides (*trans* configuration) [11]. *Cis*-monounsaturated fats, specifically oleic acid, are found in a wide variety of foods and there is no guideline for ideal consumption amounts [6, 18, 20]. *Cis*-polyunsaturated fats, including linoleic acid, are found in nuts, seeds, and oils, and are necessary in the diet to achieve health effects, such as lowering LDL and total cholesterol [6, 18, 20]. *Trans* fats are typically found in hydrogenated oils, like vegetable oil, and increase the risk of hyperlipidemia and cardiovascular disease, leading to national guidelines recommending against consumption of trans fats in any amount [18, 20].

The Food and Nutrition Board recommends that healthy adults consume 20–35% of their daily calories from fat sources, which typically results in the intake of 44 g to 77 g of fat per day [6]. Fat deficiency is rare in people who maintain these recommended amounts of daily fat, which usually signals an issue with metabolism and/or absorption. Essential fatty acid deficiency (EFAD) occurs in these specific patient populations, including patients with malabsorptive disorders, such as inflammatory bowel disease (IBD), celiac disease, and cystic fibrosis, those with a history of GI surgery or receiving parenteral nutrition, and patients with severe restriction of fat in the diet [21–23]. Patients with EFAD of any etiology usually present with rash, hair loss, impaired wound healing and immunity, increased infection risk, and growth restriction, as well as elevated liver function tests and thrombocytopenia [21, 24, 25].

Micronutrients

Fat-Soluble Vitamins

Fat-soluble vitamins, including vitamins A, D, E, and K, require the presence of fats to be absorbed. Hollander et al. described in depth the absorption of fat-soluble vitamins, initially finding that vitamin D and E are absorbed by passive diffusion, whereas vitamins A and K are absorbed by energy- and carrier-mediated transport [26–29]. However, more recent studies have suggested that both processes likely occur, with passive diffusion at high concentrations and carrier-mediated transport at dietary concentrations [30]. Regardless of the method of absorption, fat-soluble vitamins serve a wide variety of functions and are associated with classic deficiencies and even immune system regulation [31–33].

Vitamin A

Vitamin A is typically found in foods that come from animal sources, such as dairy and eggs, as well as in green, leafy vegetables and some fruits [34]. According to the Food and Nutrition Board, the RDA for vitamin A is 700–900 μg per day [6, 35]. Vitamin A deficiency is more common in resource-poor settings due to low vitamin A intake [36]. Typical symptoms of deficiency range include xeropthalmia, low-light (night) blindness, and increased susceptibility to infection [33, 36, 37].

Vitamin D

Vitamin D occurs in two forms, vitamin D_2 (ergocalciferol) and vitamin D_3 (cholecalciferol) [34]. Ergocalciferol is generally obtained from plant sources, whereas cholecalciferol is activated by direct UV radiation on the skin [34]. After ingestion, ergocalciferol and cholecalciferol undergo further activation in the body through hydroxylation in the liver to form 25-hydroxyvitamin D, and then additional hydroxylation in the kidney to the active form, 1,25-dihydroxyvitamin D [33]. This active form of vitamin D then facilitates calcium absorption and promotes calcium and phosphate homeostasis [38]. The RDA for vitamin D is 15–20 μg per day [6, 35]. Typically, groups at risk of vitamin D deficiency include breastfed infants, the elderly, people with decreased sun exposure or dark skin, and people with malabsorptive disorders [38]. Vitamin D deficiency is typically characterized by rickets, cardiomyopathy, and failure to thrive in children, as well as osteolmalacia, osteoporosis, cancers, multiple sclerosis, and cardiovascular disease in adults [38–45].

Vitamin E

Vitamin E is typically obtained through plant sources, and bioavailability is modulated by the presence of tocopherols and tocotrienols, two groups of vitamin E [33, 34]. Vitamin E is an important antioxidant in the body and is protective against aging and red blood cell destruction through neutralization of reactive oxygen species [33]. It is also anti-inflammatory and has been linked with reduction in incidence of cardiovascular disease, arthritis, and neurologic disorders [33, 46–51]. The RDA for vitamin E is 15 mg per day [6, 35]. Deficiency usually occurs in the setting malabsorption and is rare in healthy adults due to the high prevalence in the diet [33, 52]. Symptoms of vitamin E deficiency include increased risk of infection and impaired immunity, neuropathy, myopathy, and retinopathy [6, 53, 54].

Vitamin K

Vitamin K is obtained both through diet and intrinsically through metabolism via gut bacteria. Vitamin K includes two forms: vitamin K_1 (phylloquinone), which is obtained through green, leafy vegetables, and vitamin K_2 (menaquinones), which is produced by gut flora [34, 55]. The main role of vitamin K is the production of clotting factors to promote coagulation [34]. The RDA for vitamin K is 90–120 μg per day [6, 35]. Vitamin K deficiency typically occurs in infancy due to low bacterial colonization in the gut as well as in adults due to inadequate dietary intake [56]. People who take specific anticoagulants, such as warfarin, and those with malabsorptive disorders are also at risk of deficiency [55]. Vitamin K deficiency is characterized by increased propensity to bleeding as well as osteoporosis [55–57].

Water-Soluble Vitamins

Water-soluble vitamins include vitamin C and all of the B vitamins: vitamin B_1 (thiamin), vitamin B_2 (riboflavin), vitamin B_3 (niacin), vitamin B_5 (pantothenic acid), vitamin B_6 (pyridoxine), vitamin B_7 (biotin), vitamin B_9 (folate), and vitamin B_{12} (cyanocobalamin) [58]. Water-soluble vitamins are not synthesized in the body, so they must be obtained through diet or other external sources [59]. Absorption of water-soluble vitamins occurs in both the small and large intestines by carrier-mediated processes (with the exception of vitamin B_{12}, which is only absorbed in the terminal ileum), and this can be interrupted in certain malabsorptive conditions or with drug interactions that lead to characteristic deficiencies [59].

Vitamin C

Vitamin C, also known as ascorbic acid, is obtained from citrus fruits and some vegetables [58]. It is necessary for the synthesis of certain proteins, including collagen and carnitine, which support connective tissue responsible for wound healing [59, 60]. The RDA for vitamin C is 75–90 mg per day [6, 35]. Generally, people at risk of deficiency include smokers, infants, and individuals with poor diet [6, 60–63]. Vitamin C deficiency is characterized classically by scurvy, which can result in fatigue, malaise, and gingivitis, as well as poor wound healing, hyperkeratosis, petechiae, and corkscrew hair. Bleeding can also lead to iron deficiency [6, 61–65].

Thiamin

Vitamin B_1, also known as thiamin, is obtained both from the diet and from colonic bacteria [59]. It functions mainly as a cofactor in metabolic reactions, such as gluconeogenesis and the citric acid cycle [58, 59, 66]. The RDA for thiamin is 1.1–1.2 mg per day [6, 35]. People at risk of thiamin deficiency include people with alcohol use disorder, the elderly, people with HIV/AIDS, and diabetics [67–72]. Thiamin deficiency can be characterized in stages, with early symptoms including weight loss, confusion, memory loss, muscle weakness, and cardiomyopathy [66]. Worldwide, thiamin deficiency is usually the result of low dietary intake and can result in beriberi, with symptoms ranging from peripheral neuropathy to congestive heart failure and death [4, 66–68]. In the United States, deficiency is more commonly related to alcohol abuse or malabsorption, with Wernicke-Korsakoff syndrome being the most common manifestation [66, 68]. Wernicke encephalopathy is associated with the triad of nystagmus, ataxia, and confusion [73]. This can progress to Korsakoff syndrome, which includes amnesia, confabulation, and disorientation and is often irreversible [74].

Riboflavin

Vitamin B_2, also known as riboflavin, is present in milk, leafy green vegetables, and liver, to name a few [58]. Riboflavin is usually present in coenzyme forms such as flavin mononucleotide (FMN) and flavin adenine dinucleotide (FAD) that assist in cellular respiration and metabolism [58, 59, 75]. It also assists with the conversion of other vitamins into their respective coenzymes [58, 75]. The RDA for riboflavin is 1.1–1.3 mg per day [6, 35]. Vegans, pregnant women and infants, IBD patients, and patients with alcohol use disorder are at risk for riboflavin deficiency [4, 59, 76]. Riboflavin deficiency is very rare in the developed world in healthy individuals, but can result in skin disorder, hyperemia, angular stomatitis, cheilosis, hair loss, and degeneration of the liver and nervous system [4, 59, 67, 75].

Niacin

Vitamin B_3, also known as niacin, includes nicotinic acid and nicotinamide and is obtained through both endogenous and exogenous sources such as tryptophan and animal-based foods, respectively [58, 59, 77]. Niacin is converted into nicotinamide adenine dinucleotide (NAD) and nicotinamide adenine dinucleotide phosphate (NADP), both of which function as crucial components in the metabolism and formation of ATP [59, 77]. The RDA for niacin is 14–16 mg per day [6, 35]. Patients with limited diets, alcoholism, AIDS, IBD, carcinoid syndrome, and Hartnup disease are at risk of deficiency either due to decreased intake, decreased absorption of tryptophan (i.e., Hartnup disease), or shunting of tryptophan into serotonin production in carcinoid syndrome [6, 77–80]. Niacin deficiency leads to pellagra, which is associated with the 3 D's: dermatitis, diarrhea, and dementia [81]. The neurologic symptoms typically involve depression, hallucination, memory loss, and psychosis [81]. Ultimately, if unresolved, it can progress and lead to death [81].

Pantothenic Acid

Vitamin B_5, also known as pantothenic acid, is a water-soluble vitamin that supports the production of coenzyme A (CoA) and acyl carrier proteins, both of which are notably used in fatty acid synthesis and other metabolic processes [59, 82]. Pantothenic acid is acquired through both animal and plant sources [4, 82]. The RDA for vitamin B_5 is 5 mg per day [6, 35]. Deficiency is rare and typically occurs in patients with pantothenate kinase-associated neurodegeneration (PKAN), a rare genetic disorder that leads to low CoA levels [83]. Pantothenic acid deficiency is associated with neurologic symptoms, such as peripheral neuropathy, irritability, fatigue, and anorexia [4, 68, 82].

Pyridoxine

Vitamin B_6, also known as pyridoxine and its other active forms of pyridoxal and pyridoxamine, is obtained through meats, potatoes, and vegetables [6, 58, 59, 84]. Vitamin B_6 and its derivatives function in amino acid synthesis, hemoglobin synthesis, and other metabolic processes [4, 59, 84]. The RDA for vitamin B_6 is 1.3–1.7 mg per day [6, 35]. Vitamin B_6 deficiency is commonly associated with alcohol use disorder, malabsorption disorders like celiac disease, homocystinuria, and in patients on certain long-term medications, such as the tuberculosis medication isoniazid [59, 84]. Symptoms of vitamin B_6 deficiency can range widely, but often includes microcytic or sideroblastic anemia, cheilosis, glossitis, depression, peripheral neuropathy, and suppressed immunity [6, 68, 84].

Biotin

Vitamin B_7, also known as biotin, is a water-soluble vitamin that is obtained endogenously and through foods such as meats, egg, nuts, and vegetables [59, 85]. Biotin can be tightly bound to proteins (i.e., avidin, a protein found in egg whites), and requires intestinal enzymatic breakdown before absorption is possible [4, 6, 68]. Biotin is a cofactor for five carboxylases that play a role in several metabolic reactions, such as gluconeogenesis and fatty acid synthesis [4, 59, 68, 85]. The RDA for biotin is 30 μg per day [6, 35].

Deficiency is rare, typically occurring in those with biotinidase deficiency and alcohol use disorder [86–88]. Symptoms of biotin deficiency include thin hair, conjunctivitis, skin rash and infection, metabolic acidosis, and neurologic manifestations such as depression and paresthesias [4, 68].

Folate

Vitamin B_9, more commonly known as folate, is typically acquired through the diet and can be found in leafy green vegetables like spinach as well as nuts, beans, fruits, eggs, and meat products [4, 89]. Folate serves many functions, including single-carbon transfers in metabolic processes such as amino acid and DNA synthesis, as well as in the formation of methionine from homocysteine [4, 58, 59, 89]. The RDA for folate is 400 μg per day, which is often increased to 600 μg per day in pregnancy [6, 35]. Deficiency of folate is most notably found in patients with alcohol use disorder, pregnant women, people with malabsorptive disorders, and patients taking certain medications that interfere with folate absorption and metabolism, such as trimethoprim and pyrimethamine [4, 59, 68, 90, 91]. Deficiency is characterized by macrocytic anemia, depression, dementia, fatigue, stomatitis, and cardiovascular disease [4, 68, 89, 92].

Cyanocobalamin

Vitamin B_{12}, also known as cyanocobalamin, is obtained through meats, milk and other dairy products, and eggs [58, 93]. Vitamin B_{12} serves as a cofactor for methionine synthase and methylmalonyl-CoA mutase and functions in a wide array of metabolic processes, specifically the conversion of homocysteine to methionine, and in DNA and erythrocyte synthesis [6, 58, 93]. The RDA for vitamin B_{12} is 2.4 μg per day [6, 35]. There are many well-documented causes of vitamin B_{12} deficiency, including pernicious anemia, malabsorptive disorders such as celiac disease and IBD, individuals with a history of bariatric surgery, and veganism due to its unique metabolism [6, 93–96]. Vitamin B_{12} deficiency is associated with a classic constellation of symptoms such as peripheral neuropathy, paresthesia, depression, dementia, psychosis, ataxia, megaloblastic anemia, and potentially cardiovascular disease [97].

Trace Metals

Many trace metals are considered essential and must be obtained through the diet for necessary biologic functions. This section will discuss six of the trace metals that are most clinically relevant and can be associated with classic deficiency syndromes, including zinc, copper, chromium, selenium, iodine, and iron.

Zinc

Zinc is obtained primarily through meat products, but it is largely ubiquitous in nature [6, 98]. Zinc is used to stabilize enzymatic reactions and cellular structures and helps with gene expression and metabolism [99, 100]. The RDA for zinc is 8–11 mg per day [6, 35]. Individuals with malabsorptive disorders, pregnant women, sickle cell patients, diabetics, and those with acrodermatitis enteropathica are at risk of zinc deficiency [98, 99, 101, 102]. Zinc deficiency typically manifests as growth restriction, diarrhea, dermatitis, appetite suppression, weakened immunity, hair loss, and hypogonadism [98–102].

Copper

Copper is an essential trace metal found in seafood, nuts, meats, and fruits [4, 99–101, 103]. It is involved in redox reactions and is incorporated into many enzymes in the body [99–101]. The RDA for copper is 900 μg per day [6, 35]. People at risk of copper deficiency include those with celiac disease, individuals with high zinc or protein consumption (due to altered absorption/competing cofactors), or patients with Menkes disease, a genetic condition affecting the ATP7A gene, leading to decreased copper absorption [99, 103, 104]. Patients with copper deficiency present with anemia, skin and hair hypopigmentation, osteoporosis and increased fracture risk, impaired immunity, and hyperlipidemia [100, 101, 103, 105].

Chromium

Chromium is commonly found in meat products, grains, spices, and nuts [4, 100, 101, 106]. Chromium is thought to augment the actions of insulin, although the mechanism of action remains unclear [99, 100]. The RDA for chromium is 20–35 μg per day. While no definitive chromium deficiency syndrome has been well defined, it has been speculated that symptoms can include hyperglycemia, peripheral neuropathy, and weight loss [100, 106–109]. These symptoms were observed in patients on total parenteral nutrition (TPN), with subsequent improvement with chromium supplementation [100, 106–109].

Selenium

Selenium is found in seafood, liver, cereals, and dairy products [68, 100, 110]. Selenium serves as a part of glutathione peroxidase, an antioxidant enzyme, to assist with immunity, normal thyroid homeostasis, and reproduction [4, 99, 100, 110]. The RDA for selenium is 55 μg per day. Selenium deficiency occurs in those with insufficient intake, patients on dialysis, and HIV patients [110–113]. Deficiency is characterized by impaired immunity and cognition, as well as a risk of developing Keshan disease, a form of cardiomyopathy that is responsive to selenium supplementation [110, 111, 114].

Iodine

Iodine is an essential trace metal found in soil and a wide variety of foods, including seafood and seaweed, eggs, and some dairy products [6, 100, 115, 116]. The main function of iodine is its role in the synthesis of the thyroid hormones, triiodothyronine (T3) and thyroxine (T4) [99–101, 116]. The RDA for iodine is 150 μg per day [6, 35]. People who live in areas with low soil iodine concentrations, pregnant women, vegans, and those who avoid iodized salt are at risk of deficiency [6, 115, 116]. Iodine deficiency in pregnancy can result in growth restriction and cretinism, which can result in global developmental delay, motor spasticity, and other neurologic symptoms [115–117]. In adults, iodine deficiency can result in goiter and signs and symptoms of hypothyroidism, including depression, fatigue, constipation, and weight gain [100, 101, 115, 116].

Iron

Iron is an important trace metal obtained through foods such as meat, seafood, nuts, vegetables, and grains [68, 118, 119]. Iron serves as an important part of hemoglobin to carry oxygen throughout the body [4, 119]. It also functions as a component of myoglobin and in redox reactions in human metabolism [120]. The RDA for iron is 8–18 mg per day [6, 35]. Pregnant women, infants, women of reproductive age, cancer patients, chronic kidney disease patients, those with malabsorption disorders, and those with hookworm infections in the developing world are just some groups that are at risk of iron deficiency [68, 120–124]. Iron deficiency is common and leads to anemia, which can be associated with fatigue, decreased concentration, pica, restless leg syndrome, impaired immunity, and Plummer-Vinson syndrome. It may also be asymptomatic and diagnosed on routine lab testing [119, 125, 126].

Conclusion

Macronutrients and micronutrients form the foundation of dietary composition and are equally important in terms of nutritional and overall health. Certain populations may be at higher risk of deficiencies in these nutrients, especially in those with disorders of the gastrointestinal tract (Table 2.2). A balanced diet that incorporates standard RDA values for specific nutrients, with supplementation as needed in states of disease, can prevent complications and decline in health over time.

Table 2.2 Common gastrointestinal disorders and associated nutritional deficiencies

Gastrointestinal disorders	Associated deficiencies
Celiac disease	Fats Fat-soluble vitamins Vitamin B12 Folate Trace metals, namely Zn and Fe
Inflammatory bowel disease (Crohn and ulcerative colitis)	Fats Fat-soluble vitamins Certain water-soluble vitamins, namely vitamins B2, B3, B12 Certain trace metals
Gastric or intestinal surgery (i.e., gastric sleeve, Roux-en-Y, intestinal resection)	Fats Fat-soluble vitamins Folate and vitamin B12 Trace metals, namely Zn, Fe, Cu
Pancreatic exocrine insufficiency (i.e., pancreatic resection, cystic fibrosis, chronic pancreatitis)	Fats Fat-soluble vitamins Proteins
Whipple disease	Fats Fat-soluble vitamins Folate and vitamin B12 Trace metals, namely Zn and Fe
Pernicious anemia	Vitamin B12
Small intestinal bacterial overgrowth (SIBO)	Fats Fat-soluble vitamins Folate and vitamin B12 Iron
GI infection and immunodeficiency (i.e., HIV, giardiasis, cryptosporidium, helminth infections)	Certain water-soluble vitamins, such as vitamin B1 and B3 Folate and vitamin B12 Iron

References

1. Cui SW. Food carbohydrates: chemistry, physical properties, and applications. CRC Press; 2005.
2. Robyt JF. Beginnings [Internet]. In: Robyt JF, editor. Essentials of carbohydrate chemistry. New York: Springer; 1998 [cited 2021 Feb 2]. p. 1–18. Available from: https://doi.org/10.1007/978-1-4612-1622-3_1.
3. Cummings JH, Stephen AM. Carbohydrate terminology and classification. Eur J Clin Nutr. 2007;61(1):S5–18.
4. Ross AC, Caballero B, Cousins RJ, Tucker KL, Ziegler TR. Modern nutrition in health and disease. 11th ed; 2012.
5. Mann J, Cummings J, Englyst H, et al. FAO/WHO scientific update on carbohydrates in human nutrition: conclusions. Eur J Clin Nutr. 2007;61:S132–7. https://doi.org/10.1038/sj.ejcn.1602943.
6. Institute of Medicine. Food and nutrition board. Dietary reference intakes. Washington, DC: National Academy Press; 2000.
7. Wu G. Dietary protein intake and human health. Food Funct. 2016;7(3):1251–65.
8. Hoffman JR, Falvo MJ. Protein – Which is Best? J Sports Sci Med. 2004;3(3):118–30.
9. St Jeor ST, Howard BV, Prewitt TE, et al. Dietary protein and weight reduction: a statement for healthcare professionals from the Nutrition Committee of the Council on Nutrition, Physical Activity, and Metabolism of the American Heart Association. Circulation. 2001;104(15):1869–74.
10. Shams-White MM, Chung M, Fu Z, et al. Animal versus plant protein and adult bone health: A systematic review and meta-analysis from the National Osteoporosis Foundation. PLoS One [Internet] 2018 [cited 2021 Feb 8];13(2).
11. Forouhi NG, Krauss RM, Taubes G, Willett W. Dietary fat and cardiometabolic health: evidence, controversies, and consensus for guidance. The BMJ [Internet] 2018 [cited 2021 Feb 5];361.
12. Titi-Lartey OA, Gupta V. Marasmus [Internet]. In: StatPearls. Treasure Island (FL): StatPearls Publishing; 2020 [cited 2021 Feb 8].
13. Arthur SS, Nyide B, Soura AB, Kahn K, Weston M, Sankoh O. Tackling malnutrition: a systematic review of 15-year research evidence from INDEPTH health and demographic surveillance systems. Glob Health Action. 2015;8:28298.

14. Morley JE. Anorexia, weight loss, and frailty. J Am Med Dir Assoc. 2010;11(4):225–8.
15. Barltrop D, Sandhu BK. Marasmus--1985. Postgrad Med J. 1985;61(720):915–23.
16. Grover Z, Ee LC. Protein energy malnutrition. Pediatr Clin North Am. 2009;56(5):1055–68.
17. Benjamin O, Lappin SL. Kwashiorkor [Internet]. In: StatPearls. Treasure Island (FL): StatPearls Publishing; 2020 [cited 2021 Feb 8].
18. Calder PC. Functional roles of fatty acids and their effects on human health. J Parenter Enteral Nutr. 2015;39(1S):18S–32S.
19. Das UN. Essential fatty acids - a review. Curr Pharm Biotechnol. 2006;7(6):467–82.
20. Liu AG, Ford NA, Hu FB, Zelman KM, Mozaffarian D, Kris-Etherton PM. A healthy approach to dietary fats: understanding the science and taking action to reduce consumer confusion. Nutr J [Internet] 2017 [cited 2021 Feb 5];16.
21. Mogensen KM. Essential fatty acid deficiency. Pract Gastroenterol. 2017;7.
22. Siguel EN, Lerman RH. Prevalence of essential fatty acid deficiency in patients with chronic gastrointestinal disorders. Metabolism. 1996;45(1):12–23.
23. 2019 Patient Registry Annual Data Report. 2019;92.
24. Richardson TJ, Sgoutas D. Essential fatty acid deficiency in four adult patients during total parenteral nutrition. Am J Clin Nutr. 1975;28(3):258–63.
25. Gramlich L, Meddings L, Alberda C, et al. Essential fatty acid deficiency in 2015: the impact of novel intravenous lipid emulsions. JPEN J Parenter Enteral Nutr. 2015;39(1 Suppl):61S–6S.
26. Hollander D, Rim E, Muralidhara KS. Mechanism and site of small intestinal absorption of α-tocopherol in the rat. Gastroenterology. 1975;68(6):1492–9.
27. Hollander D, Truscott TC. Mechanism and site of small intestinal uptake of vitamin D3 in pharmacological concentrations. Am J Clin Nutr. 1976;29(9):970–5.
28. Hollander D. Vitamin K1 absorption by everted intestinal sacs of the rat. Am J Physiol-Leg Content. 1973;225(2):360–4.
29. Hollander D, Muralidhara KS. Vitamin A1 intestinal absorption in vivo: influence of luminal factors on transport. Am J Physiol-Endocrinol Metab. 1977;232(5):E471.
30. Reboul E, Borel P. Proteins involved in uptake, intracellular transport and basolateral secretion of fat-soluble vitamins and carotenoids by mammalian enterocytes. Prog Lipid Res. 2011;50(4):388–402.
31. Stephensen CB. Vitamin A, infection, and immune function. Annu Rev Nutr. 2001;21:167–92.
32. Holick MF. Sunlight and vitamin D for bone health and prevention of autoimmune diseases, cancers, and cardiovascular disease. Am J Clin Nutr. 2004;80(6 Suppl):1678S–88S.
33. Albahrani AA, Greaves RF. Fat-soluble vitamins: clinical indications and current challenges for chromatographic measurement. Clin Biochem Rev. 2016;37(1):27–47.
34. Health NRC (US) C on D and. Fat-Soluble Vitamins [Internet]. National Academies Press (US); 1989 [cited 2021 Feb 2].
35. Ward E. Addressing nutritional gaps with multivitamin and mineral supplements. Nutr J. 2014;13:72.
36. Office of Dietary Supplements - Vitamin A [Internet]. [cited 2021 Feb 3].
37. Sommer A, Vitamin A. Deficiency and clinical disease: an historical overview. J Nutr. 2008;138(10):1835–9.
38. Office of Dietary Supplements - Vitamin D [Internet]. [cited 2021 Feb 3].
39. Elder CJ, Bishop NJ. Rickets. Lancet Lond Engl. 2014;383(9929):1665–76.
40. Munns CF, Shaw N, Kiely M, et al. Global consensus recommendations on prevention and management of nutritional rickets. J Clin Endocrinol Metab. 2016;101(2):394–415.
41. Uday S, Högler W. Nutritional rickets and osteomalacia in the twenty-first century: revised concepts, public health, and prevention strategies. Curr Osteoporos Rep. 2017;15(4):293–302.
42. Jin J. Vitamin D and calcium supplements for preventing fractures. JAMA. 2018;319(15):1630.
43. Manson JE, Bassuk SS, Buring JE. Vitamin D, calcium, and cancer: approaching daylight? JAMA. 2017;317(12):1217–8.
44. Al Mheid I, Quyyumi AA. Vitamin D and cardiovascular disease: controversy unresolved. J Am Coll Cardiol. 2017;70(1):89–100.
45. Jagannath VA, Filippini G, Di Pietrantonj C, et al. Vitamin D for the management of multiple sclerosis. Cochrane Database Syst Rev. 2018;9:CD008422.
46. Nazrun AS, Norazlina M, Norliza M, Nirwana SI. The anti-inflammatory role of vitamin E in prevention of osteoporosis. Adv Pharmacol Sci [Internet] 2012 [cited 2021 Feb 3];2012.
47. Packer L. Protective role of vitamin E in biological systems. Am J Clin Nutr. 1991;53(4 Suppl):1050S–5S.
48. Clarke MW, Burnett JR, Croft KD. Vitamin E in human health and disease. Crit Rev Clin Lab Sci. 2008;45(5):417–50.
49. Alkhenizan A, Hafez K. The role of vitamin E in the prevention of cancer: a meta-analysis of randomized controlled trials. Ann Saudi Med. 2007;27(6):409–14.
50. Kline K, Lawson KA, Yu W, Sanders BG. Vitamin E and breast cancer prevention: current status and future potential. J Mammary Gland Biol Neoplasia. 2003;8(1):91–102.
51. Dror DK, Allen LH. Vitamin E deficiency in developing countries. Food Nutr Bull. 2011;32(2):124–43.
52. Office of Dietary Supplements - Vitamin E [Internet]. [cited 2021 Feb 3];
53. Brion LP, Bell EF, Raghuveer TS. Vitamin E supplementation for prevention of morbidity and mortality in preterm infants. Cochrane Database Syst Rev. 2003;(4):CD003665.

54. Kowdley KV, Mason JB, Meydani SN, Cornwall S, Grand RJ. Vitamin E deficiency and impaired cellular immunity related to intestinal fat malabsorption. Gastroenterology. 1992;102(6):2139–42.
55. Office of Dietary Supplements - Vitamin K [Internet]. [cited 2021 Feb 3].
56. Committee on Fetus and Newborn. Controversies concerning vitamin K and the newborn. Pediatrics. 2003;112(1):191–2.
57. Jagannath VA, Fedorowicz Z, Thaker V, Chang AB. Vitamin K supplementation for cystic fibrosis. Cochrane Database Syst Rev. 2015;1:CD008482.
58. Health NRC (US) C on D and. Water-Soluble Vitamins [Internet]. National Academies Press (US); 1989 [cited 2021 Feb 3].
59. Said HM. Intestinal absorption of water-soluble vitamins in health and disease. Biochem J. 2011;437(3):357–72.
60. Office of Dietary Supplements - Vitamin C [Internet]. [cited 2021 Feb 3].
61. Jacob RA, Sotoudeh G. Vitamin C function and status in chronic disease. Nutr Clin Care Off Publ Tufts Univ. 2002;5(2):66–74.
62. Weinstein M, Babyn P, Zlotkin S. An orange a day keeps the doctor away: scurvy in the year 2000. Pediatrics. 2001;108(3):E55.
63. Francescone MA, Levitt J. Scurvy masquerading as leukocytoclastic vasculitis: a case report and review of the literature. Cutis. 2005;76(4):261–6.
64. Li Y, Schellhorn HE. New developments and novel therapeutic perspectives for vitamin C. J Nutr. 2007;137(10):2171–84.
65. Carr AC, Frei B. Toward a new recommended dietary allowance for vitamin C based on antioxidant and health effects in humans. Am J Clin Nutr. 1999;69(6):1086–107.
66. Office of Dietary Supplements - Thiamin [Internet]. [cited 2021 Feb 3].
67. Coates PM, Blackman MR, Betz JM, Cragg GM, Levine M, Moss J, White JD, editors. Encyclopedia of dietary supplements. 2nd ed. CRC Press; 2015. https://doi.org/10.1201/b14669.
68. Bettendorff L. Thiamin. In: Erdman JW, Macdonald IA, Zeisel SH, editors. Present knowledge in nutrition. 10th ed. Washington, DC: Wiley-Blackwell; 2012. p. 261–79.
69. Boldorini R, Vago L, Lechi A, Tedeschi F, Trabattoni GR. Wernicke's encephalopathy: occurrence and pathological aspects in a series of 400 AIDS patients. Acta Bio-Medica Ateneo Parm Organo Della Soc Med E Sci Nat Parma. 1992;63(1–2):43–9.
70. Larsen TR, Dragu D, Williams M. Wernicke's encephalopathy: an unusual consequence of the acquired immune deficiency syndrome – case report and literature review. Case Rep Med. 2013;2013:709474.
71. Thornalley PJ, Babaei-Jadidi R, Al Ali H, et al. High prevalence of low plasma thiamine concentration in diabetes linked to a marker of vascular disease. Diabetologia. 2007;50(10):2164–70.
72. Al-Attas OS, Al-Daghri NM, Alfadda AA, Abd-Alrahman SH, Sabico S. Blood thiamine and its phosphate esters as measured by high-performance liquid chromatography: levels and associations in diabetes mellitus patients with varying degrees of microalbuminuria. J Endocrinol Invest. 2012;35(11):951–6.
73. Vasan S, Kumar A. Wernicke Encephalopathy [Internet]. In: StatPearls. Treasure Island (FL): StatPearls Publishing; 2020 [cited 2021 Feb 3].
74. Arts NJ, Walvoort SJ, Kessels RP. Korsakoff's syndrome: a critical review. Neuropsychiatr Dis Treat. 2017;13:2875–90.
75. Office of Dietary Supplements - Riboflavin [Internet]. [cited 2021 Feb 3].
76. Larsson CL, Johansson GK. Dietary intake and nutritional status of young vegans and omnivores in Sweden. Am J Clin Nutr. 2002;76(1):100–6.
77. Office of Dietary Supplements - Niacin [Internet]. [cited 2021 Feb 3].
78. Li R, Yu K, Wang Q, Wang L, Mao J, Qian J. Pellagra secondary to medication and alcoholism: a case report and review of the literature. Nutr Clin Pract Off Publ Am Soc Parenter Enter Nutr. 2016;31(6):785–9.
79. Crook MA. The importance of recognizing pellagra (niacin deficiency) as it still occurs. Nutr Burbank Los Angel Cty Calif. 2014;30(6):729–30.
80. Hartnup Disease [Internet]. NORD Natl. Organ. Rare Disord. [cited 2021 Feb 3].
81. Pitche PT. Pellagra. Sante Montrouge Fr. 2005;15(3):205–8.
82. Office of Dietary Supplements - Pantothenic Acid [Internet]. [cited 2021 Feb 4].
83. Hayflick SJ. Defective pantothenate metabolism and neurodegeneration. Biochem Soc Trans. 2014;42(4):1063–8.
84. Office of Dietary Supplements – Vitamin B6 [Internet]. [cited 2021 Feb 4].
85. Office of Dietary Supplements – Biotin [Internet]. [cited 2021 Feb 4].
86. Wolf B. Biotinidase deficiency and our champagne legacy. Gene. 2016;589(2):142–50.
87. Küry S, Ramaekers V, Bézieau S, Wolf B. Clinical utility gene card for: Biotinidase deficiency-update 2015. Eur J Hum Genet EJHG. 2016;24(7):3–5.
88. Srinivasan P, Kapadia R, Biswas A, Said HM. Chronic alcohol exposure inhibits biotin uptake by pancreatic acinar cells: possible involvement of epigenetic mechanisms. Am J Physiol Gastrointest Liver Physiol. 2014;307(9):G941–9.
89. Office of Dietary Supplements – Folate [Internet]. [cited 2021 Feb 4].
90. Bailey LB, Stover PJ, McNulty H, et al. Biomarkers of nutrition for development—folate review. J Nutr. 2015;145(7):1636S–80S.
91. Scholl TO, Johnson WG. Folic acid: influence on the outcome of pregnancy. Am J Clin Nutr. 2000;71(5 Suppl):1295S–303S.
92. Snow CF. Laboratory diagnosis of vitamin B12 and folate deficiency: a guide for the primary care physician. Arch Intern Med. 1999;159(12):1289–98.

93. Office of Dietary Supplements – Vitamin B12 [Internet]. [cited 2021 Feb 4].
94. Johnson MA. If high folic acid aggravates vitamin B12 deficiency what should be done about it? Nutr Rev. 2007;65(10):451–8.
95. Andrès E, Federici L, Affenberger S, et al. B12 deficiency: a look beyond pernicious anemia. J Fam Pract. 2007;56(7):537–42.
96. Sumner AE, Chin MM, Abrahm JL, et al. Elevated methylmalonic acid and total homocysteine levels show high prevalence of vitamin B12 deficiency after gastric surgery. Ann Intern Med. 1996;124(5):469–76.
97. Oh RC, Brown DL. Vitamin B12 deficiency. Am Fam Physician. 2003;67(5):979–86.
98. Office of Dietary Supplements – Zinc [Internet]. [cited 2021 Feb 7].
99. Mehri A. Trace elements in human nutrition (II) – an update. Int J Prev Med [Internet] 2020 [cited 2021 Feb 7];11.
100. WHO | Trace elements in human nutrition and health [Internet]. WHO. 1996. [cited 2021 Feb 7].
101. Chitturi R, Baddam VR, Prasad L, Prashanth L, Kattapagari K. A review on role of essential trace elements in health and disease. J Dr NTR Univ Health Sci. 2015;4(2):75.
102. Prasad AS. Zinc deficiency. BMJ. 2003;326(7386):409–10.
103. Office of Dietary Supplements – Copper [Internet]. [cited 2021 Feb 7].
104. Costa LSDA, Pegler SP, Lellis RF, et al. Menkes disease: importance of diagnosis with molecular analysis in the neonatal period. Rev Assoc Medica Bras 1992. 2015;61(5):407–10.
105. Prohaska JR. Impact of copper deficiency in humans. Ann N Y Acad Sci. 2014;1314:1–5.
106. Office of Dietary Supplements – Chromium [Internet]. [cited 2021 Feb 7].
107. Brown RO, Forloines-Lynn S, Cross RE, Heizer WD. Chromium deficiency after long-term total parenteral nutrition. Dig Dis Sci. 1986;31(6):661–4.
108. Freund H, Atamian S, Fischer JE. Chromium deficiency during total parenteral nutrition. JAMA. 1979;241(5):496–8.
109. Jeejeebhoy KN, Chu RC, Marliss EB, Greenberg GR, Bruce-Robertson A. Chromium deficiency, glucose intolerance, and neuropathy reversed by chromium supplementation, in a patient receiving long-term total parenteral nutrition. Am J Clin Nutr. 1977;30(4):531–8.
110. Office of Dietary Supplements – Selenium [Internet]. [cited 2021 Feb 7].
111. Rayman MP. Selenium and human health. Lancet Lond Engl. 2012;379(9822):1256–68.
112. Tonelli M, Wiebe N, Hemmelgarn B, et al. Trace elements in hemodialysis patients: a systematic review and meta-analysis. BMC Med. 2009;7:25.
113. Stone CA, Kawai K, Kupka R, Fawzi WW. Role of selenium in HIV infection. Nutr Rev. 2010;68(11):671–81.
114. Chen X, Yang G, Chen J, Chen X, Wen Z, Ge K. Studies on the relations of selenium and Keshan disease. Biol Trace Elem Res. 1980;2(2):91–107.
115. Zimmermann MB. Iodine deficiency. Endocr Rev. 2009;30(4):376–408.
116. Office of Dietary Supplements – Iodine [Internet]. [cited 2021 Feb 7].
117. Srivastav A, Maisnam I, Dutta D, Ghosh S, Mukhopadhyay S, Chowdhury S. Cretinism revisited. Indian J Endocrinol Metab. 2012;16(Suppl 2):S336–7.
118. 2015–2020 Dietary Guidelines | health.gov [Internet]. [cited 2021 Feb 8].
119. Office of Dietary Supplements – Iron [Internet]. [cited 2021 Feb 8].
120. Abbaspour N, Hurrell R, Kelishadi R. Review on iron and its importance for human health. J Res Med Sci Off J Isfahan Univ Med Sci. 2014;19(2):164–74.
121. Black MM, Quigg AM, Hurley KM, Pepper MR. Iron deficiency and iron-deficiency anemia in the first two years of life: strategies to prevent loss of developmental potential. Nutr Rev. 2011;69 Suppl 1:S64–70.
122. Napolitano M, Dolce A, Celenza G, et al. Iron-dependent erythropoiesis in women with excessive menstrual blood losses and women with normal menses. Ann Hematol. 2014;93(4):557–63.
123. Aapro M, Österborg A, Gascón P, Ludwig H, Beguin Y. Prevalence and management of cancer-related anaemia, iron deficiency and the specific role of i.v. iron. Ann Oncol Off J Eur Soc Med Oncol. 2012;23(8):1954–62.
124. Bayraktar UD, Bayraktar S. Treatment of iron deficiency anemia associated with gastrointestinal tract diseases. World J Gastroenterol. 2010;16(22):2720–5.
125. Camaschella C. Iron deficiency. Blood. 2019;133(1):30–9.
126. Camaschella C. Iron-deficiency anemia [Internet]. https://doi.org/10.1056/NEJMra1401038. 2015 [cited 2021 Feb 8].

Clinical Nutrition Assessment Tools

3

Jeanette N. Keith

Introduction

You have been consulted to manage a prevalent condition in your hospital and outpatient clinic, called Disease X. This disease potentially affects one of every two patients over 60 years of age in your practice. It is associated with a lower quality of life, increased morbidity as well as mortality, decreased overall survival, and significant health costs of more than 15 billion dollars annually in the United States [1]. This disorder negatively impacts the health outcomes of any chronic disease state when present, including gastrointestinal diseases. The affected patients have higher infection rates, increased muscle loss, impaired wound healing, and longer lengths of stay in the hospital [2].

Though long recognized in medicine, the clinical impact of Disease X relative to healthcare costs and hospital outcomes was first reported by Dr. Charles E. Butterworth in 1974 who termed this condition the "skeleton in the closet" [3]. At the time of Dr. Butterworth's initial report, Disease X was found to affect over 50% of hospitalized patients on both the medical and surgical wards but was under-recognized and undertreated [4, 5]. Despite its recognition as a major clinical entity over 40 years ago and the development of known effective treatment, Disease X continues to affect both pediatric and adult patient populations. Consequences can be particularly severe for older adults. In 2015, up to 50% of ambulatory senior adults in Ohio presenting to an outpatient clinic were found to have Disease X [6]. In a 2017 report, Disease X was present in 50% of adults over age 60 years at hospital admission [7]. Of concern, two of three unaffected patients at admission developed Disease X during their hospital stay, when unmonitored [8].

Disease X occurs in normal weight, underweight, and overweight or obese patients [9]. Importantly, Disease X can occur in relatively weight-stable patients. In one Italian study, more than 80% of obese adults over age 60 years who reported no significant weight loss (i.e., < 10% in the 3–6 months prior to evaluation) were negatively impacted by Disease X [10]. In a pivotal 2018 report by Dr. Silver et al. at Vanderbilt University, 30–50% of inpatients were found to have Disease X but only 11% of healthcare providers correctly documented the presence of this condition in the electronic medical record [11]. What is this clinical condition that impacts both inpatients and outpatients, regardless of specialty? Disease X is "disease-related malnutrition" (DRM). DRM is specifically defined as "undernutrition as a result of a disease process" [12].

J. N. Keith (✉)
Department of Medicine, Section of Gastroenterology, Decatur Morgan Hospital, Decatur Morgan GI and Nutrition, Decatur, AL, USA
e-mail: jeanette.keith@dmhnet.org

C. Newberry et al. (eds.), *Nutrition, Weight, and Digestive Health*,
https://doi.org/10.1007/978-3-030-94953-2_3

In your practice, how do you identify at-risk populations? How do you screen for this disorder?

Because this condition is preventable with early detection and, in most cases, responds well to treatment, it is imperative that clinicians recognize the risk factors for this disorder and screen all patients for this prevalent condition. In the clinical setting, we easily recognize starvation-related malnutrition and acute disease or injury-related malnutrition. However, too few healthcare providers understand, recognize, screen for, and treat chronic DRM, especially in the setting of obesity.

This chapter will define DRM, describe the concept of "anabolic competence," review the risk factors for DRM in adults, identify high risk populations, and discuss the important role of bedside nutrition assessment in clinical practice.

Defining the Problem

According to the World Health Organization (WHO), there are different types of malnutrition (i.e., inadequate consumption of nutrients). These include (1) undernutrition or total calorie deficit (e.g., wasting, stunting, underweight, and deficiencies in vitamins/minerals), (2) micronutrient-related malnutrition, (3) overweight (including obesity) with excess total calories but inadequate nutrients, and (4) diet-related noncommunicable diseases such as diabetes and lipid disorders [13]. The European Society of Parenteral and Enteral Nutrition (ESPEN) distinguishes cachexia and sarcopenia from "malnutrition" [14]. Cachexia is defined as a "multifactorial syndrome characterized by severe body weight, fat and muscle loss and increased catabolism due to underlying disease." Sarcopenia is the "loss of muscle mass and function." Malnutrition is the "inadequate consumption of nutrients." Disease-related malnutrition due to inadequate nutrient intake can result in the development of the more complex syndromes of cachexia or sarcopenia.

The American Society for Parenteral and Enteral Nutrition (ASPEN) expanded the definition of adult malnutrition, defining it as an "acute, subacute or chronic state of nutrition, in which a combination of varying degrees of overnutrition or undernutrition with or without inflammatory activity have led to a change in body composition and diminished function" [15]. The specific subtypes of malnutrition, as defined by ASPEN, are (1) starvation-related malnutrition and chronic starvation without inflammation (e.g., anorexia nervosa), (2) chronic disease-related malnutrition where inflammation is chronic and of mild to moderate degree (e.g., organ failure, pancreatic cancer, rheumatoid arthritis, or sarcopenic obesity), and (3) acute disease or injury-related malnutrition where inflammation is acute and of a severe degree (e.g., major infections, burns, and closed head injury). Notably, there is increasing recognition of the role of inflammation in chronic disease and malnutrition as body composition can be synergistically affected by the nutritional status and the degree of inflammation. Inflammation causes catabolic loss of muscle mass and function (i.e., sarcopenia) and decreased albumin concentration by reducing protein synthesis and increasing protein catabolism [16]. Cytokine production and the resultant inflammation are also integral to the pathogenesis of obesity and inflammatory bowel disease as well as cardiovascular disease [17, 18].

Despite the recognition of malnutrition in 1974 as a clinical condition that impacts the management of all patients, malnutrition remains under-recognized and undertreated. In a 2020 study of Dutch inpatients, 31% of the patients assessed at hospital admission were malnourished or at risk for malnutrition based on the results of the scored Patient-Generated Subjective Global Assessment© or PG-SGA©. This at-risk population increased over time. By day 5 of the hospitalization, the number of at-risk or malnourished patients increased to 56%. By day 10 of their hospital course, 66% of patients met criteria for malnutrition. For those admitted for 15 days or more, 79% of the patients were found to be malnourished. After their hospital course and treatment for the indicated diagnosis, 36% remained malnourished at the time of discharge. Because patients have persistent DRM at discharge, it behooves us to screen for nutritional risk or malnutrition in the pre-discharge, post-hospital discharge, and outpatient settings. Further, there should be an evidenced-based nutritional intervention when DRM is identified.

Of greatest concern, when nutritional status of patients was assessed at admission and pre-discharge, 30% of well-nourished patients became malnourished and 82% of malnourished patients showed no improvement in their nutritional status prior to discharge [19]. Consistent with these findings, Luong et al. found that 40% of ambulatory patients with cirrhosis presenting for care at a tertiary care metropolitan hospital outpatient clinic were malnourished based on scores from both the Patient-Generated Subjective Global Assessment (PG-SGA©) and the Subjective Global Assessment modified for liver disease (SGA-LD) [20]. These findings highlight the need to use a clinical tool such as the Scored PG-SGA© that is an effective screening tool, provides a risk assessment for malnutrition, allows for triaging of nutrition interventions (i.e., determining when to intervene with specific interventions), and has prescriptive recommended nutritional interventions based on the PG-SGA© score and that can be used for active monitoring of patients over time [21, 22].

Anabolic Competence

DRM can have devastating effects and increase the risk of complications, especially for 1 in 4 hospitalized patient and 17.5% of elderly nursing home residents [23]. Malnutrition increases hospital length of stay (LOS) by 18–34%, depending on the severity of malnutrition, and hospital costs by 31–55% [24, 25]. In addition, malnourished patients are more likely to be readmitted and have a higher mortality rate compared to non-malnourished patients with matching diagnosis-related groups (DRG). Under federal programs, hospitals that have high readmission rates are at risk for receiving reduced or no payments [26]. Specific treatment options are beyond the scope of this chapter and are reviewed elsewhere in this publication. However, it is important to recognize that a meta-analysis revealed that when malnutrition was diagnosed and treated during the hospital course, there was a two-day decrease in length of stay, 7% decrease in hospital readmission, and 20% savings in healthcare costs [27]. Using pneumonia as an example, when nutrition interventions were included as part of the hospital treatment course and the discharge planning, there was a 77% reduction in readmission rates [28]. These findings support the need for treatment plans that routinely screen for nutritional risk or malnutrition during hospital admissions, at post-hospital discharge, and in general medical clinics and nutrition clinics.

Prevention and treatment of DRM must also address the other metabolic factors that affect nutritional status. The most influential factors are physical activity (e.g., exercise) and the hormonal/metabolic (i.e., internal) environment in the body, with inflammation being a significant contributor [29]. The term "internal milieu" reflects the hormonal and metabolic influences that affect nutrition status. The internal milieu encompasses hormones, neuroendocrine regulators, inflammatory factors, the impact of the clinical disease or condition, and the potential adverse effects of treatment. Taken together, some authors suggest that the treatment of DRM should focus on achieving "anabolic competence," rather than thinking about nutritional status in isolation, with a rapidly growing evidence base regarding the importance of body composition in numerous clinical outcomes [30]. Langer et al. defined anabolic competence as "that state which optimally supports protein synthesis and lean body mass, global aspects of muscle and organ function, and immune response." This paradigm allows clinicians to address malnutrition, the changes in lean body mass, and any functional deficits due to the disease treatment (e.g., Crohn's disease exacerbation treated with corticosteroids or hypothyroidism in patients with head and neck cancer treated with chemotherapy and radiation). It also supports a research approach facilitating optimized clinical outcomes [31].

Risk Factors and High-Risk Populations

The American Dietetic Association defines nutrition risk screening as "the process of identifying patients with characteristics commonly associated with nutritional problems who may require comprehensive nutrition assessment" [32] or "the process of identifying patients, clients or groups who may have a nutrition diagnosis and benefit from nutrition assessment and intervention by a registered dietitian nutritionist (RDN)" [33]. Most often, this consists of answering validated questions using a "quick and easy" (<10 minutes) tool that predicts nutrition risk or malnutrition. Patients are identified as being "at-risk" or "minimal to no risk" for malnutrition. The initial risk assessment is usually performed by a dietitian using a tool that requires minimal training. In contrast, nutrition assessment is defined as "a comprehensive approach to defining nutritional status using medical, nutritional and medical histories; physical exam, anthropometric measures and laboratory data." The British Dietetic Association notes in their definition of nutritional assessment that it is a "systematic process of collecting and interpreting information in order to make decisions about the nature and cause of nutrition-related health issues that affect an individual" [34]. Nutrition assessment is generally performed by a trained healthcare professional including physicians, nurse practitioners, nurses, and qualified nutrition staff. Patients determined to be at risk or malnourished are referred for nutritional interventions by dietitians, nursing, and/or medical providers.

Common risk factors that increase the risk for malnutrition in clinical practice are outlined in Table 3.1 [35, 36]. Upon review of the list, it is apparent that many of the risk factors associated with DRM can be identified in the clinical history for most patients cared for in inpatient and outpatient practices. Thus, one should have a high index of suspicion that DRM may be influencing clinical outcomes.

Consistent with the published literature, the experience in our practice is that the patients with the greatest risk of an adverse outcome due to DRM are adults ≥65 years of age, those with declining health, and those with unplanned or unintentional weight loss. Clinicians often underappreciate the compounding effect of chronic inflammation of moderate to severe degree in the setting of a chronic illness. For example, a thin patient with Crohn's disease may suffer from general undernutrition, which worsens during periods of acute disease exacerbations, driven by underlying inflammation and potential corticosteroid use. These high-risk patients can also worsen the degree of their malnutrition with self-imposed food restrictions due to previous adverse food reactions, misinformation, and fear [37].

In patients presenting to the emergency department, the prevalence of malnutrition has been reported to be as high as 12% but most emergency departments do not typically screen for DRM [38]. DRM also occurs in medical and surgical patients presenting to an outpatient GI practice. As previously noted, Luong et al. found that 40% of cirrhotic patients presenting to an outpatient clinic were malnourished [20]. Sherry et al. found strikingly similar results relative to the prevalence of malnutrition in hospitalized patients with 20–50% affected in a multicenter study; however, at discharge, fewer than 10% of malnourished patients were given a nutrition recommendation or prescription for an oral supplement that could have improved outcomes, including reduced mortality. It is intuitive that when malnourished patients are discharged from the hospital without a treatment plan addressing DRM, they will subsequently present to the outpatient clinic with untreated disease [39].

Kamperidis et al. [40] used the Malnutrition Universal Screening Tool (MUST) to screen patients presenting to an outpatient clinic on initial visit. The body mass index (BMI) and percent weight loss (%WL) over a two-week period prior to the clinic visit were assessed. Among 605 adults including 316 women, 86% (519 patients) of the patients had a normal BMI and %WL. A total of 14% (n = 86) of patients screened had a BMI <20 kg/m^2 or 5% WL consistent with malnutrition as defined by the authors. Based on the MUST screening tool, 10% (n = 61) met criteria for MUST "medium risk" and 4% (n = 25) were

Table 3.1 Common risk factors for malnutrition

Advanced age	Depression	Head injury	Obesity
Alcohol intake	Difficulty walking	Hospitalization	Organ failure
Altered nutrient need	Drug metabolism	Income satisfaction	Parkinson's disease
Cognitive decline	Drug-nutrient interactions	Inflammation, acute	Polypharmacy
Constipation	Dysphagia	Inflammatory conditions, chronic	Poor dental hygiene
Corticosteroid use	Drug-nutrient interactions	Loss of appetite	Serious infection
Declining health	Eating disorders	Needing assistance with feeding	Smoking status
Decreased physical activity	Education level	Nutrient metabolism	Unplanned weight loss
Dementia	Frailty	Nutrition status	

References: [35, 36]

deemed "high risk" of malnutrition. Notably, 18% of patients with inflammatory bowel disease and 25% of patients with GI cancers were malnourished, as defined by the authors. DRM was present in 12% of the non-IBD patients and 12% of non-cancer patients. Of concern, though malnourished, 61% were not being managed by a dietitian. In another study, using the SGA within 48 hours of admission, malnourished patients were found to have increased mortality with a 34% mortality at 1 year, 42.6% mortality at 2 years, and a 48.5% mortality at 3 years [41, 42]. Despite the recognition that DRM results in longer hospital stays, early readmissions, increased healthcare costs and a higher mortality rate, and real or perceived barriers to nutrition screening in a busy practice continue to compromise nutrition care.

Bedside Nutrition Assessment

In his initial report, Dr. Butterworth listed multiple factors that contributed to iatrogenic malnutrition in hospital (see Table 3.2) and clinical practices in 1974 that compromised the nutritional health of hospitalized patients. Dr. Butterworth encouraged clinicians to understand the clinical missteps that led to the initial report of the "skeleton in the closet" [3]. These concerning behaviors persist as noted in 2011 and 2018 reviews of hospital malnutrition, which is worrisome (see Table 3.3) [2, 43]. It is imperative to revisit the importance of bedside nutrition screening or assessment in clinical practice beyond nutrition clinics. There is an educational gap between the nutrition management skills required by a physician and the nutrition education received in medical school and beyond, regardless of year of training [44]. Given the impact of DRM on healthcare outcomes and costs, nutrition screening, assessment, and treatment should be fully integrated into medical training curriculum.

There are a number of questions that should be considered in your practice to identify at-risk patients and to risk-stratify nutrition interventions in order to optimize health outcomes.

- How do you determine which screening tool is appropriate in your clinical setting?
- At what point in the clinical flow is screening or an assessment done?
- Who does the screening or assessment?
- Once the patient is screened or assessed, what do you do with the information?
- Can the tool help with determining specific nutrition interventions that are appropriate for your patient?
- Will the tool assess the effectiveness of the nutrition intervention?
- Does the tool allow you to detect subtle changes in nutrition status over time?

As you consider implementing nutrition screening in your clinical practice or a medical training curriculum, Table 3.4 outlines considerations that should be addressed as one incorporates an effective nutrition screening process into routine clinical care [45–48].

Following the initially shocking report in 1974 that documented the widespread presence of iat-

Table 3.2 The factors contributing to iatrogenic malnutrition in hospitalized patients in 1974, 2011, and 2018

Height not measured in 56% of patients at any time during the hospitalization	Body weight not recorded in the first 7 days in 26%	Of 36% in the study, 22 (or 61%) experienced weight loss (average of 6 kg)	Hypoalbuminemia (albumin <3.0 gram percent) present in 28% at admission	Anemia was present in 37% of patients at admission, with another 16% becoming anemic during the admission
Body weight not recorded in 23%, preventing the calculation of body mass index	Body weight not recorded regularly during the hospitalization in 43%	Patients not allowed food during an average of 3.1 days	Nine well-nourished patients became hypoalbuminemic during the hospital course	Patients experienced frequent blood draws during the admission that may have contributed to the anemia
Fourteen patients admitted for >3 weeks did not receive nutrition intervention, despite the presence of nutritional inadequacy	There was no nutrition intervention, despite 37% meeting criteria of treatment	During the hospitalization, 18% of meals were replaced with intravenous glucose	Patients receiving IV glucose had a calorie deficit of 2600 kcal per week during their admission	Nearly every patient underwent expensive diagnostic testing, received complex drug regimens, or had specialized surgery

References: [2, 3, 43]

Table 3.3 Practices that compromise the nutritional health of hospitalized patients in 1974, 2011, and 2018

Failure to record a measured height and weight	Failure to observe patients' food intake (not just reported intake)	Failure to recognize increased nutritional needs due to injury or illness	Lack of communication between the physician and the dietitian
Rotation of clinical staff at frequent intervals	Withholding multiple meals because of diagnostic testing, rehabilitation therapy, dialysis, etc.	Performance of surgical procedures without first making sure the patient is optimally nourished	Delay of nutrition support until the patient is in an advanced state of depletion, which is sometimes irreversible
Diffusion of responsibility for patient care	Use of tube feedings with inadequate caloric intake, of uncertain compositions and under insanitary conditions	Failure to provide nutrition support in the postoperative period	Limited availability of specialized testing to assess nutritional status
Prolonged use of glucose and saline intravenous feedings leading to caloric deficits	Ignorance of the composition of vitamin mixtures and other nutritional products	Failure to appreciate the role of nutrition in the prevention of and recovery from infection, independent of antibiotics	Failure to use specialized testing to assess nutritional status when testing is available

References: [2, 3, 43]

rogenic malnutrition in hospitalized patients, multiple nutritional screening tools were developed [49]. Early clinical screening tools included multiple components such as diet history, medical history, amount of weight loss, biochemical variables, anthropometrics, and often several calculations. The tools were too cumbersome for routine clinical use, obtained static or categorical data, had poor reproducibility in varying populations, had poor interrater reproducibility, were unable to determine the patient's nutrition status early in their clinical course, were not appropriate for a given age/patient population, or were poorly understood. Therefore, they are not currently routinely performed in clinical practice.

Newer screening and assessment tools rely primarily on clinical judgement with specific objective measures and less on precise body

Table 3.4 Considerations for an effective nutrition screening tool

Has the tool been validated in your patient population?	Who will perform the screening?	What is the clinical action that will be taken once the at-risk person is identified?	Is specialized training required prior to use of the screening tool?	Is the nutrition screening tool dynamic (assesses change in status) or static (identifies at-risk status only)?
Determine the complexity of the tool and whether calculations are required (N.B.: the more the calculations, the greater the risk for errors)	At what point in the patient assessment is the data collected?	What is the ease of use of the nutritional screening tool in clinical practice?	Is the tool cost-effective to implement?	Does the tool allow for triaging of nutritional intervention?
How sensitive is the tool? Will it identify all those at risk for malnutrition?	How can the assessment be incorporated into routine care?	What is the reproducibility of the results compared with clinical gold standards?	Is the tool noninvasive?	Can the screening be performed in a time-efficient manner?

References: [45–47]

composition analysis with few, if any, calculations. There are multiple screening and assessment tools available for clinical use. The most commonly used malnutrition screening tools are outlined in Table 3.5 [50–58]. Screening tools with a higher sensitivity are more effective in identifying the risk of malnutrition in the clinical setting. Of the screening tools listed in the table, the SGA and PG-SGA© are generally considered to be the gold standards for nutritional assessment in clinical practice.

The SGA was first reported in 1982 [59] and has been fully described elsewhere [60]. The SGA is both a screening tool and an assessment tool. It is based on the premise that clinicians are able to identify malnutrition when key historical features and pertinent physical exam features are assessed. The entire assessment is performed by the clinician [61]. Factors that most influence the SGA grade include muscle wasting, loss of subcutaneous tissue, and the pattern of weight loss [62]. The patient's weight history is assessed at 6 months and two weeks prior to the visit to allow the provider to define the degree of change in body weight. Weight loss of less than 5% in 6 months was originally considered to have a "small" effect on clinical outcomes. Weight loss of 5–10% in 6 months was considered "potentially significant." Weight loss of more than 10% in 6 months was deemed to be "definitely significant" relative to the risk for malnutrition. Ongoing weight loss at two weeks prior to assessment was indicative of a more acute state of malnutrition. It is important to note that when the weight loss is followed by weight regain, it suggests early recovery (i.e., conversion to anabolism), and often, the SGA grade improves despite a total net weight loss. The SGA also addressed functional capacity or energy level. Based on the clinical assessment, the individuals are classified into three groups: (1) well-nourished or SGA category A, (2) mild/moderately malnourished or SGA category B, and (3) severely malnourished or SGA category C. Using this grading system, individuals who would benefit from nutrition support are identified. The advantage of this clinical tool is that it is easy to use, has been validated in multiple patient populations, has good inter-observer reproducibility, requires no medical equipment or calculations, and incorporates functional status into the overall nutritional assessment [63].

In 1996 at Fox Chase Cancer Center in Philadelphia, Ottery and colleagues modified the original SGA to allow patients to provide the historical details of the patient's global history, including weight history, nutritional intake, nutrition impact score (NIS), and performance status (patient version of ECOG performance status). This modified tool became known as the PG-SGA©. The patient component of the PG-SGA© (Boxes 1–4) is known as the "PG-SGA SF" or by some authors as the abridged PG-SGA©

Table 3.5 Validated nutrition screening tools

Malnutrition screening tool	Patient population	Sensitivity	Specificity
Mini Nutritional Assessment (NMA)	Setting: acute, community, rehab, long-term care Population: geriatric Limit: low specificity in acute population	96%	98%
Mini Nutritional Assessment-Short Form (MNA-SF)	Elderly; better for sub-acute care and residential care; less optimal for acute care	97.9% (MNA) 100% (SGA)	100% (MNA) 52% (SGA)
Malnutrition Screening Tool (MST)	Acute adults: inpatient and outpatient; residental care facilities	93%	93%
Malnutrition Universal Screening Tool (MUST)	Acute care in adults; community. Note: predicts mortality risk, increased length of stay, and discharge destination in acute patients	69.7% to 80% (PG-SGA)	75.8% to 90% (PG-SGA)
Nutrition Risk Screening (NRS-2002)	Acute adults: predicts likelihood of positive outcome from nutrition support and reduced LOS among at-risk patients that receive nutrition support	62–74%	87–93%
Nutrition Risk Initiative (NRI)	Adults, inpatients	43%	89%
Subjective Global Assessment (SGA)	Settings: acute, rehab, community, and residential; populations: surgery, geriatric, oncology, renal, medical	82–100%	60–73%
Patient-Generated Subjective Global Assessment (PG-SGA)	Setting: acute, ambulatory Populations: oncology, renal, stroke	80–100%	60–80%
Scored Patient Generated Subjective Global Assessment (sPG-SGA)	Numerical score assists in monitoring changes in nutritional status and triaging nutritional interventions (i.e., dynamic versus static assessment)	98%	82%
DETERMINE (or NSI) Checklist	Elderly adults	60%	60%
Seniors in the Community: Risk Evaluation for Eating and Nutrition (SCREEN©)-I	Elderly adults, community based	94%	32%
Seniors in the Community: Risk Evaluation for Eating and Nutrition (SCREEN©)-II	Elderly adults, community based	84%	62%

References: [50–58]

[64]. Boxes 1–4 are designed so that, for a given patient, 80–90% of the total PG-SGA© score is collected by patient self-report [65].

The healthcare provider continues to complete the clinician component, addressing the patient's potential catabolic effect for the patient, with input regarding the primary and other diagnoses, and the metabolic considerations including fever (degree and duration) and the use of corticosteroids (type and dose). Each of these variables are often overlooked in terms of increased nutritional risk or deficit.

The PG-SGA© is both a categorical tool (A, B, and C), similar to the original SGA, and a dynamic or continuous measures tool (with a continuous point score). This latter aspect is important since it not only allows a "snapshot" of the patient at a given time but also facilitates real-time and granular determination of improvement or deterioration of patient variables. The point score change also is effective in terms of patient awareness and empowerment, since variables such as weight (or categorization) may take much longer to document improvement.

The scoring categories (also referred to as "stage" for the PG-SGA©) remained the same as the traditional SGA. However, the categories A and B were sub-divided into either nutritionally low-risk or nutritionally high-risk, with therapies depending on the nutrition risk associated with their disease or cancer and proposed treatment. Patients with stage C risks were considered high risk and the category was not subdivided. If a patient was in the stage A or low-risk stage B category, repeat nutritional assessment was performed at each visit in the system so that both the outpatient (i.e., oncology clinic appointments) and inpatient (i.e., admission) status were assessed. For patients in the high-risk stage B or stage C, there was a nutrition intervention performed. These patients were then reassessed two weeks after the specialized intervention to determine if the treatment was effective [66].

The PG-SGA© underwent further development to include a scoring system that transformed the tool from a static or categorical measurement to a dynamic or continuous assessment such that it reflects changes in nutritional status over time. The categorical scores were included to (1) be consistent with the legacy SGA tool, (2) to allow comparison between the two tools, and (3) to better address global outcomes across medical conditions and patient populations [21]. There is a global assessment of risk for malnutrition (i.e., well-nourished, moderately or suspected malnourished, or severely malnourished) and a scored section derived from the patient's historical information. For each component of the scored PG-SGA©, 0 to 4 points are assigned based on the impact of the symptom on the nutritional status. The total score is summed and provides a scale to determine which patients require nutritional intervention. Higher scores are associated with increased risk of malnutrition. If the score is ≥9, there is a need for an urgent nutritional intervention as this score represents a critical need for enteral or parenteral support. For scores less than 9, the recommended nutrition interventions include active monitoring, patient/family education, diet modification, and oral nutrition supplements. The scored PG-SGA© should be repeated after the nutrition intervention to assess for interval changes in nutritional status. The scored PG-SGA© has a sensitivity of 98% and a specificity of 82% in accurately predicting the SGA grade [64, 67].

There are several features that make the scored PG-SGA© an ideal tool for routine use in clinical practice. The PG-SGA© score was a major predictor of prognosis and mortality across a number of publications, with particular illustrative data in patients (n = 146) with gynecological (ovarian, endometrial, or cervical) malignancies admitted to a referral oncologic hospital. In this study, particularly critical were the following findings: (1) a score of >10 points was associated with a 30.7% increased risk of death at one year; (2) decreased survival was seen in patients categorized as B or C, and (3) the Kaplan-Meier survival data demonstrated an adverse impact that was seen regardless of disease state (early [stages I–II] or advanced [stages III–IV]) or cancer site [68].

In addition to these important clinical outcomes, the advantages of the PG-SGA© include the following: (1) prediction of increased hospital costs in severely malnourished patients in hospitalized patients screened upon admission [69], (2) prediction of changes in quality of life (QOL) due to DRM and correlates with the change in QOL as nutrition status improves or deteriorates, at baseline and following therapy in ambulatory patients [22], (3) facilitation of awareness of symptoms that adversely affect nutritional intake and status as well as monitoring of success of specific pharmacological or behavioral interventions [70], (4) facilitation of detection of early or subtle changes in nutritional status [70], and (5) identification of potentially treatable patient concerns that affect their nutritional status allowing for proactive interventions [71].

Boxes 1–4 (or the PG-SGA© SF) form a patient-centric or patient-reported outcomes (PRO) tool and can be completed prior to evaluation by the clinician; it can serve to streamline clinic flow, while providing patient self-report vital information for effective patient management, improved quality of patient-clinician interaction, and early awareness and intervention [72]. The scored PG-SGA© was originally designed by Ottery and colleagues for use across a spectrum of patient populations and was not limited for use in oncology. However, based on Ottery's oncology practice and research as well as early adoption by the American Dietetics Practice Group (ONDPG) of the Academy of

Nutrition and Dietetics (AND, previously the American Dietetic Association or ADA), it is often considered the gold standard or reference tool for nutritional screening and assessment in oncology. However, it has since been shown to perform well in other clinical settings including but not limited to (1) ambulatory inflammatory bowel disease patients [73], (2) obese cancer patients [74], (3) cirrhotic liver patients [75], and (4) renal dialysis patients [76], to name a few. Taken together, the scored PG-SGA© meets all the criteria as an effective nutrition screening tool as well as a global nutritional assessment tool. It is a 4-in-1 tool that can be used across multiple patient settings from outpatient, inpatient, home care, hospice, and clinical research. Its ease of use, cost-effectiveness, time efficiency, and clinical effectiveness make the scored PG-SGA© an ideal tool for medical student training and subsequent use in routine clinical care [57, 65].

Summary

Malnutrition in clinical practice is often underrecognized and undertreated with potentially devastating consequences, especially for older adults. Disease-related malnutrition, when unrecognized or inadequately treated, adversely affects the clinical, health, and economic outcomes across a broad spectrum of conditions and patient populations. Treatment goals for DRM should be to optimize or achieve the important interdisciplinary, multimodal concept of anabolic competence. Routine nutrition screening should be included in all patient assessments. Standardized screening tools with a scoring system such as the Scored Patient-Generated Subjective Global Assessment © allow for time-efficient, dynamic monitoring of patients. The continuous measure scoring allows for risk assessment and triaging of nutrition interventions and predicts health-related outcomes. Because DRM remains so prevalent, optimal clinical outcomes for our patients demand (mandate) that every practitioner actively incorporate nutrition screening and assessment into their routine for each and every nutritionally at-risk patient. Medical training programs are encouraged to prioritize integrated nutrition education in the medical education curriculum with emphasis on nutrition screening and assessment training as these are essential skills that lead to improved quality of care and health outcomes for patients.

References

1. Goates S, Du K, Braunscheig CA, Arensberg MB. Economic burden of disease-associated malnutrition at the state level. PLoS One. 2016;11(9):e0161833.
2. Barker LA, Gout BS, Crowe TC. Hospital malnutrition: prevalence, identification and impact on patients and the healthcare system. Int J Environ Res Public Health. 2011;8(2):514–27.
3. Butterworth CE. Skeleton in the hospital closet. Nutrition Care. 1974;9(2):4–8.
4. Bistrian BR, Blackburn GL, Vitale J, Cochran D, Naylor J. Prevalence of malnutrition in general medical patients. JAMA. 1976;235(15):1567–70.
5. Hill GL, Pickford I, Young CJ, Schorah CJ, Blackett RL, Burkinshaw L, Warren JV, Morgan DB. Malnutrition in surgical patients: an unrecognised problem. Lancet. 1977;309(8013):689–92.
6. Malone A. Malnutrition in the older adult. Todays's Geriatr Med. 2018;11(5):16. https://www.todaysgeriatricmedicine.com/archive/SO18p16.shtml. Accessed 24 June 2020.
7. Avelino-Silva T, Jaluul O. Malnutrition in hospitalized older patients: management strategies to improve patient care and clinical outcomes. Int J Gerentol. 2017;11(2):56–61.
8. Smith S, Chamblee TB, Falder-Saeed, Height K, Horbal Shuster M, Waldo MJ, Yoon HL. Manutrition in hospitalized adult patients: the role of the clinical nurse specialist. https://nacns.org/wp-content/uploads/2017/01/Malnutrition-Report.pdf. Accessed 24 June 2020.
9. W.H.O. Fact Sheet on Nutrition: The double burden of malnutrition. https://www.who.int/nutrition/double-burden-malnutrition/en/. Accessed 24 June 2020.
10. Rizzi M, Mazzuoli S, Regano N, et al. Undernutrition, risk of malnutrition and obesity in gastroenterological patients: a multicenter study. WJGO. 2016;8(7):563–72.
11. Silver HJ, Jones Pratt K, Bruno M, Lynch J, Mitchell K, McCauley SM. Effectiveness of the malnutrition quality improvement initiative on practitioner malnutrition knowledge and screening, diagnosis and timeliness of malnutrition-related care provided to older adults admitted to a tertiary care facility: a pilot study. J Acad Nutr Diet. 2018;118(1):101–9.
12. Guenter P, Jensen G, Patel V, et al. Addressing disease-related malnutrition in hospitalized patients:

a call for a national goal. Jt Comm J Qual Patient Saf. 2015;41(10):469–73.
13. Malnutrition. https://www.who.int/news-room/fact-sheets/detail/malnutrition. Accessed: 24 June 2020.
14. Muscaritoli M, Anker SD, Argiles J, Aversa Z, Bauer JM, Biolo G, Bioirie Y, Bosaeus I, Cederholm T, Costelli P, Fearon KC, Laviano A, Maggio M, Rossi Fanelli F, Schneider SM, Schols A, Sieber CC. Consensus definition of sarcopenia, cachexia and pre-cachexia: joint document elaborated by Special Interest Groups (SIG) —cachexia-anorexia in chronic wasting diseases and —nutrition in geriatrics. Clin Nutr. 2010;29:154–9.
15. White JV, Guenter P, Jensen G, et al. Consensus statement: Academy of Nutrition and Dietetics and American Society for parenteral and enteral nutrition. J Parenter Enteral Nutr. 2012;36:275–83.
16. Kaysen GA. Association between inflammation and malnutrition as risk factor of cardiovascular disease. Blood Purif. 2006;24:51–5.
17. Ellulu MS, Patimah I, Khaza'ai H, Rahmat A, Abed Y. Obesity and inflammation: the liking mechanisms and the complications. Arch Med Sci. 2017;4:851–63.
18. Rubin DC, Shaker A, Levin MS. Chronic intestinal inflammation: inflammatory bowel disease and colitis-associated colon cancer. Front Immunol. 2012;3(107):1–10.
19. van Vliet IM, Gomes-Neto AW, de Jong MFC, Jager-Wittenaar H, Navis GJ. High prevalence of malnutrition both on hospital admission and predischarge. https://european-nutrition.org/good-practices/malnutrition-before-hospital-discharge/. Accessed 24 June 2020.
20. Luong R, Kim M, Lee A, Carey S. Assessing nutritional status in a cohort of liver cirrhosis outpatients: a prospective cross-sectional study. Nutr Health. 2020;26(1):19–25.
21. Jager-Wittenaar H, Ottery FD. Assessing nutritional status in cancer: role of the patient-generated subjective global assessment. Curr Opin Clin Nutr Metab Care. 2017;20(5):322–9.
22. Isenring E, Bauer J, Capra S. The scored patient-generated subjective global assessment (PG-SGA) and its association with quality of life in ambulatory patients receiving radiotherapy. Eur J Clin Nutr. 2003;57(2):305–9.
23. Cereda E, Pedrolli C, Klersy C, et al. Clin Nutr. 2016;35(6):1282–90. https://doi.org/10.1016/j.clnu.2016.03.008. Epub 2016 Apr 6.
24. Khalatbari-Soltani S, Marques-Vidal P. The economic cost of hospital malnutrition in Europe; a narrative review. Clin Nutr ESPEN. 2015;10(3):e89–94.
25. Curtis LJ, Bernier P, Jeejeebhoy K, Allard J, Duerksen D, Gramlich L, Laporte M, Keller HH. Costs of hospital malnutrition. Clin Nutr. 2017;36(5):1391–6.
26. Hospital Readmission Risk Reduction Program (HRRP). https://www.cms.gov/Medicare/Medicare-Fee-for-Service-Payment/AcuteInpatientPPS/Readmissions-Reduction-Program. Accessed 9 July 2020.
27. Philipson TJ, Snider JT, Lakdawalla DN, et al. Impact of oral nutritional supplementation on hospital outcomes. Am J Manag Care. 2013;19(2):121–8.
28. Yang P, Lin M, Lee C, Chang N. Effect of nutritional intervention programs on nutritional status and readmission rate in malnourished older adults with pneumonia: a randomized control trial. Int J Environ Res Public Health. 2019;16(23):4758. Published online 2019 Nov 27. https://doi.org/10.3390/ijerph16234758.
29. Reckman GAR, Gomes AW, Vonk RJ, et al. Anabolic competence: assessment and integration of the multimodality interventional approach in disease-related malnutrition. Nutrition. 2019;65:179–84.
30. Kyle UG, Morabia A, Slosman DO, Mensi N, Unger P, Pichard C. Contribution of body composition to nutritional assessment at hospital admission in 995 patients: a controlled population study. Br J Nutr. 2001 Dec;86(6):725–31.
31. Langer CJ, Hoffman JP, Ottery FD. Clinical significance of weight loss in cancer patients: rationale for the use of anabolic agents in the treatment of cancer related cachexia. Nutrition. 2001;17(1Suppl):S1–21.
32. Association, A.D. Identifying patients at risk: ADA's definition for nutrition screening and nutrition assessment. J Am Diet Assoc. 1994;94(8):838–9. https://doi.org/10.1016/0002-82233(94)92357-4.
33. Nutrition Screening Adults. Academy of nutrition and dietetics. https://www.andeal.org/topic.cfm?menu=5382#:~:text=Nutrition%20screening%20is%20the%20process,registered%20dietitian%20nutritionist%20(RDN). Accessed 9 July 2020.
34. Nutritional assessment. https://www.bapen.org.uk/nutrition-support/assessment-and-planning/nutritional-assessment#:~:text=Nutritional%20assessment%20is%20the%20systematic,(BDA)%2C%202012). Accessed 9 July 2020.
35. Favaro-Moeira NC, Krausch-Hofmann S, Matthys C, Vereecken C, Vanhauwaert E, Declercq A, Bekkering GE, Duyck J. Risk factors for malnutrition in older adults: a systematic review of the literature based on longitudinal data. Adv Nutr. 2016;7(3):507–22.
36. Vafaei Z, Mokhtari H, Sadooghi Z, Meamar R, Chitsaz A, Moeini M. Malnutrition is associated with depression in rural elderly population. J Res Med Sci. 2013;18(Suppl 1):S15–9.
37. Casanova MJ, Chaparro M, Molina B, Merino O, et al. Prevalence of malnutrition and nutritional characteristics of patients with inflammatory bowel disease. J Crohns Colitis. 2017;11(12):1430–9.
38. Burks CE, Jones CW, Braz VA, Swor RA, Richmond NL, et al. Risk factors for malnutrition among older adults in the emergency department: a multicenter study. J Am Geriatr Soc. 2017;65(8):1741–7.
39. Sherry CL, Sauer AC, Thrush KE. Assessment of the nutrition care process in US hospitals using a web-based tool demonstrates the need for quality improvement in malnutrition diagnosis and discharge

care. Curr Dev Nutr. 2017;1:e001297. https://doi.org/10.3945/cdn.117.001297.eCollection.
40. Kamperidis N, Tesser L, Wolfson TP, Katechia K, Robinson D, Nightingale J. Prevalence of malnutrition in medical and surgical gastrointestinal outpatients. Clin Nutr ESPEN. 2020;35:188–93.
41. Lim SL, Ong KCB, Chan YH, Loke WC, Ferguson M, Daniels L. Malnutrition and its impact on cost of hospitalization, length of stay, readmission and 3-year mortality. Clin Nutr. 2012;31(3):345–50.
42. Gonzales CS, Lacerda MS, Chaves GV. Patient Generated Subjective Global Assessment as a prognosis tool in women with gynecologic cancer. Nutrition. 2015;31:1372–8.
43. Kang MC, Kim JH, Ryu SW, Moon JY, Park JH, et al. Prevalence of malnutrition in hospitalized patients: a multicenter cross-sectional study. J Korean Med Sci. 2018;33(2):e10–20.
44. Crowley J, Ball L, Hiddink GJ. Nutrition in medical education: a systematic review. Lancet Planet Health. 2019;3:e379–89.
45. Validated malnutrition screening and assessment tools: comparison guide. https://www.health.qld.gov.au/__data/assets/pdf_file/0021/152454/hphe_scrn_tools.pdf. Accessed 5 July 2020.
46. Reber E, Gomes F, Vasiloglou MF, Schuetz P, Stagna Z. Nutritional risk screening and assessment. J Clin Med. 2019;8(7):1065–84.
47. Harris PS, Payne L, Morrison L, Green SM, Ghio D, Hallett C, Parsons EL, Aveyard P, Roberts HC, et al. Barriers and facilitator to screening and treating malnutrition in older adults living in the community: a mixed-methods synthesis. BMC Fam Pract. 2019;20:100–10. https://doi.org/10.1186/s12875-019-0983-y.
48. de van der Schueren MAE, Keller H, GLIM Consortium, et al. Global Leadership Initiative on Malnutrition (GLIM): Guidance on validation of the operational criteria for the diagnosis of protein-energy malnutrition in adults [published online ahead of print, 2020 Jun 11]. Clin Nutr. 2020;43(1):S0261-5614(19)33208-X. https://doi.org/10.1016/j.clnu.2019.12.022.
49. Elia M, Stratton RJ. An analytic appraisal of nutrition screening tools supported by original data with particular reference to age. Nutrition. 2012;28(5):477–94.
50. National Counseling on Aging: Malnutrition and Screening Assessment Tools. https://www.health.qld.gov.au/__data/assets/pdf_file/0021/152454/hphe_scrn_tools.pdf. Accessed 5 July 2020.
51. Validity in screening tools. https://www.mna--elderly.com/validity_in_screening_tools.html#:~:text=The%20MNA%C2%AE%20is%20the,97%25%20compared%20to%20clinical%20status. Accessed 5 July 2020.
52. Secher M, Soto ME, Villars H, van Kan GA, Vellas B. The Mini Nutritional Assessment (MNA) after 20 years of research and clinical practice. Rev Clin Gerontol. 2007;17:293–310.
53. Boleo-Tome C, Monteiro-Grillo I, Ravasco P. Validation of the malnutrition universal screening tool (MUST) in cancer. Br J Nutr. 2012;108(2):343–8.
54. Kyle UG, Kossovsky MP, Karsegard VL, Pichard C. Comparison of tools for nutritional assessment and screening at hospital admission: a population study. Clin Nutr. 2006;25(3):409–17.
55. Shafiee F, Karandish M, Handianford AM, Eftekhari MH, Haghighizadeh M. Determing the ability of Subjective Global Assessment to diagnosis risk of malnutrition in hospitalized patients. J Res Med Dent Sci. 2017;5(2):48–55.
56. Bauer J, Capra S. Ferguson. Use of the scored patient-generated subjective global assessment tool in patients with cancer. Eur J Clin Nutr. 2002;56(8):779–85.
57. Keller HH, Goy R, Kane S-L. Validity and reliability of SCREEN II (Seniors in the community: risk evaluation for eating and nutrition, Version II). Eur J Clin Nutr. 2005;59:1149–57.
58. Sealy MJ, Nijholt W, Stuiver MM, van der Berg MM, Roodenburg JLN, van der Schans CP, Ottery FD, Jager-Wittenaar H. Content validity across methods of malnutrition assessment in patients with cancer is limited. J Clin Epidemiol. 2016;76:126–36.
59. Baker JP, Detsky AS, Wesson DE, et al. Nutritional assessment: a comparison of clinical judgement and objective measures. N Engl J Med. 1982;306:969–72.
60. Keith JN. Bedside nutrition assessment past, present and future: a review of the subjective global assessment. Nutr Clin Pract. 2008;23(4):410–6.
61. Detsky AS, McLaughlin JR, Baker JP, Johnston N, Whittaker S, Mendelson RA, Jeejeebhopy KN. What is subjective global assessment of nutritional status? J Parenter Enteral Nutr. 1987;11(1):8–13.
62. Makhija S, Baker J. The subjective global assessment: a review of its use in clinical practice. Nutr Clin Pract. 2008;23(4):405–9.
63. Wu B-W, Yin T, Cao W-X, Gu Z-D, Wang X-J, Yan M, Liu B-Y. Clinical application of subjective global assessment in Chinese patients with gastrointestinal cancer. World J Gastroenterol. 2009;15(28):3542–9.
64. Gabrielsen DK, Scaffidi D, Leung E, Stoyanoff L, Robinson J, Nisenbaum R, Brezden-Masley C, Darling PB. Use of an abridged scored Patient-Generated Subjective Global Assessment (abPG-SGA) as a nutritional screening tool for cancer patients in an outpatient setting. Nutr Cancer. 2013;65(2):234–9.
65. Ottery FD. Definition of standardized nutritional assessment and interventional pathways in oncology. Nutrition. 1996;12(1 Suppl):S15–9.
66. https://www.andeal.org/worksheet.cfm?worksheet_id=257021. Ottery FD. Definition of standardized nutritional assessment and interventional pathways in oncology. Nutrition. 1996;12(1 Suppl):S15–S19. Accessed 6 July 2020.
67. Bauer J, Capra S, Ferguson M. Use of the scored Patient-Generated Subjective Global Assessment (PG-SGA) as a nutrition assessment tool in patients with cancer. Eur J Clin Nutr. 2002;56:779–85.
68. Rodrigues CE, Larceda MS, Chaves GV. Patient Generated Subjective Global Assessment as a prognosis tool in women with gynecologic cancer. Nutrition. 2015;31:1372–8.

69. Guerra RS, Sousa AS, Fonseca I, Pichel F, Restivo MT, Ferreira S, Amaral TF. Comparative analysis of undernutrition screening and diagnostic tools as predictors of hospitalization costs. J Hum Nutr Diet. 2016;29:165–73.
70. Vigano AL, di Tomasso J, Kilgor RD, et al. The abridged patient-generated subjective global assessment is a useful tool for early detection and characterization of cancer cachexia. J Acad Nutr Diet. 2014;114(7):1088–98.
71. Ottery FD, Wagner K, Dixon S. Integrating routine nutritional screening for cancer patients at the point of care: pilot testing a novel care planning system plus certified professional training. https://www.carevive.com/integrating-routine-nutritional-screenings-for-cancer-patients-at-the-point-of-care/. Accessed 24 June 2020.
72. Nitichai N, Angkatavanich J, Somlaw N, Voravad N, Lertbutsayanukul C. Validation of the scored Patient-Generated Subjective Assessment (PG-SGA) and association with nutritional parameters in cancer patients. Asian Pac J Cancer Prev. 2019;20(4):1249–55.
73. Bian D, Shi Y, Jiang Y, Zhong J, Sun J, Gu Y. Combined Patient-Generated Subjective Global Assessment and body composition facilitates nutrition support in inflammatory bowel disease: an ambulatory study in Shanghai. Asia Pac J Clin Nutr. 2018;27(6):1230–8.
74. Martin L, Gioulbasanis I, Senesse P, Baracos VE. Cancer-associated malnutrition and CT-defined sarcopenia and myosteatosis and endemic in overweight and obese patients. J Parenter Enteral Nutr. 2020;44(2):227–38.
75. Luong R, Kim M, Lee A, Carey S. Assessing nutritonal status in a cohort of liver cirrhosis outpatients: a prospective cross-sectional study. Nutr Health. 2020;26(1):19–25.
76. Roach LA, Lambert K, Holt JL, Meyer BJ. Diet quality in patients with end-stage kidney disease undergoing dialysis. J Ren Care. 2017;43(4):226–34.

General Therapeutic Principles for Nutritional Support

4

Lena B. Palmer

Once an individual has been identified as being unable to meet his or her nutrition and hydration needs by oral intake alone, or is anticipated to need medical nutrition therapy (MNT) due to an upcoming procedure or therapy, planning should begin regarding the most appropriate route, timing, and setting for initiation of nutrition support. National and international societies have provided consensus guidelines which can provide decision support at each step, but rigorous evidence-based data underlying those guidelines are often lacking. Decisions will also differ depending on whether the need for MNT is acute or chronic and will further differ in the presence of critical illness. Practitioners who work in both the inpatient and outpatient setting must be familiar with many different aspects of nutrition care to help guide therapy. A table outlining major international nutrition and specialty societies with nutrition-related guidelines is provided for reference, though this list should not be considered comprehensive and is not an endorsement of any specific guideline or society (Table 4.1). Detailed concepts in nutrition support such as individual protein and caloric requirements based on disease process, oral dietary therapy and medical diets, polymeric versus specialized enteral supplements, rate of feeding, and nutrition concepts specific to individual disease states are beyond the scope of this generalized review.

Initiating Medical Nutrition Therapy – Timing

Acute care hospitals often include basic malnutrition screening questionnaires at the time of hospital admission, and in the United States, the Joint Commission mandates nutritional screen within 48 hours of admission [1]. However, the Joint Commission does not require use of any one specific screening tool, and a 2014 survey of US hospitals showed hospitals approach nutrition screening in a variety of ways, ranging from simple questions of weight loss history to complex malnutrition screening tools such as the Subjective Global Assessment (SGA) [2].

Nutrition support planning should be routinely included in the initial assessment of all critically ill hospitalized patients. Consensus guidelines from the American Society for Parenteral and Enteral Nutrition (ASPEN), the Society of Critical Care Medicine (SCCM), the Canadian Clinical Practice Guidelines, as well as the European Society for Clinical Nutrition and Metabolism (ESPEN) recommend performing a

Disclaimer: The contents of this chapter do not represent the views of the Department of Veterans Affairs or the US Government

L. B. Palmer (✉)
Medicine, Gastroenterology, Southeast Louisiana Veterans Health Care System,
New Orleans, LA, USA
e-mail: Lena.Palmer@va.gov

C. Newberry et al. (eds.), *Nutrition, Weight, and Digestive Health*,
https://doi.org/10.1007/978-3-030-94953-2_4

Table 4.1 International Nutrition and Specialty Societies, Guideline Statements and Consensus Documents[a]

Society	Subject	Year of Publication
American Society for Parenteral and Enteral Nutrition (ASPEN)	Refeeding Syndrome	2020
	Central Venous Access Devices for Home PN	2019
	Enterocutaneous Fistula[b]	2019
	EN	2017
	Critical Illness[c]	2016
	Home and Alternative Site Care	2014
European Society for Parenteral and Enteral Nutrition (ESPEN)	Home PN	2020
	Home EN	2020
	Acute and Chronic Pancreatitis	2020
	Critical Illness	2019
	Polymorbid Internal Medicine Patients	2018
	Surgery	2017
Federación Latino Americana de Terapia Nutricional, Nutrición Clínica y Metabolismo (FELANPE)	Enterocutaneous Fistula[d]	2019
American Gastroenterological Association (AGA)	Acute Pancreatitis	2018
American College of Gastroenterology (ACG)	Adult Hospitalized Patients	2016
Society for Critical Care Medicine (SCCM)	Critical Illness[d]	2016
Canadian Critical Care Society (CCCS) and the Canadian Critical Care Trials Group (CCTG)	Critical Illness	2013/2015
American Society for Gastrointestinal Endoscopy (ASGE)	Endoscopy in Enteral Feeding	2011
National Institute for Health and Clinical Excellence (NICE), United Kingdom	Nutrition Support for Adults	2006

[a]Only guidelines referenced in the text are included
[b]In conjunction with FELANPE
[c]In conjunction with SCCM
[d]In conjunction with ASPEN

standardized nutrition risk assessment and initiating nutrition support within 24–48 hours of admission to the ICU for all patients regardless of the presence or degree of malnutrition at baseline [1, 3, 4]. The ASPEN/SCCM recommendation is based on four meta-analyses comparing outcomes in early versus delayed initiation of enteral nutrition (EN) that show a clinical benefit to early EN, mostly in the form of decreased infectious complications. The meta-analyses showed mixed results regarding mortality with one showing a trend in mortality reduction [5], and two showing a clear mortality benefit [1, 6]. Reduced hospital length of stay has also been demonstrated. The quality of the evidence was considered very low, however, and a Cochrane Database Systematic Review determined that the quality of evidence was insufficient to draw consistent conclusions of clinical benefit [7]. The societies differ in regard to the method of nutrition risk screening, with ASPEN/SCCM guidelines recommending use of a validated malnutrition screening tool such as the Nutrition Risk Score (NRS-2002) and ESPEN noting that no tools have been universally validated in all critical care populations, and a broader approach was endorsed. Nutrition care for critically ill patients with burn injuries is a specialized area of nutrition support due to the extreme metabolic and physiologic derangements that occur; Abdullahi & Jeschke provide a helpful overview of key principles in the nutrition care of patients with burns [8].

If EN is contraindicated or not feasible, and parenteral nutrition (PN) is considered, studies have shown little benefit and even harm from early initiation of PN in patients who are well nourished or only mildly malnourished upon admission [9, 10]; therefore, it is recommended to wait between 3 and 7 days after admission for critical illness to begin PN in patients who are not moderately to severely malnourished and who cannot be fed orally or enterally [1, 3, 9]. In those patients who do meet criteria for moderate to severe malnutrition, MNT should begin as soon as possible and immediately after hemodynamic stabilization regardless of route. If hemodynamic instability is prolonged, the parenteral route should be considered.

There is evidence that MNT is beneficial in hospitalized patient who are not critically ill [11–13], however, there is little evident to guide timing of therapy initiation. Generally accepted principles in patients who are not critically ill stratify timing based on degree of malnutrition, and enteral or parenteral interventions are usually avoided in the first week of hospitalization when patients are well nourished or mildly malnourished at baseline [9, 14]. MNT including insertion of enteral or parenteral access devices should be considered within 48–72 hours of admission in moderate to severely malnourished patients.

Recognition of chronic malnutrition in the outpatient setting is more challenging due to fragmented episodes of care, lack of routine weight monitoring, and a lack of nutrition screening mandates from accrediting bodies. Ideally nutrition screening should be performed in most routine follow-up encounters or encounters for medical conditions where malnutrition is a common complication. General nutrition support should begin immediately when malnutrition, weight loss, or inadequate oral intake has been identified. This includes identifying the medical, emotional, social, and cultural factors that are contributing to malnutrition; considering how other comorbid illness and prior surgeries are impacting malnutrition; evaluating allergies and medications to identify those that can impact nutritional intake; and providing enhanced oral dietary advice to help prevent further decline. If rapid or severe changes are noted, it may be necessary to proceed directly to EN or PN [11].

Perioperative nutrition support has received a great deal of attention in the last decade with the increasing recognition of a concept known as "pre-habilitation" [15]. Pre-habilitation protocols use "bundles" of preoperative interventions that have collectively been shown to decrease postoperative complications, with the goal of improving postsurgical outcomes. Nutrition is an important component of perioperative risk reduction interventions. One of the earliest studies of the impact of MNT on postoperative outcomes was the 1991 Veterans Affairs Cooperative study of PN prior to elective major surgery [16]. This landmark trial demonstrated that MNT in the form of parenteral nutrition started 7–15 days prior to major surgery and continued for at least 3 days postoperatively reduced non-infectious complications by almost 90% compared to controls [5% versus 43%; $P = 0.03$; RR 0.12 (95% CI 0.02–0.91)]. There were no differences in infectious complications between the two groups. In contrast, patients who were borderline or only mildly malnourished did not show a benefit and incurred increased infectious complications. Two of the most widely applied examples of modern preoperative initiatives include the Enhanced Recovery after Surgery® or ERAS® protocol [17] and the Strong for Surgery initiative [18]. The ERAS® protocol is a distinct set of interventions that have been widely studied in many forms of surgery, mostly gastrointestinal surgery. Randomized controlled trials and meta-analyses of ERAS® protocols have shown reductions in morbidity, costs, hospital length of stay (LOS), pain, recovery times, and improved quality of life (QOL) and patient satisfaction [19]. The benefit of pre-habilitation, which can vary significantly by site and utilizes additional strategies beyond those in the ERAS® bundle, has been questioned in a recent systematic review showing no improvement in outcomes from RCTs included in the analysis [20]. The analysis included 14 RCTs, but the wide range of interventions, types of surgeries, lengths of pre-habilitation programs, and degree of compliance with protocol limit the ability to assess outcomes in a systematic or generalizable way. A separate meta-analysis that focused only on nutritional pre-habilitation in colorectal surgery did find a benefit in functional status as measured by a 6-minute walk test and hospital length of stay for ONS and/or counseling prior to surgery, or ONS with or without counseling and with exercise [21].

Initiating Medical Nutrition Therapy – Route

MNT can be delivered via one of the following three routes: orally by volitional intake, enterally through a device inserted into the intestine, or parenterally through a venous access device. Oral MNT is often the first recommendation for chronically malnourished patients in need of MNT, given it is the least invasive and least expensive option, and it preserves the natural process of consuming nutrition by mouth. Commercially available oral nutrition supplements (ONS), usually in the form of liquid beverages, are widely available and come in a variety of flavors. Studies have shown benefit from the addition of ONS when patients retain the ability to eat and drink, including decreased hospitalization rates, improved functional and nutritional status, increased weight and muscle mass, decreased length and costs of hospital stay, and reduced readmission rates [11–13, 22]. Though liquid ONS is the most common form, commercial providers have developed calorie-dense offerings in the form of solid snack bars and puddings that can provide additional variety depending on a patient's preferences and swallowing abilities. A significant downside of commercial ONS in the ambulatory setting, however, is the lack of financial resources for patients, as this route of therapy is not usually covered by insurance.

If oral intake is not adequate or possible due to factors such as an impaired ability to swallow, then the enteral route of feeding should be used except in very specific situations. Physiologic benefits of providing MNT directly to the intestine include preservation of the gut mucosal barrier, blood supply, motor function, and microbiome, and decreased secretion of inflammatory mediators [1, 9, 23]. Improved outcomes from EN over PN have been shown in numerous studies, with the most consistent benefit being in reduced infectious complications [1, 3]. In the ICU setting, reduced length of stay has also been shown. Results on mortality, though, have been inconsistent, and at present the data are not sufficient to show a mortality benefit for EN [1]. Gastrointestinal intolerance is common in acute illness, however, as is under-administration of EN. Supplemental PN is the process of adding PN when patients are failing to meet nutritional targets with EN or oral intake alone. Russell and Wischmeyer provide a comprehensive review of recent guidelines and clinical scenarios where supplemental PN may be considered [24].

There are a few specific clinical scenarios where evidence-based guidelines have been published to help guide route of therapy. ESPEN and the American Gastroenterology Association (AGA) have both recommended oral/enteral feeding over PN for patients with acute pancreatitis (Grade of Recommendation A, strong consensus, moderate quality of evidence) [25, 26]. ESPEN guidelines recommend administering EN to the level of the stomach initially and reserving post-pyloric feeding in the case of intolerance, and the AGA guidelines do not provide guidance regarding the decision to target the stomach or the small bowel. For patients with high output enterocutaneous fistula where enteral access below the level of the fistula cannot be established, ASPEN and the Federación Latino Americana de Terapia Nutricional, Nutrición Clínica y Metabolismo (FELANPE) recommend consideration of PN, at least until fistula output can be controlled [27]. There is no consensus as to whether and when to use medical diet therapy, EN, or PN in the setting of a chyle leak which is a disruption in the flow of lymphatic fluids that complicates some surgeries of the head, neck, and gastrointestinal tract [28]; the choice and timing of route generally depend on the severity of the leak [29, 30].

Enteral nutrition therapy is delivered via feeding tube, and it can be delivered to various points in the intestine. The least invasive method of EN delivery is via small bore nasoenteric tube [31]. Usually these range in size from 8 to 12 French for adults and utilize an internal stylet during insertion as opposed to larger bore tubes that lack a stylet and are inserted for medication delivery or decompression of the intestine in the event of a bowel obstruction. Large bore tubes are not recommended for EN due to the risk of sinusitis and mucosal breakdown, ulceration, necrosis, or perforation with long-term use, and oral insertion of enteric tubes is generally only used in patients who are intubated and sedated due to oropharyngeal irritation and gag reflexes [32]. Small bore tubes also carry these risks, though, and a general guideline is that nasoenteric feeding tubes should not be used beyond 4–6 weeks [33, 34]. Additional complications of nasoenteric tubes include complications from insertion such as bleeding or malpositioning which can result in serious injury or even death due to pneumothorax or perforation at any point along the insertion tract, including malpositioning into the sinuses or cranium. EN has also been infused into tubes that were not recognized to be malpositioned in the lungs, resulting in pneumonia and respiratory distress [35]. Insertion is contraindicated in patients with a basilar skull fracture, recent sinus surgery, deviated septum or other anatomical barrier to insertion through the nose, or an uncorrected coagulopathy [31]. Small bore feeding tubes are also uncomfortable for patients and are prone to clogging, migration, reflux from a small intestine segment back into the stomach, and dislodgement from accidental or deliberate removal. Meta-analysis shows that dislodgement can be reduced through the use of a nasal bridle device which is a plastic or fabric tie that is inserted through the nares, wrapped around the vomer bone, and then attached to the nasoenteric tube [36]. The nasal bridle technique was initially developed using common hospital supplies [37], but a commercial apparatus is available which simplifies the procedure [38].

Percutaneous feeding tubes can be inserted endoscopically, radiographically, or surgically directly from the outer abdominal wall into the intestine. The most common method of insertion is percutaneous endoscopic gastrostomy insertion or PEG. This technique was first described in 1980 [39], and it has been shown to be safe and effective [40]. Surgical gastrostomies are generally reserved for patients with altered anatomy in whom percutaneous or radiographic insertion is not possible. Complications are higher and success rates are lower for this technique (though selection bias confounds this comparison). Tubes can also be inserted percutaneously into the jejunum (known as direct percutaneous endoscopic jejunostomy or DPEJ); however, insertion of a PEJ tube is technically more complex, requires an experienced operator, and success rates are lower [40]. The choice of technique usually depends on local expertise and availability. Contraindications and cautions to percutaneous or surgical enteral feeding tubes include ascites, connective tissue disorders, uncorrectable coagulopathy, and varices or infiltrative disorders of the target organ.

Parenteral nutrition should be reserved for situations when use of the intestine is not medically possible. This includes anatomic issues such as intestinal obstruction or severe dysmotility, proximal or high output entero-cutaneous fistulae, and chyle leak when dietary or enteral therapy has failed. It is also appropriate to consider parenteral nutrition when MNT is needed but patients are hemodynamically unstable or where intestinal ischemia is of concern.

Ethical and practical dilemmas can occur when debating timing and route of MNT [41]. Patients may decline EN due to perceived discomfort from a feeding tube, prioritizing immediate physical comfort and downplaying the increased medical risks and costs associated with PN. Patients may refuse oral feeding or fail to meet oral feeding goals despite lack of identifiable medical conditions that would inhibit oral intake. Patients or caregivers may also insist upon MNT when providing MNT is either futile or potentially harmful, such as in the case of inserting PEG tubes for feeding in the setting of advanced dementia [41–43]. Practical dilemmas occur when insurance regulations may significantly impact the choice of route, in that insurance providers are unlikely to cover the high costs of PN if there is no medical indication for its use [44]. Insurance limitations can also impact the ability to provide EN, as some insurers may cover insertion of a feeding device but may not cover the actual EN formulation, and others may not cover EN unless a permanent medical disability exists [44]. Insurers who only cover MNT in the setting of permanent disability exclude those who need MNT for short periods of time (such as after a major intestinal surgery when oral feeding adequacy may be delayed) or when there is no obvious medical reason prohibiting intake [45]. The cost of paying out of pocket for MNT may be prohibitive for the patient, particularly if PN is needed. It is necessary to confirm that patients have adequate resources for any MNT plan prior to initiation. When patient wishes for MNT differ from best medical advice, it is very important to engage patients and caregivers in a detailed discussion of the risks, benefits, indications, costs, and monitoring requirements of the desired MNT and why an alternative is being recommended. Often providers will find that enhanced understanding of the rationale behind certain recommendations allows patients and providers to reach a mutually beneficial strategy.

Initiating Medical Nutrition Therapy – Setting

If MNT is being considered for patients who are ambulatory, providers will need to determine if MNT can be safely and practically initiated in the home, or whether safety or other parameters necessitate admission to an acute care facility for coordination of access device insertion and clinical monitoring during therapy initiation. Safety is of utmost importance, and providers must assess patients for risk of refeeding syndrome. Refeeding syndrome, first described immediately following the Second World War [46, 47], is the observed constellation of clinical symptoms experienced by those who have been deprived of nutrition for extended periods of time and are suddenly provided with nutrition. Patients who are significantly malnourished and at risk of refeeding syndrome must be hospitalized to initiate MNT so that serious potential complications can be managed or avoided. Potential complications include cardiac arrhythmias, rhabdomyolysis, seizures, coma, respiratory decompensation, extreme electrolyte abnormalities, and even death [48]. A consensus definition and guidelines regarding management of refeeding syndrome have recently been published [49]. Refeeding syndrome was defined as a decrease in one or a combination of serum sodium, magnesium, or phosphorous of at least 10% from baseline, with or without organ dysfunction, occurring within 5 days of reintroduction of feeding. Organ damage resulting from thiamin deficiency occurring within the same time frame was also included in the definition of refeeding syndrome. Tenants of anticipating and managing refeeding syndrome include frequent electrolyte monitoring, replacement of deficits prior to and during initiation of oral feeding (usually with intravenous and not oral formulations), prescribing thiamin supplementation before and during refeeding, and starting oral feeding at a fraction of anticipated needs (usually 10–25% of estimated caloric needs).

It was historically common to admit patients needing PEG tube insertion to the hospital for overnight monitoring after placement even if refeeding syndrome was not a concern, often delaying EN initiation to the next morning. Published experiences with outpatient insertion of PEG tubes, and even unsedated outpatient PEG placement in victims of stroke, have challenged this practice [50–52]. As for timing of EN initiation after PEG placement, multiple meta-analyses have shown no harm from EN started 2–4 hours after the PEG has been placed [33, 53], and delaying EN start to the next morning simply prolongs hospitalization time and decreases nutrition delivery.

Initiating parenteral nutrition is a complex process that requires frequent clinical and laboratory assessment to ensure safety, and this is not usually initiated in a home setting as daily labs and adequate clinical assessment are not readily available. However, Newton & DeLegge have discussed home-start PN and laid out a framework for conditions, checks, balances, and considerations where this could be accomplished under the management of experienced nutrition support teams [54]. Choosing the appropriate venous access device is an important part of the process, and recent guidelines have been published to help teams choose the right device for the right clinical scenario [55]. While peripherally-inserted central venous catheters (PICC) are commonly used in acute care settings, they are not ideal devices for patients who require long-term PN. Single lumen tunneled catheters are the preferred venous access device for patients who require long-term PN and when no other parenteral infusions are needed. Single lumen catheters minimize the risk of catheter-related infections which are one of the most common complications of PN.

Monitoring Medical Nutrition Therapy

After MNT has begun, it is very important to closely monitor for complications of therapy and to routinely reassess feeding tolerance and progress toward goals [33, 35]. Studies have shown clinical and economic benefit when a nutrition support team is involved in this process [33, 34, 56, 57]. Nutrition support teams are usually composed of a physician or licensed independent provider who is experienced in MNT, an expert-level registered dietitian nutritionist, a clinical pharmacist experienced with PN, and potentially specialized nutrition support nurses [34]. Unfortunately increasing financial burdens on hospital systems have resulted in a steady decline of formal NST [58]. It is still necessary, particularly when PN is used, for patients to be connected with a main team or provider who will be responsible for the frequent follow-up needed to ensure safe and effective care [33, 34, 59].

The frequency, nature, or timing of laboratory and clinical assessment needed when MNT is begun is usually based on local policy and expertise, though at least one clinical guideline has provided recommendations for follow-up assessment [9]. Inpatients are often reassessed daily or several times a week by nutrition support staff, and daily laboratory monitoring is usually available. The main concerns during initiation phase are to ensure electrolyte stability and patient tolerance of the route of therapy as well as to manage hyperglycemia if it occurs [35]. Electrolytes including magnesium and phosphorous, kidney function, liver enzymes, and triglycerides are monitored prior to initiation of parenteral therapy and after starting. Electrolytes are monitored daily in the initiation phase, but liver enzymes and triglycerides should not require daily checks unless significant abnormalities develop. Hyperglycemia is a common occurrence in hospitalized and critically ill patients even in the absence of preexisting diabetes, and it is associated with worse clinical outcomes [60]. Therefore, it is important to monitor for the development of hyperglycemia during the initiation of MNT. There is currently no standard regarding how to manage hyperglycemia in the setting of enteral or parenteral nutrition [61], but the annually updated American Diabetes Association® *Standards of Care in Diabetes* addresses glycemic control in hospitalized patients and can be used to guide therapy even in those without preexisting diabetes [62]. Acute phase proteins such as albumin and pre-albumin are not reliable markers of malnutrition and they should not be used to guide therapy, particularly in the setting of acute inflammation where the catabolic process significantly impacts serum levels [9, 63]. The measurement of gastric residual volume (the amount of fluid contained in the stomach after EN infusion, as assessed by aspiration of contents from the feeding tube) has historically been used as a marker of tolerance to EN [3]. This practice is no longer widely recommended for routine clinical care due to numerous inconsistencies in technique and the lack of association with clinical outcomes [1, 35, 64]. If it is still performed, though, recommendations are to avoid holding EN therapy unless the aspirated volume is more than 500 ml [1, 3]. Though assessment for vitamin deficiencies may be indicated depending on patient symptoms and malnutrition, several serum vitamin or mineral assays such as selenium, iron, copper, zinc, and vitamin A are highly influenced by the serum proteins to which they are complexed or by which they are measured. As many of these are acute phase reactants, monitoring during an acute care stay may not yield an accurate assessment of the body's stores [65–67]. Additionally, multivitamins that are incorporated into EN or PN formulas can confound the assessment of a patient's underlying reserve.

Assessment of daily weight is not usually needed to guide nutrition support, but weekly monitoring is helpful to establish trends. Symptoms such as abdominal fullness, bloating, nausea, vomiting, coughing/choking during feeding, regurgitation or reflux, leakage from tube sites, abdominal pain, and alteration in bowel habits should be promptly explored [35]. While EN is commonly blamed for diarrhea in hospitalized patients, there are many potential alternative causes such as hyperosmolar medications or underlying medical conditions that can be corrected with good result before altering the EN therapy itself [9, 68]. Also, villous atrophy can occur during periods of severe intestinal infections or prolonged bowel rest, and diarrhea can be seen in the first few weeks when the small intestine is rebuilding absorptive capacity [69, 70].

Ambulatory patients will not have the benefit of frequent in-person monitoring unless PN is utilized and weekly assessment for central line care and lab checks are standards of care. Ambulatory patients on oral or EN therapy are at particular risk of loss to follow-up, and patient visits should be scheduled ahead of time to ensure that patients do not lose access to care. The increasing use of telehealth and distance monitoring may improve access for ambulatory patients. An additional financial barrier, at least in the United States, may be lack of coverage for dietitian assessment and monitoring [44]. This is often a significant barrier in the assessment and initiation phase, where very few insurers will cover dietitian care outside of a physician visit.

Long-Term Management and Cessation of Medical Nutrition Therapy

Two outcomes are possible after MNT has been initiated—patients will either require long-term interventions or MNT will eventually be stopped. Some may even progress to more invasive forms of nutrition support depending on the nature of the underlying disease. This is where having a clear and transparent understanding of goals of MNT and setting realistic patient expectations are key [34, 59].

Some patients naturally come to the end of MNT through resolution of the underlying disease process – bowel obstructions resolve, patients regain swallow function, inflammatory diseases like Crohn's disease enter remission with disease-modifying regimens, appetites return after major surgery, or patients benefit from organ transplants which improve all aspects of functioning. Though patients who have attained independent and volitional oral intake are often eager to end the monitoring and devices that come with MNT, it is important that they be formally assessed for the ability to end support. For example, in patients with oropharyngeal dysphagia, a speech pathologist should officially sanction safety of the patient's swallow mechanism through bedside or fluoroscopic assessments of swallowing [59]. Ideally a registered dietitian nutritionist should have established a relationship with the patient and can attest that the patient is reliably meeting caloric and hydration needs by mouth. Input from other medical providers is often needed to confirm an end to drug therapies such as chemotherapy that dramatically impact nutrition intake or to provide an assessment of the outcome of cancer treatment. This includes providing an honest assessment of an individual's risk to return to a prior state of need. Physician input is very important so that patients can understand the disease process, anticipate the potential for regression, and to discuss the risk of discontinuing devices such as percutaneous feeding tubes in the event they may be needed in the future.

When percutaneous feeding tubes have been inserted and the risk for regression is high, it is prudent to maintain access devices for a sufficient period of time beyond their need to ensure patients are reliably obtaining nutrition by mouth. Percutaneous tubes that have been inserted into an intestine segment where no prior tube existed should not be removed before 4 weeks have passed from the initial placement in order to allow the tract to mature, and longer time periods may be necessary if conditions that can delay wound healing are present [71]. If the enterostomy tract has matured, the medical risk of removal is much less [72]. While there is no formal recommendation for how long the device should be maintained after a patient is eating orally, 4–8 weeks of independent oral intake is often sufficient to notice gross weight trends that could signal concern. If patients have underlying medical comorbidities that would make reinsertion of an access device difficult, they can be offered a low-profile feeding tube in exchange for a traditional feeding tube that can serve as a “place holder” in the event enteral access is needed in the future [32, 73]. Low-profile percutaneous tubes are often called “button” tubes because the external portion of the device resembles a clothing button in both shape and size. If patients do not have significant drainage or local complications at the enterostomy site, these low-profile devices are often unobtrusive and well tolerated. They can provide reassurance and relieve some of the pressure of oral feeding if clinical conditions deteriorate.

Feeding tubes can be manufactured from silicone, latex, or polyurethane, and they require exchange due to normal wear and tear [74]. Fungal overgrowth in enteral feeding devices can occur where fungal colonies create a biofilm on the external tube segment. This is usually manifested as “beading” of the tube extension and visible off-white or even black deposits that cannot be flushed. While this is not harmful to the patient, it can weaken the integrity of the tube itself, and it is a sign that the tube should be exchanged [9]. Manufacturer guidelines generally recommend exchanging replacement feeding tubes every 3–6 months.

Cessation of PN can occur when patients are consistently meeting most of their caloric and hydration needs by an oral or enteral route. There is usually no need to “wean” PN support in the sense that once alternative nutrition is sufficient, no further PN infusion is necessary. This milestone may be clear in patients who have transitioned to alternative means or regained bowel function, but in patients who have sustained a significant amount of intestinal loss and are suspected of having short bowel syndrome, it may be much more difficult to determine when PN support is no longer needed [75]. Additionally, the risk of maintaining central venous access, even if the device is not utilized, is higher than maintaining a non-utilized enteral feeding device as central venous catheters remain a constant risk for infection and thromboembolism. Unfortunately it can take a year or more before the intestine achieves maximal absorptive capacity in patients with short bowel syndrome [76]. This process is called intestinal adaptation. Patients with some ileum and/or colon remaining are more likely to achieve intestinal autonomy and independence from PN as the ileum has a remarkable ability to adapt to increased absorptive demands, and the colon is crucial for reabsorbing fluid and electrolytes. Patients with little ileum or only jejunum remaining, however, may not have sufficient intestine left to meet nutrition and hydration needs without parenteral support. Gross cutoffs regarding the length of remaining intestine after massive resection are often used as guides, with authors quoting 110–130 cm of small bowel alone or 70–90 cm of small bowel in continuity with the colon as being at risk for needing long-term PN [77, 78]. However, compliance with diet, environment, and other comorbidities result in a wide degree of variation in the ability of short bowel syndrome patients to achieve intestinal autonomy after a major insult [78]. The level of the amino acid citrulline has been studied as a prognostic indicator of the ability to achieve intestinal autonomy. Studies of patients with short bowel syndrome have suggested that levels above 20 μmol/L correlate with the ability to discontinue PN therapy after an initial period of adaptation with a sensitivity of 82.5% and a specificity of 82% [79, 80].

Teduglutide is a synthetic glucagon-like-peptide 2 agonist that has been FDA approved to treat short bowel syndrome. Though the main benefit of Teduglutide in randomized controlled clinical trials was a reduction in the weekly need for parenteral therapy, some patients, including some with ultra-short intestinal segments, were able to completely discontinue PN therapy [75]. This has even been demonstrated after significant time has passed from the initial insult. Teduglutide is a once daily subcutaneous injection, and it must be continued indefinitely to maintain the clinical benefit. Many of the risks of Teduglutide are related to its primary mechanisms of action as a growth factor; as such, significant increases in absorptive capacity and area can cause stomal swelling or obstruction and fluid overload. The potential to induce neoplasia is also a concern as colon polyps have been frequently seen, and there are case reports of malignancies occurring in those on Teduglutide therapy. Active GI malignancy is a contraindication to therapy, and GI endoscopy visualizing the remaining bowel is required prior to initiation and routinely thereafter to survey for the development of colon polyps [77].

Patients who are unable to return to oral feeding should maintain contact with nutrition support providers [33]. Patients requiring EN and PN should be monitored for vitamin deficiencies, particularly if EN or PN is the sole source of nutrition. Most adult patients requiring EN for the majority of nutrition needs or those on long-term PN will obtain the equivalent of a daily multivitamin, but specific deficiencies may develop due to the low levels of some nutrients in commercial EN and PN multi-vitamin formulas. Also, patients on semi-elemental EN formulations utilizing mostly medium-chain triglycerides are at risk of developing an essential fatty acid deficiency [81].

One of the most common and dreaded complications of long-term PN therapy are catheter-related infections. These can be referred to as either central line-associated blood stream infections (CLABSIs) or catheter-related blood stream infections (CRBSIs), and occur at a rate of 0.85 episodes per 1000 catheter days (CRSBI) to 1.65 episodes per 1000 catheter days (CLABSI) [82]. Both terms indicate catheter-related infections, but the definitions and clinical use are slightly different [82]. Catheter-related infections result in a significant degree of morbidity, mortality, and cost. Ethanol and taurolidine line locks are small amounts of medical-grade chemical solutions instilled into the lumen of a central venous catheter, and they have been shown to substantially reduce the incidence of CLABSI and CRBSI in patients on long-term PN [83]. Taurolidine locks are recommended for use by ESPEN [84]. However, neither therapy is approved for use in the United States, and taurolidine is not commercially available [82]. Other complications of long-term PN include hyperglycemia; micro and macronutrient deficiencies; metabolic bone disease; non-infectious venous and venous access device complications such as thrombosis, clogging, stenosis, or loss of central venous access; and intestinal failure-associated liver disease (also known as PN-associated liver disease or PN cholestasis) [85]. These are further detailed in Chap. 18.

Conclusions

This very broad overview only touches the surface of MNT, but many of the details such as tools for nutrition screening and assessment, the nature of MNT prescriptions, choices of therapy in specific disease processes, assessing and treating vitamin deficiencies, and more in-depth understanding of enteral and parenteral support are provided in other chapters. Perhaps the greatest resources, however, are the experienced practitioners of one's local nutrition support team who are indefatigable advocates for ensuring that all patients receive nutrition support as a crucial component of care and recovery.

References

1. McClave SA, Taylor BE, Martindale RG, Warren MM, Johnson DR, Braunschweig C, et al. Guidelines for the provision and assessment of nutrition support therapy in the adult critically ill patient: Society of Critical Care Medicine (SCCM) and American Society for Parenteral and Enteral Nutrition (A.S.P.E.N.). JPEN J Parenter Enteral Nutr. 2016;40(2):159–211.
2. Patel V, Romano M, Corkins MR, DiMaria-Ghalili RA, Earthman C, Malone A, et al. Nutrition screening and assessment in hospitalized patients: a survey of current practice in the United States. Nutr Clin Pract. 2014;29(4):483–90.
3. Singer P, Blaser AR, Berger MM, Alhazzani W, Calder PC, Casaer MP, et al. ESPEN guideline on clinical nutrition in the intensive care unit. Clin Nutr (Edinburgh, Scotland). 2019;38(1):48–79.
4. Dhaliwal R, Cahill N, Lemieux M, Heyland DK. The Canadian critical care nutrition guidelines in 2013: an update on current recommendations and implementation strategies. Nutr Clin Pract. 2014;29(1):29–43.

5. Heyland DK, Dhaliwal R, Drover JW, Gramlich L, Dodek P. Canadian clinical practice guidelines for nutrition support in mechanically ventilated, critically ill adult patients. JPEN J Parenter Enteral Nutr. 2003;27(5):355–73.
6. Doig GS, Heighes PT, Simpson F, Sweetman EA, Davies AR. Early enteral nutrition, provided within 24 h of injury or intensive care unit admission, significantly reduces mortality in critically ill patients: a meta-analysis of randomised controlled trials. Intensive Care Med. 2009;35(12):2018–27.
7. Fuentes Padilla P, Martínez G, Vernooij RW, Urrútia G, Roqué IFM, Bonfill Cosp X. Early enteral nutrition (within 48 hours) versus delayed enteral nutrition (after 48 hours) with or without supplemental parenteral nutrition in critically ill adults. The Cochrane database of systematic reviews. 2019;2019(10).
8. Abdullahi A, Jeschke MG. Nutrition and anabolic pharmacotherapies in the care of burn patients. Nutr Clin Pract. 2014;29(5):621–30.
9. McClave SA, DiBaise JK, Mullin GE, Martindale RG. ACG clinical guideline: nutrition therapy in the adult hospitalized patient. Off J Am Coll Gastroenterol | ACG. 2016;111(3):315–34.
10. Casaer MP, Mesotten D, Hermans G, Wouters PJ, Schetz M, Meyfroidt G, et al. Early versus late parenteral nutrition in critically ill adults. N Engl J Med. 2011;365(6):506–17.
11. Gomes F, Schuetz P, Bounoure L, Austin P, Ballesteros-Pomar M, Cederholm T, et al. ESPEN guidelines on nutritional support for polymorbid internal medicine patients. Clin Nutr (Edinburgh, Scotland). 2018;37(1):336–53.
12. Deutz NE, Matheson EM, Matarese LE, Luo M, Baggs GE, Nelson JL, et al. Readmission and mortality in malnourished, older, hospitalized adults treated with a specialized oral nutritional supplement: a randomized clinical trial. Clin Nutr (Edinburgh, Scotland). 2016;35(1):18–26.
13. Schuetz P, Fehr R, Baechli V, Geiser M, Deiss M, Gomes F, et al. Individualised nutritional support in medical inpatients at nutritional risk: a randomised clinical trial. Lancet (London, England). 2019;393(10188):2312–21.
14. National Collaborating Centre for Acute C. National Institute for Health and Clinical Excellence: Guidance. Nutrition support for adults: oral nutrition support, enteral tube feeding and parenteral nutrition. London: National Collaborating Centre for Acute Care (UK). Copyright © 2006, National Collaborating Centre for Acute Care; 2006.
15. Whittle J, Wischmeyer PE, Grocott MPW, Miller TE. Surgical prehabilitation: nutrition and exercise. Anesthesiol Clin. 2018;36(4):567–80.
16. Perioperative total parenteral nutrition in surgical patients. New Engl J Med. 1991;325(8):525–32.
17. ERAS®Society. ERAS / GUIDELINES / LIST OF GUIDELINES Stockholm, Sweden: ERAS®Society 2016. Available from: https://erassociety.org/guidelines/list-of-guidelines/.
18. Strong for Surgery Chicago, IL: American College of Surgeons (ACS); 2018. Available from: https://www.facs.org/quality-programs/strong-for-surgery.
19. Pędziwiatr M, Mavrikis J, Witowski J, Adamos A, Major P, Nowakowski M, et al. Current status of enhanced recovery after surgery (ERAS) protocol in gastrointestinal surgery. Med Oncol (Northwood, London, England). 2018;35(6):95.
20. Lyons NB, Bernardi K, Olavarria OA, Dhanani N, Shah P, Holihan JL, et al. Prehabilitation among patients undergoing non-bariatric abdominal surgery: a systematic review. J Am Coll Surg. 2020;231(4):480–9.
21. Gillis C, Buhler K, Bresee L, Carli F, Gramlich L, Culos-Reed N, et al. Effects of nutritional prehabilitation, with and without exercise, on outcomes of patients who undergo colorectal surgery: a systematic review and meta-analysis. Gastroenterology. 2018;155(2):391–410.e4.
22. Philipson TJ, Snider JT, Lakdawalla DN, Stryckman B, Goldman DP. Impact of oral nutritional supplementation on hospital outcomes. Am J Manag Care. 2013;19(2):121–8.
23. Elke G, van Zanten AR, Lemieux M, McCall M, Jeejeebhoy KN, Kott M, et al. Enteral versus parenteral nutrition in critically ill patients: an updated systematic review and meta-analysis of randomized controlled trials. Crit Care. 2016;20(1):117.
24. Russell MK, Wischmeyer PE. Supplemental parenteral nutrition: review of the literature and current nutrition guidelines. Nutr Clin Pract Off Publ Am Soc Parent Enteral Nutr. 2018;33(3):359–69.
25. Arvanitakis M, Ockenga J, Bezmarevic M, Gianotti L, Krznarić Ž, Lobo DN, et al. ESPEN guideline on clinical nutrition in acute and chronic pancreatitis. Clin Nutr (Edinburgh, Scotland). 2020;39(3):612–31.
26. Crockett SD, Wani S, Gardner TB, Falck-Ytter Y, Barkun AN. American Gastroenterological Association Institute guideline on initial management of acute pancreatitis. Gastroenterology. 2018;154(4):1096–101.
27. Kumpf VJ, de Aguilar-Nascimento JE, Diaz-Pizarro Graf JI, Hall AM, McKeever L, Steiger E, et al. ASPEN-FELANPE clinical guidelines: nutrition support of adult patients with enterocutaneous fistula. JPEN J Parenter Enteral Nutr. 2017;41(1):104–12.
28. Besselink MG, van Rijssen LB, Bassi C, Dervenis C, Montorsi M, Adham M, et al. Definition and classification of chyle leak after pancreatic operation: a consensus statement by the international study group on pancreatic surgery. Surgery. 2017;161(2):365–72.
29. Delaney SW, Shi H, Shokrani A, Sinha UK. Management of chyle leak after head and neck surgery: review of current treatment strategies. Int J Otolaryngol. 2017;2017:8362874.
30. Sriram K, Meguid RA, Meguid MM. Nutritional support in adults with chyle leaks. Nutrition (Burbank, Los Angeles County, Calif). 2016;32(2):281–6.
31. Halloran O, Grecu B, Sinha A. Methods and complications of nasoenteral intubation. JPEN J Parenter Enteral Nutr. 2011;35(1):61–6.

32. Fletcher J. Adult enteral device selection: which is the best for the patient? Br J Community Nurs. 2014;Suppl Nutrition:S19–23.
33. Bischoff SC, Austin P, Boeykens K, Chourdakis M, Cuerda C, Jonkers-Schuitema C, et al. ESPEN guideline on home enteral nutrition. Clin Nutr (Edinburgh, Scotland). 2020;39(1):5–22.
34. Ukleja A, Gilbert K, Mogensen KM, Walker R, Ward CT, Ybarra J, et al. Standards for nutrition support: adult hospitalized patients. Nutr Clin Pract. 2018;33(6):906–20.
35. Boullata JI, Carrera AL, Harvey L, Escuro AA, Hudson L, Mays A, et al. ASPEN safe practices for enteral nutrition therapy [formula: see text]. JPEN J Parenter Enteral Nutr. 2017;41(1):15–103.
36. Bechtold ML, Nguyen DL, Palmer LB, Kiraly LN, Martindale RG, McClave SA. Nasal bridles for securing nasoenteric tubes: a meta-analysis. Nutr Clin Pract. 2014;29(5):667–71.
37. Meer JA. A new nasal bridle for securing nasoenteral feeding tubes. JPEN J Parenter Enteral Nutr. 1989;13(3):331–4.
38. The AMT Bridle™ nasal tube retaining system brecksville, OH: Applied Medical Technology, Inc; 2020. Available from: https://www.appliedmedical.net/enteral/bridle/.
39. Gauderer MW, Ponsky JL, Izant RJ Jr. Gastrostomy without laparotomy: a percutaneous endoscopic technique. J Pediatr Surg. 1980;15(6):872–5.
40. Bechtold ML, Mir FA, Boumitri C, Palmer LB, Evans DC, Kiraly LN, et al. Long-term nutrition: a clinician's guide to successful long-term enteral access in adults. Nutr Clin Pract. 2016;31(6):737–47.
41. Schwartz DB, Barrocas A. Ethics and law. In: Mueller CM, editor. The ASPEN adult nutrition support core curriculum. 3rd ed. Silver Spring: American Society for Parenteral and Enteral Nutrition (ASPEN); 2017. p. 785–804.
42. Goldberg LS, Altman KW. The role of gastrostomy tube placement in advanced dementia with dysphagia: a critical review. Clin Interv Aging. 2014;9:1733–9.
43. Zelig R, Famularo PJ, Szeto M. Nutrition support for older adults. In: Mueller CM, editor. The ASPEN adult nutrition support core curriculum. 3rd ed. Silver Spring: American Society for Parenteral and Enteral Nutrition (ASPEN); 2017. p. 723–42.
44. Brill JV, August D, Delegge MH, Hegazi R, Jensen GL, Van Way CW 3rd, et al. A vision of the future for physician practice in nutrition. JPEN J Parente Enteral Nutr. 2010;34(6 Suppl):86s–96s.
45. Konrad D, Mitchell R, Hendrickson E. Home nutrition support. In: Mueller CM, editor. The ASPEN adult nutrition support core curriculum. 3rd ed. Silver Spring: American Society for Parenteral and Enteral Nutrition (ASPEN); 2017. p. 765–84.
46. Schnitker MA, Mattman PE, Bliss TL. A clinical study of malnutrition in Japanese prisoners of war. Ann Intern Med. 1951;35(1):69–96.
47. Brozek J, Chapman CB, Keys A. Drastic food restriction; effect on cardiovascular dynamics in normotensive and hypertensive conditions. JAMA. 1948;137(18):1569–74.
48. Doley J, Phillips W. Overview of enteral nutrition. In: Mueller CM, editor. The ASPEN nutrition support Core curriculum. 3rd ed. Silver Spring: American Society for Parenteral and Enteral Nutrition; 2017. p. 213–26.
49. da Silva JSV, Seres DS, Sabino K, Adams SC, Berdahl GJ, Citty SW, et al. ASPEN consensus recommendations for refeeding syndrome. Nutr Clin Pract. 2020;35(2):178–95.
50. de Souza e Mello GF, Lukashok HP, Meine GC, Small IA, de Carvalho RL, Guimarães DP, et al. Outpatient percutaneous endoscopic gastrostomy in selected head and neck cancer patients. Surg Endosc. 2009;23(7):1487–93.
51. Wilhelm SM, Ortega KA, Stellato TA. Guidelines for identification and management of outpatient percutaneous endoscopic gastrostomy tube placement. Am J Surg. 2010;199(3):396–9; discussion 9-400.
52. Tsaousi G, Stavrou G, Kapanidis K, Michalopoulos A, Kotzampassi K. Unsedated outpatient percutaneous endoscopic gastrostomy in stroke patients: is it feasible and safe? Surg Laparosc Endosc Percutan Tech. 2019;29(5):383–8.
53. Toussaint E, Van Gossum A, Ballarin A, Arvanitakis M. Enteral access in adults. Clin Nutr (Edinburgh, Scotland). 2015;34(3):350–8.
54. Newton AF, DeLegge MH. Home initiation of parenteral nutrition. Nutr Clin Pract Off Publ Am Soc Parent Enteral Nutr. 2007;22(1):57–64.
55. Kovacevich DS, Corrigan M, Ross VM, McKeever L, Hall AM, Braunschweig C. American Society for Parenteral and Enteral Nutrition guidelines for the selection and care of central venous access devices for adult home parenteral nutrition administration. JPEN J Parenter Enteral Nutr. 2019;43(1):15–31.
56. Schneider PJ. Nutrition support teams: an evidence-based practice. Nutr Clin Pract. 2006;21(1):62–7.
57. Kennedy JF, Nightingale JM. Cost savings of an adult hospital nutrition support team. Nutrition (Burbank, Los Angeles County, Calif). 2005;21(11–12):1127–33.
58. Palmer LB, Limketkai BN. Modern challenges to gastrointestinal nutrition physicians and the nutrition support team: cautionary tales and call to action. Nutr Clin Pract. 2020.
59. Durfee SM, Adams SC, Arthur E, Corrigan ML, Hammond K, Kovacevich DS, et al. A.S.P.E.N. standards for nutrition support: home and alternate site care. Nutr Clin Pract. 2014;29(4):542–55.
60. Gosmanov AR, Umpierrez GE. Management of hyperglycemia during enteral and parenteral nutrition therapy. Curr Diab Rep. 2013;13(1):155–62.
61. Laesser CI, Cumming P, Reber E, Stanga Z, Muka T, Bally L. Management of glucose control in noncritically ill, hospitalized patients receiving parenteral and/or enteral nutrition: a systematic review. J Clin Med. 2019;8(7):935.

62. Diabetes care in the hospital: standards of medical care in diabetes-2021. Diabetes Care. 2021;44(Suppl 1):S211–s20.
63. Tignanelli CJ, Bukowiec JC, editors. Hospital based nutrition support: a review of the latest evidence; 2017.
64. Reignier J, Mercier E, Le Gouge A, Boulain T, Desachy A, Bellec F, et al. Effect of not monitoring residual gastric volume on risk of ventilator-associated pneumonia in adults receiving mechanical ventilation and early enteral feeding: a randomized controlled trial. JAMA. 2013;309(3):249–56.
65. Rubin LP, Ross AC, Stephensen CB, Bohn T, Tanumihardjo SA. Metabolic effects of inflammation on vitamin A and carotenoids in humans and animal models. Adv Nutr (Bethesda, Md). 2017;8(2):197–212.
66. Salota R, Omar S, Sherwood RA, Raja K, Vincent RP. Clinical relevance of trace element measurement in patients on initiation of parenteral nutrition. Ann Clin Biochem. 2016;53(6):680–5.
67. Bresnahan KA, Tanumihardjo SA. Undernutrition, the acute phase response to infection, and its effects on micronutrient status indicators. Adv Nutr (Bethesda, Md). 2014;5(6):702–11.
68. Pitta MR, Campos FM, Monteiro AG, Cunha AGF, Porto JD, Gomes RR. Tutorial on diarrhea and enteral nutrition: a comprehensive step-by-step approach. JPEN J Parenter Enteral Nutr. 2019;43(8):1008–19.
69. Salim AF, Phillips AD, Farthing MJ. Pathogenesis of gut virus infection. Baillieres Clin Gastroenterol. 1990;4(3):593–607.
70. Santos JI. Nutritional implications and physiologic response to pediatric diarrhea. Pediatr Infect Dis. 1986;5(1 Suppl):S152–4.
71. Lohsiriwat V. Percutaneous endoscopic gastrostomy tube replacement: a simple procedure? World J Gastrointestinal Endoscopy. 2013;5(1):14–8.
72. Jain R, Maple JT, Anderson MA, Appalaneni V, Ben-Menachem T, Decker GA, et al. The role of endoscopy in enteral feeding. Gastrointest Endosc. 2011;74(1):7–12.
73. Michaud L, Guimber D, Blain-Stregloff AS, Ganga-Zandzou S, Gottrand F, Turck D. Longevity of balloon-stabilized skin-level gastrostomy device. J Pediatr Gastroenterol Nutr. 2004;38(4):426–9.
74. DeLegge RL, DeLegge MH. Percutaneous endoscopic gastrostomy evaluation of device materials: are we "failsafe"? Nutr Clin Pract. 2005;20(6):613–7.
75. Ukleja A. Weaning from parenteral nutrition. Gastroenterol Clin North Am. 2019;48(4):525–50.
76. Limketkai BN, Hurt RT, Palmer LB. Short bowel syndrome. In: Mueller CM, editor. The ASPEN adult nutrition support core curriculum. 3rd ed. Silver Spring: American Society for Parenteral and Enteral Nutrition; 2017. p. 587–601.
77. Bechtold ML, McClave SA, Palmer LB, Nguyen DL, Urben LM, Martindale RG, et al. The pharmacologic treatment of short bowel syndrome: new tricks and novel agents. Curr Gastroenterol Rep. 2014;16(7):392.
78. Thompson JS, Rochling FA, Weseman RA, Mercer DF. Current management of short bowel syndrome. Curr Probl Surg. 2012;49(2):52–115.
79. Fitzgibbons S, Ching YA, Valim C, Zhou J, Iglesias J, Duggan C, et al. Relationship between serum citrulline levels and progression to parenteral nutrition independence in children with short bowel syndrome. J Pediatr Surg. 2009;44(5):928–32.
80. Fragkos KC, Forbes A. Citrulline as a marker of intestinal function and absorption in clinical settings: a systematic review and meta-analysis. United Eur Gastroenterol J. 2018;6(2):181–91.
81. Pettei MJ, Daftary S, Levine JJ. Essential fatty acid deficiency associated with the use of a medium-chain-triglyceride infant formula in pediatric hepatobiliary disease. Am J Clin Nutr. 1991;53(5):1217–21.
82. Reitzel RA, Rosenblatt J, Chaftari AM, Raad II. Epidemiology of infectious and noninfectious catheter complications in patients receiving home parenteral nutrition: a systematic review and meta-analysis. JPEN J Parenter Enteral Nutr. 2019;43(7): 832–51.
83. Daoud DC, Wanten G, Joly F. Antimicrobial locks in patients receiving home parenteral nutrition. Nutrients. 2020;12(2):439.
84. Pironi L, Boeykens K, Bozzetti F, Joly F, Klek S, Lal S, et al. ESPEN guideline on home parenteral nutrition. Clin Nutr (Edinburgh, Scotland). 2020;39(6):1645–66.
85. Kumpf VJ, Gervasio JM. Complications of parenteral nutrition. In: Mueller CM, editor. The ASPEN adult nutrition support core curriculum. 3rd ed. Silver Spring: American Society of Parenteral and Enteral Nutrition (ASPEN); 2017. p. 345–60.

Part II

Dietary Approaches and Nutritional Considerations for GI Diseases

The Foregut 5

Anita Ganti and Matthew J. Whitson

Diseases of the Oropharynx and Esophagus

The major role of the oropharynx and esophagus is to successfully and safely transport the food we ingest to the areas of the gastrointestinal tract where digestion and absorption occur. Through a series of coordinated motions, a bolus of food is ushered by the pharyngeal muscle safely past the upper esophageal sphincter (UES), ensuring that liquid and food are not accidentally brought into the trachea and lungs. The food bolus is propelled down the esophagus by first skeletal and then smooth muscle peristaltic contractions, which places this bolus into the distal esophagus where the relaxation of the lower esophageal sphincter (LES) allows the food to enter the stomach. While the purpose of these organs may be straightforward, the disruption of this process can lead to a multitude of symptoms.

Physicians manage multiple symptoms suggestive of oropharyngeal and esophageal disorders including dysphagia, heartburn, chest pain, regurgitation, cough, and sore throat. In particular, it can be challenging to differentiate between oropharyngeal (transfer) and esophageal dysphagia. Oropharyngeal dysphagia is often a presenting symptom of central process, like stroke, or a musculoskeletal disorder, such as ALS. It is often associated with "choking while eating," chronic cough, and/or sore throat. Esophageal dysphagia typically is described as a patient sensing food or liquid getting "stuck" in the middle of the chest and/or having slow transit of bolus to the stomach. Emergencies such as food impactions, where the food bolus is stuck in the esophagus preventing the passage of saliva and food, can occur, often requiring endoscopic intervention.

Both forms of dysphagia can restrict the amount and/or types of food that are able to be ingested safely by a patient. This can lead to weight loss, nutrient and vitamin deficiencies, and generalized symptoms such as fatigue and/or weakness. This next section of the chapter focuses on esophageal disorders and dysphagia.

Eosinophilic Esophagitis

Eosinophilic esophagitis (EoE) is a chronic immune-mediated, allergic disorder that is characterized by the infiltration of eosinophils into the esophagus, resulting in esophageal dysfunction [1]. Typical symptoms of EoE may include

A. Ganti (✉)
Department of Medicine, The Donald and Barbara Zucker School of Medicine at Hofstra-Northwell, Manhasset, NY, USA
e-mail: Aganti@northwell.edu

M. J. Whitson
Division of Gastroenterology, The Donald and Barbara Zucker School of Medicine at Hofstra-Northwell, Manhasset, NY, USA
e-mail: Mwhitson1@northwell.edu

C. Newberry et al. (eds.), *Nutrition, Weight, and Digestive Health*,
https://doi.org/10.1007/978-3-030-94953-2_5

dysphagia, heartburn, and food impactions in adults. Meanwhile, children may have additional symptoms including nausea, vomiting, abdominal pain, and weight loss. Diagnosis may be suspected in the case of typical endoscopic findings including esophageal furrows, rings, exudate, and/or strictures but is only confirmed on histology with biopsies of the esophagus demonstrating at least 15 eosinophils per high-power field.

While initially diagnosed predominantly in children, there has been an increase in the overall incidence and prevalence of the disease in adults [2]. The pathophysiology of EoE is incompletely understood, but it is suspected to be a multi-hit pathway [3]. This pathway includes esophageal allergen exposures via food antigens, aeroallergens, and potentially environmental factors. This exposure, coupled with a genetic predisposition, leads to decreased barrier function in the esophagus and heightened cellular recruitment and proliferation, generating an acute inflammatory reaction. This cascade, in turn, leads to acute inflammation in the esophagus and potential for fibrostenotic progression to strictures and ultimately a small-caliber esophagus. In addition to the above, the active inflammation of EoE likely has an impact on esophageal motility. These changes can lead to difficulty in propelling food through the esophagus to the stomach and result in limited oral intake.

Standard-of-care treatments for EoE include proton pump inhibitors (PPIs), topical steroid therapy, and dietary interventions which all aim to reduce the inflammation in the esophagus [4]. A review of these dietary treatment options will be discussed here and can be found in Table 5.1.

Six-Food Elimination Diet

The six-food elimination diet (SFED) is the empiric elimination of milk, wheat, soy, eggs, tree nuts/pine nuts, and seafood/shellfish [5]. These are the most common dietary allergens and are implicated in the development of EoE. By eliminating this combination of dietary allergens, patients do not continue along the pathway of inflammation in the esophagus, leading to improved symptoms and a decrease of eosinophils to normal ranges. With adherence to the entire SFED, a 2017 meta-analysis demonstrated that patients are able to achieve histologic response rates upwards of 75–80% as well as a symptom response in upwards of 85% of patients [6]. After elimination of food groups and confirmation of histological remission on endoscopy, foods are re-added by the patient and their clinical team until specific triggers are identified. This process requires multiple endoscopies but allows patients to expand their dietary options over time, improving compliance and sustainability.

Embracing the SFED can be a daunting task for patients, as it significantly limits food options, can create social anxiety, and can be very expensive [7]. Other studies have looked at starting with more limited diets that patients may be able to tolerate. For example, a European study published in 2018 demonstrated that a twofood elimination diet of milk and wheat can lead to clinico-histologic remission in 43% of patients and a four-food elimination diet of milk, wheat, soy, and eggs can achieve remission in 62% of patients [8]. This "step-up" algorithm may be better tolerated by patients and lead to fewer endoscopies.

Elemental Diet

The purpose of this diet is similar to the six-food elimination diet in that it eliminates specific food intake to avoid allergens. Patients consume an elemental feeding formula which eliminates all ingested proteins and only delivers single amino acids. A meta-analysis published in 2014 examined the effectiveness of this approach, showing that clinico-histologic response was approximately 90% [9]. However, this diet is socially restrictive and expensive and has significant limitations with implementation in clinical practice. It is rarely used in adults.

Allergy Testing-Directed Diet

Given the pathogenesis of EoE, significant interest has been paid to allergy testing and the subse-

Table 5.1 Overview of the efficacy of elimination diet treatment options for eosinophilic esophagitis [5]

	Details of elimination diet	Limitations	Histologic remission
Elemental diet	Elemental formula with only single amino acids	Expensive Not universally covered by insurance Quality of life impairment Difficult to continue long-term	90%
Six-food elimination diet (SFED)	Milk, wheat, egg, soy, tree nuts/pine nuts, seafood/shellfish	Expensive Socially restrictive	72–80%
Two-food elimination diet	Milk, wheat	Less effective than SFED May result in delay to histologic remission	38–44%
Milk elimination	Milk	Less effective in adults	18–22% in adults 35–56% in children
Allergy testing-directed diet	Elimination diet based on results of skin prick/atopy patch allergy testing	Positive study results not reproducible Varied testing results	7–35% in adults 48% in children

quent elimination of those allergens from the diet. Typically, allergy testing is done via skin prick tests and atopy patch tests. Initial studies in the pediatric population resulted in remission in approximately 50% of patients [10]. However, subsequent studies in the pediatric population have not shown any data approaching that level of efficacy. In the adult population, remission rates have been between 22% and 33% [11]. Given these results, allergy testing-directed elimination diets are not routinely recommended as the sole therapy in EoE; however, additional studies are ongoing to see if new assays and testing of additional environmental triggers may improve efficacy.

Achalasia

Achalasia is an esophageal disorder characterized by the inability of the LES to relax and the presence of abnormal esophageal peristalsis [12]. As a result of these changes, both solid food and liquids have difficulty entering the stomach and can sit in the esophagus for an extended time. Symptoms of achalasia include dysphagia to solids and liquids, regurgitation, chest pain, and potentially weight loss.

The development of achalasia is driven by the functional loss of the myenteric plexus in the distal esophagus, predominantly at the LES [13]. Specifically, there is a loss of the inhibitory post-ganglionic neurons most commonly associated with the nitric oxide neurotransmitter. The loss of inhibitory control results in unopposed stimulation of the esophageal muscle and thus impaired relaxation of the LES. The exact trigger for the loss of the myenteric plexus is incompletely understood, but a post-infectious viral state is suspected to play a role. Chagas disease, due to the parasite *Trypanosoma cruzi*, has also been documented to cause the destruction of the myenteric plexus resulting in an achalasia-like syndrome.

Given the difficulty with swallowing and impaired passage of food from the esophagus into the stomach, it is reasonable to assume that dietary modifications may play a role in treatment. Patients often present with weight loss, and this can serve as a marker of disease severity [14]. A 2018 study examined the impact of achalasia on overall nutritional risk [15]. The researchers found that even though 69.8% of patients were characterized as obese on presentation, about 50% of patients were at moderate or high risk for malnutrition based on validated assessment tools.

Limited data is available regarding dietary modifications with achalasia. Specific foods may be triggers for individuals, and typically patients are advised to avoid them. Patients are encouraged to modify eating habits including eating in an upright position, maximizing time between last meal and laying down, and potentially using liquid chasers after each swallow of solid food if they predominantly have dysphagia to solids [16]. However, no specific dietary intervention has been shown to improve symptoms of disease and definitive therapy including surgical or endoscopic myotomy and/or dilation is usually necessary.

Gastroesophageal Reflux Disease

Gastroesophageal reflux disease (GERD) is the most common gastrointestinal complaint encountered in the outpatient setting in the United States, affecting up to a quarter of the American population [17]. GERD is defined as the exposure of esophageal mucosa to refluxed stomach contents that results in troublesome symptoms or complications for the patient. These symptoms may include heartburn, regurgitation, belching, and cough. In addition, untreated GERD can lead to complications or other disease states including stricture formation, bleeding from erosive esophagitis, Barrett's esophagus, and esophageal adenocarcinoma.

The major physiologic cause of GERD is transient lower esophageal sphincter relaxation (TLESR) [18]. The lower esophageal sphincter (LES) is not a single muscle, but rather the composite of multiple anatomical mechanisms including thickened longitudinal and circular muscles of the esophagus and the external pinch of the diaphragm. The LES has intrinsic tone that helps maintain contraction, which can be affected by oral intake. Additionally, TLESRs occur secondary to gastric distention from ingestion of food and air. Multiple factors can increase one's propensity for GERD including structural issues (i.e., hiatal hernia), patient-specific attributes (i.e., obesity), and an increase in TLESR frequency from medications or specific foods.

While PPIs have been used as first-line medical therapy for gastroesophageal reflux disease for years, new evidence concerning the harms of using long-term PPIs have prompted renewed investigation and research into lifestyle modifications, which have varying levels of supporting evidence. Weight loss, tobacco cessation, and head of bed elevation are routinely recommended and supported in the literature; however the array of recommended dietary modifications have varying and often conflicting support. This section will highlight common dietary modifications that may have a role in GERD management.

Eating Patterns

It is generally recommended that patients with GERD eat dinner at least 3 hours prior to sleeping. Several studies have looked at supine esophageal acid exposure along with symptoms of heartburn; the majority of which demonstrate that a shorter meal-to-bed time frame is associated with higher supine esophageal acid exposure and increased self-reporting of GERD symptoms [19, 20]. Therefore, in symptomatic patients, it is reasonable to suggest avoiding late-night meals in an effort to improve symptoms.

There have also been studies that have looked at meal density and its relation to GERD symptoms. A large 2017 Korean population-based survey found a positive correlation between total energy intake and reflux symptoms [21]. A smaller 2002 study of 13 patients who were fed meals with varying caloric content found that participants who ate higher-calorie meals experienced more reflux episodes and had higher esophageal acid exposure as measured by intra-esophageal pH monitoring [22]. These studies are limited but suggest that eating discrete meals with fewer total calories may be beneficial in improving reflux symptoms.

Carbohydrate Intake

Carbohydrates are only partially absorbed in the small bowel and are later fermented by colonic bacteria. This fermentation process can cause an increase in TLESR and therefore may contribute to GERD symptoms. Several recent studies have shown that a low-carbohydrate diet is associated with reductions in esophageal acid exposure time along with improvement in GERD symptoms. A 2018 study with 130 patients found that after following a low glycemic index diet for 2 weeks, participants reported statistically significant improvement in their GERD symptoms [23]. This suggests a potential role for a low-carbohydrate diet in GERD. Of note, a confounding variable in these studies may be weight loss as BMI is independently associated with reflux symptoms.

In addition to above, an increase in fiber specifically may be beneficial. There are several small studies that suggest that increased fiber intake is associated with a reduction in GERD symptoms [24, 25]. The mechanism of this clinical benefit is hypothesized to be through dietary fiber's ability to bind to nitric oxide and subsequently decrease its negative effect on LES pressure. Despite small study sample sizes, ensuring adequate fiber intake in favor of simple sugars may be of benefit.

Fat Intake

The data regarding fat intake and its relation to GERD symptoms is variable. There are a few small studies that compare isocaloric high-fat meals versus low-fat meals which have reported high-fat meals are associated with increased esophageal acid exposure. For example, in a 1996 study, 20 asymptomatic subjects underwent intra-esophageal pH monitoring during a 3-hour post-prandial period after consuming either a low-fat or high-fat diet. The researchers found that those who consumed a high-fat diet had significantly longer acid exposure time compared to the low-fat cohort [26].

Other studies contradict this. In a recent study from 2018, participants were assigned to receive a high-fat meal (50% of the calories) versus a low-fat, isocaloric meal (10% of the calories). There was no difference in the number of reflux episodes experienced among the study participants [27]. Additionally, analysis of the NHANES I database, a cohort of 12,349 nursing professionals followed from 1971 through 1993, found no correlation between dietary fat intake and reflux symptoms [28]. Given this information, more research is needed to clearly delineate the effect of increased fat on reflux symptomatology.

The Mediterranean Diet

The Mediterranean diet, which consists of whole grains, fish, vegetables, monounsaturated fats, and moderate alcohol, has been studied as an effective comprehensive diet that can both prevent and reduce the development of many chronic diseases [29]. A recent cross-sectional study conducted in Albania found that people who followed a Mediterranean diet were less likely to report GERD symptoms, even after correcting for demographic and lifestyle factors [30]. Similar findings were published in a recent Greek case-control study that found that individuals who adhered to a Mediterranean diet were less likely to have gastrointestinal diseases including GERD, Crohn's disease, ulcerative colitis, or IBS [31]. These findings suggest that a Mediterranean diet, which encompasses many of the previously mentioned dietary modifications including high intake of fiber and low intake of processed sugars, may be associated with less gastroesophageal reflux (GER) symptoms.

Caffeine

A decrease in caffeinated beverages is often recommended to patients to minimize GERD symptoms. In small studies, caffeine has been shown to decrease the resting LES pressure as well as the number of contractions of the distal esophagus – both potentially leading to GERD symptoms [32]. Despite the theoretical impact of caffeinated beverages on GERD symptoms, presented data regarding association has had mixed results. A 2014 meta-analysis of pooled data from 15 case-control studies found that there was no significant association between coffee intake and GERD based on endoscopic findings and reported symptoms [33]. In this study, no correlation was seen between the amount of caffeine consumed and the number of reported symptoms. A more recent 2019 study pooled data from the Nurses' Health Study II on almost 50,000 patients, showing consumption of coffee, tea, or soda was associated with an increase in reflux symptoms. In subsequent analysis, replacement of two servings of water for two servings of either coffee, tea, or soda was also associated with a reduced risk of GERD symptoms [34]. Interestingly, decaffeinated tea was additionally implicated, implying other substances that are found in decaffeinated and herbal teas may also induce symptoms.

Review of this data suggests that reduction of coffee, tea, and soda may be beneficial for patients who experience GERD and may reduce their symptoms. A limitation to these studies, however, is the lack of data regarding carbonated drinks alone. Further research is needed about whether carbonation itself, without caffeine, is independently related to an increase in GERD-like symptoms.

Alcohol

Alcohol has also been proposed to increase the frequency of TLESRs [35]. The most recent meta-analysis suggests that there may be a dose-dependent association between alcohol consumption and GERD symptoms, with a stronger effect noted for those patients with evidence of reflux esophagitis on endoscopy [36]. There was also a correlation between drinking alcohol frequency (greater than three to five times per week) and the presence of GERD. Of note, the included studies that relied solely on patient-reported symptoms did not find any statistically significant association between alcohol intake and GERD. Overall, recommending reduction and/or abstinence from alcohol for patients with GERD is controversial, though may have benefits in some.

Other Foods

Other foods including chocolate and mint have been associated with rapid LES relaxation and therefore thought to induce GERD symptoms [37]. However, the limited studies available have not shown a significant correlation with increased intake of these foods and reflux.

Spicy foods are thought to cause direct irritation to the esophageal mucosa and therefore can mimic heartburn symptoms. A cross-sectional study from Iran showed that men who ate spicy food more than ten times per week were almost three times as likely to have heartburn compared to men who never ate spicy food, although this effect was not seen in women [38]. In select cases, reduction of spicy food intake may be of benefit, particularly in men.

Rumination Syndrome

Rumination disorder is the repeated regurgitation of food that is consumed either during or immediately after eating, followed by the re-chewing, re-swallowing, or expulsion of the material from the mouth. It is thought that patients typically experience a pressure or discomfort in either their esophagus or stomach after eating: a sensation called the premonitory urge. This leads to habitual contraction of the abdominal wall so that food contents in the stomach travel up the esophagus into the mouth, where they are then re-chewed, re-swallowed, or spit out. The premonitory urge disappears once the abdominal wall contraction begins, and this repetitive process can begin again. Rumination disorder can lead to complications such as dental erosions, weight loss, electrolyte disturbances, and psychosocial effects [39].

While the nuances of rumination syndrome are still not well understood, there are some reports that individuals are more likely to experience regurgitation after the consumption of specific foods [40]. Rumination may occur with the ingestion of either liquids or solids, but no studies to date have looked at associations between specific foods and the trigger or alleviation of rumination symptoms.

Disease of the Stomach

The stomach plays a central role in digestion and ultimate absorption of many nutrients. While mastication begins the physical digestion of food in the oropharynx, the churning and grinding of the stomach muscles assist with further digestion via mixing with gastric and salivary secretions that aid in chemical breakdown. Chief cells secrete pepsinogen and gastric lipase to promote continued metabolism of proteins and fats, while parietal cells secrete hydrochloric acid (HCl) and intrinsic factor, which further digestion and vitamin B12 absorption. The antrum and the pylorus of the stomach work to purposefully empty these digested contents from the stomach into the small intestine where they are absorbed.

Given the multiple functions of the stomach, there are a number of presenting symptoms that may be suggestive of a gastric disorder. These include abdominal pain, nausea, vomiting, early satiety, and weight loss. The inability to properly digest both proteins and fats can contribute to malnutrition and vitamin deficiencies. In addition, the symptoms of gastric disorders may limit the amount of food a patient is able to tolerate contributing to weight loss and malnutrition. More so than other areas of the GI tract, disorders of the stomach often have dietary interventions that can minimize symptoms and maximize nutritional benefit. The next part of this chapter will review the data for these potential interventions.

Gastroparesis

Gastroparesis is characterized by objectively quantified delayed gastric emptying in the absence of any mechanical obstructive cause [41]. Symptoms include nausea, vomiting, early satiety, and bloating and less commonly abdominal pain and belching. While the pathophysiology of gastroparesis remains poorly understood, there are certain etiologies that are clearly associated including diabetes, post-viral syndromes, and post-surgical complications.

Normal functioning of the stomach depends on the coordination between smooth muscle, autonomic nerves, and the interstitial cells of Cajal (ICC) that trigger fundic and antral contractions with an associated relaxation of the pylorus – the sphincter muscle connecting the stomach and small intestine. The ICC function as the pacemakers of the gut, regulating smooth muscle contractility by interacting with enteric nerves that produce excitatory and inhibitory signals. In gastroparesis, there appears to be a loss of ICC function, possibly secondary to expression of nitric oxide related to immune injury [42]. This loss of function in turn causes delays in gastric emptying which can precipitate the aforementioned symptoms of gastroparesis. Complications of gastroparesis may include severe malnutrition secondary to the inability to tolerate food by mouth with subsequent nutritional deficiencies and inadequate hydration [43].

Treatment for gastroparesis is often multipronged. Options include dietary modifications, reversing the underlying etiology if identified (i.e., improved glycemic control), medication therapy (i.e., prokinetic agents), endosurgical procedures (i.e., pyloric myotomy), and direct gastric electrical stimulation via pacemaker. We will review the evidence behind some of the proposed dietary modifications below.

Diet Consistency

Patients with gastroparesis typically empty liquids easier than solids. This is because liquids of low caloric density empty through the pressure gradient between fundic tone and the pylorus. High-calorie liquids also rely on this pressure gradient, though emptying may be slower. Solid foods, in contrast, require antral contraction until the particle size is less than 2 mm before emptying can begin [44]. Given this information, liquid and pureed foods have been recommended to patients with gastroparesis, as they may be better tolerated. A small study in patients with gastroparesis published in 2015 found that solid meals were associated with increased and longer-lasting nausea when compared to liquid meals [45]. While this study had a small sample size ($n = 12$), it may be reasonable to recommend liquid meals either as primary or supplemental nutrition if patients are highly symptomatic and/or unable to meet their caloric needs with solid options.

Small Particle Diet

A recent study found that a "small particle size diet" significantly reduced the severity of nausea, bloating, and post-prandial fullness in patients with gastroparesis [46]. This randomized controlled trial enrolled a total of 56 patients who all had diabetic gastroparesis. The foods that were recommended in the intervention group included foods that could be easily processed into small particles, such as pureed vegetables and beans, soft fruits, and seafood. Foods that were excluded and more routinely consumed in the control group included fresh and raw vegetables, rice and pasta, and nuts. More data is needed, but this diet may be of some benefit in this patient population.

Fat Intake

Fat intake increases cholecystokinin release, which can delay the rate of gastric emptying. As such, a low-fat diet is often recommended for gastroparesis. A 2015 study looked at patient symptoms after consuming high-fat solid, low-fat solid, high-fat liquid, and low-fat liquid diets [45]. Participant surveys revealed that patients reported the most symptoms with a high-fat solid diet and the least symptoms with a low-fat liquid diet. Even among the same diet type (solid versus liquid), the high-fat diets were associated with more symptoms compared to the low-fat diets. Similar results were obtained from another 2015 study that surveyed 45 patients with gastroparesis and asked them to fill out a food toleration and aversion survey [47]. This study found that provoking foods had a higher fat content than alleviating foods on average. Despite the small study sizes, it is reasonable to include this recommendation in treatment plans.

Carbohydrate Intake

Limited research is available regarding carbohydrate intake and gastroparesis. A recent study that surveyed 45 gastroparesis patients regarding food tolerances and aversions found carbohydrate-heavy, low-fiber foods were better tolerated and less symptom provoking than other options. This diet included white potatoes, white rice, and pretzels [47]. As such, patients with gastroparesis are often recommended to avoid high-fiber foods as they slow gastric emptying and are associated with an increased risk of forming a bezoar. The same study cited above found that the fiber content among the symptom-triggering and symptom-alleviating foods was actually similar. While further data is necessary, some patients with gastroparesis may benefit from increasing their intake of low-fiber carbohydrates.

Cyclic Vomiting Syndrome

Cyclic vomiting syndrome (CVS) is characterized by recurrent episodes of nausea and vomiting, often accompanied by severe abdominal pain. In between these severe episodes of nausea and vomiting, there are symptom-free periods for an extended time. While it is still unclear what exactly causes these episodes, they are thought to be triggered by a number of factors including infections, stress, and lack of sleep [48]. It appears that CVS is caused by a dysregulation in the brain-gut neural axis resulting in nausea and vomiting. An association with migraine headaches also suggests a neurological component.

There are some reports that certain foods, such as cheese and chocolate, may provoke episodes leading to recommendations to avoid these triggers [49]. However, no trials to date have studied dietary triggers or treatment strategies in this population.

Atrophic Gastritis

Atrophic gastritis (AG) is a chronic condition of the stomach characterized by the loss of healthy gastric glands and subsequent replacement with intestinal metaplasia, pseudopyloric metaplasia, and potentially fibrosis [50]. It is typically caused either by an autoimmune reaction or by a chronic infection with *Helicobacter pylori*. Regardless of the cause, AG can lead to the malabsorption of multiple vitamins, especially iron and B12.

Autoimmune AG is the result of TH1 cytotoxic cells attacking the parietal cells of the stomach, which reduces production of hydrochloric acid and intrinsic factor [51]. When *Helicobacter pylori* infection is the cause, there is a localized destruction of gastric glands which progresses in a pathway leading initially to chronic superficial gastritis, then to gastric atrophy, and finally to intestinal metaplasia [52]. Although autoimmune AG spares the gastric antrum, while *Helicobacter pylori*-associated AG does not, they can be difficult to distinguish clinically. Dyspepsia, vitamin deficiencies, and gastric malignancies can occur in both types of AG.

Dietary interventions in this population are limited. The first major approach is to replace the vitamins lost through malabsorption – typically vitamin B12 and iron (Fig. 5.1). The destruction

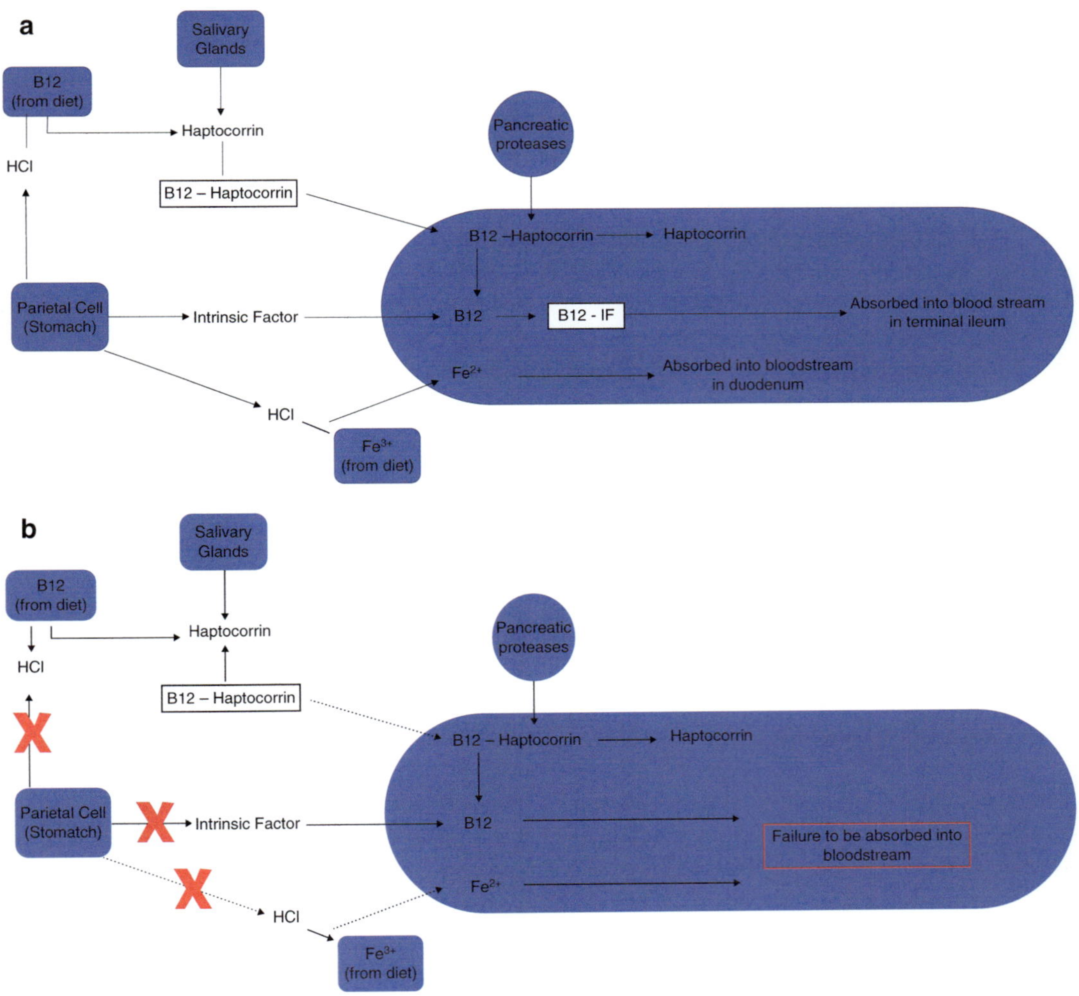

Fig. 5.1 (**a**) Pathway for normal absorption of vitamin B12 and iron. (**b**) The effect of atrophic gastric on absorption of vitamin B12 and iron. Atrophic gastritis results in destruction of parietal cell results in (1) decreased HCl secretion leading to inability to free vitamin B12 and iron from food contents for absorption and (2) loss of intrinsic factor necessary for absorption of vitamin B12 in the terminal ileum

of parietal cells and gastric glands in AG can result in B12 malabsorption in two ways. First, the destruction of parietal cells leads to reduced production of intrinsic factor, a binding protein necessary for successful B12 absorption in the terminal ileum [53]. Second, the destruction of parietal cells and gastric glands can lead to limited binding of haptocorrin to free B12 in the stomach. While B12 deficiency is classically associated with AG, studies have demonstrated iron deficiency is also present in 50% of patients [54]. The resulting achlorhydria from the destruction of parietal cells impairs the solubilization and reduction of food iron, resulting in decreased absorption.

The most feared consequence of AG is the development of gastric cancer – both adenocarcinoma and neuroendocrine tumors of the stomach have been implicated. There have been associations between salt and salt-preserved foods with gastric cancer, and therefore a low-salt diet is typically recommended in patients with risk factors for developing cancer [55]. In addition, studies demonstrate an increased risk of gastric cancer in diets rich in red and processed meats and other nitroso compounds (compounds containing an -NO group) [56]. As such, in patients with AG, a recommendation of a low-salt, limited red-meat diet may be of benefit. The impact of diet on gastrointestinal cancers is discussed in future chapters.

Other dietary interventions for patients with AG are used typically to modify the resulting symptoms such as dyspepsia. These interventions will be discussed in the next section.

Functional Dyspepsia

Functional dyspepsia (FD) is a gastrointestinal disorder that is characterized by bothersome symptoms that may or may not be associated with food ingestion and does not have evidence of an organic or structural cause [57]. FD is often divided into subtypes: postprandial dyspeptic symptoms (PDS), epigastric pain syndrome (EPS), and an overlap condition of the two. PDS primarily manifests with bloating, early satiety, nausea, vomiting, and lack of appetite, while EPS typically manifests as upper abdominal pain with stomach cramps [58]. This is a clinical diagnosis that has been associated with significant impairments in quality of life [59] and has a prevalence of approximately 10% in the general population [60]. Complications of FD may include weight loss and malnutrition secondary to poor oral intake [61].

The pathophysiology of FD is incompletely understood. Varied potential mechanisms have been suggested. There has been an association with impaired gastric motility – including both rapid and delayed emptying – and gastric compliance [62]. In addition, there is a proposed mechanism of action between FD and visceral hypersensitivity [63]. While there may be significant overlap between gastric emptying delays and hypersensitivity, there are additional studies that demonstrate patients with FD have hypersensitivity without any altered gastric motility [64].

It is suspected that FD, like many functional disorders, may be a result of an altered brain-gut axis. A 2012 population-based, telephone survey demonstrated a twofold increase in generalized anxiety disorder and a threefold increase in major depressive episodes in patients with FD as based on the Rome III criteria [65]. Older studies have reported an increased history of abuse as a child or adult in patients with FD as compared to the general population [66].

Additional data has suggested that the duodenum may also play a role in FD. Patients with FD have a higher occurrence of increased eosinophils [67] and mast cells [68] in the duodenum than the general population. A 2019 study showed that in patients with FD, as compared to both patients with non-dyspeptic abdominal symptoms and to healthy patients, there was an increase in interleukin IL-1B and a decrease in zonula occludens-1 [69]. Both are integral to the mucosal barrier function of the duodenum.

The microbiome has also been suggested as a possible cause of FD. Studies have demonstrated an increase in FD after previous bacterial infections [70] or other episodes of acute gastroenteritis. A 2013 meta-analysis demonstrated an estimated odds ratio of 2.18 of FD following an acute infectious gastroenteritis [71].

Regardless of the underlying cause, treating the symptoms of FD can be challenging and requires a multidisciplinary approach including medications such as neuromodulators, alternative interventions such as biofeedback or hypnotherapy, prokinetics, probiotics, and dietary interventions [72]. This last category of treatment will be discussed.

Eating Patterns

Several studies have looked at meal frequency in patients with FD. A 2016 cross-sectional study from Iran asked 4763 participants to report on the number of main meals and snacks they consumed daily [73]. They found that people who consumed six to seven total meals and snacks per day had lower odds of FD symptoms compared with those who ate <3 meals and snacks daily (OR 0.51). The findings of this study are similar to a 2009 case-control study which showed patients with FD eat meals less frequently as compared to healthy individuals, possibly suggesting that those with FD understand that larger meals tend to induce symptoms [74]. Therefore, it may be reasonable to recommend to patients with FD to eat smaller, more frequent meals and snacks to help alleviate their symptoms.

Caloric Intake and Dietary Volume

Small studies have suggested that the amount of calories and/or volume at meals may impact symptoms for patients with FD. The goal of this dietary modification is to address the impairment in gastric distension that may induce symptoms in patients with FD. In a small study of 62 total patients, patients with FD were found to have higher overall satiety scores with maximum satiety occurring at lower calories as compared to normal controls [75]. Additional studies have shown patients with FD to have an impaired drinking capacity as compared to healthy controls [76]. Given these studies, providers will often recommend low-volume meals to patients with FD. However, there are limited clinical studies demonstrating an improvement in symptoms with this dietary strategy.

Low-FODMAP Diet

Among the most commonly identified food triggers recognized by patients with FD are fermentable oligosaccharides, disaccharides, monosaccharides, and polyols (FODMAPs) which are carbohydrates that are poorly absorbed and osmotically active [77]. Foods high in FODMAPs include milk and certain kinds of fruits, vegetables, wheat and grain products, and soft drinks. FODMAPs have been shown to increase abdominal distension and can trigger discomfort and bloating in patients with documented visceral hypersensitivity [78], a potential mechanistic cause of FD. Multiple studies have shown that a low-FODMAP diet improves overall dyspeptic symptoms in patients [79]; however, gluten-free diets are encompassed into low-FODMAP diets, which has led to some discussion as to what the driving force truly is for patient improvement. In 2018, a systematic review concluded that a low-FODMAP diet likely has an additive benefit over just a gluten-free diet for patients with FD [80].

Gluten-Free Diet

Gluten-free diets (GFD), separate of low-FODMAP diets, also have some data as to their benefit. A retrospective study of 142 patients with dysmotility-like dyspepsia symptoms found significant improvement in their symptoms after going on a GFD [81]. It is worth noting that a little over one-third of these patients had some component of enteropathy as well, which may confound results. A separate study of definitively non-celiac patients with dyspeptic symptoms found improvement with a GFD [82]. Beyond the initial response, there was a secondary double-blind gluten or placebo capsule crossover trial, with the majority of patients reporting worsening of well-being when on the gluten capsule.

The GFD may not benefit all patients, and studies may have confounding overlap with common dietary triggers of symptoms. For example, a 2013 double-blind crossover study initially placed subjects on a gluten-free, low-FODMAP diet for 2 weeks, followed by a 1-week diet reintroducing a variable amount of gluten (high, low, or placebo – i.e., no gluten). Universally, subjects had significantly improved symptoms when on a low-FODMAP diet, but the reintroduction of gluten was not a universal cause of the return of symptoms, and the severity of symptoms recorded did not correlate to the amount of gluten ingested by the subject. The authors found gluten-specific effects only in a small number of the participants. This suggests that perhaps it is not only the gluten but other fermentable carbohydrates that are found in gluten-containing grains that may be responsible for causing functional GI symptoms [83]. Further research is necessary to help clarify this issue.

Dietary Fats

Dietary fats have been suggested as a potential trigger for FD symptoms as well. The proposed mechanism of symptoms includes the slowing of gastric emptying and the triggering CCK [84]. In multiple studies, not only was the restriction of dietary fats shown to improve symptoms of dyspepsia [85], but the introduction of dietary fat was shown to trigger those symptoms [86]. A 2016 study had 168 FD patients, and 135 health control patients fill out short-term food frequency questionnaires [87]. They found that patients with FD reported their most common symptom-triggering food was fatty foods. As such, a low-fat diet is suggested for patients with FD in those who find benefit.

Conclusion

The foregut is the initial site of food ingestion and the major driver of both chemical and mechanical digestion, ultimately serving an important function in overall nutritional status. Any dysfunction in these processes can result in major symptoms for patients as well as potential nutritional deficits. Whether it be through the elimination of specific foods, the replacement of vitamins insufficiently absorbed, or the modification of food contents or consistency, dietary interventions have a role in helping patients address diseases of the foregut.

References

1. Shaheen NJ, Mukkada V, Eichinger CS, et al. Natural history of eosinophilic esophagitis: a systematic review of epidemiology and disease course. Dis Esophagus. 2018;31(8):1–14.
2. Arias A, Perez-Martinez I, Tenias JM, et al. Systematic review with meta-analysis: the incidence and prevalence of eosinophilic oesophagitis in children and adults in population-based studies. Aliment Pharmacol Ther. 2016;43:3–15.
3. Furuta GT, Katzka DA. Eosinophilic esophagitis. N Engl J Med. 2015;373(17):1640–8.
4. Chen JW, Kao JY. Eosinophilic esophagitis: update on management and controversies. BMJ. 2017;259:j4482.
5. Molina-Infante J, Lucendo AJ. Dietary therapy for eosinophilic esophagitis. J Allergy Clin Immunol. 2018;142:41–7.
6. Cotton CC, Elhuri S, Wolf WA, et al. Six-food elimination diet and topical steroids are effective for eosinophilic esophagitis. Dig Dis Sci. 2017;62:2408–20.
7. Wang R, Hirano I, Doerfler B, et al. Assessing adherence and barriers to long-term elimination diet therapy in adults with eosinophilic esophagitis. Dig Dis Sci. 2018;63(7):1756–62.
8. Molina-Infante J, Arias A, Alcedo J, et al. Step-up empiric elimination diet for pediatric and adult eosinophilic esophagitis: The 2-4-6 study. J Allergy Clin Immunol. 2018;141:1365–72.
9. Arias A, Gonzalez-Cervera J, Tenais JM, et al. Efficacy of dietary interventions for inducing histologic remission in patients with eosinophilic esophagitis: a systematic review and meta-analysis. Gastroenterology. 2014;146:1639–48.
10. Spergel JM, Beausoleil JL, Mascarenahas M, et al. The use of skin prick tests an patch tests to identify causative foods in eosinophilic esophagitis. J Allergy Clin Immunol. 2002;109:363–8.

11. Molina-Infante J, Martin-Noguerol E, Alvarado-Arenas M, et al. Selective elimination diet based on skin testing has suboptimal efficacy for adult eosinophilic esophagitis. J Allergy Clin Immunol. 2012;130:1200–2.
12. Pandolfino JE, Gawron AJ. Achalasia: a systematic review. JAMA. 2015;313(18):1841–52.
13. Goldblum JR, Whyte RI, Orringer MB, et al. Achalasia: a morphologic study of 42 resected specimens. Am J Surg Pathol. 1994;18(4):327–37.
14. Vaezi MF, Pandolfino JE, Vela MF. ACG clinical guideline: diagnosis and management of achalasia. Am J Gastroenterol. 2013;108:1238–49.
15. Newberry C, Vajravelu RK, Pickett-Blakely O, et al. Achalasia patients are at nutritional risk regardless of presenting weight category. Dig Dis Sci. 2018;63:1243–9.
16. Krasaelep A, Kovacic K, Goday PS. Nutrition Management in Pediatric Gastrointestinal motility disorders. Nutr Clin Pract. 2020;35:265–72.
17. Richter J, Rubenstein J. Presentation and epidemiology of gastroesophageal reflux disease. Gastroenterology. 2018;154:267–76.
18. Newberry C, Lynch K. The role of diet in the development and management of gastroesophageal reflux disease: why we feel the burn. J Thorac Dis. 2019;11:S1594–601.
19. Fujiwara Y, Machida A, Watanabe Y, et al. Association between dinner-to-bed time and gastro-esophageal reflux disease. Am J Gastroenterol. 2005;100:2633–6.
20. Piesman M, Hwang I, Maydonovitch C, et al. Nocturnal reflux episodes following the Administration of a Standardized Meal. Does timing matter? Am J Gastroenterol. 2007;102:2128–34.
21. Nam SY, Park BJ, Cho Y, et al. Different effects of dietary factors on reflux esophagitis and non-erosive reflux disease in 11,690 Korean subjects. J Gastroenterol. 2017;52:818–29. https://doi.org/10.1007/s00535-016-1282-1.
22. Colombo P, Mangano M, Bianchi PA, Penagini R. Effect of calories and fat on postprandial gastro-oesophageal reflux. Scand J Gastroenterol. 2002;37(1):3–5. https://doi.org/10.1080/003655202753387266.
23. Langella C, Naviglio D, Marino M, et al. New food approaches to reduce and/or eliminate increased gastric acidity related to gastroesophageal pathologies. Nutrition. 2018;54:26–32.
24. Morozov S, Isakov V, Konovalova M. Fiber-enriched diet helps to control symptoms and improves esophageal motility in patients with non-erosive gastroesophageal reflux disease. World J Gastroenterol. 2018;24:2291–9.
25. El-Serag H, Satia JA, Rabeneck L. Dietary intake and the risk of gastro-oesophageal reflux disease: a cross sectional study in volunteers. Gut. 2005;54:11–7.
26. Becker D, Sinclair J, Castell D. A comparison of high and low-fat meals on postprandial esophageal acid exposure. Am J Gastroenterol. 1989;84:782.
27. Pehl C, Waizenhoefer A, Wendl B, et al. Effect of low and high fat meals on lower esophageal sphincter motility and gastroesophageal reflux in healthy subjects. Am J Gastroenterol. 1999;94:1192–6.
28. Ruhl C, Everhart J. Overweight, but not high dietary fat intake, increases risk of gastroesophageal reflux disease hospitalization. Ann Epidemiol. 1999;9:424–35.
29. Widmer R, Flammer A, Lerman L, et al. The Mediterranean diet, its components, and cardiovascular disease. Am J Med. 2015;128:229–38.
30. Mone I, Kraja B, Bregu A, et al. Adherence to a predominantly Mediterranean diet decreases the risk of gastroesophageal reflux disease: a cross-sectional study in a south eastern European population. Dis Esophagus. 2015;29:794–800.
31. Elmaliklis I, Liveri A, Ntelis B, et al. Increased functional foods' consumption and Mediterranean diet adherence may have a protective effect in the appearance of gastrointestinal diseases: a case–control study. Medicines. 2019;6:50.
32. Lohsiriwat S, Puengna N, Leelakusolvong S. Effect of caffeine on lower esophageal sphincter pressure in Thai healthy volunteers. Dis Esophagus. 2006;19:183–8.
33. Kim J, Oh S, Myung S, et al. Association between coffee intake and gastroesophageal reflux disease: a meta-analysis. Dis Esophagus. 2013;27:311–7.
34. Mehta R, Song M, Staller K, et al. Association between beverage intake and incidence of gastroesophageal reflux symptoms. Clin Gastroenterol Hepatol. 2020;18:2226–33.
35. Castell D, Murray J, Tutuian R, et al. Review article: the pathophysiology of gastro-oesophageal reflux disease - oesophageal manifestations. Aliment Pharmacol Ther. 2004;20:14–25.
36. Pan J, Cen L, Chen W, et al. Alcohol consumption and the risk of gastroesophageal reflux disease: a systematic review and meta-analysis. Alcohol Alcohol. 2018;54:62–9.
37. Kaltenbach T, Crockett S, Gerson L. Are lifestyle measures effective in patients with gastroesophageal reflux disease? Arch Intern Med. 2006;166:965.
38. Rajaie S, Ebrahimpour-Koujan S, Hassanzadeh Keshteli A, et al. Spicy food consumption and risk of uninvestigated heartburn in Isfahani adults. Dig Dis. 2019;38:178–87.
39. Murray H, Juarascio A, Di Lorenzo C, et al. Diagnosis and treatment of rumination syndrome. Am J Gastroenterol. 2019;114:562–78.
40. Halland M, Pandolfino J, Barba E. Diagnosis and treatment of rumination syndrome. Clin Gastroenterol Hepatol. 2018;16:1549–55.
41. Liu N, Abell T. Gastroparesis updates on pathogenesis and management. Gut Liver. 2017;11:579–89.
42. Grover M, Farrugia G. And Stanghellini. Gastroparesis: a turning point in understanding and treatment. Gut. 2019;68(12):2238–50.

43. Camilleri M, Parkman H, Shafi M, et al. Clinical guideline: Management of Gastroparesis. Am J Gastroenterol. 2013;108:18–37.
44. Camilleri M. Novel diet, drugs, and gastric interventions for gastroparesis. Clin Gastroenterol Hepatol. 2016:1072–80.
45. Homko C, Duffy F, Friedenberg F, et al. Effect of dietary fat and food consistency on gastroparesis symptoms in patients with gastroparesis. Neurogastroenterol Motil. 2015;27:501–8.
46. Olausson E, Störsrud S, Grundin H, et al. A small particle size diet reduces upper gastrointestinal symptoms in patients with diabetic gastroparesis: a randomized controlled trial. Am J Gastroenterol. 2014;109:375–85.
47. Wytiaz V, Homko C, Duffy F, et al. Foods provoking and alleviating symptoms in gastroparesis: patient experiences. Dig Dis Sci. 2015;60:1052–8.
48. Abell T, Adams K, Boles R, et al. Cyclic vomiting syndrome in adults. Neurogastroenterol Motil. 2008;20:269–84.
49. Chepyala P, Svoboda R, Olden K. Treatment of cyclic vomiting syndrome. Curr Treat Options Gastroenterol. 2007;10:273–82.
50. Lahner E, Conti L, Annibale B, et al. Current perspectives in atrophic gastritis. Curr Gastroenterol Rep. 2020;22:38.
51. D'Elios MM, Bergman MP, Azzurri A, et al. H{+}, K[+]-atpase [proton pump] is the target autoantigen of Th1-type cytotoxic T cells in autoimmune gastritis. Gastroenterology. 2001;120:377–86.
52. Uemura N, Okamoto S, Yamamoto S, et al. Helicobacter pylori infection and the development of gastric cancer. N Engl J Med. 2001;345(11):784.
53. Marignani M, Delle Fave G, Mecarocci S, et al. High prevalence of atrophic body gastritis in patients with unexplained microcytic and macrocytic anemia: a prospective screening study. Am J Gastroenterol. 1999;94:766–72.
54. Hershko C, Ronson A, Souroujon M, et al. Variable hematologic presentation of autoimmune gastritis: age-related progression from iron deficiency to cobalamin depletion. Blood. 2006;107:1673–9.
55. Tsugane S, Sasazuki S. Diet and the risk of gastric cancer: review of epidemiological evidence. Gastric Cancer. 2007;10(2):75.
56. Bouvard V, Loomis D, Guyton KZ, et al. Carcinogenicity of consumption of red and processed meat. Lancet Oncol. 2015;16(16):1599.
57. Talley NJ, Walker MM, and Holtmann G. Functional dyspepsia, Curr Opin Gastroenterol 2016; 32(6): 467–473.
58. Enck P, Azpiroz F, Boeckxstaens G, et al. Functional dyspepsia. Nat Rev Dis Primers. 2017;3:17081.
59. Hantoro IF, Syam AF, Mudjaddid E, et al. Factors associated with health-related quality of life in patients with functional dyspepsia. Health Qual Life Outcomes. 2018;16(1):83.
60. Aziz I, Palsson OS, Tornblom H, et al. Epidemiology, clinical characteristics, and associations for symptom-based Rome IV functional dyspepsia in adults in the USA, Canada, and the UK: a cross-sectional population-based study. Lancet Gastroenterol Hepatol. 2018;3(4):252.
61. Hassanzadeh S, Saneei P, Keshteli A, et al. Meal frequency in relation to prevalence of functional dyspepsia among Iranian adults. Nutrition. 2016;32:242–8.
62. Vanheel H, Carbone F, Valvekens L, et al. Pathophysiological abnormalities in functional dyspepsia subgroups according to the Rome III criteria. Am J Gastroenterol. 2017;112(1):132.
63. Farre R, Vanheel H, Vanuytsel T, et al. In functional dyspepsia, hypersensitivity to postprandial distension correlates with meal-related symptom severity. Gastroenterology. 2013;145(3):566–73.
64. Mertz H, Fullerton S, Naliboff SB, et al. Symptoms and visceral perception in severe functional and organic dyspepsia. Gut. 1998;42(6):814.
65. Mak AD, Wu JC, Chan Y, et al. Dyspepsia is strongly associated with major depression and generalized anxiety disorder – a community study. Aliment Pharmacol Ther. 2012;36(8):800.
66. Talley NJ, Fett SL, Zinsmeister AR, et al. Gastrointestinal tract symptoms and self-reported abuse: a population-based study. Gastroenterology. 1994;107(4):1040.
67. Talley NJ, Walker MM, Aro P, et al. Non-ulcer dyspepsia and duodenal eosinophilia: an adult endoscopic population-based case-control study. Clin Gastroenterol Hepatol. 2007;5(10):1175.
68. Walker MM, Talley NJ, Prabhakar M, et al. Duodenal mastocytosis, eosinophilia and intraepithelial lymphocytosis as possible disease markers in the irritable bowel syndrome and functional dyspepsia. Aliment Pharmacol Ther. 2009;29(7):765.
69. Komori K, Ihara E, Minoda Y, et al. The altered mucosal barrier function in the duodenum plays a role in the pathogenesis of functional dyspepsia. Dig Dis Sci. 2019;64(11):3228–39.
70. Mearin F, Perez-Oliveras M, Perello A, et al. Dyspepsia and irritable bowel syndrome after a salmonella gastroenteritis outbreak: one-year follow-up cohort study. Gastroenterology. 2005;129(1):98.
71. Pike BL, Porter CK, Sorrell TJ, et al. Acute gastroenteritis and the risk of functional dyspepsia: a systematic review and meta-analysis. Am J Gastroenterol. 2013;108(10):1558.
72. Lacy BE, Cangemi D, and Vazquez-Roque M. Management of chronic abdominal distension and bloating. Clin Gastroenterol Hepatol. 2020; E-pub ahead of print.
73. Hassanzadeh S, Saneei P, Keshteli A, et al. Meal frequency in relation to prevalence of functional dyspepsia among Iranian adults. Nutrition. 2016;32:242–8.
74. Pilichiewicz A, Horowitz M, Holtmann G, et al. Relationship between symptoms and dietary patterns in patients with functional dyspepsia. Clin Gastroenterol Hepatol. 2009;7:317–22.
75. Tack J, Caenepeel P, Piessevaux H, et al. Assessment of meal induced gastric accommodation by a satiety

drinking test in health and in severe functional dyspepsia. Gut. 2003;52(9):1271–7.
76. Boeckxstaens GE, Hirsch DP, van den Elzen BD, et al. Impaired drinking capacity in patients with functional dyspepsia: relation with proximal stomach function. Gastroenterology. 2001;121:1054–63.
77. Carvalho RV, Lorena SL, Almeida JR, et al. Food intolerance, diet composition, and eating patterns in functional dyspepsia patients. Dig Dis Sci. 2010;55:60–5.
78. Eswaran S, Farida JP, Green J, et al. Nutrition in the management of gastrointestinal diseases and disorders: the evidence for the low FODMAP diet. Curr Opin Pharmacol. 2017;37:151–7.
79. Gibson PR, Shepherd SJ. Evidence-based dietary management of functional gastrointestinal symptoms: the FODMAP approach. J Gastroenterol Hepatol. 2010;25(2):252–8.
80. Duncanson KR, Talley NJ, Walker MM, et al. Food and functional dyspepsia: a systematic review. J Hum Nutr Diet. 2018;31:390–407.
81. Santolaria S, Alcedo J, Cuartero B, et al. Spectrum of gluten-sensitive enteropathy in patients with dysmotility-like dyspepsia. Gastroenterol Hepatol. 2013;36(1):11–20.
82. Elli L, Tomba C, Branchi F, et al. Evidence for the presence of non-celiac gluten sensitivity in patients with functional gastrointestinal symptoms: results from a multicenter randomized double-blind placebo-controlled gluten challenge. Nutrients. 2016;8:84.
83. Biesiekierski JR, Peters SL, Newnham ED, Rosella O, Muir JG, Gibson PR. No effects of gluten in patients with self-reported non-celiac gluten sensitivity after dietary reduction of fermentable, poorly absorbed, short-chain carbohydrates. Gastroenterology. 2013;145(2):320–8.e1–3. https://doi.org/10.1053/j.gastro.2013.04.051. Epub 2013 May 4. PMID: 23648697
84. Feinle C, Meier O, Otto B, et al. Role of duodenal lipid and cholecystokinin a receptors in the pathophysiology of functional dyspepsia. Gut. 2001;48:347–55.
85. Carvalho RV, Lorena SL, Almeida JR, et al. Food intolerance, diet composition, and eating patterns in functional dyspepsia patients. Dig Dis Sci. 2010;55:60–5.
86. Pilichiewicz AN, Feltrin KL, Horowitz M, et al. Functional dyspepsia is associated with great symptomatic response to fat but not carbohydrate, increased fasting and postprandial CCK, and diminished PYY. Am J Gastroenterol. 2008;103:2613–23.
87. Göktaş Z, Köklü S, Dikmen D, et al. Nutritional habits in functional dyspepsia and its subgroups: a comparative study. Scand J Gastroenterol. 2016;51:903–7.

6 Small Bowel and Colon

Parita Patel and Dejan Micic

Introduction

Dietary modifications are important considerations in patients who suffer from gastrointestinal disorders, especially those that affect the small intestine and colon. The role of diet in the pathogenesis and management of gastrointestinal disorders is an area of ongoing research. While conditions such as celiac disease (CeD) have a clear association with dietary antigens [1, 2], other gastrointestinal conditions such as inflammatory bowel disease (IBD) and diverticulitis lack clear improvements with alterations in diet. As both patients and medical providers seek guidance on natural and less-invasive management strategies, further study of both the role of diet in the pathogenesis and management of gastrointestinal conditions is an area of utmost priority.

This chapter describes the role diet can play in the pathogenesis and treatment of several intestinal disorders, namely CeD, diverticular disease, short bowel syndrome (SBS), IBD, and irritable bowel syndrome (IBS).

P. Patel · D. Micic (✉)
Department of Internal Medicine, Section of Gastroenterology, Hepatology and Nutrition, University of Chicago, Chicago, IL, USA
e-mail: dmicic@medicine.bsd.uchicago.edu

Celiac Disease

Introduction

Celiac disease (CeD) is an autoimmune disorder triggered by the ingestion of gluten in genetically susceptible individuals. This disease primarily affects the small intestine, but there is a broad spectrum of extra-intestinal clinical manifestations. Pathologically, the ongoing ingestion of gluten (wheat, barley, rye) results in intestinal damage, characterized by villous blunting and increased intraepithelial lymphocytes, ultimately resulting in intestinal malabsorption [3]. Celiac disease affects approximately 1% of the general population, although the proportion of diagnosed patients varies between countries [3–5]. For example, Germany (0.3%) has a lower prevalence compared to Sweden and Finland (2.4%). Celiac disease is also increasingly prevalent in northern India, where wheat consumption is higher compared to other regions in the country [4]. Throughout the world, prevalence of the disease continues to increase due to multiple factors including westernization of diet, changes in wheat production, and increased awareness of the disease [6].

Pathogenesis

Both genetic and environmental factors play a large role in the predisposition to CeD. The HLA

C. Newberry et al. (eds.), *Nutrition, Weight, and Digestive Health*,
https://doi.org/10.1007/978-3-030-94953-2_6

DQ2 haplotype is expressed in 90% of patients with CeD compared to a 33% prevalence in the general population; the HLA DQ8 haplotype is expressed in another 5% of patients with CeD [6]. Once consumed, large, undigested gluten peptides enter the lamina propria of the small bowel in these genetically susceptible individuals. Tissue transglutaminase (TTG), the predominant autoantigen of CeD, deaminates these large gluten peptides and thereby "activates" the peptides, allowing for binding to antigen presenting cells with DQ2 and DQ8 haplotypes [6]. This leads to stimulation of T cells and initiates the innate inflammatory cascade in the intestinal epithelium mediated by additional immune signals that further recruit intraepithelial lymphocytes [3, 4, 7, 8].

Clinical Presentation

Although CeD is a disease that results in small bowel enteropathy, it has a wide spectrum of intestinal and extra-intestinal manifestations. Clinical features result from the malabsorption of electrolytes, vitamins, and minerals within the proximal small bowel including iron, folic acid, calcium, and fat-soluble vitamins. Table 6.1 shows the various nutrient and mineral deficiencies reported in CeD at diagnosis and clinical follow-up after treatment with a gluten-free diet (GFD).

Intestinal inflammation and associated malabsorption can lead to abdominal pain, gas/bloating, diarrhea, and weight loss. Other manifestations include iron deficiency anemia, elevated aminotransferases, hypocalcemia, reduced bone mineral density, and fatigue [3, 6]. Dermatitis herpetiformis, the primary skin manifestation of CeD, commonly occurs over the elbows, knees, buttocks, and scalp due to IgA deposition. Other extra-intestinal manifestations include arthritis [9] and neurologic or psychiatric symptoms (headache, peripheral neuropathy, ataxia, or depression) [10].

Table 6.1 Prevalence of nutrient deficiencies at the time of diagnosis and follow-up after a gluten-free diet in patients with celiac disease

	Prevalence of deficiency	
Nutrient	Diagnosis	Follow-up
Iron	11%–46% [143–145]	4.6% [145][a]
Vitamin B12	7.7%–41% [145, 146]	2.8–22.2% [147][b]
Folic acid	7.5% [145]	1.4% [145][a]
Zinc	18.6%- 67% [145, 148]	18.2% [145][a]

[a]Follow-up of 18 months

[b]Median follow-up of 7.8 years (1–22 years)

Nutritional Changes as the Mainstay Treatment

Currently, no medications can effectively prevent duodenal mucosal damage and, therefore, a lifelong GFD remains the only effective long-term treatment for CeD [1]. A GFD entails strict avoidance of all products containing the gluten proteins from wheat, barley, and rye [1]. Although the term gluten free implies complete elimination of all sources of gluten, this is extremely difficult. Even with a strict diet, individuals may consume products with "hidden" gluten (sausages, soups, soy sauce, ice cream) or consume foods that are cross-contaminated with gluten secondary to storage or processing considerations [11]. Therefore, a GFD is defined as a diet that contains gluten at such a low level as to be considered harmless to a patient with CeD [1, 11]. This precise level is unknown, but studies have suggested that less than 10 mg of gluten per day is safe in most patients [12].

The primary benefit of a GFD is repair of the intestinal damage and resolution of the symptoms of malabsorption [1], ultimately leading to an increase in body weight, body mass index, and bone mineralization [1, 2, 13]. A study by Rubio Tapia et al. demonstrated mucosal recovery in 35% of patients over two years after starting a GFD and in 66% after five years [14]. In addition, the institution of a GFD restores vitamin B12, folic acid, calcium, and magnesium levels in most patients (Table 6.1) [15]. Ingestion of oats and other alternative grains can further improve the nutrient content of a GFD by increasing the consumption of fiber, B vitamins, magnesium, and iron [16]. However, given the high likelihood of cross contamination with gluten-containing products, close clinical follow-up should be employed when these products are reintroduced into a diet.

Adherence to a GFD can also have protective effects against possible complications from CeD. Slightly higher rates of malignancy, particularly lymphoproliferative malignancies, have been noted in patients with untreated CeD. Enteropathy associated T-cell lymphoma is a rare form of high-grade, T-cell non-Hodgkin lymphoma of the upper small intestine that derives from a clonal proliferation of intraepithelial lymphocytes, often arising among individuals with refractory CeD [3, 17]. Although firm evidence is lacking, some studies suggest that a GFD is protective against lymphoproliferative malignancies in CeD [18, 19]. Other complications of untreated CeD include infertility [20], neuropathy [21], nonalcoholic fatty liver disease [22], and metabolic bone disease [3]. Small studies have shown that the institution of a GFD can increase bone mineral density [23, 24] and decrease rates of infertility, spontaneous abortions, preterm deliveries, and delivery of low birth weight infants [25–28].

Although difficult, strict compliance to a GFD is clearly essential in CeD. Noncompliance has been associated with an inability to correctly prepare meals, poor satisfaction with gluten-free products, and lack of confidence in treatment information relayed by providers [29, 30]. While it is important for patients to establish close follow-up with a gastroenterologist, establishing care with a registered dietitian is also important and can significantly improve adherence [31]. The Academy of Nutrition and Dietetics has established several evidence-based practice guidelines to help serve as a general framework to provide care to patients. Registered dietitians can provide education and counseling on the initiation and maintenance of a GFD, recommend alternatives to gluten, and monitor for nutrient deficiencies, fiber intake, and weight gain/loss [1].

Nutrition in Refractory Celiac Disease

Non-responsive CeD is defined as persistent signs, symptoms, or serologic abnormalities typical of CeD despite 6–12 months of a strict GFD and can occur in 7–30% of patients [1, 32, 33]. Causes include inadvertent gluten ingestion, lactose or fructose intolerance, small intestinal bacterial overgrowth, pancreatic insufficiency, microscopic colitis, irritable bowel syndrome (IBS), or refractory CeD [1]. Given that inadvertent gluten ingestion is the most common cause of non-responsive CeD, a thorough and careful evaluation of a patient's diet by a registered dietitian is necessary. Prior algorithms have been proposed and published in guidelines for management and workup of non-responsive CeD [1].

Refractory celiac disease (RCD) is defined as persistent or recurrent symptoms with signs of malabsorption despite a GFD of 12 months duration and exclusion of other potential disorders, including overt lymphoma [1]. There are two types of RCD (type I and type II), of which type II is more severe and associated with a worse prognosis. Malnutrition in RCD can be quite severe and may require parenteral nutrition support. While there are no published randomized, controlled trials of therapy for type II RCD, systemic corticosteroids, azathioprine, methotrexate, cyclosporine, and anti-TNF antibodies are commonly utilized to suppress the intestinal intraepithelial lymphocytosis and associated villous atrophy [1].

Diverticular Disease

Introduction

An intestinal diverticulum, most commonly encountered in the colon, is a protrusion of intestinal mucosa and submucosa through the muscularis layer at the site of blood vessel penetration through the muscle wall [34]. Diverticulitis occurs when there is inflammation of these outpouchings and can be associated with complications such as fistula formation, abscess, or perforation and peritonitis (diverticular disease).

The prevalence of diverticulosis is age dependent, increasing from 5–20% at age 40 to 50% by age 60 [35]. Among patients with diverticulosis, 4–15% will ultimately develop diverticulitis [36] with an overall rising incidence of diverticulitis as demonstrated by an increase in hospital admissions by 26% from 1998 to 2005 [37].

Clinical Presentation

The clinical presentation of diverticular disease can be variable and is dependent on the specific complications associated with the disease. Abdominal pain is the most common symptom in patients with acute diverticulitis, generally in the left lower quadrant when involving the sigmoid colon. While patients may have a low-grade fever, hemodynamic instability and shock are rare presentations often associated with perforation or peritonitis. Acute diverticulitis can present with altered bowel movements, with diarrhea in 25–35% of patients and constipation in 50% of patients [38]. Approximately 25% of patients will experience a complication from acute diverticulitis [39] such as abscess, obstruction, bleeding, fistula, or perforation [40]. Location of diverticula can be variable; studies have shown that distribution often varies by geography. In Western and industrialized nations, the majority of patients have left-sided disease, particularly in the sigmoid. In contrast, the disease is predominantly right-sided in Asian countries [41, 42].

Dietary Risk Factors in Diverticular Disease

Several clinical risk factors have been identified for diverticulitis including obesity [43], smoking [44], and the use of medications such as nonsteroidal anti-inflammatory drugs [45]. Population-based studies of diet and diverticular disease have also found an inverse relationship between fiber intake and symptomatic diverticular disease and a positive relationship with red meat consumption and symptomatic diverticular disease [46–50]. Vegetarians and those with low consumption of red meat (after adjustment of fiber intake) were shown to be at a decreased risk for diverticular disease [48]. In a prospective cohort study of over 47,000 men, the risk of symptomatic diverticular disease was two times higher (RR 2.35, 95% CI 1.38–3.98) in diets low in fiber and high in total fat and three times higher (RR 3.32, 95% CI 1.46–7.53) in diets high in total red meat and low in total fiber [46]. Additionally, recent dietary intake (within 1 to 4 years) was more strongly associated with risk of incident diverticulitis than long-term, cumulative intake, reflecting that relatively short-term dietary interventions may modify risk [47].

The impact of red meat on the development of diverticulitis is likely multifactorial. Red meat may promote chronic low-grade inflammation and is associated with higher levels of inflammatory markers [36, 51]. As such, consumption of red meat is also associated with increased risk of chronic diseases associated with elevated levels of circulating inflammatory markers such as type 2 diabetes mellitus and cardiovascular disease [52, 53]. Red meat contains specific compounds such as N-nitroso and heterocyclic amines which can affect colon epithelial homeostasis and have been proposed as risk factors for other colonic diseases such as colorectal cancer [54]. Consumption of red meat has also been associated with obesity, which in itself is a risk factor for diverticulitis [43, 47].

Fiber intake may decrease the risk of diverticulitis by altering the intestinal microbiota [55]. Studies have shown that a Western diet is associated with decreased microbial diversity in the intestine, whereas diets high in fiber increase gut microbiome diversity. Furthermore, dietary fiber is an important source of energy for the intestinal microbiome, which metabolizes complex carbohydrates into short-chain fatty acids. These short-chain fatty acids, in turn, increase the production of mucus and antimicrobial peptides and help mediate intestinal barrier function [40, 56]. By serving as a bulking agent, dietary fiber decreases colon pressure and stool transit time [47]. Dietary fiber has also been associated with lower levels of inflammatory markers [57] and healthy weight maintenance [58], both of which may be risk factors for development of diverticulitis [47].

In addition to fiber and red meat consumption, medical professionals have historically advised patients to avoid nuts, popcorn, corn, and other high-residue foods [59] as it was believed that these foods could lodge into diverticula, erode the colonic mucosa, and incite luminal trauma resulting in diverticulitis [60]. This commonly held belief was disproven in a large, prospective study that found no increased risk of diverticular complications with the ingestion of corn, nuts, or popcorn, and instead found a protective effect of nut and popcorn intake with diverticular disease [60]. While this protective mechanism has not been clearly elucidated, there are several possible associations that may play a role. Nuts contain fats with anti-inflammatory properties, and as such, consumption is inversely correlated with inflammatory markers, including C-reactive protein (CRP) and interleukin-6 [61]. Additionally, the high mineral content in nuts may reduce the oxidative stress in the colon, which is also thought to decrease the risk of colon cancer [60, 62, 63].

Short Bowel Syndrome

Introduction

Short bowel syndrome (SBS) is a rare gastrointestinal condition arising from a variety of gastrointestinal disorders and resulting in a reduction in the absorptive surface area of the small bowel and colon. Most often, SBS is secondary to extensive surgical resection in the setting of Crohn's disease (CD), mesenteric ischemia, and intestinal volvulus in adult patients, or from congenital defects and necrotizing enterocolitis in the pediatric patient. The underlying etiology of SBS is slowing evolving with postoperative causes and malignancy/radiation enteritis becoming the primary cause of SBS in adults at US centers [64]. Ultimately, understanding the underlying present anatomy is critical to predicting and identifying vitamin and mineral deficiencies as SBS can present with a variety of intestinal anatomical configurations.

The small intestinal length in an adult, measured from the duodenojejunal flexure, can range from 275 cm to 875 cm [65, 66]. Short bowel syndrome is defined when the small intestine in continuity is reduced to less than 200 cm [67]. Intestinal failure can result when the reduction in intestinal absorption requires intravenous supplementation to maintain health and/or growth [65], for which SBS is the leading cause [68].

Clinical Presentation

The principal cause of SBS is a reduction in the net intestinal absorptive surface area. As a result, the clinical presentation depends on a variety of mechanisms to include the residual small intestinal length, presence or absence of an ileocecal valve and colon, and integrity and adaptive potential of the remaining small intestine. Following resection, the small bowel adapts by increasing in villous height in response to growth hormones and pancreatic and biliary secretions over a period of one to two years [69, 70]. While intestinal adaptation is variable and can be reduced in individuals with an end jejunostomy, the ability of the colon to participate in net fluid and calorie absorption is critical to achieving independence from parenteral support [71]. Small intestinal lengths less than 100 cm to an end-jejunostomy, less than 65 cm to a jejunocolic anastomosis, and less than 30 cm to a jejunoileocolic anastomosis predicts as opposed to predicted to transient intestinal failure in the setting of SBS, demonstrating the adaptive capacity of the distal small bowel and role of the colon in maintaining enteral independence [72].

Individuals with an end-jejunostomy can present with high volume losses and nutrient and vitamin malabsorption as a result of rapid intestinal transit and poor intestinal adaptation. In the setting of ileal resection, bile salt and vitamin B12 malabsorption can be present resulting in diarrhea and neurologic consequences in the setting of prolonged and profound vitamin B12 deficiency. Resection over 100 cm of ileum results in a loss of enterohepatic circulation of bile acids, steatorrhea, and severe fat malabsorption [73]. Whereas the ileum has the best adaptive capacity, proximal loss of small intestine can result in calcium, zinc, copper, iron, and folate malabsorption. Therefore, a clear understanding of the resulting intestinal anatomy, resections, and future adaptive capacity is required in the management of individuals with SBS in order to tailor supplements and medical therapies aimed at reducing the risk of intestinal failure.

Dietary Modifications

The management of SBS includes a combination of medical therapies aimed at reducing intestinal transit time and secretions and dietary modifications aimed at improving intestinal absorption. When indicated for failure to maintain nutrient, mineral, or vitamin absorption, parenteral nutrition or intravenous hydration may be required. Recently developed glucagon-like peptide 2 (GLP-2) agonists have demonstrated an ability to improve the adaptation of the small intestine in intestinal failure with SBS and have resulted in a decreased need for parenteral nutrition support [74].

Appropriate and adequate dietary interventions are an integral part of the management of patients with SBS, both in an effort to reduce the need for parenteral nutrition support and in order to reduce complications of altered intestinal anatomy (i.e., calcium oxalate kidney stones, D-lactic acidosis). Adequate calorie supplementation can help reduce the risk of requiring prolonged parenteral support. Individual patients can adapt to decreased intestinal absorption through an increase in oral food intake (hyperphagia). Jeppesen et al. previously demonstrated that individuals absorbing less than one-half of consumed calories could avoid parenteral nutrition support through an intake of nearly 2000–5000 calories per day [75].

As patients with end jejunostomies have not been demonstrated to have increased ostomy losses with high fat intake [76], the optimal diet includes generous intake of complex carbohydrates and fats with a macronutrient distribution of 50% complex carbohydrates, 40% fats, and 20–30% protein [73]. Alternatively, in the presence of a colon-in-continuity, patients benefit from increased complex carbohydrates in the diet (50–60% complex carbohydrates, 20–30% protein, 20–30% fat) as the reduced fat intake results in lower fecal energy losses and the complex carbohydrates can be further metabolized by the colonic bacteria into short-chain fatty acids, resulting in a salvage of calories by the colon [73]. Additionally, the reduced fat intake in the setting of a colon-in-continuity reduces the displacement of oxalate from calcium and therefore reduces the absorption of oxalate in the colon, the primary contributor to calcium oxalate kidney stones in SBS.

Maintenance of adequate hydration is imperative to reduce the risk of dehydration and requirement of parenteral volume support. Avoidance of simple sugars and poorly absorbed sugars (lactose) reduces the dumping of hypertonic chime into the small intestine which can be associated with rapid transit through the small intestine. Fluid uptake in the small intestine can be improved with the liberal use of balanced oral rehydration solutions which utilize the sodium-glucose cotransport into the epithelial cell which subsequently drives net water absorption across the small intestinal epithelium.

Routine monitoring of electrolytes, minerals, and vitamins is required in individuals with SBS due to the wide variety of deficiencies that they can experience based on intestinal anatomy and underlying residual function. Patients with a history of ileal resection or small bowel bacterial overgrowth require routine monitoring and replacement of vitamin B12, while the divalent cations calcium, magnesium, and zinc are often deficient secondary to the reductions in intestinal absorptive surface, rapid transit, and binding with unabsorbed fats in the diet [73]. Adequate supplementation is required in order to reduce the risk of osteoporosis in SBS, which can be further compounded by fat-soluble vitamin deficiencies (vitamin D) [77]. The frequent monitoring and anticipation of deficiencies in SBS require specialized nutrition support teams including registered dietitians, nurses, and pharmacists in order to manage the wide variety of presentations and individualized patient needs.

Inflammatory Bowel Disease

Introduction

Inflammatory bowel disease (IBD) is a chronic inflammatory condition that includes Crohn's disease (CD) and ulcerative colitis (UC). Crohn's disease is a transmural inflammatory disease that can affect any part of the gastrointestinal tract from the mouth to the anus, whereas UC is a mucosal disease process that only affects the colon. Although IBD can occur at any age, there is a predominant age distribution of onset between 15 and 30 years [78]. Signs and symptoms of CD can be variable with patients experiencing chronic diarrhea, abdominal pain, intestinal fistulas, stricturing disease, or extra-intestinal manifestations such as joint pain, fatigue, and inflammatory skin disorders. Patients with UC most commonly present with signs and symptoms of rectal inflammation such as bleeding, fecal urgency, and tenesmus [78].

With the growing incidence of IBD, the number of medications utilized as first-line therapies has also increased. The main classes of medications for the treatment of IBD include 5-aminosalicylates, corticosteroids, immunomodulators (i.e., azathioprine, 6-mercaptopurine, methotrexate, and cyclosporine), and biologic therapies (i.e., anti-tumor necrosis factor, anti-integrin, and IL-12/-23 antagonists) [79]. Surgery is now reserved for patients who are refractory or intolerant to medical therapy [79].

Many studies have explored the role diet can play in the pathogenesis and treatment of IBD, but this still remains an area of active research, with limited current data to guide practitioners and patients. Although some guidelines acknowledge that dietary therapies can be effective (Table 6.2), these benefits are not thought to be durable and, therefore, are recommended to be only used in conjunction with medical management [80].

Although limited evidence-based data exists on diet-based therapies in IBD, up to 71% of patients believe that diet affects their symptoms and up to 77% of patients report avoidance of particular foods due to their disease [81]. Such avoidance of foods can lead to decreased intake of carbohydrates, monounsaturated fat, fiber, calcium, and vitamins [79, 82]. Therefore, although there is limited data on diet-based therapies, there is a clear need to investigate the role diet can play in IBD management.

Diet and the Risk of IBD

The pathogenesis of IBD is complex, involving the interaction of disease susceptibility genes, immune responses, gut microbiota, and environmental factors such as dietary intake [83, 84]. One proposed mechanism for how diet contributes to the development of CD is through the individual components of a "Western diet" (animal fat, sugar, wheat proteins, emulsifiers, maltodextrin, low fiber) leading to defects in localized bacterial clearance, promoting bacterial adhesion/penetration and subsequent intestinal inflammation [85, 86]. This has been demonstrated in murine studies in which a high-fat and high-salt diet decreased intestinal mucous layer, increased intestinal permeability, and increased the ability of bacteria to colonize the intestinal mucosa and induce inflammation [86–88]. While an increased risk of IBD is seen in populations that consume a Western diet, lower risk has been noted in patients who consume prudent diets with high intake of fiber from fruits and vegetables and low intake of animal fat, dairy, and processed foods [89–91].

Diet for Induction Therapy of Active IBD

Enteral Nutrition

Exclusive enteral nutrition (EEN) consists of intake of liquid formulas without the intake of solid foods for at least 6–8 weeks. Exclusive enteral nutrition, either in the form of elemental (amino acid based), semi-elemental (oligopeptides), or polymeric (whole protein based) formulas, is one of the most effective diets for induction of remission in CD [92] but does not demonstrate efficacy in UC [93]. Although classifying the evi-

Table 6.2 Proposed diets and nutritional supplements for induction and maintenance of inflammatory bowel disease

Induction		
Diet	Components	Types of inflammatory bowel disease
Exclusive enteral nutrition	Can be elemental (amino acid based), semi-elemental (oligopeptide), or polymeric (whole protein based)	Crohn's disease
Specific carbohydrate diet	Elimination of complex carbohydrates, processed foods, food additives, and most dairy products while maintaining consumption of almost all fruit, some vegetables, nuts, meats and eggs	Crohn's disease
Autoimmune diet	Elimination of grains, legumes, nightshade vegetables, dairy, eggs, coffee, alcohol, nuts/seeds, processed sugars, oils, and food additives while increasing consumption of nutrient-dense fresh foods and bone broth	Crohn's disease
Maintenance		
Low FODMAP diet	Limits the ingestion of single and double sugar molecules which when poorly absorbed in the small intestinal lumen	Crohn's disease/ ulcerative colitis
Anti-inflammatory diet	Five phases including modification of specific carbohydrate, ingestion of pre- and pro-biotics, separation of saturated, trans-, mono-, and polyunsaturated fats, identification of missing nutrients, and modification of texture of foods	Crohn's disease/ ulcerative colitis
Curcumin	Used as an adjunctive therapy to reduce symptoms and maintain remission due to its anti-inflammatory properties	Ulcerative colitis
Vitamin D	May decrease symptoms due to immunosuppressive properties	Crohn's disease

dence as very low quality, a recent Cochrane meta-analysis demonstrated that EEN may be more effective than steroids for induction of remission in children with active CD [86, 94]. Similar results were seen in a prospective study of 147 pediatric patients with mild-moderate CD, which demonstrated that use of EEN was associated with higher remission rates and a trend toward better growth when compared to steroid treatment [86, 95].

Despite these promising studies in pediatric populations, EEN poses more challenges in adults. Its poor taste leads to decreased tolerability and its long-term efficacy is equivalent to steroid use in recent studies [89, 96]. Partial enteral nutrition (PEN) has been suggested as an alternate treatment modality. The goal of PEN regimens is to allow oral food intake while supplementing calories with enteral formulas. Although this poses an attractive option, remission rates with PEN remain inadequate, correlating with the percentage of enteral nutrition support provided [97]. Studies assessing PEN formulas supplementing 50% of total daily calories demonstrated reduced effectiveness with lower remission rates and higher fecal calprotectin measurements compared to EEN [98, 99].

As a result, PEN regimens with restricted oral diets have been created in order to limit exposure to foods with potential contributions to inflammation or alterations in the microbiota [86]. In the Crohn's Disease Elimination Diet (CDED), potentially inflammatory foods such as wheat, dairy, emulsifiers, maltodextrins, carrageenans, and sulfites, are excluded as they are hypothesized to alter the microbiome and/or intestinal permeability [89]. Prior case series have demonstrated effectiveness of the CDED when used with polymeric PEN (Modulen, Nestle, or Pediasure, Abbott Nutrition) in CD with respect to clinical symptoms and markers of inflammation [100, 101]. Most recently, Levine et al. evaluated the CDED with PEN in a study of 74 pediatric patients with mild-moderate CD randomized to either EEN or the combination of CDED with PEN. PEN accounted for 50% of total calories in the first six weeks of the trial and 25% of calories in the second six weeks of the 12-week trial. The CDED with PEN was better tolerated and resulted in a significantly higher rate of corticosteroid-free remission at 12 weeks (76.6% vs. 45.1%, P = 0.01) [102]. Further studies are ongoing (CDED-ADULTS – NCT02231814) to extend these results to adult populations [86].

Specific Carbohydrate Diet

The specific carbohydrate diet (SCD) is thought to be effective in CD due to its elimination of complex carbohydrates, processed foods, food additives, and most dairy products while maintaining consumption of almost all fruit, some vegetables, nuts, meats, and eggs [86]. Although difficult to maintain, several retrospective studies demonstrated improvement of clinical disease activity scores, normalization of albumin, and improvement in inflammatory markers [89, 103, 104]. In a prospective pediatric cohort study, 12 patients with IBD (9 with CD) were initiated on a SCD diet without any alteration in medications. Mean pediatric Crohn's disease activity index (PCDAI) scores for participants decreased from 28.1 ± 8.8 to 4.6 ± 10.3, and an elevated CRP decreased from 70% of individuals at baseline to 20% of individuals after 12 weeks of dietary therapy [105]. Current ongoing studies are further comparing the efficacy of the SCD to a Mediterranean diet in adults with CD (DINE-CD study; ClinicalTrials.gov Identifier: NCT03058679).

Autoimmune Diet

The autoimmune diet is an extension of the Paleolithic diet while also incorporating changes described in the SCD and CDED with elimination of grains, legumes, nightshade vegetables, dairy, eggs, coffee, alcohol, nuts/seeds, processed sugars, oils, and food additives while increasing consumption of nutrient-dense fresh foods and bone broth [86]. Following an elimination phase and once clinical symptoms and inflammation are controlled, a 5-week maintenance phase is employed, followed by a reintroduction of food items one at a time. In a single-center open-label study including 15 patients with IBD (9 with CD), clinical remission was achieved in 11 patients by week 6, and among patients with CD, the mean Harvey-Bradshaw Index (HBI) (well-being, abdominal pain, number of liquid or soft stools, presence of abdominal mass, and presence of complications) improved from 6.7 (SD 1.5) to 3.3 (SD 1.8, $P = 0.001$) at week 6 and 3.4 (SD 2.6, $P = 0.004$) at week 11 [86, 106].

Diet for Maintenance of Remission and Symptom Control

Low FODMAP Diet

The FODMAP (fermentable oligosaccharides, disaccharides, monosaccharides, and polyols) diet limits the ingestion of single and double sugar molecules which, when poorly absorbed in the small intestinal lumen, lead to osmotic shifts in fluid and subsequent distension of the small bowel and colon [86, 107]. Although the low FODMAP diet was initially developed for patients with irritable bowel syndrome (IBS), some studies have demonstrated a positive impact in patients with IBD with concurrent IBS or IBS-like symptoms [108–110]. Prince et al. studied 88 patients with IBD and functional gastrointestinal symptoms. Seventy-eight percent of patients reported an improvement in symptoms from baseline following a dietary intervention of a strict low FODMAP diet over 6 weeks followed by reintroduction [108]. In a meta-analysis of six studies (two randomized controlled studies, four before–after studies) in patients with quiescent IBD, a low FODMAP diet was found to be beneficial in reducing the symptoms of diarrhea, bloating, abdominal pain, fatigue, and nausea [111]. While these studies show improvement in clinical symptoms with a low FODMAP diet, there is very little data to demonstrate any improvement in intestinal inflammation. In a small study of nine patients with clinically quiescent CD, there was no difference in fecal calprotectin in those on a low FODMAP diet compared to those on a typical "Australian" diet [112]. Future studies are needed to evaluate the long-term efficacy and impact on inflammation of a low FODMAP diet in patients with IBD.

Anti-inflammatory Diet

The anti-inflammatory diet (IBD-AID) is a recently described diet developed with the intent to reduce the frequency and severity of disease flares and maintain remission in IBD. The five basic components of this diet include modification of specific carbohydrates followed by ingestion of pre- and probiotics (soluble fiber, leeks, onions), which are thought to help restore the intestinal flora. The third phase distinguishes between saturated, trans-, mono-, and polyunsaturated fats, while the fourth phase entails review of overall dietary intake with the goal of identifying missing nutrients and possible intolerances. The fifth and final phase modifies the texture of foods (cooked, ground, blenderized) depending on the ongoing symptoms as a means to improve absorption and minimize intact fiber [113]. Unfortunately, data supporting the use of this diet in IBD is limited to a small case series evaluating symptomatic control over a period of four weeks [113].

Curcumin

Curcumin is derived from the turmeric plant and is used as an adjunctive therapy to reduce symptoms and maintain remission due to its anti-inflammatory properties [89, 114]. Although several case reports have been published, very few randomized controlled trials have examined the role of curcumin in IBD. In one multicenter, randomized, placebo-controlled study, 50 mesalamine-treated patients with mild-moderate active UC were randomly assigned to curcumin capsules (3 g/day) or placebo. Fifty-four percent of patients receiving curcumin achieved clinical remission at week 4 compared with no patients in the placebo group (OR: 42, 95% CI 2.3–760, $P = 0.01$). Endoscopic remission was seen in 38% of patients receiving curcumin compared with no patients in the placebo group, with comparable adverse events between two groups [115]. However, in a subsequent systematic review including four trials assessing adjuvant curcumin in UC, no benefit of curcumin was demonstrated in an intention-to-treat analysis [114]. Therefore, further large randomized controlled trials are needed to fully elucidate the role curcumin may play in patients with both active UC and UC in remission.

Vitamin D

Vitamin D is a potent immunostimulatory and immunosuppressive secosteroid hormone. Deficiency of vitamin D has been suggested to play a role in multiple chronic diseases including CD [86, 116]. Narula et al. conducted a randomized, double-blind, placebo-controlled trial of high-dose (10,000 IU daily) vitamin D3 supplementation compared to 1000 IU daily in CD patients in remission. At 12-month follow-up, high-dose vitamin D3 repletion led to significant improvements in 25-hydroxyvitmain D levels (increase from mean 73.5 nmol/L to 160.8 nmol/L, $P = 0.02$). An associated lower rate of clinical relapse among those on high-dose vitamin D3 supplementation was demonstrated in a per-protocol analysis but not statistically significant on an intention-to-treat basis [116]. Further studies are needed to fully understand the role vitamin D may play in patients with IBD.

Irritable Bowel Syndrome

Introduction

Irritable bowel syndrome (IBS) is a functional gastrointestinal disorder characterized by chronic abdominal pain and altered bowel habits without an identifiable organic cause. The prevalence of IBS in the United States is 7–16% among adults [117], with an overall prevalence higher in women compared with men [118]. While clinical manifestations may vary from patient to patient, the diagnosis of IBS has been standardized using the consensus Rome Criteria. The various IBS subtypes (IBS with predominant constipation, IBS with predominant diarrhea, IBS with mixed bowel habits, and unclassified IBS) have also been defined for clinical practice.

Pathogenesis of Disease

Although the pathophysiology of IBS remains uncertain, multiple factors have been thought to play a role. Alteration in gastrointestinal motility

[119, 120], visceral hypersensitivity [121], alterations in the gut microbiota [122], genetic factors [123], psychosocial factors, and infections [124] may be the possible contributing factors to the development of IBS [125]. The role of diet is not clearly understood in the development of IBS, but it may play an important role in disease management, with up to 84% of patients reporting food-related symptoms [126]. Several studies have suggested an overlap between CeD and IBS [127] as well as carbohydrate malabsorption as a cause of symptoms. As a result, many of the treatment modalities in IBS revolve around dietary modifications, although the heterogeneity of symptoms in IBS makes it difficult to have a standardized treatment protocol for all patients. Despite significant interest in using dietary treatment approaches, quality study designs are limited. The following subsections describe different diets that are often employed for treatment of IBS symptoms.

Dietary Treatment Approaches in IBS

Low FODMAP Diet

Fermentable oligosaccharides, disaccharides, monosaccharides and polyols (FODMAPs) are single and short-chain carbohydrates that are characterized by limited small bowel absorption. When poorly absorbed in the small intestinal lumen, osmotic shifts of fluid and colonic bacterial fermentation lead to distension of the small bowel and colon [86, 107], thereby causing symptoms in IBS. There are three distinct phases within the low FODMAP diet: a restriction/elimination phase, a rechallenge/reintroduction phase, and a maintenance phase. During the elimination phase, patients restrict FODMOPs from their diet for 2–6 weeks. Next, gradual reintroduction of foods containing individual FODMAPs should be employed, with the goal of identifying specific trigger carbohydrates. This phase can take several weeks as foods are slowly reintroduced. Knowing a patient's trigger foods, a personalized low FODMAP diet can be designed for the patient to carry forward (i.e., maintenance phase) [128].

The American College of Gastroenterology reviewed seven randomized controlled trials that compared outcomes for a low FODMAP diet versus alternative diets (Table 6.3). There was an overall effect of the low FODMAP diet in reducing IBS symptoms with a relative risk of remaining symptomatic on a low FODMAP diet of 0.69 (95% CI 0.54–0.88) with a number needed to

Table 6.3 Randomized controlled trials examining the role of a low FODMAP diet in irritable bowel syndrome

Title	Author	Population studied	Intervention and Control Groups	Primary Outcome	Results
A randomized controlled trial comparing the low FODMAP diet vs. modified NICE guidelines in US adults with IBS-D [149]	Eswaran S et al.	IBS-D	IBS-D vs. mNICE diet[a]	Relief of IBS-D symptoms >50%	52% vs. 41% of mNICE group reported adequate relief of IBS-D symptoms ($p = 0.13$)
Diet low in FODMAPs reduces symptoms of irritable bowel syndrome as well as traditional dietary advice: a randomized controlled trial [150]	Bohn L, et al.	Not specified	Low FODMAP diet vs. diet recommended for IBS (regular meal pattern, reduced intake of fat, insoluble fibers, caffeine, and gas-producing products)	Severity of IBS symptoms using IBS severity scale (IBS-SSS[b])	Severity of symptoms reduced in both groups. 50% in low FODMAP group had reduction in IBS severity group ≥50 compared with baseline compared to 46% in traditional IBS diet ($p = 0.72$)

(continued)

Table 6.3 (continued)

Title	Author	Population studied	Intervention and Control Groups	Primary Outcome	Results
FODMAPs alter symptoms and the metabolome of patients with IBS: a randomized controlled trial [151]	McIntosh K et al.	Not specified	Low FODMAP vs high FODMAP diet	IBS-SSS[b]	The IBS-SSS was reduced in the low FODMAP diet group ($p < 0.001$) but not in the high FODMAP group
Fermentable carbohydrate restriction reduces luminal bifidobacteria and gastrointestinal symptoms in patients with irritable bowel syndrome [152]	Staudacher HM, et al.	Not specified	Low FODMAP vs. habitual diet	Fecal microbiota and symptom response using a global symptom question	More patients in the interventional group (low FODMAP diet) reported adequate control of symptoms (68%) compared with controls (23%), $p = 0.005$)
Diet low in FODMAPs reduces symptoms in patients with irritable bowel syndrome and probiotic restores bifidobacterium species: a randomized controlled trial [153]	Staudacher HM, et al.	Not specified	Sham diet vs. low FODMAP diet +/− placebo/ probiotic	IBS-SSS[b]	A higher proportion of patients in the low FODMAP diet had adequate symptom relief (57%) than in the sham diet group (38%) ($P = 0.051$). Total mean IBS-SSS was significantly lower for patients on the low FODMAP diet (173 ± 95) than the sham diet (224 ± 89) (P = 0.001), but not different between those given probiotic (207 ± 98) or placebo (192 ± 93) ($P = 0.721$)
A diet low in FODMAPs reduces symptoms of irritable bowel syndrome [154]	Halmos EP, et al.	IBS and healthy individuals	Low FODMAP diet vs. typical Australian diet, crossover to alternate diet after 21 days	Symptoms using visual analogue scale (0–100; 0 = no symptoms, 100 = most severe) and stool samples	Subjects with IBS had lower overall gastrointestinal symptom scores (22.8; 95% confidence interval, 16.7–28.8) while on a diet low in FODMAPs compared with the Australian diet (44.9; 95% confidence interval, 36.6–53.1; $P < 0.001$)
Effects of varying dietary content of fermentable short-chain carbohydrates on symptoms, fecal microenvironment, and cytokine profiles in patients with irritable bowel syndrome [155]	Hustoft TN, et al.	IBS-D or mixed IBS	Low FODMAP for 3 weeks, followed by FODMAP vs. placebo for 10 days, followed by crossover	IBS-SSS[b] and interleukin 6,8 and tumor necrosis factor alpha	Symptoms improved after 3 weeks of low FODMAP diet, and significantly more participants reported symptom relief in response to placebo (80%) than FODMAP (30%)

[a]*mNICE* diet based upon modified National Institute for Health and Care Excellence guidelines
[b]IBS-SSS IBS Severity Scale

treat of 5 [129], albeit with low quality of evidence given a high risk of bias among the included studies.

With any restrictive diet, there is always a concern for nutritional deficiencies. However, the data related to nutritional deficiencies related to a low FODMAP diet are varied and controversial. In a small study of 26 patients with IBS, nutritional status and body composition were evaluated. Although there were statistically significant changes in albumin and lipids after the introduction of a low FODMAP diet for 8 weeks, the differences were small and laboratory values remained within the normal range [130, 131]. Given the expanding role of dietary interventions in the management of IBS, it has become increasingly important for clinicians to work alongside registered dietitians to ensure appropriate maintenance of the recommended nutrient and vitamin intakes and avoidance of nutritional deficiencies [125].

Gluten-Free Diet

The effect of gluten in patients with IBS was studied in a randomized controlled trial of 34 patients with previously noted gluten sensitivity. Patients were randomized to a high-gluten diet (16 g/day) or a GFD for a total of 6 weeks. Sixty-eight percent of patients in the high-gluten diet reported uncontrolled symptoms compared to 40% among those randomized to a GFD ($P = 0.001$) [132]. In a study by Vasquez-Roque et al., 45 patients with diarrhea-predominant IBS (and no prior diagnosis of CeD) were randomized to a gluten-containing diet and a GFD. Those on a gluten-containing diet had more bowel movements per day ($P = 0.04$) and a greater small bowel permeability when compared to those on a GFD [133]. Such data has led some to conclude that gluten is the cause of gastrointestinal symptom after ingestion of wheat [125]. However, further studies have shown that the sugar components found in wheat (i.e., fructans) may play a primary role in patients who find relief from a GFD in IBS [134, 135], supporting the role of the FODMAP diet in the management of IBS. Further well-controlled studies are needed to better understand the specific components of the GFD that may provide benefit to some individuals with IBS.

Lactose-Free Diet

Lactose intolerance is a clinical syndrome where patients develop bloating, flatulence, abdominal discomfort, and diarrhea after the consumption of lactose-containing foods. Symptom development in patients with lactose intolerance may be related to the amount of lactose consumed, intestinal hypersensitivity, and intestinal transit of lactose. As such, individuals with IBS may have increased symptoms at lower levels of lactose consumption resulting in increased self-reported lactose intolerance and lactose restriction [136, 137]. However, very few studies have investigated the actual role of lactose-free diet in patients with IBS [138–140]. Based on small trials, the British Dietetic Association states that no specific IBS symptom profiles were associated with lactose intolerance or responded better to a low lactose diet (< 9 g/day) and as such lactose restriction may only provide marginal symptom benefits [141].

While symptoms of IBS and lactose intolerance can overlap, they are two separate clinical entities [142]. It is crucial to consider and rule out lactose intolerance prior to diagnosing IBS. As such, lactose-free diets may not be helpful in all patients with IBS; a low lactose diet can be expected to improve abdominal symptoms in those with both concomitant IBS and lactose intolerance [140, 141].

Conclusion

Diet and nutrition play an integral and complex role in the pathogenesis and management of intestinal disorders, but many questions still remain unanswered. As popular diets are emerging, it is imperative to understand the nutritional consequences and benefits in various disease states. This chapter summarizes the limited evidence available on nutritional implications and common dietary therapies used in CeD, diverticular disease, SBS, IBD, and IBS. While future clinical trials are still needed to investigate the consequences of various dietary strategies in these disorders, steps such as including registered dieticians in the management of patients can lead to successful and safe dietary modifications with improved long-term adherence [1].

Disclosures No expressed conflicts of interest with respect to the submitted work

References

1. Rubio-Tapia A, et al. ACG clinical guidelines: diagnosis and management of celiac disease. Am J Gastroenterol. 2013;108(5):656–76; quiz 677.
2. Bardella MT, et al. Body composition and dietary intakes in adult celiac disease patients consuming a strict gluten-free diet. Am J Clin Nutr. 2000;72(4):937–9.
3. Micic D, Rao VL, Semrad CE. Celiac disease and its role in the development of metabolic bone disease. J Clin Densitom. 2019.
4. Lebwohl B, Sanders DS, Green PHR. Coeliac disease. Lancet. 2018;391(10115):70–81.
5. Ludvigsson JF, Murray JA. Epidemiology of celiac disease. Gastroenterol Clin N Am. 2019;48(1):1–18.
6. Fasano A, Catassi C. Clinical practice. Celiac disease. N Engl J Med. 2012;367(25):2419–26.
7. Molberg O, et al. Tissue transglutaminase selectively modifies gliadin peptides that are recognized by gut-derived T cells in celiac disease. Nat Med. 1998;4(6):713–7.
8. Lundin KE, et al. Gliadin-specific, HLA-DQ(alpha 1*0501,beta 1*0201) restricted T cells isolated from the small intestinal mucosa of celiac disease patients. J Exp Med. 1993;178(1):187–96.
9. Lubrano E, et al. The arthritis of coeliac disease: prevalence and pattern in 200 adult patients. Br J Rheumatol. 1996;35(12):1314–8.
10. Cicarelli G, et al. Clinical and neurological abnormalities in adult celiac disease. Neurol Sci. 2003;24(5):311–7.
11. Itzlinger A, et al. Gluten-free diet in celiac disease-forever and for all? Nutrients. 2018;10(11).
12. Akobeng AK, Thomas AG. Systematic review: tolerable amount of gluten for people with coeliac disease. Aliment Pharmacol Ther. 2008;27(11):1044–52.
13. Barera G, et al. Body composition in children with celiac disease and the effects of a gluten-free diet: a prospective case-control study. Am J Clin Nutr. 2000;72(1):71–5.
14. Rubio-Tapia A, et al. Mucosal recovery and mortality in adults with celiac disease after treatment with a gluten-free diet. Am J Gastroenterol. 2010;105(6):1412–20.
15. Kreutz JM, et al. Narrative review: nutrient deficiencies in adults and children with treated and untreated celiac disease. Nutrients. 2020;12(2).
16. Kemppainen TA, et al. Nutrient intakes during diets including unkilned and large amounts of oats in celiac disease. Eur J Clin Nutr. 2010;64(1):62–7.
17. Catassi C, Bearzi I, Holmes GK. Association of celiac disease and intestinal lymphomas and other cancers. Gastroenterology. 2005;128(4 Suppl 1):S79–86.
18. Ludvigsson JF. Mortality and malignancy in celiac disease. Gastrointest Endosc Clin N Am. 2012;22(4):705–22.
19. Silano M, et al. Effect of a gluten-free diet on the risk of enteropathy-associated T-cell lymphoma in celiac disease. Dig Dis Sci. 2008;53(4):972–6.
20. Collin P, et al. Infertility and coeliac disease. Gut. 1996;39(3):382–4.
21. Thawani SP, et al. Risk of neuropathy among 28,232 patients with biopsy-verified celiac disease. JAMA Neurol. 2015;72(7):806–11.
22. Reilly NR, et al. Increased risk of non-alcoholic fatty liver disease after diagnosis of celiac disease. J Hepatol. 2015;62(6):1405–11.
23. Ciacci C, et al. Effects of dietary treatment on bone mineral density in adults with celiac disease: factors predicting response. Am J Gastroenterol. 1997;92(6):992–6.
24. Kemppainen T, et al. Osteoporosis in adult patients with celiac disease. Bone. 1999;24(3):249–55.
25. Choi JM, et al. Increased prevalence of celiac disease in patients with unexplained infertility in the United States. J Reprod Med. 2011;56(5–6):199–203.
26. Ciacci C, et al. Celiac disease and pregnancy outcome. Am J Gastroenterol. 1996;91(4):718–22.
27. Nørgård B, et al. Birth outcomes of women with celiac disease: a nationwide historical cohort study. Am J Gastroenterol. 1999;94(9):2435–40.
28. Ludvigsson JF, Montgomery SM, Ekbom A. Celiac disease and risk of adverse fetal outcome: a population-based cohort study. Gastroenterology. 2005;129(2):454–63.
29. Anson O, Weizman Z, Zeevi N. Celiac disease: parental knowledge and attitudes of dietary compliance. Pediatrics. 1990;85(1):98–103.
30. Lamontagne P, West GE, Galibois I. Quebecers with celiac disease: analysis of dietary problems. Can J Diet Pract Res. 2001;62(4):175–81.
31. Løvik A, et al. Diet among patients with celiac disease. Do patients comply with a gluten-free diet? Tidsskr Nor Laegeforen. 1989;109(11):1153–5.
32. Abdulkarim AS, et al. Etiology of nonresponsive celiac disease: results of a systematic approach. Am J Gastroenterol. 2002;97(8):2016–21.
33. Leffler DA, et al. Etiologies and predictors of diagnosis in nonresponsive celiac disease. Clin Gastroenterol Hepatol. 2007;5(4):445–50.

34. Young-Fadok TM. Diverticulitis. N Engl J Med. 2018;379(17):1635–42.
35. Weizman AV, Nguyen GC. Diverticular disease: epidemiology and management. Can J Gastroenterol. 2011;25(7):385–9.
36. Strate LL, et al. Diverticular disease as a chronic illness: evolving epidemiologic and clinical insights. Am J Gastroenterol. 2012;107(10):1486–93.
37. Etzioni DA, et al. Diverticulitis in the United States: 1998-2005: changing patterns of disease and treatment. Ann Surg. 2009;249(2):210–7.
38. Yamada T. Textbook of gastroenterology. 5th ed. Chichester, West Sussex; Hoboken, NJ: Wiley-Blackwell; 2009.
39. Parks TG. Natural history of diverticular disease of the colon. A review of 521 cases. Br Med J. 1969;4(5684):639–42.
40. Strate LL, Morris AM. Epidemiology, pathophysiology, and treatment of diverticulitis. Gastroenterology. 2019;156(5):1282–1298.e1.
41. Chan CC, et al. Colonic diverticulosis in Hong Kong: distribution pattern and clinical significance. Clin Radiol. 1998;53(11):842–4.
42. Parks TG. Natural history of diverticular disease of the colon. Clin Gastroenterol. 1975;4(1):53–69.
43. Strate LL, et al. Obesity increases the risks of diverticulitis and diverticular bleeding. Gastroenterology. 2009;136(1):115–122.e1.
44. Hjern F, Wolk A, Håkansson N. Smoking and the risk of diverticular disease in women. Br J Surg. 2011;98(7):997–1002.
45. Strate LL, et al. Use of aspirin or nonsteroidal anti-inflammatory drugs increases risk for diverticulitis and diverticular bleeding. Gastroenterology. 2011;140(5):1427–33.
46. Aldoori WH, et al. A prospective study of diet and the risk of symptomatic diverticular disease in men. Am J Clin Nutr. 1994;60(5):757–64.
47. Strate LL, et al. Western dietary pattern increases, and prudent dietary pattern decreases, risk of incident diverticulitis in a prospective cohort study. Gastroenterology. 2017;152(5):1023–1030.e2.
48. Crowe FL, et al. Diet and risk of diverticular disease in Oxford cohort of European prospective investigation into cancer and nutrition (EPIC): prospective study of British vegetarians and non-vegetarians. BMJ. 2011;343:d4131.
49. Crowe FL, et al. Source of dietary fibre and diverticular disease incidence: a prospective study of UK women. Gut. 2014;63(9):1450–6.
50. Aldoori WH, et al. A prospective study of dietary fiber types and symptomatic diverticular disease in men. J Nutr. 1998;128(4):714–9.
51. Ley SH, et al. Associations between red meat intake and biomarkers of inflammation and glucose metabolism in women. Am J Clin Nutr. 2014;99(2):352–60.
52. Micha R, Michas G, Mozaffarian D. Unprocessed red and processed meats and risk of coronary artery disease and type 2 diabetes--an updated review of the evidence. Curr Atheroscler Rep. 2012;14(6):515–24.
53. Pan A, et al. Red meat consumption and risk of type 2 diabetes: 3 cohorts of US adults and an updated meta-analysis. Am J Clin Nutr. 2011;94(4):1088–96.
54. Kim E, Coelho D, Blachier F. Review of the association between meat consumption and risk of colorectal cancer. Nutr Res. 2013;33(12):983–94.
55. Cummings JH, et al. The effect of meat protein and dietary fiber on colonic function and metabolism. II. Bacterial metabolites in feces and urine. Am J Clin Nutr. 1979;32(10):2094–101.
56. Koh A, et al. From dietary fiber to host physiology: short-chain fatty acids as key bacterial metabolites. Cell. 2016;165(6):1332–45.
57. Qi L, et al. Whole-grain, bran, and cereal fiber intakes and markers of systemic inflammation in diabetic women. Diabetes Care. 2006;29(2):207–11.
58. Bertoia ML, et al. Changes in intake of fruits and vegetables and weight change in United States men and women followed for up to 24 years: analysis from three prospective cohort studies. PLoS Med. 2015;12(9):e1001878.
59. Horner JL. Natural history of diverticulosis of the colon. Am J Dig Dis. 1958;3(5):343–50.
60. Strate LL, et al. Nut, corn, and popcorn consumption and the incidence of diverticular disease. JAMA. 2008;300(8):907–14.
61. Jiang R, et al. Nut and seed consumption and inflammatory markers in the multi-ethnic study of atherosclerosis. Am J Epidemiol. 2006;163(3):222–31.
62. Folsom AR, Hong CP. Magnesium intake and reduced risk of colon cancer in a prospective study of women. Am J Epidemiol. 2006;163(3):232–5.
63. van den Brandt PA, et al. Magnesium intake and colorectal cancer risk in the Netherlands cohort study. Br J Cancer. 2007;96(3):510–3.
64. Thompson JS, et al. Risk of intestinal malignancy in patients with short bowel syndrome. JPEN J Parenter Enteral Nutr. 2017;41(4):562–5.
65. Pironi L, et al. ESPEN endorsed recommendations. Definition and classification of intestinal failure in adults. Clin Nutr. 2015;34(2):171–80.
66. Weaver LT, Austin S, Cole TJ. Small intestinal length: a factor essential for gut adaptation. Gut. 1991;32(11):1321–3.
67. Buchman AL, Scolapio J, Fryer J. AGA technical review on short bowel syndrome and intestinal transplantation. Gastroenterology. 2003;124(4):1111–34.
68. Pironi L, et al. Candidates for intestinal transplantation: a multicenter survey in Europe. Am J Gastroenterol. 2006;101(7):1633–43; quiz 1679.
69. Dowling RH, Booth CC. Functional compensation after small-bowel resection in man. Demonstration by direct measurement. Lancet. 1966;2(7455):146–7.
70. Buchman AL. Etiology and initial management of short bowel syndrome. Gastroenterology. 2006;130(2 Suppl 1):S5–S15.

71. Jeppesen PB, Mortensen PB. The influence of a preserved colon on the absorption of medium chain fat in patients with small bowel resection. Gut. 1998;43(4):478–83.
72. Messing B, et al. Long-term survival and parenteral nutrition dependence in adult patients with the short bowel syndrome. Gastroenterology. 1999;117(5):1043–50.
73. Wall EA. An overview of short bowel syndrome management: adherence, adaptation, and practical recommendations. J Acad Nutr Diet. 2013;113(9):1200–8.
74. Puello F, et al. Long-term outcomes with Teduglutide from a single center. JPEN J Parenter Enteral Nutr. 2020.
75. Jeppesen PB, Mortensen PB. Intestinal failure defined by measurements of intestinal energy and wet weight absorption. Gut. 2000;46(5):701–6.
76. Nordgaard I, Hansen BS, Mortensen PB. Colon as a digestive organ in patients with short bowel. Lancet. 1994;343(8894):373–6.
77. Fan S, et al. High prevalence of suboptimal vitamin D status and bone loss in adult short bowel syndrome even after weaning off parenteral nutrition. Nutr Clin Pract. 2017;32(2):258–65.
78. Rubin DT, et al. ACG clinical guideline: ulcerative colitis in adults. Am J Gastroenterol. 2019;114(3):384–413.
79. Haskey N, Gibson DL. An examination of diet for the maintenance of remission in inflammatory bowel disease. Nutrients. 2017;9(3).
80. Lichtenstein GR, et al. ACG clinical guideline: Management of Crohn's disease in adults. Am J Gastroenterol. 2018;113(4):481–517.
81. Holt DQ, Strauss BJ, Moore GT. Patients with inflammatory bowel disease and their treating clinicians have different views regarding diet. J Hum Nutr Diet. 2017;30(1):66–72.
82. Aghdassi E, et al. Adequacy of nutritional intake in a Canadian population of patients with Crohn's disease. J Am Diet Assoc. 2007;107(9):1575–80.
83. Limketkai BN, et al. Dietary interventions for induction and maintenance of remission in inflammatory bowel disease. Cochrane Database Syst Rev. 2019;2:CD012839.
84. Abraham C, Cho JH. Inflammatory bowel disease. N Engl J Med. 2009;361(21):2066–78.
85. Pfeffer-Gik T, Levine A. Dietary clues to the pathogenesis of Crohn's disease. Dig Dis. 2014;32(4):389–94.
86. Goens D, Micic D. Role of diet in the development and Management of Crohn's disease. Curr Gastroenterol Rep. 2020;22(4):19.
87. Martinez-Medina M, et al. Western diet induces dysbiosis with increased E coli in CEABAC10 mice, alters host barrier function favouring AIEC colonisation. Gut. 2014;63(1):116–24.
88. Agus A, et al. Western diet induces a shift in microbiota composition enhancing susceptibility to adherent-Invasive E. coli infection and intestinal inflammation. Sci Rep. 2016;6:19032.
89. Damas OM, Garces L, Abreu MT. Diet as adjunctive treatment for inflammatory bowel disease: review and update of the latest literature. Curr Treat Options Gastroenterol. 2019;17(2):313–25.
90. Ananthakrishnan AN, et al. High school diet and risk of Crohn's disease and ulcerative colitis. Inflamm Bowel Dis. 2015;21(10):2311–9.
91. Racine A, et al. Dietary patterns and risk of inflammatory bowel disease in Europe: results from the EPIC study. Inflamm Bowel Dis. 2016;22(2):345–54.
92. Borrelli O, et al. Polymeric diet alone versus corticosteroids in the treatment of active pediatric Crohn's disease: a randomized controlled open-label trial. Clin Gastroenterol Hepatol. 2006;4(6):744–53.
93. Wedrychowicz A, et al. Serum concentrations of VEGF and TGF-β1 during exclusive enteral nutrition in IBD. J Pediatr Gastroenterol Nutr. 2011;53(2):150–5.
94. Narula N, et al. Enteral nutritional therapy for induction of remission in Crohn's disease. Cochrane Database Syst Rev. 2018;4:CD000542.
95. Cohen-Dolev N, et al. Differences in outcomes over time with exclusive enteral nutrition compared with steroids in children with mild to moderate Crohn's disease: results from the GROWTH CD study. J Crohns Colitis. 2018;12(3):306–12.
96. Levine A, Sigall Boneh R, Wine E. Evolving role of diet in the pathogenesis and treatment of inflammatory bowel diseases. Gut. 2018;67(9):1726–38.
97. Yamamoto T, et al. Enteral nutrition for the maintenance of remission in Crohn's disease: a systematic review. Eur J Gastroenterol Hepatol. 2010;22(1):1–8.
98. Johnson T, et al. Treatment of active Crohn's disease in children using partial enteral nutrition with liquid formula: a randomised controlled trial. Gut. 2006;55(3):356–61.
99. Lee D, et al. Comparative effectiveness of nutritional and biological therapy in north American children with active Crohn's disease. Inflamm Bowel Dis. 2015;21(8):1786–93.
100. Sigall-Boneh R, et al. Partial enteral nutrition with a Crohn's disease exclusion diet is effective for induction of remission in children and young adults with Crohn's disease. Inflamm Bowel Dis. 2014;20(8):1353–60.
101. Sigall Boneh R, et al. Dietary therapy with the Crohn's disease exclusion diet is a successful strategy for induction of remission in children and adults failing biological therapy. J Crohns Colitis. 2017;11(10):1205–12.
102. Levine A, et al. Crohn's disease exclusion diet plus partial enteral nutrition induces sustained remission in a randomized controlled trial. Gastroenterology. 2019;157(2):440–450.e8.
103. Obih C, et al. Specific carbohydrate diet for pediatric inflammatory bowel disease in clinical practice within an academic IBD center. Nutrition. 2016;32(4):418–25.

104. Burgis JC, et al. Response to strict and liberalized specific carbohydrate diet in pediatric Crohn's disease. World J Gastroenterol. 2016;22(6):2111–7.
105. Suskind DL, et al. Clinical and fecal microbial changes with diet therapy in active inflammatory bowel disease. J Clin Gastroenterol. 2018;52(2):155–63.
106. Konijeti GG, et al. Efficacy of the autoimmune protocol diet for inflammatory bowel disease. Inflamm Bowel Dis. 2017;23(11):2054–60.
107. Major G, et al. Colon hypersensitivity to distension, rather than excessive gas production, produces carbohydrate-related symptoms in individuals with irritable bowel syndrome. Gastroenterology. 2017;152(1):124–133.e2.
108. Prince AC, et al. Fermentable carbohydrate restriction (low FODMAP diet) in clinical practice improves functional gastrointestinal symptoms in patients with inflammatory bowel disease. Inflamm Bowel Dis. 2016;22(5):1129–36.
109. Maagaard L, et al. Follow-up of patients with functional bowel symptoms treated with a low FODMAP diet. World J Gastroenterol. 2016;22(15):4009–19.
110. Pedersen N, et al. Low-FODMAP diet reduces irritable bowel symptoms in patients with inflammatory bowel disease. World J Gastroenterol. 2017;23(18):3356–66.
111. Zhan YL, Zhan YA, Dai SX. Is a low FODMAP diet beneficial for patients with inflammatory bowel disease? A meta-analysis and systematic review. Clin Nutr. 2018;37(1):123–9.
112. Halmos EP, et al. Consistent prebiotic effect on gut microbiota with altered FODMAP intake in patients with Crohn's disease: a randomised, controlled cross-over trial of well-defined diets. Clin Transl Gastroenterol. 2016;7:e164.
113. Olendzki BC, et al. An anti-inflammatory diet as treatment for inflammatory bowel disease: a case series report. Nutr J. 2014;13:5.
114. Grammatikopoulou MG, et al. Oral adjuvant curcumin therapy for attaining clinical remission in ulcerative colitis: a systematic review and meta-analysis of randomized controlled trials. Nutrients. 2018;10(11).
115. Lang A, et al. Curcumin in combination with Mesalamine induces remission in patients with mild-to-moderate ulcerative colitis in a randomized controlled trial. Clin Gastroenterol Hepatol. 2015;13(8):1444–9.e1.
116. Narula N, et al. Impact of high-dose vitamin D3 supplementation in patients with Crohn's disease in remission: a pilot randomized double-blind controlled study. Dig Dis Sci. 2017;62(2):448–55.
117. Lovell RM, Ford AC. Global prevalence of and risk factors for irritable bowel syndrome: a meta-analysis. Clin Gastroenterol Hepatol. 2012;10(7):712–721.e4.
118. Lovell RM, Ford AC. Effect of gender on prevalence of irritable bowel syndrome in the community: systematic review and meta-analysis. Am J Gastroenterol. 2012;107(7):991–1000.
119. Simrén M, et al. Abnormal propagation pattern of duodenal pressure waves in the irritable bowel syndrome (IBS) [correction of (IBD)]. Dig Dis Sci. 2000;45(11):2151–61.
120. Schmidt T, et al. Ambulatory 24-hour jejunal motility in diarrhea-predominant irritable bowel syndrome. Scand J Gastroenterol. 1996;31(6):581–9.
121. Bouin M, et al. Rectal distention testing in patients with irritable bowel syndrome: sensitivity, specificity, and predictive values of pain sensory thresholds. Gastroenterology. 2002;122(7):1771–7.
122. Kassinen A, et al. The fecal microbiota of irritable bowel syndrome patients differs significantly from that of healthy subjects. Gastroenterology. 2007;133(1):24–33.
123. Saito YA, et al. The genetics of irritable bowel syndrome. Clin Gastroenterol Hepatol. 2005;3(11):1057–65.
124. Zanini B, et al. Incidence of post-infectious irritable bowel syndrome and functional intestinal disorders following a water-borne viral gastroenteritis outbreak. Am J Gastroenterol. 2012;107(6):891–9.
125. Chey WD, Kurlander J, Eswaran S. Irritable bowel syndrome: a clinical review. JAMA. 2015;313(9):949–58.
126. Böhn L, et al. Self-reported food-related gastrointestinal symptoms in IBS are common and associated with more severe symptoms and reduced quality of life. Am J Gastroenterol. 2013;108(5):634–41.
127. Sanders DS, et al. Association of adult coeliac disease with irritable bowel syndrome: a case-control study in patients fulfilling ROME II criteria referred to secondary care. Lancet. 2001;358(9292):1504–8.
128. Chey WD. Diet and irritable bowel syndrome. Gastroenterol Hepatol (N Y). 2018;14(5):309–12.
129. Ford AC, et al. American College of Gastroenterology monograph on management of irritable bowel syndrome. Am J Gastroenterol. 2018;113(Suppl 2):1–18.
130. Bellini M, et al. Bioelectrical impedance vector analysis in patients with irritable bowel syndrome on a low FODMAP diet: a pilot study. Tech Coloproctol. 2017;21(6):451–9.
131. Werlang ME, Palmer WC, Lacy BE. Irritable bowel syndrome and dietary interventions. Gastroenterol Hepatol (N Y). 2019;15(1):16–26.
132. Biesiekierski JR, et al. Gluten causes gastrointestinal symptoms in subjects without celiac disease: a double-blind randomized placebo-controlled trial. Am J Gastroenterol. 2011;106(3):508–14. quiz 515.
133. Vazquez-Roque MI, et al. A controlled trial of gluten-free diet in patients with irritable bowel syndrome-diarrhea: effects on bowel frequency and intestinal function. Gastroenterology. 2013;144(5):903–911.e3.
134. Biesiekierski JR, et al. No effects of gluten in patients with self-reported non-celiac gluten sensitivity after dietary reduction of fermentable, poorly absorbed, short-chain carbohydrates. Gastroenterology. 2013;145(2):320-8.e1–3.

135. Skodje GI, et al. Fructan, rather than gluten, induces symptoms in patients with self-reported non-celiac gluten sensitivity. Gastroenterology. 2018;154(3):529–539.e2.
136. Micic D, Rao VL, Rubin DT. Clinical approach to lactose intolerance. JAMA. 2019.
137. Zhu Y, et al. Bloating and distention in irritable bowel syndrome: the role of gas production and visceral sensation after lactose ingestion in a population with lactase deficiency. Am J Gastroenterol. 2013;108(9):1516–25.
138. Böhmer CJ, Tuynman HA. The effect of a lactose-restricted diet in patients with a positive lactose tolerance test, earlier diagnosed as irritable bowel syndrome: a 5-year follow-up study. Eur J Gastroenterol Hepatol. 2001;13(8):941–4.
139. Parker TJ, et al. Irritable bowel syndrome: is the search for lactose intolerance justified? Eur J Gastroenterol Hepatol. 2001;13(3):219–25.
140. Böhmer CJ, Tuynman HA. The clinical relevance of lactose malabsorption in irritable bowel syndrome. Eur J Gastroenterol Hepatol. 1996;8(10):1013–6.
141. McKenzie YA, et al. British dietetic association systematic review and evidence-based practice guidelines for the dietary management of irritable bowel syndrome in adults (2016 update). J Hum Nutr Diet. 2016;29(5):549–75.
142. Szilagyi A, Ishayek N. Lactose intolerance, dairy avoidance, and treatment options. Nutrients. 2018;10(12).
143. Tursi A, et al. Prevalence and clinical presentation of subclinical/silent celiac disease in adults: an analysis on a 12-year observation. Hepato-Gastroenterology. 2001;48(38):462–4.
144. Haapalahti M, et al. Nutritional status in adolescents and young adults with screen-detected celiac disease. J Pediatr Gastroenterol Nutr. 2005;40(5):566–70.
145. Deora V, et al. Serum vitamins and minerals at diagnosis and follow-up in children with celiac disease. J Pediatr Gastroenterol Nutr. 2017;65(2):185–9.
146. Dahele A, Ghosh S. Vitamin B12 deficiency in untreated celiac disease. Am J Gastroenterol. 2001;96(3):745–50.
147. Burger JPW, et al. Low yield for routine laboratory checks in follow-up of coeliac disease. J Gastrointestin Liver Dis. 2018;27(3):233–9.
148. Wierdsma NJ, et al. Vitamin and mineral deficiencies are highly prevalent in newly diagnosed celiac disease patients. Nutrients. 2013;5(10):3975–92.
149. Eswaran SL, et al. A randomized controlled trial comparing the low FODMAP diet vs. modified NICE guidelines in US adults with IBS-D. Am J Gastroenterol. 2016;111(12):1824–32.
150. Böhn L, et al. Diet low in FODMAPs reduces symptoms of irritable bowel syndrome as well as traditional dietary advice: a randomized controlled trial. Gastroenterology. 2015;149(6):1399–1407.e2.
151. McIntosh K, et al. FODMAPs alter symptoms and the metabolome of patients with IBS: a randomised controlled trial. Gut. 2017;66(7):1241–51.
152. Staudacher HM, et al. Fermentable carbohydrate restriction reduces luminal bifidobacteria and gastrointestinal symptoms in patients with irritable bowel syndrome. J Nutr. 2012;142(8):1510–8.
153. Staudacher HM, et al. A diet low in FODMAPs reduces symptoms in patients with irritable bowel syndrome and a probiotic restores Bifidobacterium species: a randomized controlled trial. Gastroenterology. 2017;153(4):936–47.
154. Halmos EP, et al. A diet low in FODMAPs reduces symptoms of irritable bowel syndrome. Gastroenterology. 2014;146(1):67–75.e5.
155. Hustoft TN, et al. Effects of varying dietary content of fermentable short-chain carbohydrates on symptoms, fecal microenvironment, and cytokine profiles in patients with irritable bowel syndrome. Neurogastroenterol Motil. 2017;29(4).

7 Pancreas and Hepatobiliary Tract

Raj Shah, Sagarika Satyavada, and Perica Davitkov

Acute Pancreatitis (AP): Introduction, Pathophysiology, and Clinical Presentations

The worldwide incidence of acute pancreatitis is estimated to be 34 per 100,000 person-years and is rising. The obesity epidemic may be playing a role in the rise given the concomitant rise in incidence of associated obesity-related complications such as cholelithiasis, hypertriglyceridemia, and diabetes. It is also one of the most common gastrointestinal diseases implicated in hospitalizations and costs the US healthcare system up to $9.3 billion every year. Despite the increasing incidence of acute pancreatitis, mortality related to this condition has decreased in the last 10 years from 1.6% to 0.8% [2].

The pathophysiology of AP involves the activation of trypsinogen to trypsin within the acinar cell rather than the duct lumen. This leads to localized destruction of the pancreas and a systemic inflammatory response. Common etiologies include gallstone pancreatitis, which elevates ductal pressures, and alcohol abuse, which may disrupt calcium homeostasis. The resulting inflammatory cascade induces systemic manifestations such as endothelial dysfunction that can eventually lead to multi-organ system failure. Although alcohol and gallstones are the most common causes of acute pancreatitis, genetics may also play a role in pathogenesis and can lead to recurrent episodes. The genes implicated are those that also affect trypsin activation, i.e., cystic fibrosis transmembrane conductance regulator (CFTR), serine protease 1 (PRSS1), serine protease inhibitor Kazal type 1 (SPINK1), and chymotrypsin C (CTRC) [3].

Clinical Presentation

The majority of patients present with severe acute epigastric pain with associated nausea and vomiting [4]. Along with epigastric abdominal tenderness, hypoactive bowel sounds with abdominal distension may also be noted on physical examination owing to the presence of ileus. Additionally, fever, tachypnea, hypoxemia, or hypotension may be seen [5]. When it is severe, patients can present with dyspnea due to either diaphragmatic inflammation, pleural effusions, or acute respiratory distress syndrome (ARDS) [6]. In a small

R. Shah (✉) · S. Satyavada
Department of Gastroenterology and Hepatology, Digestive Health Institute, University Hospitals Cleveland Medical Center, Case Western Reserve University School of Medicine, Cleveland, OH, USA
e-mail: raj.shah@uhhospitals.org; Sagarika.Satyavada@UHhospitals.org

P. Davitkov
Department of Gastroenterology and Hepatology, Digestive Health Institute, VA Northeast Ohio Healthcare System, Case Western Reserve University School of Medicine, Cleveland, OH, USA
e-mail: pxd97@case.edu

C. Newberry et al. (eds.), *Nutrition, Weight, and Digestive Health*,
https://doi.org/10.1007/978-3-030-94953-2_7

percentage of patients, ecchymosis may be seen either in the periumbilical or flank region, termed Cullen's sign and Grey Turner's sign, respectively, indicating retroperitoneal bleeding [7, 8]. The diagnosis of acute pancreatitis is based on at least two of three following criteria: classic abdominal pain, amylase or lipase greater than three times the upper limit of normal, and evidence of pancreatitis on radiographic imaging. Lipase values are preferred over amylase given the enhanced specificity of the test [9–11].

Acute Pancreatitis: Nutritional Management

Research over the last several years has resulted in a shift in nutritional management from parenteral to enteral nutrition in the treatment of acute pancreatitis [12]. Due to the catabolic nature of AP, patients with severe pancreatitis are particularly at risk for nutritional deficiencies [13]. Comorbid conditions such as alcohol use disorder place patients with mild or moderate pancreatitis also at risk since these patients are frequently malnourished [1, 14]. The Nutritional Risk Screening 2002 (NRS-2002) is a scoring system commonly used in hospitalized patients that may be helpful in AP; however, such scoring systems have not been validated in this population [1].

Based on moderate quality of evidence, the American Gastroenterological Association (AGA) 2018 guidelines gave a strong recommendation for oral feeding as tolerated within 24 hours over nothing by mouth as there was a higher risk of interventions for necrosis associated with delayed feeding when compared to early feeding [11]. Basing the initiation of oral feeds on serum lipase levels has not been shown to improve postprandial abdominal pain [15]. When oral feeding cannot be tolerated, enteral nutrition is recommended over parenteral nutrition (PN) as this has been hypothesized to maintain the integrity of the gut and reduce bacterial translocation [11, 16]. Meta-analysis has shown a decrease in death, infection rates, multi-organ system failure, and need for operations when using enteral nutrition compared to initial use of total PN [13]. Timing of enteral nutrition is usually within 24 to 72 hours of presentation. With regard to the type of enteral nutrition, a standard polymeric formula is recommended; however, semi-elemental formulas may also be safe and well tolerated [1]. No significant differences have been shown in the ability to tolerate, complication rates, or mortality with the use of nasojejunal compared to nasogastric routes of feeding in those with severe AP [17–19]. In patients who develop intolerance to nasogastric feeding, due to delayed gastric emptying or gastric outlet obstruction, nasojejunal feeding may be preferred [1]. Parenteral nutrition may be used when patients are not able to tolerate oral or enteral feeding. Examples of these scenarios include bowel obstruction, ileus, or abdominal compartment syndrome [20]. In severe AP, if intra-abdominal pressure is less than 20 mmHg, then nasojejunal feeding may be cautiously initiated with frequent monitoring of clinical condition with adjustment of rate accordingly. However, if greater than 20 mmHg or with abdominal compartment syndrome, parenteral nutrition should be started with enteral nutrition temporarily held. It is estimated that about 10–20% of patients with AP will go on to develop pancreatic necrosis which may necessitate necrosectomy. When minimally invasive necrosectomy is planned, oral food intake or enteral (when oral food cannot be tolerated) can be started within 24 hours of the procedure. It should be noted that specific data on nutrition-related outcomes are not present in this cohort of patients, and thus the aforementioned guidance is based on a consensus recommendation. In severe forms of compartment syndrome which require surgical intervention with decompressive laparostomy, patients are in a hypermetabolic state with high nitrogen losses due to open abdomen [21, 22]. Several studies have suggested that enteral nutrition can be successfully started in these patients and may be associated with higher fascial closure rates [23].

In regard to immunonutrition therapy, it has been evaluated in AP and has shown value in decreasing complications and reducing hospital stay, but these results are limited to glutamine, and the studies assessed may have a significant risk of bias [24, 25]. Thus, glutamine can be considered in parenteral form at 0.20 g/kg per day when enteral nutrition is not feasible [1]. Probiotics have been evaluated in patients with AP; however, no benefits have been derived from their use either on infection rate, length of stay, operation rate, or mortality.

Chronic Pancreatitis: Introduction, Pathophysiology, and Clinical Presentation

Chronic pancreatitis (CP) can be defined as progressive inflammatory changes resulting in fibrosis of the pancreas and permanent damage which can lead to exocrine and/or endocrine dysfunction [26–30]. The prevalence of this condition has been reported to be between 13 and 52 per 100,000. Alcohol is the most common cause of chronic pancreatitis and can also make the pancreas vulnerable when exposed to other insults such as smoking and in those patients with a genetic predisposition to pancreatitis. Genetic etiologies of chronic pancreatitis include mutations in the PRSS1 and SPINK1 genes. In patients with idiopathic CP, CFTR gene mutations have been reported to be commonly seen. While medications may be the culprit in acute pancreatitis, they do not play a role in CP [31]. Less commonly, CP may also be seen in those with autoimmune pancreatitis (AIP), particularly type 2 over type 1 [31, 32]. Pancreatic ductal abnormalities such as inflammatory strictures or tumors may lead to CP. On the other hand, the congenital anatomic variant where the larger dorsal pancreas drains through the minor papilla, pancreatic divisum, is a rare cause of CP. Its presence with CFTR mutation may increase the risk of developing CP [33]. The diagnosis is made in patients with clinical symptoms of abdominal pain, exocrine or endocrine insufficiency, and specific features on imaging. Computed tomography (CT) or magnetic resonance imaging (MRI) may be used as first-line diagnostic testing. Alternatively, endoscopic ultrasound (EUS) is pursued if the former modes are not able to establish the diagnosis of CP. Owing to cost, invasiveness, availability, and objectivity, EUS is reserved for cases of uncertainty in diagnosis [30, 34]. Pancreatic exocrine insufficiency (PEI) results when most pancreatic function (>90%) is lost and clinical signs and symptoms include steatorrhea, azotorrhea, vitamin deficiencies, and weight loss [35, 36]. In general, pancreatic function tests such as fecal elastase, secretin stimulation test, or ^{13}C-mixed triglyceride test are not sufficient in establishing the diagnosis of CP; rather their roles are supportive since no clinical trials or systematic reviews/meta-analyses exist to recommend their routine use [37–40].

Nutritional Assessment and Malnutrition

The daily caloric intake of lipids is up to 40% in the Western diet. Lipase is secreted in small amounts from gastric and salivary glands, but it comes primarily from the pancreas. Since lipase is not secreted by the intestinal brush border, pancreatic lipase is essential to lipid digestion and requires an acidic environment. Bicarbonate is reduced in CP causing the intraduodenal pH to fall to <4 potentiating lipase breakdown and resulting in fat malabsorption [41].

Malnutrition is a late manifestation of CP, and causes include pancreatic insufficiency and common comorbid conditions: alcohol abuse, smoking, abdominal pain leading to decreased oral intake, and diabetes mellitus [1]. Weight loss can lead to sarcopenia, which may be present in up to 17% of CP patients, possibly resulting in reduced functional capacity, reduction in quality of life, and decreased survival [42, 43]. Pancreatic insufficiency can lead to loss of fat-soluble vitamins, A, D, E, and K, increasing the risk of bone loss and the development of osteoporosis. Resting energy expenditure (REE) is variable in CP; however, small studies have shown that it may be increased in those that are underweight since weight loss coincides with increased metabolism. However, the exact etiology and mechanism for the increased metabolism is still unclear [44].

Nutritional assessment in CP should be assessed in a multimodal way to identify micronutrient deficiencies, sarcopenia, or simple malnutrition. The categories evaluated may include anthropometry, biochemistry, symptoms, and body composition. Examples of anthropometric assessment include change in body weight, handgrip strength, or mid-arm muscle circumference. Biochemical assessment consists of measurements of fat-soluble vitamins, parathyroid hormone, trace elements (magnesium, selenium, zinc), anemia (B12, folate), and glycemic control (hemoglobin A1c and blood glucose) [1, 45].

Nutritional Management

Micronutrient Deficiencies

Deficiency in each of the fat-soluble vitamins varies, but the most prevalent is vitamin D and vitamin K deficiency [46–49]. Patients with CP with or without proven PEI are at risk for deficiencies in these vitamins [46, 50]. These vitamins should be monitored and supplemented in CP. Other trace elements such as zinc, selenium, and magnesium may also be low, and evaluation and supplementation should be considered [51]. Alcoholism may coexist in a cohort of CP patients; thus, thiamine deficiency should be assessed and replaced as needed [52]. Vitamin D deficiency, smoking, and minimal physical activity contribute to the development of osteoporosis in CP, and dual-energy X-ray absorptiometry (DEXA) scan can be used to identify those who are at high risk [26, 53]. In addition to recommending the avoidance of smoking and increasing physical activity, periodic testing for vitamin D deficiency and calcium and vitamin D supplementation should be considered [30, 54]. It has been suggested that DEXA scan can be repeated every 2 years in those with osteopenia, but no specific recommendations exist for those with osteoporosis in this population [26].

Diet

While in the past, low-fat diet was encouraged, this dogma is changing to recommending a balanced diet and avoiding excessive restriction of fat [26, 55–58]. High-fat diets may be associated with earlier diagnosis and persistent abdominal pain. No significant association has been found with development of PEI, diarrhea, or diabetes [59]. Modest dietary fat restriction can be considered if steatorrhea is not well controlled or abdominal pain is persistent [36, 57]. The use of medium-chain triglycerides (MCTs) in PEI has been proposed since these are less dependent on lipase for absorption compared to long-chain fatty acids. However, MCTs have not shown any added benefit with concomitant pancreatic enzyme use, have a lower energy density, and are associated with adverse effects such as pain and diarrhea, limiting use [36, 48, 60]. In regard to a high-fiber diet, it is possible this may lead to increased fecal fat losses due to inhibition of pancreatic enzyme replacement therapy (PERT); however, this is based on limited and weak evidence [36, 57, 61]. Practitioners may consider suggesting lower-fiber diets to patients with excessive weight loss or symptoms [1]. Oral nutritional supplements may be beneficial in a subset of patients to improve overall caloric intake, but no single formula is recommended in CP [36]. Enteral nutrition may be considered in those not responding to oral nutrition and is used in up to 5% of CP patients. Clinical scenarios where oral nutritional supplementation may be insufficient can be seen in those with pain, delayed gastric emptying, and persistent nausea, vomiting, and weight loss [36, 62]. Nasogastric or nasojejunal tubes can be considered, with limited data on the type of enteral formulation to use; however, semi-elemental or elemental options may be best suited for jejunal nutrition [63]. Parenteral nutrition (PN) may be used when enteral nutrition is unsuccessful. Enteral nutrition is preferred when feasible as it preserves mucosal immune function [11]. The use of PN increases the risk of catheter-associated infections but may be unavoidable in cases where a tube cannot be placed successfully such as in cases complicated by obstruction, stenosis, and fistulizing disease [36, 58, 64]. It is generally used as a short-term modality of nutrition in CP [1].

Pancreatic Enzyme Replacement Therapy (PERT)

PERT is used in CP and PEI to promote weight gain via enhanced macronutrient and fat-soluble vitamin absorption as well as to improve quality of life. It should be started when clinical, anthropometric, and/or biochemical signs of malnutrition are present [30, 36, 51, 65–67]. The coefficient of fat absorption (CFA) is the outcome that the FDA utilizes for approval of these products. Normal CFA is >93%, and clinically meaningful decrease in fat is 30% or more, particularly in those with CFA <40% prior to the use of PERT. Enzyme use may reduce fecal fat, thereby improving weight gain and quality of life; however, it may not be useful in treating abdominal pain [30, 68]. The enzymes can be taken before, during, or after meals as no significant difference has been observed in fat malabsorption and timing of administration, except with enteric coated mini-microsphere-type enzymes where dosing just after or with a meal compared to before the meal may enhance fat digestion [69]. Vitamin supplementation with PERT may additionally improve serum vitamin levels [70]. With regard to monitoring efficacy of PERT, symptom improvement and improvement in nutritional parameters (anthropometric or biochemical) are often used [71, 72]. If these parameters have not improved, then compliance may be poor, and pancreatic function tests, such as fecal fat, may be obtained [73]. Other considerations for ineffectiveness include PERT dosage. The usual dose is 20,000–50,000 pharmacology units (PhU) of lipase with meals and half the dosage with snacks [73]. A recent guideline suggests ensuring adequate dosage which may be 40,000–50,000 USP units of lipase with each meal [30]. Dosing for children is outside the scope of this chapter. However, high doses should be avoided in children, specifically, as there is risk of fibrosing colonopathy [74]. The addition of a proton pump inhibitor (PPI) is thought to improve fat digestion, but this is controversial and has not been shown to consistently decrease fat malabsorption except in non-enteric coated formulations of enzymes [75]. When symptoms are persistent despite adequate doses of PERT, small intestinal bacterial overgrowth may be the culprit, as this condition can be present in up to 15% of patients with CP [76].

Role of Surgery

The surgical treatment of chronic pancreatitis can range from endoscopic sphincterotomy and/or pancreatic duct stenting to surgical drainage procedures such as pancreaticoduodenectomy and Frey, Beger, Puestow, and Berne procedure. For pain in obstructive chronic pancreatitis, surgery is recommended when first-line endoscopic pancreatic drainage options are unsuccessful. Anatomic changes causing changes in bile transit and extent of pancreatic resection should be considered, and postoperative PERT may be required and/or diabetes mellitus may develop [30, 64]. Additionally, some centers may perform total pancreatectomy with islet cell autotransplantation to prevent diabetes mellitus. Up to 40% of patients receiving islet cell autotransplantation are independent of insulin, having implications on nutrition. Those that do not achieve insulin independence require small amounts of insulin to achieve appropriate glycemic control [77].

Post-cholecystectomy (CCY): Introduction, Pathophysiology, and Clinical Presentation

Gallstone disease is a significant health concern in the American population affecting up to 10–15% of adults. Surgery for cholelithiasis has increased since 1950 with further increases after 1989 due to the introduction of laparoscopic cholecystectomy. In the United States, cholecystectomy is one of the most commonly performed elective abdominal surgeries [78]. While the gallbladder is not a vital organ, it plays an important role in digestion, and its removal results in nutritional consequences. The post-cholecystectomy state has been associated with altered gastrointestinal motility leading to diarrhea, possible changes to glut flora, and metabolic effects [79]. These consequences can present with diarrhea, abdominal pain, and bloating, termed post-cholecystectomy syndrome occurring in 5–40% of people [79, 80]. Additionally, patients are at risk for an increased body mass index and fat-soluble vitamin deficiencies [79].

The liver makes 1000 milliliters of bile every day, and bile acids are the final products of cholesterol metabolism. These are involved in fat digestion but may also play a part in regulating glucose metabolism and energy expenditure. The bile is stored in the gallbladder until hormones such as cholecystokinin and fibroblast growth factor (FGF) stimulate gallbladder contraction [79]. Cholecystectomy alters this physiology by causing unregulated secretion of secondary bile acids resulting in altered gastrointestinal motility and diarrhea. Metabolic consequences such as the onset of non-alcoholic fatty liver disease (NAFLD) may occur from the increased rate of bile acid enterohepatic circulation after cholecystectomy [79].

Post-cholecystectomy (CCY): Nutritional Management

Immediately post-cholecystectomy, a low-fat diet is recommended for two reasons. Lipid digestion requires more bile acids than can be provided in the acute absence of a gallbladder leading to a decrease in gastric emptying and stasis-associated gastritis. Additionally, diarrhea can occur from bile salt irritation of the colon. Cholestyramine, a bile acid sequestrant, may be used to mitigate these effects. Simultaneous administration of fat-soluble vitamins (A, D, E, K) may be useful if using this medication as cholestyramine can affect absorption [79]. The post-cholecystectomy syndrome may occur more often with certain food choices such as animal protein, cholesterol, or eggs and less so with vegetable intake 3 months after cholecystectomy, but future clinical trials are needed to confirm this relationship [81].

Chronic Liver Disease: Introduction

The most common causes of cirrhosis are viral hepatitis (chronic hepatitis B and C), non-alcoholic steatohepatitis (NASH), and alcohol-related liver disease [82, 83]. Less common causes include genetic causes of liver disease such as autoimmune hepatitis, primary biliary cholangitis, primary sclerosing cholangitis, Wilson's disease, and alpha-1 antitrypsin deficiency [83–85].

The prevalence of chronic liver disease has changed over time due to advances in treatment in hepatitis C and the rise in obesity. In the United States, the prevalence of chronic hepatitis B and alcoholic liver disease has remained largely stable from 1988 to 2016 at 0.3–0.4% and 0.8–1.0%, respectively. Presumably due to advances in hepatitis C treatment, the prevalence of chronic hepatitis C has decreased from 1.6% to 0.9% during this time period. Conversely, the prevalence of NAFLD has increased from 20% to 31.9% [86]. Globally, in 2017, there were 10.6 million cases of decompensated cirrhosis and 112 million cases of compensated cirrhosis [87].

Symptoms of compensated cirrhosis may be nonspecific such as anorexia, weight loss, or fatigue, while those with decompensated cirrhosis may present with variceal bleeding, ascites, or hepatic encephalopathy (HE) [83]. The prevalence of hepatic encephalopathy may be higher in cirrhotic patients with malnourishment; however, this is controversial [88]. Physical exam findings of progressive cirrhosis include jaundice, spider angiomata, splenomegaly, ascites, caput medusa, or asterixis [83]. The pathophysiology of hepatic encephalopathy is complex involving factors such as ammonia, cytokines, and GABA with recent studies also citing relationships with microbiota and aromatic amino acids. In cirrhosis, ammonia-rich blood is shunted to the systemic circulation and crosses the blood-brain barrier where glutamine synthetase converts ammonia and glutamate to glutamine. Excess glutamine creates an osmotic gradient leading to swelling of astrocytes, which contributes to cerebral dysfunction. Intestinal dysbiosis may also contribute to HE as cirrhotic patients tend to have increased *Bacteroides*/*Firmicutes* ratio and increased *Enterobacteriaceae*. Treatment with lactulose and rifaximin results in the decrease in ammonia load and/or production and alteration in microbiota composition. Malnutrition also plays a key role in the pathophysiology of HE since the muscle is an important site for nitrogen metabolism. Malnutrition and sarcopenia occur in cirrhotic patients for numerous reasons such as anorexia, early satiety, and ascites, and muscle loss is associated with an increased risk of hepatic encephalopathy and overall mortality [89].

Nutritional Considerations in Chronic Liver Disease (CLD)

Malnutrition is a prevalent condition in patients with liver cirrhosis, estimated to occur in about 20–50% of patients. It is often recognized more in those with decompensated cirrhosis than in compensated cirrhosis and is associated with progression to liver failure [90]. Malnutrition in cirrhosis relates to the accelerated loss of both fat and muscle. Excessive muscle loss is implicated in sarcopenia [91]. Severe malnutrition is associated with complications of chronic liver disease including infections, hepatic encephalopathy (HE), and ascites [92–94]. Furthermore, nutrition assessment in cirrhotic patients serves a prognostic role in cirrhosis. An example of a nutritional assessment tool is the Royal Free Hospital-Nutritional Prioritizing Tool which may be useful to predict disease progression and outcomes [95]. In addition to undernutrition, obesity is also observed in cirrhotic and post-transplant patients. When obesity is seen in the setting of enhanced skeletal muscle loss, it is called sarcopenic obesity [96–98].

Patients diagnosed with cirrhosis are at increased risk of malnutrition secondary to a variety of factors. Cirrhosis is a state of hastened starvation where metabolism changes from using carbohydrates as its primary fuel to fatty acids (i.e., ketosis). In this state, protein synthesis is also decreased, and gluconeogenesis from amino acids is increased. This process requires proteolysis and subsequent breakdown of muscle tissue, contributing to sarcopenia. External factors such as parageusia, fasting, and decreased absorption from impaired gut motility due to portal hypertension compound the state of accelerated starvation in this population [99–103].

Decompensated cirrhosis may affect REE as suggested by a small study where ascites was shown to increase rates of energy expenditure [104]. However, there have been conflicting results in regard to the correlation between REE and different levels of disease severity and fluid retention [105–107]. The process of gluconeogenesis may also be implicated, as this is an energy-dense process [99, 102, 108, 109].

The general daily caloric requirements in liver cirrhosis are at least 35 kcal/kg/day [110, 111]. This is in comparison to the average daily caloric requirement in a healthy individual of 25–35 kcal/kg/day [112]. It is thought that frequent feeding can prevent accelerated starvation and proteolysis by reducing fasting time, for example, by implementing an early morning breakfast and a late evening snack [113]. A snack containing protein is recommended. Protein intake in cirrhosis has been previously controversial, particularly as a precipitant of hepatic encephalopathy (HE). However, studies have shown that normal to high-protein intake does not precipitate HE [114, 115]. Ideal protein intake in cirrhotic patients is 1.2–1.5 g/kg of body weight/day, which is also higher than the standard recommendation of 0.8–1.0 g/kg body weight/day [100, 111, 116].

Nutrition supplementation plays an integral role in the management of various stages of liver disease. Micronutrient deficiencies are common in cirrhosis, namely, zinc, vitamin A, and selenium. Supplementation with zinc or replacement therapy with vitamin A may improve dysgeusia and thereby improve nutritional state [117, 118].

Malnutrition in Patients Undergoing Liver Transplantation and Liver Surgery

Malnourished cirrhotic patients have a high risk of post-op morbidity and mortality; however, the use of ERAS (enhanced recovery after surgery) protocols which focus on avoidance of prolonged pre-operative fasting with the addition of carbohydrate loading 2 hour prior to surgery, early postoperative feeding, and mobilization postoperatively may improve morbidity and length of stay [119–124]. A goal of 30–35 kcal/kg/day and a protein intake 1.2–1.5 grams/kg/day should be achieved preoperatively. Standard enteral supplementation can be used since a specific regimen has not been shown to be superior with regard to morbidity and mortality. Targets for obese patients include a reduced intake of 25 kcal/kg body weight/day and enhanced protein intake of 2.0–2.5 g/kg body weight/day [88, 110, 125, 126]. After liver transplantation, enteral nutrition or oral diet should be started within 12–24 hours [88, 125, 126]. Early nutrition postoperatively may reduce complication rate, length of mechanical ventilation, and stay in intensive care unit [88, 126].

Management of Specific Disease States

Chronic Cholestasis

Cholestasis is defined by impaired bile flow or production; however, bile is needed for the digestion of macronutrients, especially fat. This condition is common in patients with infections, infiltrative liver disease, and congenital diseases such as primary biliary cirrhosis [127, 128]. Clinically, cholestasis presents as jaundice, dark urine, pruritus, and steatorrhea. Since bile flow is impaired, fat is not absorbed, including fat-soluble vitamins, A, D, E, and K. If bilirubin levels are >2 mg/dl, then nutritional modifications should be considered [128]. A fat-restricted diet of <20 grams/day can be useful in managing symptoms of steatorrhea; however, medium-chain triglycerides (MCTs) can be added to the diet to prevent weight loss and improve tolerability [128, 129]. The bile is not required for absorption of MCTs as they are absorbed via the portal system by passive diffusion [128]. A fat-restricted diet lasting more than 3 weeks will also require replacement of essential fatty acids from sources such as flaxseed, sunflower, or corn oils to avoid deficiencies [128, 129]. Metabolic bone disease can result from poor absorption of vitamin D and the direct effect of hyperbilirubinemia on osteoblast function, though this mechanism is not well elucidated. DEXA scans should be done every 2 to 4 years with supplementation of calcium and vitamin D in those who require it [128, 130]. In chronic cholestasis conditions, all fat-soluble vitamins should be checked and then repleted appropriately [128].

Hepatic Encephalopathy

Malnourished cirrhotic patients tend to suffer more from hepatic encephalopathy (HE) compared to those who are not. An association between HE and zinc deficiency has been described in case reports; however, randomized controlled trials (RCTs) have not shown marked clinical benefit with zinc supplementation [131–133].

Sarcopenia is an independent risk factor for encephalopathy after transjugular intrahepatic portosystemic shunt (TIPS) placement as the muscle plays a crucial role in ammonia removal via synthesis of glutamine [134–136]. Protein restriction was previously thought to be helpful in prevention of HE; however, this dogma has been debunked by a number of studies [137–140]. Protein recommendations for cirrhotic patients are 1.2–1.5 g/kg of body weight/day. A randomized controlled trial by Cordoba et al. showed that protein restriction may increase catabolism and has no benefit on the course of HE when compared to normal protein diets [111, 141]. If the patient has refractory HE, then a lower protein goal of 0.8–1.0 g/kg/day may be considered [142].

The branched-chain amino acids (BCAA), valine, leucine, and isoleucine, act as substrates for protein synthesis and regulate nutrient pathways in metabolism [143]. Dysregulation in metabolic pathways can result in hepatic encephalopathy as evident in patients with liver disease. The ratio of BCAA to aromatic amino acids (AAA) may be decreased with BCAA supplementation allowing for less aromatic amino acids to cross the blood-brain barrier. Supplementation is hypothesized to also improve the detoxification of ammonia. A systematic review and meta-analysis showed oral BCAA seems to have benefit on HE but may be associated with nausea and diarrhea. No high-quality evidence could be found to support the use for or against BCAA in regard to the outcomes of mortality, quality of life, or nutritional status, and further trials are needed to guide therapy [144].

Alcoholic Steatohepatitis

Malnourished alcoholic steatohepatitis (ASH) patients have poorer survival compared to non-malnourished patients [145]. Deficiency in trace elements is expected given poor oral intake in patients with severe ASH. Common micronutrient deficiencies include B vitamins, zinc, vitamin D, and thiamine. High-quality evidence is lacking in regard to whether screening and replenishment of all micronutrient deficiencies result in clinical improvement; however, guidance documents have suggested in doing so [103, 146].

Supplemental oral nutrition may be beneficial for improving infection rates. No definitive benefit on mortality for this population has been found, and further trials for both outcomes are needed [147–149]. Reduced caloric intake has been associated with higher mortality in severe ASH [150]. Data in support of nocturnal supplemental calories in cirrhotic patients has been reported to reduce duration of starvation [113]. Though patients with ASH have not been specifically studied, this recommendation may be extrapolated to include this patient population since alcoholic cirrhosis is a state of accelerated starvation similar to cirrhosis [113, 151]. Because reduced caloric intake is associated with higher mortality in severe ASH, supplemental enteral nutrition should be considered when oral nutrition alone does not suffice [150].

Parenteral nutrition (PN) is recommended in this population when moderate or severe malnutrition is present and patients cannot achieve adequate nutrition via enteral route [151]. This can come in different forms, and supplemental amino acids with or without glucose infusions are often recommended. If the fasting period is anticipated to be greater than 12 hours, then infusion of glucose or peripheral hypocaloric PN can be used to avoid prolonged periods of starvation [88, 152–156]. If fasting is required more than 72 hours, total parenteral nutrition may be required, which also includes provision of lipids [156]. Parenteral nutrition is usually short term; nevertheless, fat-soluble vitamins and trace elements should be administered concomitantly. To prevent Wernicke's encephalopathy in malnourished patients, thiamine should be administered prior to starting PN [156–159].

Acute Liver Failure

Acute liver failure (ALF), a clinical entity characterized by severe rapid decline in hepatic metabolic function presenting as encephalopathy and coagulopathy, causes derangements in metabolism. Unlike liver cirrhosis, these patients typically do not have baseline malnutrition as a result of chronic liver disease [160]. Energy expenditure is increased in patients with ALF, up to 18–30%, similar to other critically ill patients. Because of significant loss of hepatic function, there are alterations in metabolism for carbohydrates, proteins, and lipids. This may manifest as impairments in glucose production, clearance in lactate, and breakdown of protein, the latter of which is associated with hyperammonemia. Just as in malnourished cirrhotic patients, there is a decrease in branched-chain amino acids in this population [88, 160–163].

An alteration between glucose release and net glucose uptake is also commonly present in this population. Hypoglycemia is a sequela of ALF resulting from depletion in hepatic glycogen, impaired gluconeogenesis, and hyperinsulinemia because of increased secretion and reduced degradation [160, 164–166]. Hypoglycemia monitoring should occur frequently, approximately every 2 hours. In the intensive care unit, it can be managed with continuous glucose infusions. Enteral nutrition and parenteral nutrition are a means to prevent hypoglycemia. Hyperglycemia should be avoided due to the risk of exacerbating intracranial hypertension [160].

Micronutrient derangements in ALF include phosphate, magnesium, and potassium levels, and it is important to treat underlying etiology. Examples of etiology include ischemia and kidney injury [160]. Vitamin and mineral deficiencies should also be considered based on etiology of acute liver failure. Information obtained in the clinical setting such as history suggestive of alcohol or drug abuse may signal concomitant risk of vitamin B12, thiamine, and fat-soluble vitamin deficiency. Zinc plays a role in the conversion of ammonia to urea and may have a link in the pathophysiology of hepatic encephalopathy; however, the benefit of empiric treatment for HE with zinc is not clear as previously discussed [160]. Aside from management of micronutrient deficiencies, assessing a patient's baseline metabolic status is important. For example, obese patients with ALF are at a higher risk of death (OR 1.6–1.9) or need for transplantation (OR 3.4) compared to those who are not obese [167].

It has been suggested that nutrition support may positively impact the length of stay and severity of ALF; thus these critically ill patients should be screened for malnutrition. One such screening tool that may be used is the Nutrition Risk in the Critically Ill (NUTRIC) score. Practitioners should remember that a multidisciplinary team-based approach, including a dietician, is important when treating patients with ALF [160]. Oral nutrition is ideal; however, as altered mental status is part of the definition of acute liver failure, HE may limit oral nutrition intervention. In these cases, other modes such as enteral or parenteral nutrition should be considered. Enteral is preferred over parenteral because bacterial translocation may occur and feeding the bowel enhances recovery and reduces infection risk. If enteral therapy is not feasible, then parenteral nutrition (TPN) should be considered 5–7 days after presentation [168]. There is no clear benefit of starting before this in regard to mortality when data was extrapolated from a general critically ill patient population [11, 169, 170]. With regard to choice of TPN, lipid preparations seem safe; however, in those with marked mitochondrial dysfunction, lipid metabolism may be impaired and leads to liver insult [168]. Fat-related liver injury has been associated with the use of propofol for sedation; thus, a fat profile, with a triglyceride level <3 mmol/L, should be targeted [168].

Non-alcoholic Fatty Liver Disease (NAFLD) and Non-alcoholic Steatohepatitis (NASH)

NAFLD is a diagnosis of exclusion characterized by ≥5% of hepatic fat accumulation. Its prevalence has increased over the last 20 years, and the global prevalence is estimated to be as high as 1 billion [171]. Fibrosis stage in NAFLD is independently associated with mortality, liver transplantation, and decompensation events. Patients with fibrosis have shorter survival compared to patients without fibrosis [172]. The cardiovascular mortality and risk of developing diabetes are higher in NAFLD patients [173–176]. The progression from NAFLD to NASH involves dysbiosis and alterations in the gut-liver axis [177]. A weight loss of 10% of total body weight (TBW) in NASH patients has shown to improve fibrosis and even results in resolution of NASH [178–187]. Weight loss of 5–7% TBW may result in improvement in steatosis but may not affect fibrosis [186–191]. Lifestyle interventions with hypocaloric diet and exercise should be implemented to achieve weight loss [181, 186, 190, 192, 193]. With regard to the type of low-calorie diet, either a low-carbohydrate or low-fat diet can result in loss of intrahepatic lipids [188]. There is ongoing research with regard to fructose metabolism and insulin resistance which suggests a low-carbohydrate diet may have treatment implications in NAFLD [194]. Exercise has also been shown to improve hepatic triglyceride content independent of weight loss and should be additive to diet changes [195–198]. High-protein diets (animal or plant protein) have been shown to reduce intrahepatic fat and improve insulin resistance [199]. A Mediterranean-based diet has shown to be beneficial in reducing body weight, improving insulin sensitivity, and reducing hepatic steatosis and fibrosis in NAFLD patients, and this is the diet currently recommended by the European Association for the Study of the Liver (EASL) [200–212]. Guidance documents have additionally suggested to avoid processed and high-fructose-based food and beverages, which are also tenets common to the Mediterranean diet [213].

A pilot trial was conducted with the interventions of vitamin E and pioglitazone for the treatment of NASH when Sanyal and colleagues described that both insulin resistance and oxidative stress played a pathophysiologic role in NASH [214]. A little over a decade later, a meta-analysis based on high-quality evidence showed that vitamin E compared to placebo improved ballooning degeneration in patients with NASH [215]. However, there have been concerns in regard to the dosage of vitamin E and safety. A large meta-analysis suggested that a dosage >400 IU per day was associated with increased mortality; however, the population studied were patients with chronic diseases, and thus the ability to extrapolate this to healthy adults is unclear [216]. With regard to other antioxidants such as vitamin C, resveratrol, bayberries, or omega-3 fatty acids, not enough data is available with regard to efficacy for the treatment of NAFLD/NASH [217–220].

Conclusion

Considering the importance of hepatic and pancreaticobiliary function on overall nutrition, it is not surprisingly dysfunction in these organ systems can result in nutritional deficiencies, malnutrition, and sarcopenic obesity. Understanding underlying etiology of disease and treating concomitant nutritional complications can improve patient symptoms, morbidity, and mortality (Figs. 7.1 and 7.2).

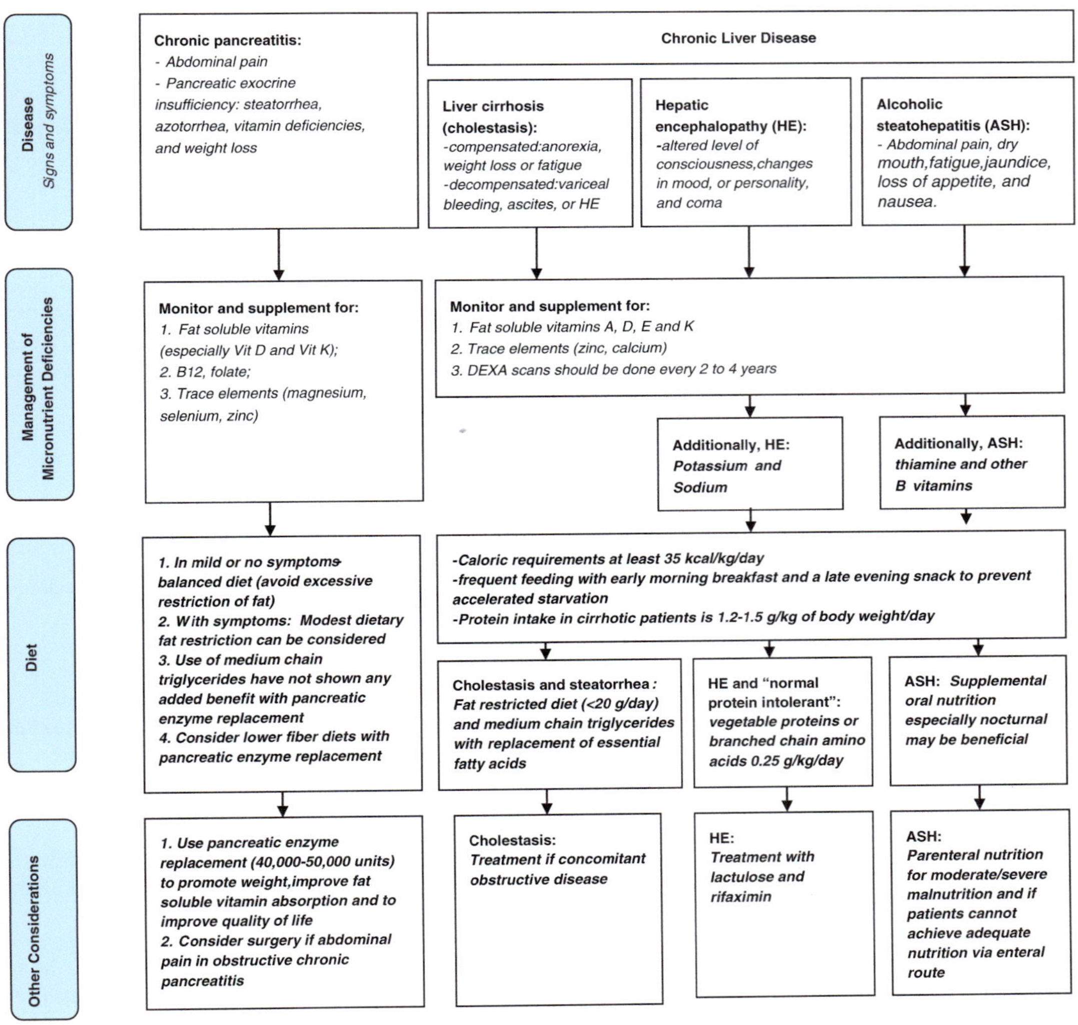

Fig. 7.1 Summary of nutritional considerations in chronic pancreatic and hepatic disorders. (Refer to text for details and references)

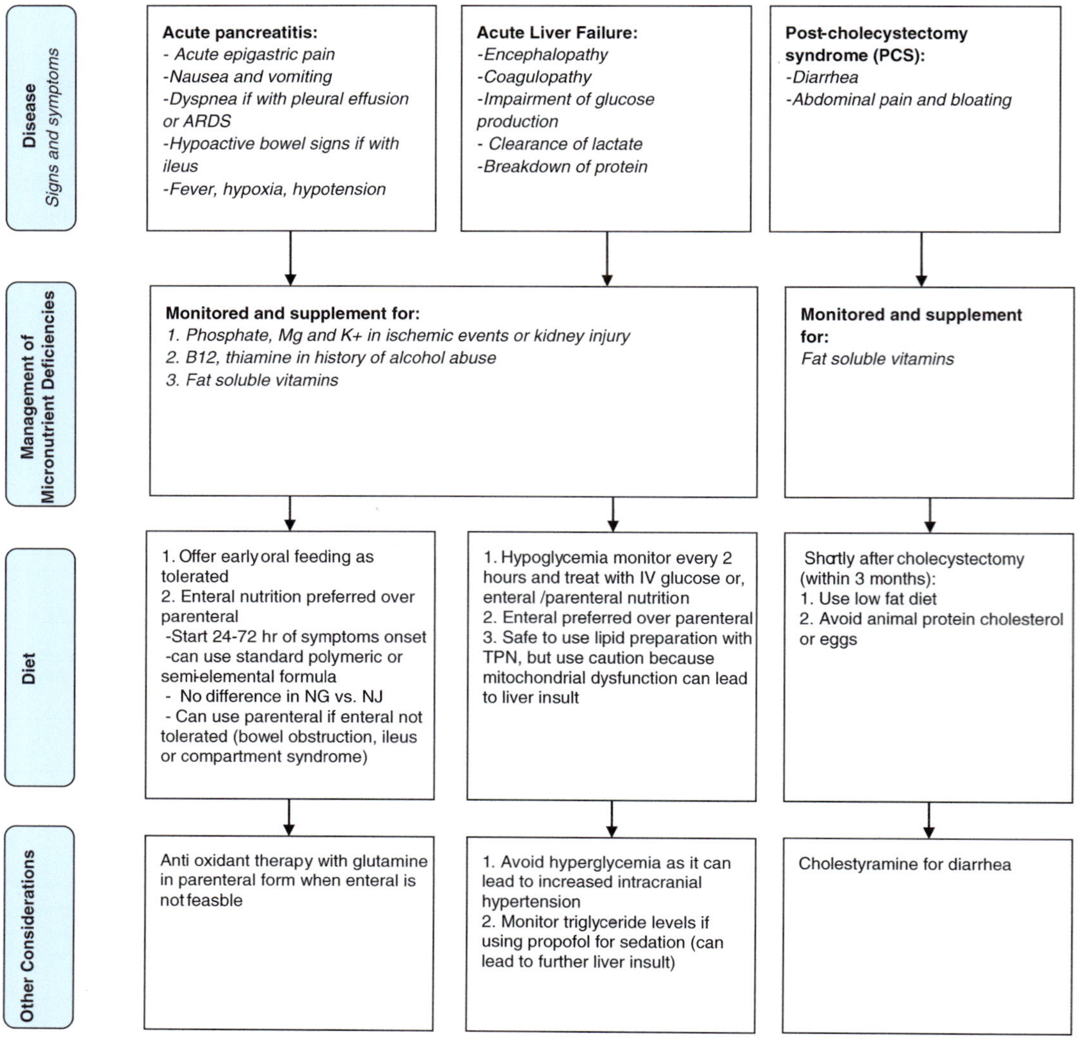

Fig. 7.2 Summary of nutritional considerations in acute pancreatic and hepatic disorders and post-cholecystectomy. (Rdefer to text for details and references)

References

1. Arvanitakis M, Ockenga J, Bezmarevic M, Gianotti L, Krznarić Ž, Lobo DN, et al. ESPEN guideline on clinical nutrition in acute and chronic pancreatitis. Clin Nutr. 2020;39(3):612–31.
2. Lee PJ, Papachristou GI. New insights into acute pancreatitis. Nat Rev Gastroenterol Hepatol. 2019;16(8):479–96.
3. StatPearls. 2020.
4. Swaroop VS, Chari ST, Clain JE. Severe acute pancreatitis. JAMA. 2004;291(23):2865–8.
5. Quinlan JD. Acute pancreatitis. Am Fam Physician. 2014;90(9):632–9.
6. Browne GW, Pitchumoni CS. Pathophysiology of pulmonary complications of acute pancreatitis. World J Gastroenterol. 2006;12(44):7087–96.
7. Mookadam F, Cikes M. Images in clinical medicine. Cullen's and Turner's signs. N Engl J Med. 2005;353(13):1386.
8. Dickson AP, Imrie CW. The incidence and prognosis of body wall ecchymosis in acute pancreatitis. Surg Gynecol Obstet. 1984;159(4):343–7.
9. Banks PA, Bollen TL, Dervenis C, Gooszen HG, Johnson CD, Sarr MG, et al. Classification of acute pancreatitis--2012: revision of the Atlanta classification and definitions by international consensus. Gut. 2013;62(1):102–11.
10. Tenner S, Baillie J, DeWitt J, Vege SS, Gastroenterology ACo. American College of

Gastroenterology guideline: management of acute pancreatitis. Am J Gastroenterol. 2013;108(9):1400–15; 16.
11. Crockett SD, Wani S, Gardner TB, Falck-Ytter Y, Barkun AN, Committee AGAICG. American gastroenterological association institute guideline on initial management of acute pancreatitis. Gastroenterology. 2018;154(4):1096–101.
12. Trikudanathan G, Wolbrink DRJ, van Santvoort HC, Mallery S, Freeman M, Besselink MG. Current concepts in severe acute and necrotizing pancreatitis: an evidence-based approach. Gastroenterology. 2019;156(7):1994–2007.e3.
13. Al-Omran M, Albalawi ZH, Tashkandi MF, Al-Ansary LA. Enteral versus parenteral nutrition for acute pancreatitis. Cochrane Database Syst Rev. 2010;(1):CD002837.
14. Sobral-Oliveira MB, Faintuch J, Guarita DR, Oliveira CP, Carrilho FJ. Nutritional profile of asymptomatic alcoholic patients. Arq Gastroenterol. 2011;48(2):112–8.
15. Teich N, Aghdassi A, Fischer J, Walz B, Caca K, Wallochny T, et al. Optimal timing of oral refeeding in mild acute pancreatitis: results of an open randomized multicenter trial. Pancreas. 2010;39(7):1088–92.
16. Wu LM, Sankaran SJ, Plank LD, Windsor JA, Petrov MS. Meta-analysis of gut barrier dysfunction in patients with acute pancreatitis. Br J Surg. 2014;101(13):1644–56.
17. Eatock FC, Chong P, Menezes N, Murray L, McKay CJ, Carter CR, et al. A randomized study of early nasogastric versus nasojejunal feeding in severe acute pancreatitis. Am J Gastroenterol. 2005;100(2):432–9.
18. Kumar A, Singh N, Prakash S, Saraya A, Joshi YK. Early enteral nutrition in severe acute pancreatitis: a prospective randomized controlled trial comparing nasojejunal and nasogastric routes. J Clin Gastroenterol. 2006;40(5):431–4.
19. Singh N, Sharma B, Sharma M, Sachdev V, Bhardwaj P, Mani K, et al. Evaluation of early enteral feeding through nasogastric and nasojejunal tube in severe acute pancreatitis: a noninferiority randomized controlled trial. Pancreas. 2012;41(1):153–9.
20. Smit M, Buddingh KT, Bosma B, Nieuwenhuijs VB, Hofker HS, Zijlstra JG. Abdominal compartment syndrome and intra-abdominal ischemia in patients with severe acute pancreatitis. World J Surg. 2016;40(6):1454–61.
21. van Brunschot S, Schut AJ, Bouwense SA, Besselink MG, Bakker OJ, van Goor H, et al. Abdominal compartment syndrome in acute pancreatitis: a systematic review. Pancreas. 2014;43(5):665–74.
22. Tsuei BJ, Magnuson B, Swintosky M, Flynn J, Boulanger BR, Ochoa JB, et al. Enteral nutrition in patients with an open peritoneal cavity. Nutr Clin Pract. 2003;18(3):253–8.
23. Burlew CC, Moore EE, Cuschieri J, Jurkovich GJ, Codner P, Nirula R, et al. Who should we feed? Western Trauma Association multi-institutional study of enteral nutrition in the open abdomen after injury. J Trauma Acute Care Surg. 2012;73(6):1380–7; discussion 7-8.
24. Jeurnink SM, Nijs MM, Prins HA, Greving JP, Siersema PD. Antioxidants as a treatment for acute pancreatitis: A meta-analysis. Pancreatology. 2015;15(3):203–8.
25. Yong L, Lu QP, Liu SH, Fan H. Efficacy of glutamine-enriched nutrition support for patients with severe acute pancreatitis: a meta-analysis. JPEN J Parenter Enteral Nutr. 2016;40(1):83–94.
26. Löhr JM, Dominguez-Munoz E, Rosendahl J, Besselink M, Mayerle J, Lerch MM, et al. United European Gastroenterology evidence-based guidelines for the diagnosis and therapy of chronic pancreatitis (HaPanEU). United European Gastroenterol J. 2017;5(2):153–99.
27. Fernandez M, Arvanitakis M, Musala C, Devière J, Van Steenbergen W, Putzeys V, et al. The Belgian national registry on chronic pancreatitis: A prospective multi-centre study covering more than 800 patients in one year. Pancreatology. 2017;17(4):572–9.
28. Hao L, Wang LS, Liu Y, Wang T, Guo HL, Pan J, et al. The different course of alcoholic and idiopathic chronic pancreatitis: A long-term study of 2,037 patients. PLoS One. 2018;13(6):e0198365.
29. Ewald N, Hardt PD. Diagnosis and treatment of diabetes mellitus in chronic pancreatitis. World J Gastroenterol. 2013;19(42):7276–81.
30. Gardner TB, Adler DG, Forsmark CE, Sauer BG, Taylor JR, Whitcomb DC. ACG clinical guideline: chronic pancreatitis. Am J Gastroenterol. 2020;115(3):322–39.
31. Machicado JD, Yadav D. Epidemiology of recurrent acute and chronic pancreatitis: similarities and differences. Dig Dis Sci. 2017;62(7):1683–91.
32. Sah RP, Pannala R, Chari ST, Sugumar A, Clain JE, Levy MJ, et al. Prevalence, diagnosis, and profile of autoimmune pancreatitis presenting with features of acute or chronic pancreatitis. Clin Gastroenterol Hepatol. 2010;8(1):91–6.
33. Pham A, Forsmark C. Chronic pancreatitis: review and update of etiology, risk factors, and management. F1000Res. 2018;7
34. Gardner TB, Levy MJ. EUS diagnosis of chronic pancreatitis. Gastrointest Endosc. 2010;71(7):1280–9.
35. DiMagno EP, Go VL. Exocrine pancreatic insufficiency. Current concepts of pathophysiology. Postgrad Med. 1972;52(1):135–40.
36. Meier R, Ockenga J, Pertkiewicz M, Pap A, Milinic N, Macfie J, et al. ESPEN guidelines on enteral nutrition: pancreas. Clin Nutr. 2006;25(2):275–84.
37. Schneider A, Löhr JM, Singer MV. The M-ANNHEIM classification of chronic pancreatitis: introduction of a unifying classification system based on a review of previous classifications of the disease. J Gastroenterol. 2007;42(2):101–19.

38. Conwell DL, Lee LS, Yadav D, Longnecker DS, Miller FH, Mortele KJ, et al. American pancreatic association practice guidelines in chronic pancreatitis: evidence-based report on diagnostic guidelines. Pancreas. 2014;43(8):1143–62.
39. Ramesh H. Proposal for a new grading system for chronic pancreatitis: the ABC system. J Clin Gastroenterol. 2002;35(1):67–70.
40. Bagul A, Siriwardena AK. Evaluation of the Manchester classification system for chronic pancreatitis. JOP. 2006;7(4):390–6.
41. Rasmussen HH, Irtun O, Olesen SS, Drewes AM, Holst M. Nutrition in chronic pancreatitis. World J Gastroenterol. 2013;19(42):7267–75.
42. Wehler M, Nichterlein R, Fischer B, Farnbacher M, Reulbach U, Hahn EG, et al. Factors associated with health-related quality of life in chronic pancreatitis. Am J Gastroenterol. 2004;99(1):138–46.
43. Olesen SS, Büyükuslu A, Køhler M, Rasmussen HH, Drewes AM. Sarcopenia associates with increased hospitalization rates and reduced survival in patients with chronic pancreatitis. Pancreatology. 2019;19(2):245–51.
44. Hébuterne X, Hastier P, Péroux JL, Zeboudj N, Delmont JP, Rampal P. Resting energy expenditure in patients with alcoholic chronic pancreatitis. Dig Dis Sci. 1996;41(3):533–9.
45. Weimann A, Braga M, Harsanyi L, Laviano A, Ljungqvist O, Soeters P, et al. ESPEN guidelines on enteral nutrition: surgery including organ transplantation. Clin Nutr. 2006;25(2):224–44.
46. Duggan SN, Smyth ND, O'Sullivan M, Feehan S, Ridgway PF, Conlon KC. The prevalence of malnutrition and fat-soluble vitamin deficiencies in chronic pancreatitis. Nutr Clin Pract. 2014;29(3):348–54.
47. Sikkens EC, Cahen DL, Koch AD, Braat H, Poley JW, Kuipers EJ, et al. The prevalence of fat-soluble vitamin deficiencies and a decreased bone mass in patients with chronic pancreatitis. Pancreatology. 2013;13(3):238–42.
48. Caliari S, Benini L, Sembenini C, Gregori B, Carnielli V, Vantini I. Medium-chain triglyceride absorption in patients with pancreatic insufficiency. Scand J Gastroenterol. 1996;31(1):90–4.
49. Klapdor S, Richter E, Klapdor R. Vitamin D status and per-oral vitamin D supplementation in patients suffering from chronic pancreatitis and pancreatic cancer disease. Anticancer Res. 2012;32(5):1991–8.
50. Girish BN, Rajesh G, Vaidyanathan K, Balakrishnan V. Zinc status in chronic pancreatitis and its relationship with exocrine and endocrine insufficiency. JOP. 2009;10(6):651–6.
51. Lindkvist B, Domínguez-Muñoz JE, Luaces-Regueira M, Castiñeiras-Alvariño M, Nieto-Garcia L, Iglesias-Garcia J. Serum nutritional markers for prediction of pancreatic exocrine insufficiency in chronic pancreatitis. Pancreatology. 2012;12(4):305–10.
52. Lindkvist B, Phillips ME, Domínguez-Muñoz JE. Clinical, anthropometric and laboratory nutritional markers of pancreatic exocrine insufficiency: Prevalence and diagnostic use. Pancreatology. 2015;15(6):589–97.
53. Uc A, Andersen DK, Bellin MD, Bruce JI, Drewes AM, Engelhardt JF, et al. Chronic pancreatitis in the 21st century - research challenges and opportunities: summary of a national institute of diabetes and digestive and kidney diseases workshop. Pancreas. 2016;45(10):1365–75.
54. Duggan S, O'Sullivan M, Feehan S, Ridgway P, Conlon K. Nutrition treatment of deficiency and malnutrition in chronic pancreatitis: a review. Nutr Clin Pract. 2010;25(4):362–70.
55. de Madaria E, Abad-González A, Aparicio JR, Aparisi L, Boadas J, Boix E, et al. The Spanish Pancreatic Club's recommendations for the diagnosis and treatment of chronic pancreatitis: part 2 (treatment). Pancreatology. 2013;13(1):18–28.
56. Delhaye M, Van Steenbergen W, Cesmeli E, Pelckmans P, Putzeys V, Roeyen G, et al. Belgian consensus on chronic pancreatitis in adults and children: statements on diagnosis and nutritional, medical, and surgical treatment. Acta Gastroenterol Belg. 2014;77(1):47–65.
57. Frulloni L, Falconi M, Gabbrielli A, Gaia E, Graziani R, Pezzilli R, et al. Italian consensus guidelines for chronic pancreatitis. Dig Liver Dis. 2010;42(Suppl 6):S381–406.
58. Mirtallo JM, Forbes A, McClave SA, Jensen GL, Waitzberg DL, Davies AR, et al. International consensus guidelines for nutrition therapy in pancreatitis. JPEN J Parenter Enteral Nutr. 2012;36(3):284–91.
59. Castiñeira-Alvariño M, Lindkvist B, Luaces-Regueira M, Iglesias-García J, Lariño-Noia J, Nieto-García L, et al. The role of high fat diet in the development of complications of chronic pancreatitis. Clin Nutr. 2013;32(5):830–6.
60. Caliari S, Benini L, Bonfante F, Brentegani MT, Fioretta A, Vantini I. Pancreatic extracts are necessary for the absorption of elemental and polymeric enteral diets in severe pancreatic insufficiency. Scand J Gastroenterol. 1993;28(8):749–52.
61. Dutta SK, Hlasko J. Dietary fiber in pancreatic disease: effect of high fiber diet on fat malabsorption in pancreatic insufficiency and in vitro study of the interaction of dietary fiber with pancreatic enzymes. Am J Clin Nutr. 1985;41(3):517–25.
62. Gianotti L, Meier R, Lobo DN, Bassi C, Dejong CH, Ockenga J, et al. ESPEN guidelines on parenteral nutrition: pancreas. Clin Nutr. 2009;28(4):428–35.
63. Silk DB. Formulation of enteral diets for use in jejunal enteral feeding. Proc Nutr Soc. 2008;67(3):270–2.
64. O'Brien SJ, Omer E. Chronic pancreatitis and nutrition therapy. Nutr Clin Pract. 2019;34(Suppl 1):S13–26.
65. Regan PT, Malagelada JR, DiMagno EP, Glanzman SL, Go VL. Comparative effects of antacids, cimetidine and enteric coating on the therapeutic response to oral enzymes in severe pancreatic insufficiency. N Engl J Med. 1977;297(16):854–8.

66. Layer P, von der Ohe MR, Holst JJ, Jansen JB, Grandt D, Holtmann G, et al. Altered postprandial motility in chronic pancreatitis: role of malabsorption. Gastroenterology. 1997;112(5):1624–34.
67. Wooldridge JL, Heubi JE, Amaro-Galvez R, Boas SR, Blake KV, Nasr SZ, et al. EUR-1008 pancreatic enzyme replacement is safe and effective in patients with cystic fibrosis and pancreatic insufficiency. J Cyst Fibros. 2009;8(6):405–17.
68. Shafiq N, Rana S, Bhasin D, Pandhi P, Srivastava P, Sehmby SS, et al. Pancreatic enzymes for chronic pancreatitis. Cochrane Database Syst Rev. 2009;(4):CD006302.
69. Domínguez-Muñoz JE, Iglesias-García J, Iglesias-Rey M, Figueiras A, Vilariño-Insua M. Effect of the administration schedule on the therapeutic efficacy of oral pancreatic enzyme supplements in patients with exocrine pancreatic insufficiency: a randomized, three-way crossover study. Aliment Pharmacol Ther. 2005;21(8):993–1000.
70. Greer JB, Greer P, Sandhu BS, Alkaade S, Wilcox CM, Anderson MA, et al. Nutrition and inflammatory biomarkers in chronic pancreatitis patients. Nutr Clin Pract. 2019;34(3):387–99.
71. Ramesh H, Reddy N, Bhatia S, Rajkumar JS, Bapaye A, Kini D, et al. A 51-week, open-label clinical trial in India to assess the efficacy and safety of pancreatin 40000 enteric-coated minimicrospheres in patients with pancreatic exocrine insufficiency due to chronic pancreatitis. Pancreatology. 2013;13(2):133–9.
72. Gubergrits N, Malecka-Panas E, Lehman GA, Vasileva G, Shen Y, Sander-Struckmeier S, et al. A 6-month, open-label clinical trial of pancrelipase delayed-release capsules (Creon) in patients with exocrine pancreatic insufficiency due to chronic pancreatitis or pancreatic surgery. Aliment Pharmacol Ther. 2011;33(10):1152–61.
73. de la Iglesia-García D, Huang W, Szatmary P, Baston-Rey I, Gonzalez-Lopez J, Prada-Ramallal G, et al. Efficacy of pancreatic enzyme replacement therapy in chronic pancreatitis: systematic review and meta-analysis. Gut. 2017;66(8):1354–5.
74. FitzSimmons SC, Burkhart GA, Borowitz D, Grand RJ, Hammerstrom T, Durie PR, et al. High-dose pancreatic-enzyme supplements and fibrosing colonopathy in children with cystic fibrosis. N Engl J Med. 1997;336(18):1283–9.
75. Sander-Struckmeier S, Beckmann K, Janssen-van Solingen G, Pollack P. Retrospective analysis to investigate the effect of concomitant use of gastric acid-suppressing drugs on the efficacy and safety of pancrelipase/pancreatin (CREON®) in patients with pancreatic exocrine insufficiency. Pancreas. 2013;42(6):983–9.
76. Ní Chonchubhair HM, Bashir Y, Dobson M, Ryan BM, Duggan SN, Conlon KC. The prevalence of small intestinal bacterial overgrowth in non-surgical patients with chronic pancreatitis and pancreatic exocrine insufficiency (PEI). Pancreatology. 2018;18(4):379–85.
77. Ong SL, Gravante G, Pollard CA, Webb MA, Illouz S, Dennison AR. Total pancreatectomy with islet autotransplantation: an overview. HPB (Oxford). 2009;11(8):613–21.
78. Stinton LM, Shaffer EA. Epidemiology of gallbladder disease: cholelithiasis and cancer. Gut Liver. 2012;6(2):172–87.
79. Altomare DF, Rotelli MT, Palasciano N. Diet after cholecystectomy. Curr Med Chem. 2019;26(19):3662–5.
80. Marcason W. What medical nutrition therapy guideline is recommended post-cholecystectomy? J Acad Nutr Diet. 2014;114(7):1136.
81. Shin Y, Choi D, Lee KG, Choi HS, Park Y. Association between dietary intake and postlaparoscopic cholecystectomic symptoms in patients with gallbladder disease. Korean J Intern Med. 2018;33(4):829–36.
82. Ge PS, Runyon BA. Treatment of patients with cirrhosis. N Engl J Med. 2016;375(21):2104–5.
83. Heidelbaugh JJ, Bruderly M. Cirrhosis and chronic liver failure: part I. Diagnosis and evaluation. Am Fam Physician. 2006;74(5):756–62.
84. Karlsen TH, Folseraas T, Thorburn D, Vesterhus M. Primary sclerosing cholangitis - a comprehensive review. J Hepatol. 2017;67(6):1298–323.
85. Hirschfield GM, Liu X, Han Y, Gorlov IP, Lu Y, Xu C, et al. Variants at IRF5-TNPO3, 17q12-21 and MMEL1 are associated with primary biliary cirrhosis. Nat Genet. 2010;42(8):655–7.
86. Younossi ZM, Stepanova M, Younossi Y, Golabi P, Mishra A, Rafiq N, et al. Epidemiology of chronic liver diseases in the USA in the past three decades. Gut. 2020;69(3):564–8.
87. Collaborators GC. The global, regional, and national burden of cirrhosis by cause in 195 countries and territories, 1990-2017: a systematic analysis for the Global Burden of Disease Study 2017. Lancet Gastroenterol Hepatol. 2020;5(3):245–66.
88. Plauth M, Bernal W, Dasarathy S, Merli M, Plank LD, Schütz T, et al. ESPEN guideline on clinical nutrition in liver disease. Clin Nutr. 2019;38(2):485–521.
89. Elwir S, Rahimi RS. Hepatic encephalopathy: an update on the pathophysiology and therapeutic options. J Clin Transl Hepatol. 2017;5(2):142–51.
90. Nutritional status in cirrhosis. Italian multicenter cooperative project on nutrition in liver cirrhosis. J Hepatol. 1994:317–25.
91. Dasarathy S. Consilience in sarcopenia of cirrhosis. J Cachexia Sarcopenia Muscle. 2012;3(4):225–37.
92. Merli M, Lucidi C, Giannelli V, Giusto M, Riggio O, Falcone M, et al. Cirrhotic patients are at risk for health care-associated bacterial infections. Clin Gastroenterol Hepatol. 2010;8(11):979–85.
93. Merli M, Giusto M, Lucidi C, Giannelli V, Pentassuglio I, Di Gregorio V, et al. Muscle depletion increases the risk of overt and minimal hepatic encephalopathy: results of a prospective study. Metab Brain Dis. 2013;28(2):281–4.
94. Huisman EJ, Trip EJ, Siersema PD, van Hoek B, van Erpecum KJ. Protein energy malnutrition predicts

complications in liver cirrhosis. Eur J Gastroenterol Hepatol. 2011;23(11):982–9.
95. Borhofen SM, Gerner C, Lehmann J, Fimmers R, Görtzen J, Hey B, et al. The royal free hospital-nutritional prioritizing tool is an independent predictor of deterioration of liver function and survival in cirrhosis. Dig Dis Sci. 2016;61(6):1735–43.
96. Montano-Loza AJ, Angulo P, Meza-Junco J, Prado CM, Sawyer MB, Beaumont C, et al. Sarcopenic obesity and myosteatosis are associated with higher mortality in patients with cirrhosis. J Cachexia Sarcopenia Muscle. 2016;7(2):126–35.
97. Carias S, Castellanos AL, Vilchez V, Nair R, Dela Cruz AC, Watkins J, et al. Nonalcoholic steatohepatitis is strongly associated with sarcopenic obesity in patients with cirrhosis undergoing liver transplant evaluation. J Gastroenterol Hepatol. 2016;31(3):628–33.
98. Choudhary NS, Saigal S, Saraf N, Mohanka R, Rastogi A, Goja S, et al. Sarcopenic obesity with metabolic syndrome: a newly recognized entity following living donor liver transplantation. Clin Transplant. 2015;29(3):211–5.
99. Dasarathy S, Merli M. Sarcopenia from mechanism to diagnosis and treatment in liver disease. J Hepatol. 2016;65(6):1232–44.
100. Dasarathy S. Nutrition and alcoholic liver disease: effects of alcoholism on nutrition, effects of nutrition on alcoholic liver disease, and nutritional therapies for alcoholic liver disease. Clin Liver Dis. 2016;20(3):535–50.
101. Dasarathy S. Cause and management of muscle wasting in chronic liver disease. Curr Opin Gastroenterol. 2016;32(3):159–65.
102. Dasarathy J, McCullough AJ, Dasarathy S. Sarcopenia in alcoholic liver disease: clinical and molecular advances. Alcohol Clin Exp Res. 2017;41(8):1419–31.
103. Rossi RE, Conte D, Massironi S. Diagnosis and treatment of nutritional deficiencies in alcoholic liver disease: Overview of available evidence and open issues. Dig Liver Dis. 2015;47(10):819–25.
104. Dolz C, Raurich JM, Ibáñez J, Obrador A, Marsé P, Gayá J. Ascites increases the resting energy expenditure in liver cirrhosis. Gastroenterology. 1991;100(3):738–44.
105. Madden AM, Morgan MY. Resting energy expenditure should be measured in patients with cirrhosis, not predicted. Hepatology. 1999;30(3):655–64.
106. Tajika M, Kato M, Mohri H, Miwa Y, Kato T, Ohnishi H, et al. Prognostic value of energy metabolism in patients with viral liver cirrhosis. Nutrition. 2002;18(3):229–34.
107. Knudsen AW, Krag A, Nordgaard-Lassen I, Frandsen E, Tofteng F, Mortensen C, et al. Effect of paracentesis on metabolic activity in patients with advanced cirrhosis and ascites. Scand J Gastroenterol. 2016;51(5):601–9.
108. Glass C, Hipskind P, Tsien C, Malin SK, Kasumov T, Shah SN, et al. Sarcopenia and a physiologically low respiratory quotient in patients with cirrhosis: a prospective controlled study. J Appl Physiol (1985). 2013;114(5):559–65.
109. Glass C, Hipskind P, Cole D, Lopez R, Dasarathy S. Handheld calorimeter is a valid instrument to quantify resting energy expenditure in hospitalized cirrhotic patients: a prospective study. Nutr Clin Pract. 2012;27(5):677–88.
110. Iwasa M, Iwata K, Hara N, Hattori A, Ishidome M, Sekoguchi-Fujikawa N, et al. Nutrition therapy using a multidisciplinary team improves survival rates in patients with liver cirrhosis. Nutrition. 2013;29(11-12):1418–21.
111. Plauth M, Cabré E, Riggio O, Assis-Camilo M, Pirlich M, Kondrup J, et al. ESPEN guidelines on enteral nutrition: liver disease. Clin Nutr. 2006;25(2):285–94.
112. Masuda K, Aoki K, Kawaguchi J, Yamakawa T, Matsuba I, Terauchi Y. Effect of caloric intake 25 or 30 kcal/kg/day on the glycemic control in obese patients with type 2 diabetes. J Clin Med Res. 2013;5(5):368–75.
113. Tsien CD, McCullough AJ, Dasarathy S. Late evening snack: exploiting a period of anabolic opportunity in cirrhosis. J Gastroenterol Hepatol. 2012;27(3):430–41.
114. Fenton JC, Knight EJ, Humpherson PL. Milk-and-cheese diet in portal-systemic encephalopathy. Lancet. 1966;1(7430):164–6.
115. Bianchi GP, Marchesini G, Fabbri A, Rondelli A, Bugianesi E, Zoli M, et al. Vegetable versus animal protein diet in cirrhotic patients with chronic encephalopathy. A randomized cross-over comparison. J Intern Med. 1993;233(5):385–92.
116. Wu G. Dietary protein intake and human health. Food Funct. 2016;7(3):1251–65.
117. Garrett-Laster M, Russell RM, Jacques PF. Impairment of taste and olfaction in patients with cirrhosis: the role of vitamin A. Hum Nutr Clin Nutr. 1984;38(3):203–14.
118. Weismann K, Christensen E, Dreyer V. Zinc supplementation in alcoholic cirrhosis. A double-blind clinical trial. Acta Med Scand. 1979;205(5):361–6.
119. Garrison RN, Cryer HM, Howard DA, Polk HC. Clarification of risk factors for abdominal operations in patients with hepatic cirrhosis. Ann Surg. 1984;199(6):648–55.
120. Merli M, Nicolini G, Angeloni S, Riggio O. Malnutrition is a risk factor in cirrhotic patients undergoing surgery. Nutrition. 2002;18(11-12):978–86.
121. Weimann A, Braga M, Carli F, Higashiguchi T, Hübner M, Klek S, et al. ESPEN guideline: clinical nutrition in surgery. Clin Nutr. 2017;36(3):623–50.
122. Coolsen MM, Wong-Lun-Hing EM, van Dam RM, van der Wilt AA, Slim K, Lassen K, et al. A systematic review of outcomes in patients undergoing liver surgery in an enhanced recovery after surgery pathways. HPB (Oxford). 2013;15(4):245–51.

123. Hughes MJ, McNally S, Wigmore SJ. Enhanced recovery following liver surgery: a systematic review and meta-analysis. HPB (Oxford). 2014;16(8):699–706.
124. Sánchez CA, Papapietro VK. Perioperative nutrition in ERAS Protocols. Rev Med Chil. 2017;145(11):1447–53.
125. Plevak DJ, DiCecco SR, Wiesner RH, Porayko MK, Wahlstrom HE, Janzow DJ, et al. Nutritional support for liver transplantation: identifying caloric and protein requirements. Mayo Clin Proc. 1994;69(3):225–30.
126. Reilly J, Mehta R, Teperman L, Cemaj S, Tzakis A, Yanaga K, et al. Nutritional support after liver transplantation: a randomized prospective study. JPEN J Parenter Enteral Nutr. 1990;14(4):386–91.
127. Hilscher MB, Kamath PS, Eaton JE. Cholestatic liver diseases: a primer for generalists and subspecialists. Mayo Clin Proc. 2020;95(10):2263–79.
128. Send SR. Nutritional management of cholestasis. Clin Liver Dis (Hoboken). 2020;15(1):9–12.
129. Mccray S, Parrish C. When chyle leaks: nutrition management options. 2004:68–72.
130. Assis DN. Chronic complications of cholestasis: evaluation and management. Clin Liver Dis. 2018;22(3):533–44.
131. Bresci G, Parisi G, Banti S. Management of hepatic encephalopathy with oral zinc supplementation: a long-term treatment. Eur J Med. 1993;2(7):414–6.
132. Reding P, Duchateau J, Bataille C. Oral zinc supplementation improves hepatic encephalopathy. Results of a randomised controlled trial. Lancet. 1984;2(8401):493–5.
133. Riggio O, Ariosto F, Merli M, Caschera M, Zullo A, Balducci G, et al. Short-term oral zinc supplementation does not improve chronic hepatic encephalopathy. Results of a double-blind crossover trial. Dig Dis Sci. 1991;36(9):1204–8.
134. Nardelli S, Lattanzi B, Torrisi S, Greco F, Farcomeni A, Gioia S, et al. Sarcopenia is risk factor for development of hepatic encephalopathy after transjugular intrahepatic portosystemic shunt placement. Clin Gastroenterol Hepatol. 2017;15(6):934–6.
135. Olde Damink SW, Jalan R, Deutz NE, Redhead DN, Dejong CH, Hynd P, et al. The kidney plays a major role in the hyperammonemia seen after simulated or actual GI bleeding in patients with cirrhosis. Hepatology. 2003;37(6):1277–85.
136. Chatauret N, Desjardins P, Zwingmann C, Rose C, Rao KV, Butterworth RF. Direct molecular and spectroscopic evidence for increased ammonia removal capacity of skeletal muscle in acute liver failure. J Hepatol. 2006;44(6):1083–8.
137. Kearns PJ, Young H, Garcia G, Blaschke T, O'Hanlon G, Rinki M, et al. Accelerated improvement of alcoholic liver disease with enteral nutrition. Gastroenterology. 1992;102(1):200–5.
138. Morgan TR, Moritz TE, Mendenhall CL, Haas R. Protein consumption and hepatic encephalopathy in alcoholic hepatitis. VA Cooperative Study Group #275. J Am Coll Nutr. 1995;14(2):152–8.
139. Kondrup J, Nielsen K, Juul A. Effect of long-term refeeding on protein metabolism in patients with cirrhosis of the liver. Br J Nutr. 1997;77(2):197–212.
140. Cabre E, Gonzalez-Huix F, Abad-Lacruz A, Esteve M, Acero D, Fernandez-Bañares F, et al. Effect of total enteral nutrition on the short-term outcome of severely malnourished cirrhotics. A randomized controlled trial. Gastroenterology. 1990;98(3):715–20.
141. Córdoba J, López-Hellín J, Planas M, Sabín P, Sanpedro F, Castro F, et al. Normal protein diet for episodic hepatic encephalopathy: results of a randomized study. J Hepatol. 2004;41(1):38–43.
142. Krenitsky J. Nutrition for patients with hepatic failure. Pract Gastroenterol. 2003;6:23–42.
143. Kawaguchi T, Taniguchi E, Sata M. Effects of oral branched-chain amino acids on hepatic encephalopathy and outcome in patients with liver cirrhosis. Nutr Clin Pract. 2013;28(5):580–8.
144. Gluud LL, Dam G, Les I, Marchesini G, Borre M, Aagaard NK, et al. Branched-chain amino acids for people with hepatic encephalopathy. Cochrane Database Syst Rev. 2017;5:CD001939.
145. Mendenhall CL, Moritz TE, Roselle GA, Morgan TR, Nemchausky BA, Tamburro CH, et al. A study of oral nutritional support with oxandrolone in malnourished patients with alcoholic hepatitis: results of a Department of Veterans Affairs cooperative study. Hepatology. 1993;17(4):564–76.
146. Paternostro R, Wagner D, Reiberger T, Mandorfer M, Schwarzer R, Ferlitsch M, et al. Low 25-OH-vitamin D levels reflect hepatic dysfunction and are associated with mortality in patients with liver cirrhosis. Wien Klin Wochenschr. 2017;129(1-2):8–15.
147. Koretz RL, Avenell A, Lipman TO. Nutritional support for liver disease. Cochrane Database Syst Rev. 2012;(5):CD008344.
148. Antar R, Wong P, Ghali P. A meta-analysis of nutritional supplementation for management of hospitalized alcoholic hepatitis. Can J Gastroenterol. 2012;26(7):463–7.
149. Fialla AD, Israelsen M, Hamberg O, Krag A, Gluud LL. Nutritional therapy in cirrhosis or alcoholic hepatitis: a systematic review and meta-analysis. Liver Int. 2015;35(9):2072–8.
150. Moreno C, Deltenre P, Senterre C, Louvet A, Gustot T, Bastens B, et al. Intensive enteral nutrition is ineffective for patients with severe alcoholic hepatitis treated with corticosteroids. Gastroenterology. 2016;150(4):903–10.e8.
151. John WJ, Phillips R, Ott L, Adams LJ, McClain CJ. Resting energy expenditure in patients with alcoholic hepatitis. JPEN J Parenter Enteral Nutr. 1989;13(2):124–7.
152. Verboeket-van de Venne WP, Westerterp KR, van Hoek B, Swart GR. Energy expenditure and substrate metabolism in patients with cirrhosis of the liver: effects of the pattern of food intake. Gut. 1995;36(1):110–6.

153. Zillikens MC, van den Berg JW, Wattimena JL, Rietveld T, Swart GR. Nocturnal oral glucose supplementation. The effects on protein metabolism in cirrhotic patients and in healthy controls. J Hepatol. 1993;17(3):377–83.
154. Swart GR, Zillikens MC, van Vuure JK, van den Berg JW. Effect of a late evening meal on nitrogen balance in patients with cirrhosis of the liver. BMJ. 1989;299(6709):1202–3.
155. Plank LD, Gane EJ, Peng S, Muthu C, Mathur S, Gillanders L, et al. Nocturnal nutritional supplementation improves total body protein status of patients with liver cirrhosis: a randomized 12-month trial. Hepatology. 2008;48(2):557–66.
156. Plauth M, Cabré E, Campillo B, Kondrup J, Marchesini G, Schütz T, et al. ESPEN guidelines on parenteral nutrition: hepatology. Clin Nutr. 2009;28(4):436–44.
157. Hu J, Juan W, Sahyoun NR. Intake and biomarkers of folate and risk of cancer morbidity in older adults, NHANES 1999-2002 with Medicare Linkage. PLoS One. 2016;11(2):e0148697.
158. Demir R, Acar G, Tanriover G, Seval Y, Kayisli UA, Agar A. Effects of excess vitamin B6 intake on cerebral cortex neurons in rat: an ultrastructural study. Folia Histochem Cytobiol. 2005;43(3):143–50.
159. Kaur P, Mishra SK, Mithal A. Vitamin D toxicity resulting from overzealous correction of vitamin D deficiency. Clin Endocrinol (Oxf). 2015;83(3):327–31.
160. Kappus MR. Acute hepatic failure and nutrition. Nutr Clin Pract. 2020;35(1):30–5.
161. Clemmesen JO, Kondrup J, Ott P. Splanchnic and leg exchange of amino acids and ammonia in acute liver failure. Gastroenterology. 2000;118(6):1131–9.
162. Record CO, Buxton B, Chase RA, Curzon G, Murray-Lyon IM, Williams R. Plasma and brain amino acids in fulminant hepatic failure and their relationship to hepatic encephalopathy. Eur J Clin Invest. 1976;6(5):387–94.
163. Rosen HM, Yoshimura N, Hodgman JM, Fischer JE. Plasma amino acid patterns in hepatic encephalopathy of differing etiology. Gastroenterology. 1977;72(3):483–7.
164. Bernuau J, Rueff B, Benhamou JP. Fulminant and subfulminant liver failure: definitions and causes. Semin Liver Dis. 1986;6(2):97–106.
165. R S, C T, A T, S S. Fulminating hepatitis with recurrent hypoglycemia and hemorrhage. Gastroenterology. 1967:291–300.
166. Vilstrup H, Iversen J, Tygstrup N. Glucoregulation in acute liver failure. Eur J Clin Invest. 1986;16(3):193–7.
167. Rutherford A, Davern T, Hay JE, Murray NG, Hassanein T, Lee WM, et al. Influence of high body mass index on outcome in acute liver failure. Clin Gastroenterol Hepatol. 2006;4(12):1544–9.
168. Wendon J, Cordoba J, Dhawan A, Larsen FS, Manns M, Samuel D, et al. EASL clinical practical guidelines on the management of acute (fulminant) liver failure. J Hepatol. 2017;66(5):1047–81.
169. Harvey SE, Parrott F, Harrison DA, Bear DE, Segaran E, Beale R, et al. Trial of the route of early nutritional support in critically ill adults. N Engl J Med. 2014;371(18):1673–84.
170. Casaer MP, Mesotten D, Hermans G, Wouters PJ, Schetz M, Meyfroidt G, et al. Early versus late parenteral nutrition in critically ill adults. N Engl J Med. 2011;365(6):506–17.
171. Perumpail BJ, Khan MA, Yoo ER, Cholankeril G, Kim D, Ahmed A. Clinical epidemiology and disease burden of nonalcoholic fatty liver disease. World J Gastroenterol. 2017;23(47):8263–76.
172. Angulo P, Kleiner DE, Dam-Larsen S, Adams LA, Bjornsson ES, Charatcharoenwitthaya P, et al. Liver fibrosis, but no other histologic features, is associated with long-term outcomes of patients with nonalcoholic fatty liver disease. Gastroenterology. 2015;149(2):389–97.e10.
173. Caldwell S, Argo C. The natural history of non-alcoholic fatty liver disease. Dig Dis. 2010;28(1):162–8.
174. Musso G, Gambino R, Cassader M, Pagano G. Meta-analysis: natural history of non-alcoholic fatty liver disease (NAFLD) and diagnostic accuracy of non-invasive tests for liver disease severity. Ann Med. 2011;43(8):617–49.
175. Targher G, Day CP. Liver enzymes, nonalcoholic fatty liver disease, and incident cardiovascular disease. Hepatology. 2011;53(1):375.
176. Armstrong MJ, Adams LA, Canbay A, Syn WK. Extrahepatic complications of nonalcoholic fatty liver disease. Hepatology. 2014;59(3):1174–97.
177. Pierantonelli I, Svegliati-Baroni G. Nonalcoholic fatty liver disease: basic pathogenetic mechanisms in the progression from NAFLD to NASH. Transplantation. 2019;103(1):e1–e13.
178. Barker KB, Palekar NA, Bowers SP, Goldberg JE, Pulcini JP, Harrison SA. Non-alcoholic steatohepatitis: effect of Roux-en-Y gastric bypass surgery. Am J Gastroenterol. 2006;101(2):368–73.
179. Caiazzo R, Lassailly G, Leteurtre E, Baud G, Verkindt H, Raverdy V, et al. Roux-en-Y gastric bypass versus adjustable gastric banding to reduce nonalcoholic fatty liver disease: a 5-year controlled longitudinal study. Ann Surg. 2014;260(5):893–8; discussion 8-9.
180. Dixon JB, Bhathal PS, O'Brien PE. Weight loss and non-alcoholic fatty liver disease: falls in gamma-glutamyl transferase concentrations are associated with histologic improvement. Obes Surg. 2006;16(10):1278–86.
181. Harrison SA, Fecht W, Brunt EM, Neuschwander-Tetri BA. Orlistat for overweight subjects with nonalcoholic steatohepatitis: A randomized, prospective trial. Hepatology. 2009;49(1):80–6.
182. Harrison SA, Fincke C, Helinski D, Torgerson S, Hayashi P. A pilot study of orlistat treatment in obese, non-alcoholic steatohepatitis patients. Aliment Pharmacol Ther. 2004;20(6):623–8.
183. Lassailly G, Caiazzo R, Buob D, Pigeyre M, Verkindt H, Labreuche J, et al. Bariatric surgery reduces fea-

tures of nonalcoholic steatohepatitis in morbidly obese patients. Gastroenterology. 2015;149(2):379–88; quiz e15-6.
184. Stratopoulos C, Papakonstantinou A, Terzis I, Spiliadi C, Dimitriades G, Komesidou V, et al. Changes in liver histology accompanying massive weight loss after gastroplasty for morbid obesity. Obes Surg. 2005;15(8):1154–60.
185. Tendler D, Lin S, Yancy WS, Mavropoulos J, Sylvestre P, Rockey DC, et al. The effect of a low-carbohydrate, ketogenic diet on nonalcoholic fatty liver disease: a pilot study. Dig Dis Sci. 2007;52(2):589–93.
186. Vilar-Gomez E, Martinez-Perez Y, Calzadilla-Bertot L, Torres-Gonzalez A, Gra-Oramas B, Gonzalez-Fabian L, et al. Weight loss through lifestyle modification significantly reduces features of nonalcoholic steatohepatitis. Gastroenterology. 2015;149(2):367–78.e5; quiz e14-5.
187. Miller EF. Nutrition management strategies for nonalcoholic fatty liver disease: treatment and prevention. Clin Liver Dis (Hoboken). 2020;15(4):144–8.
188. Haufe S, Engeli S, Kast P, Böhnke J, Utz W, Haas V, et al. Randomized comparison of reduced fat and reduced carbohydrate hypocaloric diets on intrahepatic fat in overweight and obese human subjects. Hepatology. 2011;53(5):1504–14.
189. Huang MA, Greenson JK, Chao C, Anderson L, Peterman D, Jacobson J, et al. One-year intense nutritional counseling results in histological improvement in patients with non-alcoholic steatohepatitis: a pilot study. Am J Gastroenterol. 2005;100(5):1072–81.
190. Promrat K, Kleiner DE, Niemeier HM, Jackvony E, Kearns M, Wands JR, et al. Randomized controlled trial testing the effects of weight loss on nonalcoholic steatohepatitis. Hepatology. 2010;51(1):121–9.
191. Zelber-Sagi S, Kessler A, Brazowsky E, Webb M, Lurie Y, Santo M, et al. A double-blind randomized placebo-controlled trial of orlistat for the treatment of nonalcoholic fatty liver disease. Clin Gastroenterol Hepatol. 2006;4(5):639–44.
192. Hickman IJ, Jonsson JR, Prins JB, Ash S, Purdie DM, Clouston AD, et al. Modest weight loss and physical activity in overweight patients with chronic liver disease results in sustained improvements in alanine aminotransferase, fasting insulin, and quality of life. Gut. 2004;53(3):413–9.
193. Nobili V, Manco M, Devito R, Di Ciommo V, Comparcola D, Sartorelli MR, et al. Lifestyle intervention and antioxidant therapy in children with nonalcoholic fatty liver disease: a randomized, controlled trial. Hepatology. 2008;48(1):119–28.
194. Lim JS, Mietus-Snyder M, Valente A, Schwarz JM, Lustig RH. The role of fructose in the pathogenesis of NAFLD and the metabolic syndrome. Nat Rev Gastroenterol Hepatol. 2010;7(5):251–64.
195. Houghton D, Thoma C, Hallsworth K, Cassidy S, Hardy T, Burt AD, et al. Exercise reduces liver lipids and visceral adiposity in patients with nonalcoholic steatohepatitis in a randomized controlled trial. Clin Gastroenterol Hepatol. 2017;15(1):96–102.e3.
196. Johnson NA, Sachinwalla T, Walton DW, Smith K, Armstrong A, Thompson MW, et al. Aerobic exercise training reduces hepatic and visceral lipids in obese individuals without weight loss. Hepatology. 2009;50(4):1105–12.
197. Sullivan S, Kirk EP, Mittendorfer B, Patterson BW, Klein S. Randomized trial of exercise effect on intrahepatic triglyceride content and lipid kinetics in nonalcoholic fatty liver disease. Hepatology. 2012;55(6):1738–45.
198. Thomas EL, Brynes AE, Hamilton G, Patel N, Spong A, Goldin RD, et al. Effect of nutritional counselling on hepatic, muscle and adipose tissue fat content and distribution in non-alcoholic fatty liver disease. World J Gastroenterol. 2006;12(36):5813–9.
199. Markova M, Pivovarova O, Hornemann S, Sucher S, Frahnow T, Wegner K, et al. Isocaloric diets high in animal or plant protein reduce liver fat and inflammation in individuals with type 2 diabetes. Gastroenterology. 2017;152(3):571–85.e8.
200. Gelli C, Tarocchi M, Abenavoli L, Di Renzo L, Galli A, De Lorenzo A. Effect of a counseling-supported treatment with the Mediterranean diet and physical activity on the severity of the non-alcoholic fatty liver disease. World J Gastroenterol. 2017;23(17):3150–62.
201. Katsagoni CN, Georgoulis M, Papatheodoridis GV, Fragopoulou E, Ioannidou P, Papageorgiou M, et al. Associations between lifestyle characteristics and the presence of nonalcoholic fatty liver disease: a case-control study. Metab Syndr Relat Disord. 2017;15(2):72–9.
202. Misciagna G, Del Pilar DM, Caramia DV, Bonfiglio C, Franco I, Noviello MR, et al. Effect of a low glycemic index mediterranean diet on non-alcoholic fatty liver disease. a randomized controlled clinici trial. J Nutr Health Aging. 2017;21(4):404–12.
203. Pérez-Guisado J, Muñoz-Serrano A. The effect of the Spanish Ketogenic Mediterranean Diet on nonalcoholic fatty liver disease: a pilot study. J Med Food. 2011;14(7-8):677–80.
204. Ryan MC, Itsiopoulos C, Thodis T, Ward G, Trost N, Hofferberth S, et al. The Mediterranean diet improves hepatic steatosis and insulin sensitivity in individuals with non-alcoholic fatty liver disease. J Hepatol. 2013;59(1):138–43.
205. Shai I, Schwarzfuchs D, Henkin Y, Shahar DR, Witkow S, Greenberg I, et al. Weight loss with a low-carbohydrate, Mediterranean, or low-fat diet. N Engl J Med. 2008;359(3):229–41.
206. Trovato GM, Catalano D, Martines GF, Pace P, Trovato FM. Mediterranean diet: Relationship with anxiety and depression. Ann Neurol. 2014;75(4):613.
207. Aller R, Izaola O, de la Fuente B, De Luis Román DA. Mediterranean diet is associated with liver histology in patients with non alcoholic fatty liver disease. Nutr Hosp. 2015;32(6):2518–24.
208. Della Corte C, Mosca A, Vania A, Alterio A, Iasevoli S, Nobili V. Good adherence to the Mediterranean diet reduces the risk for NASH and diabetes in pediatric patients with obesity: the results of an Italian Study. Nutrition. 2017;39-40:8–14.

209. Kontogianni MD, Tileli N, Margariti A, Georgoulis M, Deutsch M, Tiniakos D, et al. Adherence to the Mediterranean diet is associated with the severity of non-alcoholic fatty liver disease. Clin Nutr. 2014;33(4):678–83.
210. Trovato FM, Martines GF, Brischetto D, Trovato G, Catalano D. Neglected features of lifestyle: Their relevance in non-alcoholic fatty liver disease. World J Hepatol. 2016;8(33):1459–65.
211. Tzima N, Pitsavos C, Panagiotakos DB, Chrysohoou C, Polychronopoulos E, Skoumas J, et al. Adherence to the Mediterranean diet moderates the association of aminotransferases with the prevalence of the metabolic syndrome; the ATTICA study. Nutr Metab (Lond). 2009;6:30.
212. Plaz Torres MC, Aghemo A, Lleo A, Bodini G, Furnari M, Marabotto E, et al. Mediterranean diet and NAFLD: what we know and questions that still need to be answered. Nutrients. 2019;11(12)
213. EASL) EAftSotL, (EASD) EAftSoD, (EASO) EAftSoO. EASL-EASD-EASO Clinical Practice Guidelines for the management of non-alcoholic fatty liver disease. J Hepatol. 2016;64(6):1388–402.
214. Sanyal AJ, Mofrad PS, Contos MJ, Sargeant C, Luketic VA, Sterling RK, et al. A pilot study of vitamin E versus vitamin E and pioglitazone for the treatment of nonalcoholic steatohepatitis. Clin Gastroenterol Hepatol. 2004;2(12):1107–15.
215. Singh S, Khera R, Allen AM, Murad MH, Loomba R. Comparative effectiveness of pharmacological interventions for nonalcoholic steatohepatitis: a systematic review and network meta-analysis. Hepatology. 2015;62(5):1417–32.
216. Miller ER, Pastor-Barriuso R, Dalal D, Riemersma RA, Appel LJ, Guallar E. Meta-analysis: high-dosage vitamin E supplementation may increase all-cause mortality. Ann Intern Med. 2005;142(1):37–46.
217. Chachay VS, Kirkpatrick CM, Hickman IJ, Ferguson M, Prins JB, Martin JH. Resveratrol--pills to replace a healthy diet? Br J Clin Pharmacol. 2011;72(1):27–38.
218. Guo H, Zhong R, Liu Y, Jiang X, Tang X, Li Z, et al. Effects of bayberry juice on inflammatory and apoptotic markers in young adults with features of non-alcoholic fatty liver disease. Nutrition. 2014;30(2):198–203.
219. Ipsen DH, Tveden-Nyborg P, Lykkesfeldt J. Does vitamin C deficiency promote fatty liver disease development? Nutrients. 2014;6(12):5473–99.
220. Musa-Veloso K, Venditti C, Lee HY, Darch M, Floyd S, West S, et al. Systematic review and meta-analysis of controlled intervention studies on the effectiveness of long-chain omega-3 fatty acids in patients with nonalcoholic fatty liver disease. Nutr Rev. 2018;76(8):581–602.

Gastrointestinal Malignancies

8

Ryan Fecteau and AnnMarie Kieber-Emmons

Diet and Gastrointestinal Malignancy

Diet can influence tumorigenesis through pro-inflammatory and carcinogenic pathways from tumor initiation to malignant conversion and cancer progression [1–4]. There are many studies that aim to identify dietary components that modulate cancer risk. While all studies try to limit bias, residual confounding factors from other dietary constituents and lifestyle habits can be difficult to eliminate. Most studies are observational in nature, although there have been a few randomized controlled trials. While the data can be inconsistent, there are certain dietary factors that have been positively correlated with gastrointestinal malignancies. The next sections will focus specifically on dietary risks in regard to the most common gastrointestinal malignancies: colon cancer, gastric cancer, and esophageal cancer.

R. Fecteau
Department of Radiation Oncology, NewYork-Presbyterian Hospital, New York City, NY, USA
e-mail: ref61@case.edu

A. Kieber-Emmons (✉)
Department of Medicine, Division of Gastroenterology and Hepatology, Weill Cornell Medical College, New York City, NY, USA
e-mail: alk2059@med.cornell.edu

Colorectal Cancer

Colorectal cancer (CRC) is the second leading cause of cancer death in the United States. Approximately 1 in 25 people will be diagnosed with colon cancer during their lifetime [5]. Globally, the highest incidence and death rates are found in Australia, high-income Asia Pacific, and Western Europe, while the lowest rates are in South Asia, Central Sub-Saharan Africa, and Western Sub-Saharan Africa [6]. Plausible explanations of geographical differences in rates, both between and within countries, include socioeconomic factors such as access to healthcare and preventative services, environmental and dietary exposure, and genetic predisposition. It is often a combination of the aforementioned factors and population-based studies have attempted to define these complex interactions. An analysis of 10 years of prospective data from over 500,000 participants in the National Institutes of Health-AARP Diet and Health report found that differences in heath behaviors such as dietary intake, activity levels, and smoking each accounted for 8–20% of the associations seen between the risk of colorectal cancer and socioeconomic status or education level. When these health behaviors are combined with BMI, they found this accounted for 36% of the association [7]. Genome-wide association studies (GWAS) have also examined whether inheritable genetic variants may interact with dietary factors to modulate the individual risk with inconclusive results.

C. Newberry et al. (eds.), *Nutrition, Weight, and Digestive Health*,
https://doi.org/10.1007/978-3-030-94953-2_8

Red Meat and Colorectal Cancer

The International Agency for Research on Cancer (IARC) regularly evaluates and reviews the carcinogenic risk associated with red meat. They define red meat to include any unprocessed mammalian muscle tissue such as beef, veal, pork, lamb, mutton, horse, and goat [8, 9]. Geographical and cultural influences dictate the proportion of the population that consumes red meat and varies from less than 5% up to 100%, with an estimated average daily intake of 50–100 g per person [8, 9].

Per the most recent IARC monograph assessing the current body of evidence on red meat and its association with cancer, they classified red meat consumption as a Group 2A carcinogen or "probably carcinogenic to humans." This recommendation is based on mixed epidemiological data showing what is felt to be a positive association between red meat consumption and CRC, which is further supported by mechanistic data in animal models [8, 9].

The epidemiological data supporting the association between red meat consumption and CRC is mostly observational and includes cohort and case-control studies from around the globe. The IARC review lends more weight to prospective cohort studies, with population-based case-control studies and meta-analyses providing additional support. About half of the studies examined showed a positive association between red meat consumption and CRC. However, since several of the case-control studies did not show a clear association, the conclusion was that there is limited evidence to support the carcinogenicity of red meats [8–10].

The mechanistic data from animal models is felt to be strong in support of the carcinogenic potential of red meat. Heterocyclic aromatic amines (HAAs) are converted to genotoxic metabolites that induce DNA damage and similarly, alkylating N-nitroso compounds (NOCs) induce DNA adducts that promote carcinogenesis in animal models (Table 8.1) [11, 12]. Additionally, there is mechanistic data supporting the carcinogenic potential of ingested heme iron by acting either through direct cytotoxic damage on mucosal epithelium or by peroxidation of lipids with resultant NOC formation [13].

The individualized risk of red meat consumption and colorectal malignancy may be dependent on underlying genetics. A study examining approximately 2.7 million genetic variants in over 9000 cases and controls of colorectal cancer annotated with associated dietary intake variables found a significant interaction between a variant in the gene *GATA3* and processed red meat consumption. In individuals harboring this variant, the odds ratio (OR) for colon cancer associated with red meat consumption was 1.20 for heterozygous and 1.39 for homozygous individuals, indicating genetics may play a role in pathogenesis [14].

In addition to genetic and socioeconomic factors that influence dietary habits and modulate risk, certain preparations of red meat have also been shown to have variable attributable risk. High-temperature cooking techniques such as pan-frying and barbequing, which enhance digestibility as well as improve taste and texture of meat, also lead to production of carcinogenic compounds such as heterocyclic aromatic amines (HAAs) and polycyclic aromatic hydrocarbons (PAHs) (Table 8.1) [8, 9].

Processed Meat and Colorectal Cancer

Processed meat includes any meat or meat by-product such as blood that has been externally processed to improve flavor or preservation via

Table 8.1 Summary of carcinogenic compounds found in red meat, processed meat, and cooking method

Meat/cooking method	Carcinogenic components	References
Red meat	*N*-nitroso compounds (NOCs), heme iron, heterocyclic aromatic amines (HAA)	[8–12]
Processed meat	*N*-nitroso compounds (NOCs), polycyclic aromatic hydrocarbons (PAHs)	[8–10]
High-temperature cooking/charring (barbecuing, pan-frying)	Increased levels of heterocyclic aromatic amines (HAAs), polycyclic aromatic hydrocarbons (PAHs)	[8, 9]

smoking, salting, fermenting, or curing [8]. Common processed meats include sausage, bacon, ham, beef jerky, and corned beef. This processing can result in the formation of *N*-nitroso compounds (NOCs) and polycyclic aromatic hydrocarbons (PAHs) which have been shown to cause DNA damage and promote carcinogenesis in animal models [8, 9]. Geographical and cultural influences dictate the proportion of the population that consumes processed meat and varies worldwide from less than 2% to greater than 90%. In the United States, 65% of the population consume processed beef meat, while a mere 0.07% consume processed goat meat [8, 9].

The IARC has classified processed meat as a Group 1 carcinogen or "carcinogenic to humans." This recommendation is based on substantial epidemiological data including positive associations with CRC in 12 of 18 cohort studies, 6 out of 9 case-control studies [9], and a meta-analysis that defined a dose-dependent relationship in risk for each 50 g per day of processed meat consumed (RR, 1.18; 95% CI = 1.10–1.28) up until approximately 140 g/day [15].

Whole Grains, Fruits, Vegetables, and Colorectal Cancer

Evidence suggests that diets rich in whole grains, fruits, and vegetables may be beneficial in the prevention of CRC. A recent meta-analysis found that whole grain ingestion reduces the risk of CRC by 11% (RR, 0.89; 95% CI, 0.84–0.93; $P < 0.001$) but cites slight heterogeneity and lack of high-quality epidemiological studies as limitations [16]. Although more high-quality studies are needed, there are several postulated mechanisms whereby whole grain intake reduces malignancy risk. Whole grains contain several phytochemicals that may exert an antiproliferative effect, and they are a rich source of dietary fiber. Whole grains such as oats and barley are rich in soluble fiber, which is fermented in the gastrointestinal tract to produce short-chain fatty acids (SCFAs) such as butyrate. These SCFAs have tumor suppressor properties through proapoptotic and antineoplastic processes. Whole grains also contain insoluble fiber which dilutes carcinogens by increasing fecal volume and shortening intestinal transit time, leading to less mucosal apposition with toxins. Finally, whole grains regulate glycemic response, obesity, and metabolic syndrome, thereby further reducing cancer risk [1, 16, 17].

Other sources of soluble and insoluble fiber include fruits and vegetables. Fruits and vegetables also contain vitamins, minerals, phytochemicals, antioxidants, and anti-inflammatory agents that may mitigate the risk of CRC. Data to support these findings is mixed. In 2018 the World Cancer Research Fund International/American Institute for Cancer Research published an update on the effect of lifestyle factors on the risk of developing colon cancer. They concluded that there is probable evidence that the consumption of dietary fiber and calcium supplements decreases the risk of CRC. They also reported there is limited but suggestive evidence that ingesting foods containing certain antioxidants (such as vitamin C) as well as vitamin D in the form of fruits and non-starchy vegetables decreases the risk. Evidence for vitamins A and E and certain B vitamins as well as lycopene was less conclusive [18].

Gastric Cancer

Gastric cancer is the fifth most common malignancy worldwide with roughly one million new cases reported in 2018 [19]. The highest incidence of stomach cancer can be found in Eastern Asia, Central and Eastern Europe, and South America, whereas the lowest rates are in North America and much of Africa. Variation in rates is felt to reflect differences in dietary practices and/or the prevalence of *Helicobacter pylori* infection [20]. Dietary factors associated with gastric cancer risk include diets rich in red and processed meats, high-salt intake, alcohol consumption, and diets deficient in fruits and vegetables.

The link between high-salt intake and gastric cancer may be related to both a direct damaging effect on stomach mucosa and a synergistic interaction with *Helicobacter pylori* (conflicting studies), with *H. pylori* itself designated as a class I carcinogen by the World Health Organization. A meta-analysis from 2015 (consisting of prospective studies) found that more than 6 mg/day of salt intake drastically increases the risk for gastric cancer [21]. The same study found a protective effect from fruits and white vegetables, but not total intake of vegetables. The rationale for this protective effect was postulated to be related to high vitamin C content, an antioxidant that has been associated with the decreased risk of gastric cancer (RR, 0.89; 95% CI, 0.85–0.93). In terms of meat and fish consumption, the main risk categories include processed or salted meats. High-salt-containing food in general had the highest relative risk of 1.55 (95% CI, 1.17–2.05). No association between wine, coffee, black tea, green tea, milk, and juice was found, but the authors noted that beer and liquor consumption conferred a relative risk greater than 1 [21]. Though commonly cited as a risk factor, data for regular alcohol consumption and its association with gastric cancer risk is conflicting [22–24].

Esophageal Cancer

Esophageal cancer is the seventh most common malignancy worldwide with 572,034 new cases diagnosed in 2018. Although esophageal adenocarcinoma (EAC) has now become the predominant subtype in the United States and Western Europe, squamous cell carcinoma remains the most common form of esophageal cancer worldwide [19]. Dietary factors associated with the elevated risk of esophageal cancer include N-nitroso-containing foods, betel leaf, areca nut, and high-temperature beverages, while fruits and vegetables have been found to be protective. In contrast to colon and gastric cancer, there is inconsistent data on the association between red or processed meat and cancers of the esophagus.

Chewing “quid mixtures” is an accepted risk factor for oral and esophageal squamous cell cancers and should be limited. These quid mixtures include various combinations of betel leaf, areca nut, and tobacco among other substances such as slaked lime, spices, or sweeteners. It is estimated that 600 million people worldwide chew these products [25]. This practice is prevalent in the Asia-Pacific region and their respective migrant communities across the globe. The prevalence of chewing quid and its association with cancer has prompted initiatives for evidence-based global policies to reduce the use of these products [26].

In terms of food preparation, the absolute temperature of food may be a risk factor for esophageal squamous cell cancer (ESCC) due to the proximity of the esophagus to the oropharynx. There are multiple studies assessing the connection between high-temperature beverages or foods and ESCC due to thermal injury. The best evidence relates to maté, a South American caffeinated beverage made by soaking the leaves of a yerba plant in hot water. Maté consumption has been shown to be associated with ESCC development, while there is inconsistent evidence for the association of cancer incidence with hot tea or coffee consumption. Some studies even show a reduction in the risk with drinking coffee or tea, highlighting the complicated relationship between food preparation and food composition. Proposed explanations for the heterogeneity of this data include variation between beverage components which may contain mutagenic or antineoplastic constituents [27].

In contrast, fruits and vegetables likely have a protective effect against development of both EAC and ESCC. Multiple meta-analyses support a reduced risk for esophageal squamous cell carcinoma in individuals with a diet high in fruits and vegetables [28]. Additionally, a prospective study in Europe showed the importance of diversity in the diet, as an increased variety of fruits and vegetables ingested was independently associated with a lower risk of esophageal cancer in general [27]. The mechanism behind the protective effects of fruits and vegetables may be related to micronutrients such as antioxidants, as high levels of antioxidants in foods are inversely correlated with upper GI malignancies. Alternatively, the anti-carcinogenesis effect may be related to flavones contained within fruits and vegetables [27].

Table 8.2 The International Agency for Research on Cancer working group results on cancer preventative effect of the absence of excess body fatness by cancer site

Compilation of the IARC results on relative risks of BMI verse cancer site [29]			
Cancer	Strength	Relative risk of the highest BMI category evaluated versus normal BMI (95% CI)	Reference article
Esophageal adenocarcinoma	Sufficient	4.8 (3.0–7.7)	[30]
Gastric cardia	Sufficient	1.8 (1.3–2.5)	[31]
Liver	Sufficient	1.8 (1.6–2.1)	[32]
Pancreas	Sufficient	1.5 (1.2–1.8)	[33]
Colon and rectum	Sufficient	1.3 (1.3–1.4)	[34, 35]
Gallbladder	Sufficient	1.3 (1.2–1.4)	[36]
Esophageal squamous cell carcinoma	Inadequate	N/A	
Gastric non-cardia	Inadequate	N/A	
Extrahepatic biliary tract	Inadequate	N/A	

The relative risk is taken from meta-analysis or pooled analysis, with the reference article listed in the right-hand column

Obesity and Gastrointestinal Malignancy

Obesity is often cited as a risk factor for cancer. In 2016 the IARC convened to analyze the preventative effect that weight control has on cancer risk [29]. Specifically, they examined data from meta-analyses and pooled analyses to assess the relative risks of BMI versus cancer site and classified the strength of evidence as sufficient, limited, or inadequate. For cancers of the colon, gastric cardia, liver, gallbladder, pancreas, and lower esophagus, they found sufficient evidence of an increased relative risk in individuals with obesity (BMI >30) as compared to a normal BMI (range 18.5–24.9) (Table 8.2).

Further supporting the association between obesity and cancer is evidence suggesting weight loss as a protective factor. The prospective Swedish Obese Subjects (SOS) study assessed whether intentional weight loss in obese patients might protect against malignancy by comparing cancer incidence rates between patients who had bariatric surgery and those that had received nonsurgical weight loss management. The group with nonsurgical management had stable weight over the study period, whereas the bariatric surgery group had a mean weight loss of 19.9 kg over 10 years. The bariatric surgery group was found to have a lower risk of cancer when compared to the nonsurgical weight loss management group. Interestingly, the protective effect was limited to women for unclear reasons [37].

The duration of obesity also appears to have an effect on cancer risk. Data from the Women's Health Initiative, a large cohort of postmenopausal women, was examined in a US-based longitudinal study to assess the duration of adulthood obesity on cancer risk. The conclusion was that a longer duration of obesity is associated with an increased risk of developing several forms of cancer, including gastrointestinal malignancies [38]. While limited to women and observational in nature, the study suggests that increasing rates of childhood obesity may affect future population cancer risk.

Nutritional Considerations in Patients with Cancer

Terminology

In 2016 the oncology expert group from the European Society for Clinical Nutrition and Metabolism (ESPEN) convened to define the appropriate terminology for malignancy-related malnutrition (Table 8.3). Ultimately there is overlap between the conditions and definitions, but it is helpful to examine the broadly accepted terms such as malnutrition, anorexia, cachexia, sarcopenia, and others. Making distinctions between

Table 8.3 Terminology with definitions used to define nutritional states in cancer patients

Term	Definition	References
Disease-related malnutrition	Condition that results from activation of systemic inflammation which results in anorexia and tissue breakdown	[39, 40]
Anorexia	Limited food intake associated with altered CNS appetite signals, symptoms from cancer or treatments (nausea, pain), physical or mechanical limitations to food intake (GI obstructions, mucositis)	[39]
Precachexia	Early clinical and metabolic signs such as anorexia and impaired glucose tolerance that precede the involuntary loss of weight (<5%) and muscle mass	[39, 41]
Cachexia	Multifactorial wasting syndrome, loss of skeletal muscle mass with or without loss of fat mass; cannot be fully reversed by conventional nutrition care and can lead to functional impairment. Negative protein and energy balance often driven by reduced food intake and abnormal metabolism/systemic inflammation. Prior criteria included weight loss >5%, BMI < 20 and weight loss >2%, or sarcopenia and weight loss >2%	[39, 41, 42]
Refractory cachexia	Results from advanced cancer (preterminal) or presence of rapidly progressive cancer that is unresponsive to therapy. Associated with active catabolism, management of weight loss not possible or appropriate, low-performance status, and life expectancy <3 months. Burden and risks of artificial support > benefits	[42]
Sarcopenia	Low lean body mass. Common characteristics include fatigue, decreased strength, and limited physical function. Associated with lower quality of life and dependent living situations	[39, 41]
Sarcopenic obesity	Low lean body mass in a person that is obese	[39]

nutritional characterizations can help delineate diagnosis and treatment strategies, with the goal to identify and treat underlying nutritional deficits found in cancer patients. Additionally, these definitions highlight the fact that single anthropometric measurements such as BMI may not accurately reflect overall nutritional status [39].

Nutritional Risk Stratification

Patients who carry a cancer diagnosis often have concurrent malnutrition which is further exacerbated by systemic therapy, surgery, cancer-related symptoms limiting oral intake (i.e., pain or obstruction), and an overall catabolic state. There are various indices to assist clinicians with determining nutritional status in cancer patients (Table 8.4). At the time of initial cancer diagnosis, 15–50% of patients will have had recent weight loss, and upwards of 80% will ultimately develop clinical malnutrition during the course of their disease [43].

Rates of malignancy-associated malnutrition will vary at diagnosis depending on disease stage and cancer origin. Unsurprisingly, patients with advanced disease and/or obstructing tumors in the head, neck, or digestive tract are more likely to present with malnutrition at diagnosis. Hospitalized patients also have a higher likelihood of malnutrition, reflecting more severe or advanced disease stage at the time of diagnosis [43]. Conversely, hematologic malignancies such as acute lymphoblastic leukemia (ALL) are associated with lower rates of cancer-related malnutrition as they often present in young or previously healthy patients [44]. Not unexpectedly, disease progression itself is a risk factor for nutritional decline, with malnutrition rates in terminal cancer patients reaching 80–90% [45].

Table 8.4 Commonly used tools for nutritional risk screening and nutrition assessment [49]

Nutritional tools in cancer patients			
Nutrition risk screening tools		Nutritional assessment tools	
Name	*Abbreviation*	*Name*	*Abbreviation*
Nutrition Risk Screening 2002	NRS-2002	Subjective Global Assessment	SGA
Malnutrition Universal Screening Tool	MUST	Patient-Generated Subjective Global Assessment	PG-SGA
Malnutrition Screening Tool	MST	Mini Nutritional Assessment	MNA
Mini Nutritional Assessment-Short Form Revised	MNA-SF		

Despite differences in rates upon diagnosis, all cancer patients should have their nutritional statuses continuously monitored throughout their clinical course as various factors including therapeutic interventions, local and systemic effects of the malignancy, and psychiatric conditions (concurrent depression, anxiety, etc.) may lead to acute deterioration of nutrition indices and adversely affect outcomes. This is especially pertinent in patients with digestive tract malignancies, who are already at higher risk for nutritional complications. European studies have shown only 30–60% of eligible hospitalized cancer patients actually receive nutritional assessment and support and 40% are misclassified in terms of nutritional risk [39]. Thus, heightened clinical awareness to appropriately diagnose and address nutritional deficits is needed.

Frequent nutritional assessment identifies at-risk patients who would most benefit from early intervention, as malnutrition has been associated with worse outcomes and prognosis. Muscle wasting (i.e., sarcopenia) is associated with reduced quality of life, poor response to treatment modalities, an increase in chemotherapy toxicity, and decrease in survival [46, 47]. Importantly, roughly 10–20% of cancer patient mortality can be attributed to malnutrition [39]. Malignancy-related malnutrition may also pose a non-trivial financial burden on health systems. Findings from the PREDyCES study, a nationwide, prospective case-controlled study conducted in Spain, show that an elevated nutritional risk in admitted patients is associated with significantly longer hospital stays and consequently higher costs [48].

Mechanisms for Malnutrition in Cancer Patients

Mechanisms for malnutrition in cancer patients can be broadly classified into local or systemic effects. Tumor-related local effects include tissue infiltration and obstruction, especially in cancers affecting the gastrointestinal tract or head and neck. Proximally located tumors (i.e., head, neck, esophageal and gastric cardia) can invade and encroach on the luminal gastrointestinal tract leading to dysphagia and mechanical obstruction. In a similar manner, gastric cancer can progress to cause gastric outlet obstruction which may lead to post-prandial pain, nausea, and vomiting. Further intestinal blockage from a primary bowel tumor or extrinsic compression from a metastatic lesion can cause symptoms of bloating, pain, nausea, vomiting, or constipation depending on the location. Primary bowel tumors may disrupt proper nutrient uptake by causing symptomatic diarrhea from either secretory pathways, malabsorption, or infections [39].

The systemic mechanisms that affect nutritional status include altered host metabolism and a cachectic state in which there is an increase in muscle protein catabolism, inflammation, and insulin resistance. Cancer cachexia is clinically characterized by loss of muscle mass with or without a loss of fat mass [50]. In cachexia, cytokine-driven dysregulation of hormones such as leptin and ghrelin [50] is associated with decreased oral intake and increased resting energy expenditure, leading to caloric deficit and weight loss [46].

Given this complex and multifactorial nature, nutritional support as a unimodal therapy is usually ineffective in treating cancer cachexia as it fails to address the full extent of the problem. Instead, to combat cancer cachexia, a multimodal approach is required, and while the therapeutic tactic should include targeting the anorexia with nutritional support, there has also been much effort to concomitantly address the inflammation-mediated metabolic derangements [46].

Nutritional Support Planning

Though there is limited data to define the optimal time for initiating nutritional support, it stands to reason that nutritional therapy should be initiated during early stages of malnutrition while it remains in the patient's goals of care. As discussed above, systemic treatment and therapeutic interventions will be better tolerated in healthier individuals, and thus promptly addressing nutritional deficits in the malnourished patient carries prognostic significance. Furthermore, it can prove challenging to revert malnutrition in the setting of a severe metabolic imbalance accompanying disease progression. It is generally agreed upon that nutritional status should be assessed immediately upon cancer diagnosis and proper intervention commenced early in the oncologic course. It is prudent to address even the mildest of deficiencies, especially in patients who are likely to develop disease- or therapy-related side effects that may negatively affect outcomes [49].

Once a patient is deemed at nutritional risk, specialized oral intake in association with dedicated and repeated nutrition counseling is the first step in management. Typically, a diet of calorically dense and protein-rich foods is the preferred first line. If intake remains inadequate, oral nutritional supplements can be added to augment standard food intake [49]. It is generally advised that vitamins and minerals be supplied in the recommend daily allowances and not to use high-dose micronutrients if there is no indication [49]. In a prospective study on colon cancer patients with stage III disease enrolled in a clinical trial of adjuvant chemotherapy, multivitamin use was not associated with a statistically significant difference in disease-free survival nor overall survival [51]. This held true even when total dietary and supplemental intake of individual vitamins was examined [51]. Excess antioxidant vitamin intake may also decrease efficacy of commonly used chemotherapies and radiation therapy and should be avoided [52].

In addition to modifying food content to meet energy and nutritional requirements, the textural quality of the food is also important, especially in gastrointestinal malignancies or head and neck cancer patients. For example, in esophageal cancer, switching to a soft or liquid diet can improve tolerability and therefore quality of per oral nutritional intake. Changing frequency or distribution of meals can also help minimize symptoms of early satiety, bloating, and nausea.

Restrictive diets are typically contraindicated for malnourished patients or patients who are at risk for malnourishment. Often patients will present with questions regarding fad diets derived from non-peer-reviewed or anecdotal sources. It is worth noting that there is no reproducible strong evidence to suggest specific diets are effective in treating cancer or preventing recurrence. Conversely, many of these diets are restrictive and may exacerbate nutritional deficiencies, placing patients at further risk for frank malnutrition [49]. Interestingly, there is a small amount of data to suggest that intermittent dietary changes, such as short-term fasting, can improve tolerability and effectiveness of chemotherapy, but this requires further study [49, 53].

In addition to addressing diet, medications can be used to help meet nutritional goals by stimulating appetite, improving gut motility, decreasing inflammation, and/or managing symptoms such as nausea. Medications to address mucositis can improve per oral tolerability. Proton pump inhibitors can help with ulcerations and reflux symptoms. Anti-secretory agents can be used to decrease excessive saliva production or gastric secretions, especially if recurrent vomiting arises from issues with intestinal transport. Alternatively, salivary stimulating agents such as pilocarpine or cevimeline may be indicated in patients suffering from xerostomia that is not responsive to lifestyle modifications or saliva substitutes. There are weak recommendations for corticosteroids and progestin to stimulate appetite, though both have potential side effects limiting their generalized use [49].

If volitional intake with oral nutrition remains inadequate to meet caloric demands, other options include supplementary or complete nutritional support by enteral or parenteral routes. Distal enteral feeding tubes are often used to bypass mechanical obstruction in the proximal alimentary canal, such as lesions obstructing the gastro-esophageal junction, gastric outlet, and even the duodenum or proximal jejunum. Parenteral support is often required in cases of inability to establish enteral access due to anatomical issues or malabsorption due to intestinal insufficiency from short gut syndrome, radiation enteritis, or peritoneal carcinomatosis. The specifics of these modalities are discussed in other chapters; however, a careful assessment of the goals of nutritional support should be considered in relation to any competing risk. Procedures for enteral feeding are not without complications, and parenteral nutrition poses a significant risk of infection and requires careful titration to minimize metabolic derangements. Clinical practice can often differ due to economic, ethical, and cultural factors; however, the risks of parenteral nutrition will likely outweigh the benefits for patients with a life expectancy of less than 2 months [54]. In the majority of cases, any benefits continue to weaken during the weeks preceding death [49].

Physical therapy is a sometimes overlooked but important treatment modality in addressing malnutrition and cachexia. Routine activity may counteract the physical deconditioning often seen in cancer patients and help promote anabolism and utilization of nutrients. Nutritional societies recommend that cancer patients increase or maintain their level of physical activity after diagnosis, which should include both resistance and aerobic exercise [49].

As with all interventions, the goals of therapy and patient preference need to be considered on a case-by-case basis. Patients requiring nutritional support early on in their oncologic course might have more transient circumstances, as in the case of a medically operable patient with a resectable tumor causing obstruction. Here nutritional supplementation or enteral nutrition bypassing obstruction could provide temporary support until definitive intervention, at which point patients may resume normal or near-normal intake. This is in stark contrast to the diffusely metastatic patient suffering from both obstructing and metabolic complications, where nutritional support is mainly to provide comfort and improve quality of life [49, 55]. Whereas in the first scenario nutritional support has prognostic importance, in the latter, it is primarily palliative, a distinction that should be discussed in detail with the patient and/or caregivers.

Conclusion

Diet is a modifiable lifestyle factor that influences tumorigenesis through both local and systemic effects. However, heterogeneity in data and constraints in study design limit our full understanding of the complex interaction between diet and cancer pathogenesis. This hinders our ability to recommend specific cancer-preventing diets beyond general recommendations but does not diminish the importance of diet in modulating cancer risk. Continued high-quality studies for further clarification on cancer prevention are subsequently needed. For patients who already have a cancer diagnosis, the focus shifts from prevention to management, highlighting the importance of early nutritional risk stratification to identify patients in most need of support.

References

1. Anand P, Kunnumakara AB, Sundaram C, Harikumar KB, Tharakan ST, Lai OS, et al. Cancer is a preventable disease that requires major lifestyle changes. Pharm Res. 2008;25(9):2097–116.
2. O'Keefe SJD. Diet, microorganisms and their metabolites, and colon cancer. Nat Rev Gastroenterol Hepatol. 2016;13(12):691–706.
3. Aguirre-Portolés C, Fernández LP, Ramírez de Molina A. Precision nutrition for targeting lipid metabolism in colorectal cancer. Nutrients [Internet]. 2017 Sep

28 [cited 2020 Dec 27];9(10). Available from: https://www.ncbi.nlm.nih.gov/pmc/articles/PMC5691693/
4. Goncalves MD, Lu C, Tutnauer J, Hartman TE, Hwang S-K, Murphy CJ, et al. High-fructose corn syrup enhances intestinal tumor growth in mice. Science. 2019;363(6433):1345–9.
5. Siegel RL, Miller KD, Jemal A. Cancer statistics, 2020. CA Cancer J Clin. 2020;70(1):7–30.
6. Global, regional, and national cancer incidence, mortality, years of life lost, years lived with disability, and disability-adjusted life-years for 32 Cancer Groups, 1990 to 2015. JAMA Oncologia. 2017;3(4):524–548.
7. Doubeni CA, Major JM, Laiyemo AO, Schootman M, Zauber AG, Hollenbeck AR, et al. Contribution of behavioral risk factors and obesity to socioeconomic differences in colorectal cancer incidence. JNCI J Natl Cancer Inst. 2012;104(18):1353–62.
8. Bouvard V, Loomis D, Guyton KZ, Grosse Y, Ghissassi FE, Benbrahim-Tallaa L, et al. Carcinogenicity of consumption of red and processed meat. Lancet Oncol. 2015;16(16):1599–600.
9. International Agency for Research on Cancer, Working Group on the Evaluation of the Carcinogenic Risks to Humans. Red meat and processed meat this publication represents the views and expert opinions of an IARC Working Group on the Evaluation of Carcinogenic Risks to Humans, which met in Lyon, 6-13 October 2015 [Internet]. 2018 [cited 2020 Oct 26]. Available from: https://www.ncbi.nlm.nih.gov/books/NBK507971/.
10. Aune D, Chan DSM, Vieira AR, Navarro Rosenblatt DA, Vieira R, Greenwood DC, et al. Red and processed meat intake and risk of colorectal adenomas: a systematic review and meta-analysis of epidemiological studies. Cancer Causes Control. 2013;24(4):611–27.
11. Leu RKL, Winter JM, Christophersen CT, Young GP, Humphreys KJ, Hu Y, et al. Butyrylated starch intake can prevent red meat-induced O6-methyl-2-deoxyguanosine adducts in human rectal tissue: a randomised clinical trial. Br J Nutr. 2015;114(2):220–30.
12. Lewin MH, Bailey N, Bandaletova T, Bowman R, Cross AJ, Pollock J, et al. Red meat enhances the colonic formation of the DNA adduct *O* [6] -Carboxymethyl guanine: implications for colorectal cancer risk. Cancer Res. 2006;66(3):1859–65.
13. Fiorito V, Chiabrando D, Petrillo S, Bertino F, Tolosano E. The multifaceted role of Heme in cancer. Front Oncol [Internet] 2020 [cited 2020 Oct 26];9. Available from: https://www.frontiersin.org/articles/10.3389/fonc.2019.01540/full.
14. Figueiredo JC, Hsu L, Hutter CM, Lin Y, Campbell PT, Baron JA, et al. Genome-wide diet-gene interaction analyses for risk of colorectal cancer. PLoS Genet [Internet] 2014 Apr 17 [cited 2020 Aug 5];10(4). Available from: https://www.ncbi.nlm.nih.gov/pmc/articles/PMC3990510/.
15. Chan DSM, Lau R, Aune D, Vieira R, Greenwood DC, Kampman E, et al. Red and processed meat and colorectal cancer incidence: meta-analysis of prospective studies. PLoS One. 2011;6(6):e20456.
16. Zhang X-F, Wang X-K, Tang Y-J, Guan X-X, Guo Y, Fan J-M, et al. Association of whole grains intake and the risk of digestive tract cancer: a systematic review and meta-analysis. Nutr J [Internet] 2020 Jun 3 [cited 2020 Dec 21];19. Available from: https://www.ncbi.nlm.nih.gov/pmc/articles/PMC7271550/.
17. Soliman GA. Dietary fiber, atherosclerosis, and cardiovascular disease. Nutrients [Internet]. 2019 May 23 [cited 2020 Dec 26];11(5). Available from: https://www.ncbi.nlm.nih.gov/pmc/articles/PMC6566984/.
18. World Cancer Research Fund / American Institute for Cancer Research. Continuous Update Project Expert Report. Diet, nutrition, physical activity and colorectal cancer [Internet]. 2018 [cited 2020 Dec 26]. Available from: dietandcancerreport.org
19. Worldwide cancer data [Internet]. World Cancer Research Fund. 2018 [cited 2020 Oct 26]. Available from: https://www.wcrf.org/dietandcancer/cancer-trends/worldwide-cancer-data.
20. Jemal A, Bray F, Center MM, Ferlay J, Ward E, Forman D. Global cancer statistics. CA Cancer J Clin. 2011;61(2):69–90.
21. Fang X, Wei J, He X, An P, Wang H, Jiang L, et al. Landscape of dietary factors associated with risk of gastric cancer: a systematic review and dose-response meta-analysis of prospective cohort studies. Eur J Cancer. 2015;51(18):2820–32.
22. Wang S, Freedman ND, Loftfield E, Hua X, Abnet CC. Alcohol consumption and risk of gastric cardia adenocarcinoma and gastric noncardia adenocarcinoma: a 16-year prospective analysis from the NIH-AARP diet and health cohort. Int J Cancer. 2018;143(11):2749–57.
23. Tramacere I, Negri E, Pelucchi C, Bagnardi V, Rota M, Scotti L, et al. A meta-analysis on alcohol drinking and gastric cancer risk. Ann Oncol. 2012;23(1):28–36.
24. Barstad B, Sørensen TIA, Tjønneland A, Johansen D, Becker U, Andersen IB, et al. Intake of wine, beer and spirits and risk of gastric cancer. Eur J Cancer Prev. 2005;14(3):239–43.
25. Humans IWG on the E of CR to. Betel-quid and Areca-nut Chewing [Internet]. Betel-quid and Areca-nut Chewing and Some Areca-nut-derived Nitrosamines. International Agency for Research on Cancer; 2004 [cited 2020 Oct 20]. Available from: https://www.ncbi.nlm.nih.gov/books/NBK316574/.
26. Mehrtash H, Duncan K, Parascandola M, David A, Gritz ER, Gupta PC, et al. Defining a global research and policy agenda for betel quid and areca nut. Lancet Oncol. 2017;18(12):e767–75.
27. Abnet CC, Corley DA, Freedman ND, Kamangar F. Diet and upper gastrointestinal malignancies. Gastroenterology. 2015;148(6):1234–1243.e4.
28. Liu J, Wang J, Leng Y, Lv C. Intake of fruit and vegetables and risk of esophageal squamous cell carcinoma: a meta-analysis of observational studies. Int J Cancer. 2013;133(2):473–85.
29. Lauby-Secretan B, Scoccianti C, Loomis D, Grosse Y, Bianchini F, Straif K. Body fatness and cancer — viewpoint of the IARC Working Group [internet]. https://doi.org/10.1056/NEJMsr1606602.

Massachusetts Medical Society; 2016 [cited 2020 Sep 16]. Available from: https://www.nejm.org/doi/https://doi.org/10.1056/NEJMsr1606602.
30. Hoyo C, Cook MB, Kamangar F, Freedman ND, Whiteman DC, Bernstein L, et al. Body mass index in relation to oesophageal and oesophagogastric junction adenocarcinomas: a pooled analysis from the International BEACON Consortium. Int J Epidemiol. 2012;41(6):1706–18.
31. Chen Y, Liu L, Wang X, Wang J, Yan Z, Cheng J, et al. Body mass index and risk of gastric cancer: a meta-analysis of a population with more than ten million from 24 prospective studies. Cancer Epidemiol Prev Biomark. 2013;22(8):1395–408.
32. Chen Y, Wang X, Wang J, Yan Z, Luo J. Excess body weight and the risk of primary liver cancer: An updated meta-analysis of prospective studies. Eur J Cancer. 2012;48(14):2137–45.
33. Genkinger JM, Spiegelman D, Anderson KE, Bernstein L, van den Brandt PA, Calle EE, et al. A pooled analysis of 14 cohort studies of anthropometric factors and pancreatic cancer risk. Int J Cancer J Int Cancer. 2011;129(7):1708–17.
34. Ma Y, Yang Y, Wang F, Zhang P, Shi C, Zou Y, et al. Obesity and risk of colorectal cancer: a systematic review of prospective studies. PLoS ONE [Internet]. 2013 Jan 17 [cited 2020 Sep 16];8(1). Available from: https://www.ncbi.nlm.nih.gov/pmc/articles/PMC3547959/.
35. Renehan AG, Tyson M, Egger M, Heller RF, Zwahlen M. Body-mass index and incidence of cancer: a systematic review and meta-analysis of prospective observational studies. Lancet. 2008;371(9612):569–78.
36. Gallbladder-Cancer-2015-Report.pdf [Internet]. [cited 2020 Sep 16]. Available from: https://www.wcrf.org/sites/default/files/Gallbladder-Cancer-2015-Report.pdf
37. Sjöström L, Gummesson A, Sjöström CD, Narbro K, Peltonen M, Wedel H, et al. Effects of bariatric surgery on cancer incidence in obese patients in Sweden (Swedish Obese Subjects Study): a prospective, controlled intervention trial. Lancet Oncol. 2009;10(7):653–62.
38. Arnold M, Jiang L, Stefanick ML, Johnson KC, Lane DS, LeBlanc ES, et al. Duration of adulthood overweight, obesity, and cancer risk in the women's health initiative: a longitudinal study from the United States. PLoS Med. 2016;13(8):e1002081.
39. Arends J, Baracos V, Bertz H, Bozzetti F, Calder PC, Deutz NEP, et al. ESPEN expert group recommendations for action against cancer-related malnutrition. Clin Nutr. 2017;36(5):1187–96.
40. Cederholm T, Barazzoni R, Austin P, Ballmer P, Biolo G, Bischoff SC, et al. ESPEN guidelines on definitions and terminology of clinical nutrition. Clin Nutr. 2017;36(1):49–64.
41. Ryan AM, Power DG, Daly L, Cushen SJ, Ní Bhuachalla E, Prado CM. Cancer-associated malnutrition, cachexia and sarcopenia: the skeleton in the hospital closet 40 years later. Proc Nutr Soc. 2016;75(2):199–211.
42. Fearon K, Strasser F, Anker SD, Bosaeus I, Bruera E, Fainsinger RL, et al. Definition and classification of cancer cachexia: an international consensus. Lancet Oncol. 2011;12(5):489–95.
43. Nitenberg G, Raynard B. Nutritional support of the cancer patient: issues and dilemmas. Crit Rev Oncol Hematol. 2000;34(3):137–68.
44. Uderzo C, Rovelli A, Bonomi M, Barzaghi A, Strada S, Balduzzi A, et al. Nutritional status in untreated children with acute leukemia as compared with children without malignancy. J Pediatr Gastroenterol Nutr. 1996;23(1):34–7.
45. Virizuela JA, Camblor-Álvarez M, Luengo-Pérez LM, Grande E, Álvarez-Hernández J, Sendrós-Madroño MJ, et al. Nutritional support and parenteral nutrition in cancer patients: an expert consensus report. Clin Transl Oncol. 2018;20(5):619–29.
46. Fearon K, Arends J, Baracos V. Understanding the mechanisms and treatment options in cancer cachexia. Nat Rev Clin Oncol. 2013;10(2):90–9.
47. Aoyagi T, Terracina KP, Raza A, Matsubara H, Takabe K. Cancer cachexia, mechanism and treatment. World J Gastrointest Oncol. 2015;7(4):17–29.
48. Planas M, Álvarez-Hernández J, León-Sanz M, Celaya-Pérez S, Araujo K, García de Lorenzo A, et al. Prevalence of hospital malnutrition in cancer patients: a sub-analysis of the PREDyCES® study. Support Care Cancer. 2016;24(1):429–35.
49. Arends J, Bachmann P, Baracos V, Barthelemy N, Bertz H, Bozzetti F, et al. ESPEN guidelines on nutrition in cancer patients. Clin Nutr. 2017;36(1):11–48.
50. Mantovani G, Madeddu C. Cancer cachexia: medical management. Support Care Cancer. 2009;18(1):1.
51. Ng K, Meyerhardt JA, Chan JA, Niedzwiecki D, Hollis DR, Saltz LB, et al. Multivitamin use is not associated with cancer recurrence or survival in patients with stage III colon cancer: findings from CALGB 89803. J Clin Oncol. 2010;28(28):4354–63.
52. Harvie M. Nutritional supplements and cancer: potential benefits and proven harms. Am Soc Clin Oncol Educ Book Am Soc Clin Oncol Annu Meet. 2014;2014:e478–86.
53. de Groot S, Vreeswijk MP, Welters MJ, Gravesteijn G, Boei JJ, Jochems A, et al. The effects of short-term fasting on tolerance to (neo) adjuvant chemotherapy in HER2-negative breast cancer patients: a randomized pilot study. BMC Cancer. 2015;15(1):652.
54. Bozzetti F. Home total parenteral nutrition in incurable cancer patients: a therapy, a basic humane care or something in between? Clin Nutr. 2003;22(2):109–11.
55. Baldwin C, Spiro A, Ahern R, Emery PW. Oral nutritional interventions in malnourished patients with cancer: a systematic review and meta-analysis. JNCI J Natl Cancer Inst. 2012;104(5):371–85.

Surgical Nutrition and Post-Surgical Management

9

Jessica Schucht, W. Aaron Marshall, Christian Brown, Nicholas Caminiti, and Martin Rosenthal

Introduction

The perioperative patient has clear nutritional needs beyond maintaining homeostasis which include providing adequate energy and substrates to enter an anabolic state and recover from the insult of surgery. The caloric needs of a surgical patient are estimated at 25 kcal/kg of body weight/day, and the protein requirements of the post-operative patient can be as high as 1–1.5 g/kg of body weight/day. Although these values are estimates, they provide the foundation to meet the nutritional needs in most surgical patients. In many post-operative patients, these needs can be met through an unrestricted, oral diet. When augmentation of oral intake is necessary, a variety of supplements are satisfactory, and when initiation of tube feeding is required, most whole peptide formulations are appropriate. Although rarely required, there are a variety of tube feeding formulations with various alterations for use in situations such as renal failure or diminished GI tract absorbing capacity [1–4]. If patients are unable to meet nutritional needs with enteral provisions or have absolute contraindications to enteral feeding, parenteral nutrition can be considered.

J. Schucht (✉) · W. A. Marshall · N. Caminiti
M. Rosenthal
University of Louisville, Department of Surgery, Louisville, KY, USA
e-mail: jeschu03@louisville.edu; william.marshall@louisville.edu; nicolas.caminiti@louisville.edu; martin.rosenthal@surgery.ufl.edu

C. Brown
University of Florida, UF Health, Department of Surgery, Gainesville, FL, USA
e-mail: christian.brown@surgery.ufl.edu

Enteral Nutrition

The role of enteral nutrition (EN) in the critically ill surgical patient is widely studied [1]. Multisystem organ failure in the post-surgical patient is often the end manifestation of hypermetabolic changes throughout the body, which often lead to lipid mobilization and myocyte catabolism to augment adequate cell regeneration [2]. This process supports adequate wound healing in the nutritionally replete patient. Critically ill surgical patients, in contrast, often need additional nutritional support. Pre-existing malnutrition is a widely recognized contributing factor in the morbidity and mortality of surgical patients, as they lack the metabolic substrates necessary for anabolic processes required for wound healing [3]. Understanding this mechanism and attempting to interrupt this state of hypermetabolism have been the goal of researchers for the last several decades.

EN remains the preferred method for nutritional delivery in the surgical patient who maintains competent gastrointestinal function, but cannot meet nutritional needs via oral diet [4].

C. Newberry et al. (eds.), *Nutrition, Weight, and Digestive Health*,
https://doi.org/10.1007/978-3-030-94953-2_9

Though more recent studies have attempted to prove non-inferiority of parenteral nutrition (PN), the benefits of EN are well-established [2].

Caloric Benefits

While specific methodologies for optimal nutritional delivery continue to be debated, it is well-established that malnutrition is an independent risk factor for morbidity and mortality for patients in the intensive care unit [5]. To combat this, most international societies (including the American Society for Parenteral and Enteral Nutrition (ASPEN)) recommend initiation of EN as early as possible to avoid large cumulative caloric deficits over prolonged stays in the ICU.

Gastrointestinal Integrity

The well-being of the critically ill surgical patient is largely dependent on maintenance of gastrointestinal tract integrity and function. There is the conventional belief that early administration of enteral feeds maintains gastrointestinal integrity and reduces intestinal ischemia, thereby reducing the incidence of sepsis and end-organ failure. This phenomenon was studied in rat models in the 1990s, where suffusion of glucose solution onto ileal mucosa was shown to reverse the effect of mesenteric ischemia, mimicking the physiologic effect of early EN in critically ill patients with hemorrhagic or septic shock [6]. Furthermore, there is evidence to support that delayed luminal transit and gut dysmotility could contribute to delayed end-organ failure even after adequate resuscitation and stabilization, which has been proven in various animal models over the last 25 years [7]. These studies demonstrated an inverse relationship between intestinal motility and bacterial translocation in mice and pigs in physiologic shock and low-flow states. As such, maintenance of a competent GI tract is thought to be of utmost importance, and though this mechanism is not widely understood, there is a consensus that early administration of enteral feedings will ameliorate some of these delayed deleterious effects.

Immunologic Benefits

Administration of nutrition in critically ill patients improves the efficacy of innate host defenses both within the GI tract and other organ systems. EN is superior to PN in maintaining gut-associated lymphoid tissue within Peyer's patches, which is necessary for stimulation of B-lymphocytes and production of systemic secretory IgA, an antibody found in high quantities across multiple mucosal surfaces and bodily secretions [8, 9]. The absence of stimulation to the GI mucosa, even while supplying nutritional substrates via PN, has shown to cause atrophy of lymphoid tissue within the GI tract, leading to extraintestinal disruption of innate mucosal immunity. This is hypothesized to be related to impaired IgA production, which predisposes these patients to bacterial invasion and sepsis [10–12].

Adverse immunologic effects also occur in the absence of EN. Atrophy of lymphoid tissue within Peyer's patches in the small intestine results in reduced production of IL-4 and IL-10, which drop in proportion with IgA levels [12]. These cytokines normally decrease expression of ICAM-1, an important protein required for recruitment and adherence of neutrophils to sites of injury. In the absence of EN, neutrophil recruitment to the endothelium in the gastrointestinal vasculature is markedly increased, resulting in upregulation of the inflammation cascade that can both directly damage the GI tract and magnify the damage caused in times of intestinal stress [12].

Microbiome Considerations

In recent years, the gut microbiome of the surgery patient has been extensively studied. Composed of more than a thousand of different species, the gut microbiome serves a multitude of physiologic purposes, including roles in macronutrient metabolism, intestinal homeostasis, and immunologic defense against a multitude of pathogens [13]. The microbiome becomes profoundly altered in critical illness, leading to proliferation of gram-negative *Proteobacteria* phyla and decreased prevalence of the preferred *Firmicutes* and *Bacteroidetes* phyla, forming the aptly named "pathobiome" of critical illness. This shift in prevalence in the microbiome has profound effects on normal intestinal function, including decreased epithelial integrity, decreased absorption of nutrients, atrophy of functional mucosa, and increased systemic inflammation. Many measures that are implemented in the critical care of a surgery patient, such as the use of systemic antibiotics, vasopressor agents, and empiric proton pump inhibitor therapy, compromise the healthy microbiome further, leading to increased overall morbidity and mortality in the ICU setting [13].

PN and starvation have both been shown to have deleterious effects on the bacterial diversity of the microbiome, and previous studies in mice using PN have shown it promotes proliferation of *Proteobacteria* and increases production of pro-inflammatory cytokines [14]. The compromise of a healthy microbiome in those receiving PN predisposes the surgical patient to a host of deleterious immunologic consequences, such as surgical site infections, pneumonia, urinary tract infections, and blood stream infections not associated with the use of intravenous catheter. These infectious complications are likely the result of decreased expression of cytoskeletal elements leading to increased bacterial translocation across the mucosal barrier [14]. Early EN, meanwhile, appears to have the opposite effect, as studies have shown that levels of pro-inflammatory cytokines produced while on EN are considerably decreased.

Special Considerations: Feeding in Gastrointestinal Surgery

Given the benefits of EN, there has been an ongoing research as to when to initiate feeds following gastrointestinal surgery. Traditionally, oral feeding is initiated in the post-operative period after observance of GI function, such as flatus or bowel movements. While initiation of gastric feeds in the setting of recent foregut surgery is typically initiated after a mandatory period of healing, more recent research supports early EN for most small and large bowel surgeries even in the setting of resection and anastomosis. A recent systematic review of 17 randomized controlled trials failed to demonstrate a difference in the incidence of post-operative complications, including wound infection, anastomotic breakdown, or intra-abdominal infection, in patients who received EN within 24 hours of lower gastrointestinal surgery when compared with the more traditional management of waiting for the return of bowel function [15]. In this context, classic surgical dogma of waiting to feed post-operative patients until the return of bowel function continues to be challenged, and preliminary data seems to support initiation of early enteral feeding in the post-surgical period.

Risks/Contraindications/ Complications of Enteral Feeding

Not all surgical patients are candidates for EN. Patients with disruption of gastrointestinal continuity, as in the case of anastomotic leakage or proximal gastrointestinal diversion, have absolute contraindications to EN [16]. Those requiring the use of high-dosage vasopressors to maintain hemodynamic stability should also forego early EN, as these agents intrinsically lead to redistribution of blood flow away from the GI tract, which can induce intestinal ischemia in the fed state. This can also lead to the development of nonocclusive bowel necrosis (NOBN), a phenomenon that is rarely encountered in patients who receive strictly PN in times of severe metabolic stress [17]. While the pathogenesis of NOBN is not entirely understood, it is likely the result of increased energy requirements in already stressed enterocytes, bowel dysmotility resulting in ischemic injury, and toxic metabolite buildup within the enterocytes [17, 18]. Massive gastrointestinal hemorrhage should halt any attempts at enteral feeding until this source is found and corrected [16].

Enteral Access

Enteral access for EN is an important consideration in patients with a functioning gastrointestinal tract who are unable to reach nutrition goals through oral intake alone. The choice of enteral access depends on many factors, first and foremost, the expected duration the access will be needed. Oroenteric/nasoenteric tubes (NETs), such as nasogastric and nasojejunal tubes (orogastric/orojejunal), are the simplest mode of enteral access and are typically reserved for short-term feeding, defined as less than 4–6 weeks [19]. They are usually passed nasally but may be passed orally if desired or in the case of mechanical ventilation. Placement of post-pyloric tubes in the small intestine can be more technically challenging than gastric placement [20]. For simplicity, this chapter will refer to these temporary tubes as NETs. Although they are cost-efficient and have low morbidity, their use is limited in conscious patients due to discomfort. The risk of complications associated with NET use generally increases the longer the tubes are in place. The most common complications are pharyngitis, otitis media, nasal mucosal ulceration, pneumothorax, sinusitis, aspiration, or tracheal, esophageal, or gastroenteric ulceration [19]. To minimize the risk of aspiration and improper positioning, plain radiographs can be obtained following bedside placement and prior to initiating feeds. Because of the discomfort and complications associated with long-term use of NETs, once it is determined, a patient will need long-term nutritional support (i.e., >4–6 weeks), more permanent access should be established [21].

For patients requiring long-term access, more permanent feeding tubes are preferred. These may be placed endoscopically, radiologically, or surgically. The choice of placement method depends on several factors including local resources and expertise, hospital policy, and patient anatomy.

Surgical gastrostomy tubes can be placed open or laparoscopically. They are the preferred option if patient anatomy or body habitus precludes safe endoscopic or radiologic placement. Surgical tubes may also be placed in conjunction with another already scheduled procedure [22]. Surgical gastrostomy or jejunostomy creation involves placement of an enteric tube or red rubber catheter into the stomach or small intestine under direct visualization. Current research shows no difference in morbidity and mortality when comparing PEGs and surgical gastrostomy tubes [19, 23, 24]. However, PEGs may not require general anesthesia, require less procedure time, and are overall much less expensive than surgically placed tubes. Hybrid procedures using laparoscopic instrumentation to confirm apposition of the stomach to the abdominal wall during endoscopic PEG tube placement have also been described [19].

The two options for non-surgical gastrostomy tube placement are percutaneous endoscopic gastrostomy (PEG)/jejunostomy (PEJ) and radiologically inserted gastrostomy (RIG) or jejunostomy (RIJ) tube. Jejunal extensions may also be placed through gastrostomy tubes if this is desired and/or indicated [19]. There is no clear evidence favoring one technique over the other; the decision is made based on preference and local expertise and availability [19]. PEG tubes can be placed at bedside or in the endoscopy suite. They are rather quick procedures and are associated with limited major complications. The most common complications of these procedures include dislodgement, peristomal infections, and peri-procedural issues (i.e., aspiration). An abdominal binder and continued evaluation of proper bumper placement can prevent inadvertent tension and dislodgement of the PEG tube, and a dose of antibiotics given prior to the procedure has been shown to minimize the risk of wound infections [21, 22]. The risk of orotracheal aspiration is minimized by appropriate patient positioning, suction, and avoiding over-sedation. RIG tubes are placed under fluoroscopic guidance either in the radiology suite or at bedside.

The most common complication is dislodgement of the tube. These tubes also clog more frequently due to decreased diameter compared to PEG tubes [19, 22].

Parenteral Nutrition

Malnutrition is a well-established risk factor for post-operative complications and increased mortality among surgical patients [25, 26]. Because of this, it is important to consider peri-operative nutritional therapy in high-risk or malnourished patients as assessed by nutritional risk scores. Nutrition therapy can be provided orally, enterally, parenterally, or through a combination of methods. As previously discussed, oral/enteral nutrition is preferred; however, patients with intestinal failure or those who cannot meet nutritional goals through these methods may require parenteral supplementation (Table 9.1). PN is a mixture of solutions including dextrose, amino acids, vitamins and minerals, trace elements, and lipid emulsions given intravenously (typically centrally) to supplement nutrition. The use of PN in surgical patients has evolved significantly since its initial widespread use in the 1970s when the late Stanley Dudrick revolutionized nutritional supplementation with his early studies on Beagles [27–29]. Since this time, numerous prospective randomized control trials have failed to demonstrate the benefit of routine perioperative PN, and some have even demonstrated poorer outcomes. Because of this, the use of PN has diminished significantly over time and is typically reserved for patients with inadequate enteral intake or contraindication. Although there have been numerous advances in PN formulations and stricter glycemic control in patients on PN (a proposed contributing factor of previously reported complications), it is still thought to be inferior to EN [30]. However, when used in the appropriate patients, PN can improve nitrogen balance, augment immune recovery and wound healing, and improve post-operative outcomes [31–34]. The most common indication for PN in surgical patients is contraindication to EN. Contraindications to feeding the gut include intestinal failure, intestinal obstruction, significant malabsorption, proximal or high-output fistula, intestinal ischemia, severe shock with impaired splanchnic perfusion, and fulminant septic shock [26, 28, 34, 35]. Other indications are less well-defined but generally involve a significant deficiency in the ability to tolerate enteral intake in combination with malnutrition or high-risk nutritional status.

Table 9.1 Contraindications to enteral nutrition

Absolute	Relative
Lack of GI tract continuity	Poor intestinal absorption
GI hemorrhage	GI tract fistula
Bowel obstruction/paralytic ileus	Vasopressor requirement
Hemodynamic instability with end-organ malperfusion	Abdominal distension/ evidence of intolerance of feeds

Pre-operative Parenteral Nutrition

The routine use of pre-operative PN in healthy patients is not beneficial and is potentially harmful. Therefore, this practice should be reserved for patients already at risk for surgical complications due to poor nutritional status. Malnourished or high-risk nutritional patients unable to meet energy requirements by EN alone should be given supplemental pre-operative PN. Pre-operative PN should be initiated at least 7–14 days prior to surgery and continued post-operatively. If deemed appropriate, pre-operative PN can be administered by trained nurses at the patient's home, with close follow-up [26, 34, 36].

Post-operative Parenteral Nutrition

Routine post-operative use of PN is not beneficial and may increase morbidity up to 10%; therefore, it is not recommended [26, 34, 36, 37]. Malnourished patients, deemed appropriate for pre-operative PN, should continue PN post-operatively for at least 9 days to see the full benefit of supportive therapy. If a patient is unable to tolerate post-operative EN and is not at increased nutritional risk, PN should be held until 5–7 days post-operatively. PN should be initiated in these patients at this time if they are unable to receive >50% of estimated nutritional requirements enterally. Even then, PN should only be initiated if a patient will likely require >7 days of nutritional support. If able to tolerate it, a combination of EN and supplementary PN is preferred. In nutritionally at-risk patients that are not severely malnourished, PN may be started after 3–5 days of insufficient nutrition via EN (Fig. 9.1) [36].

Intestinal Failure

Apart from providing caloric benefit to high-risk nutritional patients perioperatively, most other indications for PN in surgical patients are related to intestinal failure. This may be acute in the setting of recent surgery or illness which only required brief parenteral support, or chronic, necessitating long-term PN with gut rehabilitation and/or intestinal transplantation. In general, intestinal failure (IF) is defined as loss of enterocyte cell mass or physiologic function secondary to surgical resection, dysmotility, obstruction, congenital defects, or disease, resulting in the loss of absorptive capabilities [27, 36, 38]. It is estimated that 40,000 patients in the USA currently depend on PN for nutrition due to IF. The most common cause is post-operative short gut syndrome (SGS) after extensive small bowel resections related to inflammatory bowel diseases [39]. High-output fistulas, malignant obstructions, and post-bariatric surgery complications are other notable causes of IF that may necessitate PN support.

Short Gut Syndrome

SGS can result from significant bowel resections, which leave less than 1.5 m of the small intestine. These patients are usually unable to meet nutritional needs through enteral nutrition alone secondary to limited absorptive capacity. If possible, referral to nutritional and intestinal rehab can significantly increase the quality of life in these

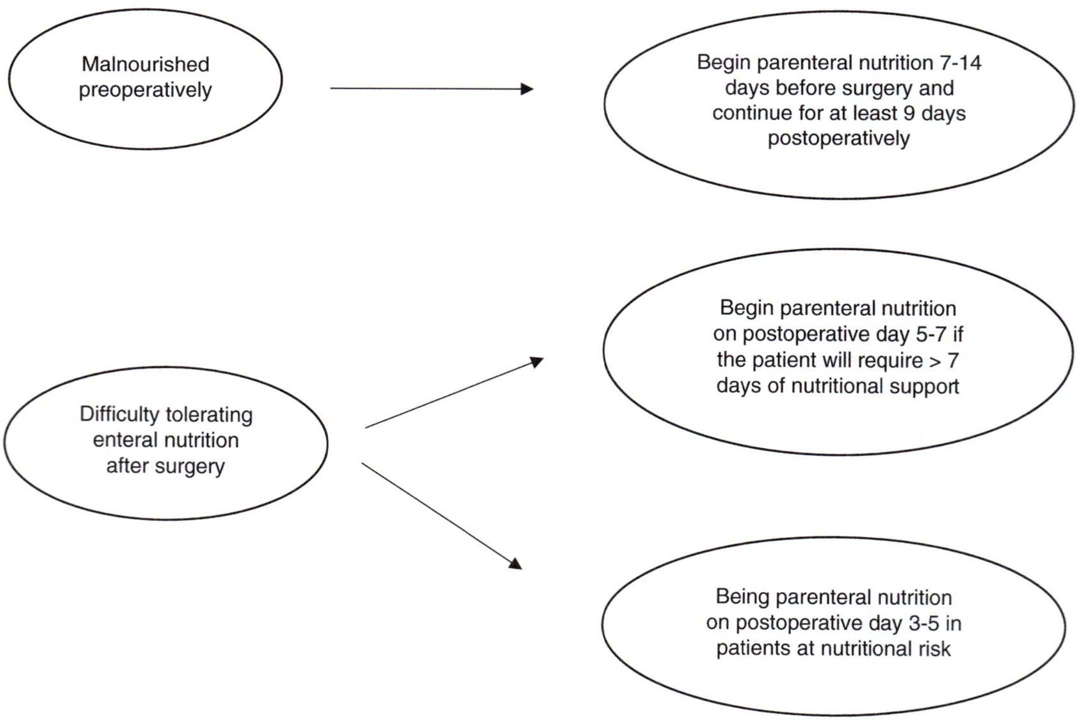

Fig. 9.1 Decision tree regarding perioperative parenteral nutrition

patients. If unable to reach nutritional autonomy, long-term PN is indicated. The total length of bowel necessary to avoid long-term PN is variable and ultimately depends on the functionality and nature of the remaining bowel. In general, patients with >100 cm of the small bowel can often avoid long-term PN dependence regardless of colon presence, while those with an intact colon can often meet their nutritional needs with >50 cm of the remaining small bowel. Although outside the scope of this review, it is important to note that the development of significant complications resulting from PN is an indication for referral for intestinal transplant [39–41].

Inflammatory Bowel Disease

As previously stated, inflammatory bowel diseases, Crohn's disease (CD), and ulcerative colitis (UC) represent a significant subset of surgical patients requiring PN. In general, the indications for PN in these patients are the same as those for the general population and already discussed in this chapter. However, especially in the most severe CD cases, patients are at high nutritional risk and commonly require supplemental PN at some point during their disease course. PN is considered when patients demonstrate an inability to meet nutritional needs via an enteral route. In cases of SGS secondary to repeated bowel resections, obstruction where enteral access distal to the obstruction cannot be obtained, or prolonged ileus, this is especially common [42]. Additionally, PN is generally used in CD patients with proximal or high-output fistulas in an attempt to control output [42]. Notably many patients with severe CD are chronically malnourished, and PN may be recommended 2–3 weeks perioperatively to improve surgical outcomes [43]. There is some evidence that the role of PN in patients with CD extends beyond simple caloric and nutrient supplementation to actual improvement in disease course. A recent meta-analysis demonstrated some benefit in improving the disease process of CD when patients are on PN [44]. It has been theorized that the combination of complete gut rest and PN allows for adequate nutrition while reducing antigenic mucosal stimulation during acute CD flairs, thereby improving outcomes [42]. However, there is no convincing evidence for overall benefit from this treatment plan, and EN remains the preferred route of nutrition in IBD when possible [45, 46]. Compared to UC which does not involve the small intestine, CD patients are more likely to require long-term PN due to repeated resections resulting in SGS, persistent high-output fistulas or stomas, and prolonged incomplete bowel obstructions. Studies have shown that although home PN does decrease quality of life, it is still a safe and a preferred alternative to prolonged hospitalizations or early surgery in patients with complicated CD [42, 47].

Critically Ill Patients

Critically ill surgical patients, like those with acute IBD, experience a hypermetabolic state. Indications for PN in these patients include feeding intolerance, prolonged ileus, peritonitis or obstruction (>3 days), abdominal distension on EN, severe malabsorption, splanchnic ischemia, or > 5 days of failure to reach full EN requirements. Careful attention should be paid to avoiding overfeeding with PN in these patients. When possible, a combination of EN and PN is recommended to reach goal calorie and protein delivery. PN may also be indicated in patients who are at high risk for aspiration and are not candidates for post-pyloric feeding [36, 48].

High-Output Fistulas

Enterocutaneous fistulas (ECFs), abnormal connections between the GI tract and skin, can occur due to radiation exposure, IBD, malignancy, obstruction, or post-operatively. Due to the underlying pathophysiology of ECFs, these patients are often malnourished and can suffer from severe electrolyte and fluid imbalances. Because of their tenuous nutritional status, these patients should be cared for by a multidisciplinary team that is able to carefully monitor and adjust treatment as necessary [49, 50]. Typical management of these patients includes wound care/fistula management with careful monitoring and optimization of fluid, electrolyte, and nutritional status. Depending on the etiology, location, and output of the ECF, patients may require

PN. In general, ECFs with output less than 500 mL per day (i.e., low-output fistulas) are more likely to close spontaneously and less likely to require PN than high-output fistulas (i.e., >500 mL/day). Entero-atmospheric fistulas, those with intestinal mucosa exposed to the atmosphere, are also unlikely to close spontaneously and may require PN support. Indications for PN in patients with ECF include output >500 ml per day, bowel obstruction, and/or wound care difficulties secondary to fistula output. Patients can be started on PN during their hospitalization and transitioned to home PN with close monitoring once medically stable [49, 50]. Surgical intervention to repair the fistula should be delayed at least 3–6 months after the initial development of the ECF, following resolution of the acute inflammatory response and optimization of nutritional status. In addition to PN and the cessation of enteral intake, ASPEN recommends the use of somatostatin or somatostatin analogues as well as oral glutamine supplementation, in patients with output >500 ml/day [50, 51] [52]. Somatostatin may decrease fistula output and promote closure. Glutamine supplementation should not be given to patients with evidence of hepatic or renal failure, but has been shown to enhance fistula closure and improve mortality in those without contraindication.

Bariatric Surgery

Bariatric surgery provides a complicated nutritional picture. Although patients are obese, sarcopenia is common and increases the risk of post-operative complications [53]. PN is not universally recommended for patients following uncomplicated surgery; instead early post-operative EN is preferred. Post-bariatric surgery complications do, however, represent a subset of patients who may require PN due to inadequate absorption or intolerance of EN. Most of these patients only require PN in the short term until a corrective operation is performed [54–56].

Malignant Bowel Obstruction

The mainstay of treatment for malignant bowel obstruction (MBO) is prompt cessation of enteral intake, nasogastric aspiration, and the use of anti-secretory agents. Most patients will have recurrence of symptoms upon resuming oral intake, necessitating the need to defer enteral intake indefinitely. The role of PN in these patients is controversial, and supplementation remains palliative and should be given in consultation with medical providers, patients, and caregivers. The most recent data suggests that the administration of PN in patients with MBO is associated with longer survival than patients who did not receive PN. According to the most recent ESPEN guidelines in cancer patients, PN is indicated if patients are unable to tolerate any oral intake for >1 week or are meeting less than 60% of nutritional goals for >1–2 weeks [57, 58]. Overall, in patients with MBO, it is reasonable to consider PN, when life expectancy depends on delivery of nutrients and not on the disease process itself [57, 59, 60].

Amino Acid Supplementation

Glutamine

Glutamine is a key amino acid in gastrointestinal function. Some studies suggest that supplementation in times of stress may decrease infections and improve glycemic control. Supplementation may also aid in preservation of positive nitrogen balance. Because of its important metabolic role in GI function, when used in PN, it is hypothesized to attenuate villous atrophy and associated intestinal permeability that may result from long-term parenteral support. However, a recent study found an increase in mortality in critically ill ICU patients who received glutamine supplementation; further research may be necessary to optimize the use of glutamine in the critically ill [61]. In its latest report, ESPEN recommends considering glutamine supplementation in standard doses; however, there is not enough evidence of positive effects to give a strong recommendation for use [35].

Arginine

Arginine is essential in would healing, T cell function and contributes to endothelial function. Some data suggests that parenteral arginine may decrease fistula occurrence and improve outcomes in patients with head and neck cancer [62, 63]. One study also suggested a decrease in recurrence of malignancy, but it is not clear whether this correlates with a decrease in mortality. Because of the uncertainty, there are not clear recommendations regarding arginine supplementation in the surgical population [35].

Special Circumstances in Surgical Nutrition

Since the late 1980s, nutritional therapy has gained significant attention from surgeon scientists. Increasingly rigorous studies occurring in translational animal models and at clinical bedsides have yielded significant advances in the understanding of nutritional support, particularly in critically ill and surgical patients. As a result, specialized metabolic care has become common and crucial to optimal perioperative management and pre-habilitation. As previously discussed, EN improves perioperative outcomes and decreases morbidity and mortality. This improvement is driven by both caloric and non-caloric benefits extending from improved enteric mucosal integrity, innate and adaptive immune responses, and the diversity and dynamics of the microbiome [8, 10–12]. Nutrition as a primary therapeutic intervention should both be considered during prehabilitation in elective surgeries and early in the perioperative period to promote wound healing and decrease septic morbidity. In this section, we discuss specific considerations useful for nutritional optimization.

Immune-Enhancing Diets

Traditionally, the provision of early EN was thought to mitigate the acute protein malnutrition associated with major elective surgery and trauma. More recently, there have also been increasing efforts to curb innate and adaptive immune dysfunction occurring after physical insult, thus decreasing the subsequent inflammatory-driven catabolic response. Immune-enhancing diets, also known as pharmaconutrition or immunonutrition, were popularized after demonstration that supraphysiologic doses of certain micronutrients exhibit immune-altering pharmacologic properties [64–66]. Commonly studied nutrients include specific amino acids (e.g., arginine, glutamine, leucine), omega-3 fatty acids, and vitamins.

Of the micronutrients, the effects of arginine have been most widely scrutinized. Arginine is an amino acid integral in human metabolism. Metabolic processes involving arginine include polypeptide anabolism and catabolism, islet secretion of insulin, and nitric oxide-mediated vasodilation [67–69]. With activation of the hypothalamic-pituitary-adrenocortical (HPA) axis – as occurs with major surgery or trauma – the endogenous production of non-essential arginine is significantly suppressed, resulting in a conditional deficiency [70]. Of interest, supplementation of arginine in stressed murine populations has been shown to promote positive nitrogen balance and enhanced peripheral lymphocyte response dynamics to cellular mitogens [71]. These findings have been reproduced in humans [72] and fueled optimism for dietary manipulation and commercial nutritional formulations that might broadly improve morbidity and mortality associated with trauma and oncologic and abdominal surgeries. Additionally, arginine serves as an intermediate amino acid during proline synthesis, which is required for wound healing and collagen synthesis [73–75]. Arginine also has a role in immune competence as it serves as an intra-cellular substrate for nitric oxide production allowing macrophages to improve bactericidal activity and improves T cell function, proliferation, and maturation [72, 76–81]. This is of great importance for the post-operative, convalescing surgical patient.

Optimism for immunonutrition has historically also extended beyond arginine. Scientific studies have evaluated a wide range of additives, including glutamine, Ω-3 fatty acids, minerals (such as selenium), and nucleotides. Broadly, these individual studies have demonstrated statistically significant results, including reducing the incidence of perioperative deep space and nosocomial infections and supporting fewer ventilator days and shorter intensive care unit and hospital length of stays by a mean difference of 2 days [82–84]. Despite these initial positive findings, meta-analyses suggest that although immune-enhancing diets containing one or more of the aforementioned additives may benefit specific cohorts, clinical benefits are modest with no effect on mortality rates [85]. Additionally, most of the articles analyzed demonstrate selection, reporting, and industry bias. Consequently, lack of high-quality evidence precludes generalized provision of immune-enhancing diets to surgical patients. Scientific substantiation – in the form of high-quality, investigator-initiated studies which take measures to mitigate methodological flaws and bias – will be required to define putative benefits of immunonutrition in the perioperative or peri-traumatic period.

Pre-, Pro-, and Synbiotics

Although it continues to improve, critical care continues to have limitations, which has led to interest in novel approaches to treatment during critical illness, such as manipulation of the microbiome. Since 1907, when Nobel Laureate Elie Metchnikoff first described the concept of probiotics, the overarching opinion has been that probiotics are safe and have a role in treating gastrointestinal diseases; however, routine use has not been supported by literature [86]. Over the past several decades, research has provided insight into how the stresses of ICU care, critical illness, and surgery all negatively impact the microbiome giving rise to virulent organisms collectively called the pathobiome [87–95]. Various strategies have been reported to reduce the burden the pathobiome with variable results. Probiotics are of increased interest in this domain, and research is forthcoming in use in critically ill populations.

The science of probiotics has evolved in a supplementary fashion like seen in immunonutrition. Probiotics are live microbial mixtures administered pharmacologically to improve a patient's gastrointestinal microbiome and confer health benefits. These microbes can be administered concurrently with non-digestible food ingredients (i.e., fiber) called prebiotics that promote the growth of beneficial microorganisms. When a formulation contains both a live beneficial microbe and a prebiotic ingredient, it is known as a synbiotic or symbiotic mixture.

Clinical interest in probiotics continues due to the beneficial microorganisms' metabolic abilities, which include the production of essential vitamins, hydrolysis of indigestible oligosaccharides, competitive inhibition of nosocomial infections, improvement in host immune function, improvement in gut integrity, decrease in inflammation, reduction in surgical site infections, shortening of hospital length of stay, reduction in septic episodes, and even improvement in anastomotic leak rates [96–104]. Over the last decade, probiotics have been shown to reduce inflammatory biomarkers and oxidative stress while improving lipid profiles, glycemic control, dysbiosis, and clinical outcomes [105–112]. Regardless of the amounting research that has shown a benefit, supplementing probiotics is still not considered standard of care in all ICU settings. Nevertheless, the idea of "bioecological control" has blossomed in the critically ill and polytrauma patients defined as supplying viable beneficial bacteria or substrate to enhance these specific beneficial bacteria instead of eliminating the pathogen [113–115].

Despite the promising nature of these results, some attested benefits are plagued by the same major study limitations affecting the quality of surgical immunonutrition data – bias and heterogeneity. For example, meta-analysis of 20 studies demonstrated a decrease in post-operative infections with perioperative use of syn- and probiotic formulations. Of these, however, more than half did not report their randomization methods, allocation concealment, or blinding methods. Nineteen of the twenty studies also had missing participant data, the highest percentage of which was 42.4% [116]. There is even trouble validating and providing the exact bacterial strain advertised on the product label due to lack of standardization [117]. Of the 16 total probiotic products evaluated, only one perfectly matched the bifidobacterial label claims on pill-to-pill and lot-to-lot bases. Both further studies and quality control of offered products are required before the perioperative use of syn- and probiotics can be routinely recommended, despite its promise.

Enhanced Recovery After Surgery (ERAS) Protocols and Applications Within Nutrition

With the progression of surgical science, technique, and instrumentation, it has become increasingly safe and common to reintroduce enteral feeds early in the post-operative course. Enhanced recovery after surgery (ERAS) protocols are standardized perioperative care pathways specifically designed to minimize post-surgical systemic inflammatory response (SIR), improve glycemic control, and overall shorten hospital length of stay [118–126]. This is achieved through a multimodal approach with components consisting of pre-operative optimization and immunonutrition shakes twice a day for 1 week, anesthesia, goal-directed fluid resuscitation, mobilization, chemoprophylaxis, and importantly early enteral feeding [126–130]. ERAS protocols are safe and cost-effective and are proven to lower recovery time and complication frequency [131, 132]. Minimizing the length of enteric starvation is important to recovery programs and runs counter to historical surgical dogma recommending return of bowel function prior to feeding, as alluded to earlier in this chapter. Early EN is theorized to minimize enteric mucosal atrophy, normalize peristalsis, maintain the intestinal flora, and may reduce the physiologic hypermetabolism associated with surgery and the stress response.

Conclusion

Surgical fields continue to recognize the importance of nutritional provision as an adjunctive, therapeutic modality within surgical populations. The consideration of nutritional state in the perioperative period and adjunctive supplements are, in general, safe, feasible, and useful. As larger randomized controlled trials are performed within surgical populations, the consideration of individualized nutritional plans and operation-tailored protocols will be important in improving surgical outcomes and minimizing healthcare costs.

References

1. Cerra FB. Hypermetabolism, organ failure, and metabolic support. Surgery. 1987;101(1):1–14.
2. Kott M, Hartl WH, Elke G. Enteral vs. parenteral nutrition in septic shock: are they equivalent? Curr Opin Crit Care. 2019;25(4):340–8.
3. Elke G, van Zanten AR, Lemieux M, McCall M, Jeejeebhoy KN, Kott M, et al. Enteral versus parenteral nutrition in critically ill patients: an updated systematic review and meta-analysis of randomized controlled trials. Crit Care. 2016;20(1):117.
4. Fukatsu K. Role of nutrition in gastroenterological surgery. Ann Gastroenterol Surg. 2019;3(2): 160–8.
5. Yeh DD, Fuentes E, Quraishi SA, Cropano C, Kaafarani H, Lee J, et al. Adequate nutrition may get you home: effect of caloric/protein deficits on the discharge destination of critically ill surgical patients. JPEN J Parenter Enteral Nutr. 2016;40(1):37–44.
6. Grossie VB Jr, Weisbrodt NW, Moore FA, Moody F. Ischemia/reperfusion-induced disruption of rat small intestine transit is reversed by total enteral nutrition. Nutrition. 2001;17(11–12):939–43.
7. Flynn WJ Jr, Gosche JR, Garrison RN. Intestinal blood flow is restored with glutamine or glucose suffusion after hemorrhage. J Surg Res. 1992;52(5):499–504.
8. Alverdy J, Chi HS, Sheldon GF. The effect of parenteral nutrition on gastrointestinal immunity. The importance of enteral stimulation. Ann Surg. 1985;202(6):681–4.
9. Fukatsu K. Impact of the feeding route on gut mucosal immunity. Curr Opin Clin Nutr Metab Care. 2014;17(2):164–70.
10. Kang W, Kudsk KA. Is there evidence that the gut contributes to mucosal immunity in humans? JPEN J Parenter Enteral Nutr. 2007;31(3):246–58.
11. Kudsk KA. Beneficial effect of enteral feeding. Gastrointest Endosc Clin N Am. 2007;17(4):647–62.
12. Kudsk KA. Effect of route and type of nutrition on intestine-derived inflammatory responses. Am J Surg. 2003;185(1):16–21.
13. Moron R, Galvez J, Colmenero M, Anderson P, Cabeza J, Rodriguez-Cabezas ME. The importance of the microbiome in critically ill patients: role of nutrition. Nutrients. 2019;11(12):3002.
14. Demehri FR, Barrett M, Ralls MW, Miyasaka EA, Feng Y, Teitelbaum DH. Intestinal epithelial cell apoptosis and loss of barrier function in the setting

of altered microbiota with enteral nutrient deprivation. Front Cell Infect Microbiol. 2013;3:105.
15. Levett-Jones T. Early enteral nutrition within 24 hours of lower gastrointestinal surgery versus later commencement for length of hospital stay and postoperative complications. Clin Nurse Spec. 2019;33(5):212–3.
16. Xu L, Wang T, Chen T, Yang WQ, Liang ZP, Zhu JC. Identification of risk factors for enteral feeding intolerance screening in critically ill patients. Saudi Med J. 2017;38(8):816–25.
17. Marvin RG, McKinley BA, McQuiggan M, Cocanour CS, Moore FA. Nonocclusive bowel necrosis occurring in critically ill trauma patients receiving enteral nutrition manifests no reliable clinical signs for early detection. Am J Surg. 2000;179(1):7–12.
18. Kozar RA, Schultz SG, Hassoun HT, Desoignie R, Weisbrodt NW, Haber MM, et al. The type of sodium-coupled solute modulates small bowel mucosal injury, transport function, and ATP after ischemia/reperfusion injury in rats. Gastroenterology. 2002;123(3):810–6.
19. DeLegge MH. Enteral access and associated complications. Gastroenterol Clin N Am. 2018;47(1): 23–37.
20. Pash E. Enteral nutrition: options for short-term access. Nutr Clin Pract. 2018;33(2):170–6.
21. Blumenstein I, Shastri YM, Stein J. Gastroenteric tube feeding: techniques, problems and solutions. World J Gastroenterol. 2014;20(26):8505–24.
22. Phillips MS, Ponsky JL. Overview of enteral and parenteral feeding access techniques: principles and practice. Surg Clin North Am. 2011;91(4):897–911. ix
23. Leeds JS, McAlindon ME, Grant J, Robson HE, Lee FK, Sanders DS. Survival analysis after gastrostomy: a single-centre, observational study comparing radiological and endoscopic insertion. Eur J Gastroenterol Hepatol. 2010;22(5):591–6.
24. Wollman B, D'Agostino HB, Walus-Wigle JR, Easter DW, Beale A. Radiologic, endoscopic, and surgical gastrostomy: an institutional evaluation and meta-analysis of the literature. Radiology. 1995;197(3):699–704.
25. McClave SA, Snider HL, Spain DA. Preoperative issues in clinical nutrition. Chest. 1999;115(5 Suppl):64S–70S.
26. Abunnaja S, Cuviello A, Sanchez JA. Enteral and parenteral nutrition in the perioperative period: state of the art. Nutrients. 2013;5(2):608–23.
27. Lappas BM, Patel D, Kumpf V, Adams DW, Seidner DL. Parenteral nutrition: indications, access, and complications. Gastroenterol Clin N Am. 2018;47(1):39–59.
28. Dudrick SJ, Pimiento JM. Parenteral nutrition and nutritional support of surgical patients: reflections, controversies, and challenges. Surg Clin North Am. 2011;91(3):675–92.
29. Nakayama DK. The development of total parenteral nutrition. Am Surg. 2017;83(1):36–8.
30. Rosenthal MD, Vanzant EL, Martindale RG, Moore FA. Evolving paradigms in the nutritional support of critically ill surgical patients. Curr Probl Surg. 2015;52(4):147–82.
31. Compher CW, Spencer C, Kinosian BP. Perioperative parenteral nutrition: impact on morbidity and mortality in surgical patients. Nutr Clin Pract. 2005;20(4):460–7.
32. Torosian MH. Perioperative nutrition support for patients undergoing gastrointestinal surgery: critical analysis and recommendations. World J Surg. 1999;23(6):565–9.
33. Bozzetti F. Peri-operative nutritional management. Proc Nutr Soc. 2011;70(3):305–10.
34. Braga M, Ljungqvist O, Soeters P, Fearon K, Weimann A, Bozzetti F, et al. ESPEN guidelines on parenteral nutrition: surgery. Clin Nutr. 2009;28(4):378–86.
35. Weimann A, Braga M, Carli F, Higashiguchi T, Hubner M, Klek S, et al. ESPEN guideline: clinical nutrition in surgery. Clin Nutr. 2017;36(3):623–50.
36. Worthington P, Balint J, Bechtold M, Bingham A, Chan LN, Durfee S, et al. When is parenteral nutrition appropriate? JPEN J Parenter Enteral Nutr. 2017;41(3):324–77.
37. Howard L, Ashley C. Nutrition in the perioperative patient. Annu Rev Nutr. 2003;23:263–82.
38. Pironi L, Arends J, Bozzetti F, Cuerda C, Gillanders L, Jeppesen PB, et al. Corrigendum to "ESPEN guidelines on chronic intestinal failure in adults" [Clin Nutr 35 (2) (2016) 247–307]. Clin Nutr. 2017;36(2):619.
39. Bharadwaj S, Tandon P, Rivas JM, Furman A, Moccia L, Ratliff A, et al. Update on the management of intestinal failure. Cleve Clin J Med. 2016;83(11):841–8.
40. Gotthardt DN, Gauss A, Zech U, Mehrabi A, Weiss KH, Sauer P, et al. Indications for intestinal transplantation: recognizing the scope and limits of total parenteral nutrition. Clin Transpl. 2013;27(Suppl 25):49–55.
41. Carroll RE, Benedetti E, Schowalter JP, Buchman AL. Management and complications of short bowel syndrome: an updated review. Curr Gastroenterol Rep. 2016;18(7):40.
42. Triantafillidis JK, Papalois AE. The role of total parenteral nutrition in inflammatory bowel disease: current aspects. Scand J Gastroenterol. 2014;49(1):3–14.
43. Forbes A, Escher J, Hebuterne X, Klek S, Krznaric Z, Schneider S, et al. ESPEN guideline: clinical nutrition in inflammatory bowel disease. Clin Nutr. 2017;36(2):321–47.
44. Comeche JM, Comino I, Altavilla C, Tuells J, Gutierrez-Hervas A, Caballero P. Parenteral nutrition in patients with inflammatory bowel disease systematic review, meta-analysis and meta-regression. Nutrients. 2019;11(12):2865.
45. Jones VA. Comparison of total parenteral nutrition and elemental diet in induction of remission of

Crohn's disease. Long-term maintenance of remission by personalized food exclusion diets. Dig Dis Sci. 1987;32(12 Suppl):100S–7S.
46. Kleinman RE, Baldassano RN, Caplan A, Griffiths AM, Heyman MB, Issenman RM, et al. Nutrition support for pediatric patients with inflammatory bowel disease: a clinical report of the north American Society for Pediatric Gastroenterology, Hepatology And Nutrition. J Pediatr Gastroenterol Nutr. 2004;39(1):15–27.
47. Schwartz E. Perioperative parenteral nutrition in adults with inflammatory bowel disease: a review of the literature. Nutr Clin Pract. 2016;31(2):159–70.
48. McClave SA, Taylor BE, Martindale RG, Warren MM, Johnson DR, Braunschweig C, et al. Guidelines for the provision and assessment of nutrition support therapy in the adult critically ill patient: Society of Critical Care Medicine (SCCM) and American Society for Parenteral and Enteral Nutrition (A.S.P.E.N.). JPEN J Parenter Enteral Nutr. 2016;40(2):159–211.
49. Gribovskaja-Rupp I, Melton GB. Enterocutaneous fistula: proven strategies and updates. Clin Colon Rectal Surg. 2016;29(2):130–7.
50. Kumpf VJ, de Aguilar-Nascimento JE, Diaz-Pizarro Graf JI, Hall AM, McKeever L, Steiger E, et al. ASPEN-FELANPE Clinical Guidelines. JPEN J Parenter Enteral Nutr. 2017;41(1):104–12.
51. Compher C, Winkler MF, Guenter P, Steiger E. Nutrition management of home parenteral nutrition among patients with enterocutaneous fistula in the sustain registry. JPEN J Parenter Enteral Nutr. 2018;42(2):412–7.
52. Fekaj E, Salihu L, Morina A. Treatment of enterocutaneous fistula with total parenteral feeding in combination with octreotide: a case report. Cases J. 2009;2:177.
53. Olmos MA, Vazquez MJ, Gorria MJ, Gonzalez PP, Martinez IO, Chimeno IM, et al. Effect of parenteral nutrition on nutrition status after bariatric surgery for morbid obesity. JPEN J Parenter Enteral Nutr. 2005;29(6):445–50.
54. Chen Y. Acute bariatric surgery complications: managing parenteral nutrition in the morbidly obese. J Am Diet Assoc. 2010;110(11):1734–7.
55. Van Gossum A, Pironi L, Chambrier C, Dreesen M, Brandt CF, Santarpia L, et al. Home parenteral nutrition (HPN) in patients with post-bariatric surgery complications. Clin Nutr. 2017;36(5):1345–8.
56. Mundi MS, Vallumsetla N, Davidson JB, McMahon MT, Bonnes SL, Hurt RT. Use of home parenteral nutrition in post-bariatric surgery-related malnutrition. JPEN J Parenter Enteral Nutr. 2017;41(7):1119–24.
57. Bozzetti F. The role of parenteral nutrition in patients with malignant bowel obstruction. Support Care Cancer. 2019;27(12):4393–9.
58. Arends J, Bachmann P, Baracos V, Barthelemy N, Bertz H, Bozzetti F, et al. ESPEN guidelines on nutrition in cancer patients. Clin Nutr. 2017;36(1):11–48.
59. Sowerbutts AM, Lal S, Sremanakova J, Clamp AR, Jayson GC, Teubner A, et al. Palliative home parenteral nutrition in patients with ovarian cancer and malignant bowel obstruction: experiences of women and family caregivers. BMC Palliat Care. 2019;18(1):120.
60. Bozzetti F. Parenteral nutrition. Nutrition. 2019;66:101–7.
61. Heyland D, Muscedere J, Wischmeyer PE, Cook D, Jones G, Albert M, et al. A randomized trial of glutamine and antioxidants in critically ill patients. N Engl J Med. 2013;368(16):1489–97.
62. Buijs N, van Bokhorst-de van der Schueren MA, Langius JA, Leemans CR, Kuik DJ, Vermeulen MA, et al. Perioperative arginine-supplemented nutrition in malnourished patients with head and neck cancer improves long-term survival. Am J Clin Nutr. 2010;92(5):1151–6.
63. Vidal-Casariego A, Calleja-Fernandez A, Villar-Taibo R, Kyriakos G, Ballesteros-Pomar MD. Efficacy of arginine-enriched enteral formulas in the reduction of surgical complications in head and neck cancer: a systematic review and meta-analysis. Clin Nutr. 2014;33(6):951–7.
64. Barbul A, Wasserkrug HL, Sisto DA, Seifter E, Rettura G, Levenson SM, et al. Thymic stimulatory actions of arginine. J Parenter Enter Nutr. 1980;4(5):446–9.
65. Alexander NJ, Smythe NL. Dietary fat modulation of in vitro lymphocyte function. Ann Nutr Metab. 1988;32(4):192–9.
66. Kulkarni AD, Fanslow WC, Rudolph FB, Van Buren CT. Effect of dietary nucleotides on response to bacterial infections. J Parenter Enter Nutr. 1986;10(2):169–71.
67. Henningsson R, Lundquist I. Arginine-induced insulin release is decreased and glucagon increased in parallel with islet NO production. Am J Physiol Endocrinol Metab. 1998;275(3):E500–E6.
68. Moncada S, Higgs A. The L-arginine-nitric oxide pathway. N Engl J Med. 1993;329(27):2002–12.
69. Morris SM Jr. Regulation of enzymes of the urea cycle and arginine metabolism. Annu Rev Nutr. 2002;22(1):87–105.
70. Furst P, editor. Conditionally indispensable amino acids (glutamine, cyst (e) ine, tyrosine, arginine, ornithine, taurine) in enteral feeding and the dipeptide concept. Nestle Nutr Workshop Ser Clin Perform Programme; 2000.
71. Barbul A, Wasserkrug HL, Seifter E, Rettura G, Levenson SM, Efron G. Immunostimulatory effects of arginine in normal and injured rats. J Surg Res. 1980;29(3):228–35.
72. Barbul A, Sisto D, Wasserkrug H, Efron G. Arginine stimulates lymphocyte immune response in healthy human beings. Surgery. 1981;90(2):244–51.
73. Barbul A, Rettura G, Levenson SM, Seifter E. Wound healing and thymotropic effects of arginine: a pituitary mechanism of action. Am J Clin Nutr. 1983;37(5):786–94.

74. Alexander JW, Supp DM. Role of arginine and omega-3 fatty acids in wound healing and infection. Adv Wound Care (New Rochelle). 2014;3(11):682–90.
75. Albina JE, Mills CD, Barbul A, Thirkill CE, Henry WL Jr, Mastrofrancesco B, et al. Arginine metabolism in wounds. Am J Phys. 1988;254(4 Pt 1):E459–67.
76. Bansal V, Ochoa JB. Arginine availability, arginase, and the immune response. Curr Opin Clin Nutr Metab Care. 2003;6(2):223–8.
77. Zhu X, Pribis JP, Rodriguez PC, Morris SM Jr, Vodovotz Y, Billiar TR, et al. The central role of arginine catabolism in T-cell dysfunction and increased susceptibility to infection after physical injury. Ann Surg. 2014;259(1):171–8.
78. Daly JM, Reynolds J, Thom A, Kinsley L, Dietrick-Gallagher M, Shou J, et al. Immune and metabolic effects of arginine in the surgical patient. Ann Surg. 1988;208(4):512–23.
79. Morris SM Jr. Arginine: master and commander in innate immune responses. Sci Signal. 2010;3(135):e27.
80. Barbul A, Rettura G, Levenson SM, Seifter E. Arginine: a thymotropic and wound-healing promoting agent. Surg Forum. 1977;28:101–3.
81. Barbul A, Wasserkrug HL, Sisto DA, Seifter E, Rettura G, Levenson SM, et al. Thymic stimulatory actions of arginine. JPEN J Parenter Enteral Nutr. 1980;4(5):446–9.
82. Marimuthu K, Varadhan KK, Ljungqvist O, Lobo DN. A meta-analysis of the effect of combinations of immune modulating nutrients on outcome in patients undergoing major open gastrointestinal surgery. LWW; 2012.
83. Zheng Y-M, Li F, Zhang M-M, Wu X-T. Glutamine dipeptide for parenteral nutrition in abdominal surgery: a meta-analysis of randomized controlled trials. World J Gastroenterol: WJG. 2006;12(46):7537.
84. Beale RJ, Bryg DJ, Bihari DJ. Immunonutrition in the critically ill: a systematic review of clinical outcome. Crit Care Med. 1999;27(12):2799–805.
85. Probst P, Ohmann S, Klaiber U, Huttner FJ, Billeter AT, Ulrich A, et al. Meta-analysis of immunonutrition in major abdominal surgery. Br J Surg. 2017;104(12):1594–608.
86. Williams MD, Ha CY, Ciorba MA. Probiotics as therapy in gastroenterology: a study of physician opinions and recommendations. J Clin Gastroenterol. 2010;44(9):631–6.
87. Alverdy J, Zaborina O, Wu L. The impact of stress and nutrition on bacterial-host interactions at the intestinal epithelial surface. Curr Opin Clin Nutr Metab Care. 2005;8(2):205–9.
88. Alverdy JC. During critical illness the gut does not pass the acid test. Crit Care. 2012;16(5):150.
89. Carlisle EM, Poroyko V, Caplan MS, Alverdy J, Morowitz MJ, Liu D. Murine gut microbiota and transcriptome are diet dependent. Ann Surg. 2013;257(2):287–94.
90. Long J, Zaborina O, Holbrook C, Zaborin A, Alverdy J. Depletion of intestinal phosphate after operative injury activates the virulence of P aeruginosa causing lethal gut-derived sepsis. Surgery. 2008;144(2):189–97.
91. Morowitz MJ, Carlisle EM, Alverdy JC. Contributions of intestinal bacteria to nutrition and metabolism in the critically ill. Surg Clin North Am. 2011;91(4):771–85, viii
92. Zaborina O, Zaborin A, Romanowski K, Babrowski T, Alverdy J. Host stress and virulence expression in intestinal pathogens: development of therapeutic strategies using mice and C. elegans. Curr Pharm Des. 2011;17(13):1254–60.
93. Alverdy J, Holbrook C, Rocha F, Seiden L, Wu RL, Musch M, et al. Gut-derived sepsis occurs when the right pathogen with the right virulence genes meets the right host: evidence for in vivo virulence expression in Pseudomonas aeruginosa. Ann Surg. 2000;232(4):480–9.
94. Babrowski T, Romanowski K, Fink D, Kim M, Gopalakrishnan V, Zaborina O, et al. The intestinal environment of surgical injury transforms Pseudomonas aeruginosa into a discrete hypervirulent morphotype capable of causing lethal peritonitis. Surgery. 2013;153(1):36–43.
95. Laughlin RS, Musch MW, Hollbrook CJ, Rocha FM, Chang EB, Alverdy JC. The key role of Pseudomonas aeruginosa PA-I lectin on experimental gut-derived sepsis. Ann Surg. 2000;232(1):133–42.
96. Shogan BD, Belogortseva N, Luong PM, Zaborin A, Lax S, Bethel C, et al. Collagen degradation and MMP9 activation by Enterococcus faecalis contribute to intestinal anastomotic leak. Sci Transl Med. 2015;7(286):286ra68.
97. Kotzampassi K, Giamarellos-Bourboulis EJ, Voudouris A, Kazamias P, Eleftheriadis E. Benefits of a synbiotic formula (Synbiotic 2000Forte) in critically ill trauma patients: early results of a randomized controlled trial. World J Surg. 2006;30(10):1848–55.
98. Kotzampassi K, Stavrou G, Damoraki G, Georgitsi M, Basdanis G, Tsaousi G, et al. A four-probiotics regimen reduces postoperative complications after colorectal surgery: a randomized, double-blind, placebo-controlled study. World J Surg. 2015;39(11):2776–83.
99. Hempel S, Newberry SJ, Maher AR, Wang Z, Miles JN, Shanman R, et al. Probiotics for the prevention and treatment of antibiotic-associated diarrhea: a systematic review and meta-analysis. JAMA. 2012;307(18):1959–69.
100. Johnston BC, Ma SS, Goldenberg JZ, Thorlund K, Vandvik PO, Loeb M, et al. Probiotics for the prevention of Clostridium difficile-associated diarrhea: a systematic review and meta-analysis. Ann Intern Med. 2012;157(12):878–88.
101. Goldenberg JZ, Ma SS, Saxton JD, Martzen MR, Vandvik PO, Thorlund K, et al. Probiotics for the prevention of Clostridium difficile-associated diar-

rhea in adults and children. Cochrane Database Syst Rev. 2013;5:CD006095.
102. Morrow LE, Kollef MH, Casale TB. Probiotic prophylaxis of ventilator-associated pneumonia: a blinded, randomized, controlled trial. Am J Respir Crit Care Med. 2010;182(8):1058–64.
103. Custodero C, Mankowski RT, Lee SA, Chen Z, Wu S, Manini TM, et al. Evidence-based nutritional and pharmacological interventions targeting chronic low-grade inflammation in middle-age and older adults: a systematic review and meta-analysis. Ageing Res Rev. 2018;46:42–59.
104. Miyauchi E, O'Callaghan J, Butto LF, Hurley G, Melgar S, Tanabe S, et al. Mechanism of protection of transepithelial barrier function by Lactobacillus salivarius: strain dependence and attenuation by bacteriocin production. Am J Physiol Gastrointest Liver Physiol. 2012;303(9):G1029–41.
105. Mazloom Z, Yousefinejad A, Dabbaghmanesh MH. Effect of probiotics on lipid profile, glycemic control, insulin action, oxidative stress, and inflammatory markers in patients with type 2 diabetes: a clinical trial. Iran J Med Sci. 2013;38(1):38–43.
106. Mohamadshahi M, Veissi M, Haidari F, Javid AZ, Mohammadi F, Shirbeigi E. Effects of probiotic yogurt consumption on lipid profile in type 2 diabetic patients: a randomized controlled clinical trial. J Res Med Sci. 2014;19(6):531–6.
107. Mohamadshahi M, Veissi M, Haidari F, Shahbazian H, Kaydani GA, Mohammadi F. Effects of probiotic yogurt consumption on inflammatory biomarkers in patients with type 2 diabetes. Bioimpacts. 2014;4(2):83–8.
108. Morrow LE, Gogineni V, Malesker MA. Probiotics in the intensive care unit. Nutr Clin Pract. 2012;27(2):235–41.
109. Petrof EO, Dhaliwal R, Manzanares W, Johnstone J, Cook D, Heyland DK. Probiotics in the critically ill: a systematic review of the randomized trial evidence. Crit Care Med. 2012;40(12):3290–302.
110. Rajkumar H, Mahmood N, Kumar M, Varikuti SR, Challa HR, Myakala SP. Effect of probiotic (VSL#3) and omega-3 on lipid profile, insulin sensitivity, inflammatory markers, and gut colonization in overweight adults: a randomized, controlled trial. Mediat Inflamm. 2014;2014:348959.
111. Valentini L, Pinto A, Bourdel-Marchasson I, Ostan R, Brigidi P, Turroni S, et al. Impact of personalized diet and probiotic supplementation on inflammation, nutritional parameters and intestinal microbiota – the "RISTOMED project": randomized controlled trial in healthy older people. Clin Nutr. 2015;34(4):593–602.
112. Watkinson PJ, Barber VS, Dark P, Young JD. The use of pre- pro- and synbiotics in adult intensive care unit patients: systematic review. Clin Nutr. 2007;26(2):182–92.
113. Bengmark S. Bioecologic control of inflammation and infection in critical illness. Anesthesiol Clin. 2006;24(2):299–323. vi
114. Bengmark S. The bioecological medicine is here to stay. About microflora, synbiotics, immunity and resistance against disease. Lakartidningen. 2006;103(5):293–7.
115. Bommiasamy AK, Connelly C, Moren A, Dodgion C, Bestall K, Cline A, et al. Institutional review of the implementation and use of a Clostridium difficile infection bundle and probiotics in adult trauma patients. Am J Surg. 2018;215(5):825–30.
116. Lytvyn L, Quach K, Banfield L, Johnston BC, Mertz D. Probiotics and synbiotics for the prevention of postoperative infections following abdominal surgery: a systematic review and meta-analysis of randomized controlled trials. J Hosp Infect. 2016;92(2):130–9.
117. Lewis ZT, Shani G, Masarweh CF, Popovic M, Frese SA, Sela DA, et al. Validating bifidobacterial species and subspecies identity in commercial probiotic products. Pediatr Res. 2016;79(3):445–52.
118. Azhar RA, Bochner B, Catto J, Goh AC, Kelly J, Patel HD, et al. Enhanced recovery after urological surgery: a contemporary systematic review of outcomes, key elements, and research needs. Eur Urol. 2016;70(1):176–87.
119. Cerantola Y, Valerio M, Persson B, Jichlinski P, Ljungqvist O, Hubner M, et al. Guidelines for perioperative care after radical cystectomy for bladder cancer: enhanced recovery after surgery (ERAS((R))) society recommendations. Clin Nutr. 2013;32(6):879–87.
120. Collins JW, Patel H, Adding C, Annerstedt M, Dasgupta P, Khan SM, et al. Enhanced recovery after robot-assisted radical cystectomy: EAU robotic urology section scientific working group consensus view. Eur Urol. 2016;70(4):649–60.
121. Patel HD, Semerjian A. Enhanced recovery after surgery protocols to reduce morbidity in the aging patient. Eur Urol Focus. 2017;3(4–5):313–5.
122. Patel HR, Cerantola Y, Valerio M, Persson B, Jichlinski P, Ljungqvist O, et al. Enhanced recovery after surgery: are we ready, and can we afford not to implement these pathways for patients undergoing radical cystectomy? Eur Urol. 2014;65(2):263–6.
123. Smith MD, McCall J, Plank L, Herbison GP, Soop M, Nygren J. Preoperative carbohydrate treatment for enhancing recovery after elective surgery. Cochrane Database Syst Rev. 2014;8:CD009161.
124. Taylor SJ, Fettes SB, Jewkes C, Nelson RJ. Prospective, randomized, controlled trial to determine the effect of early enhanced enteral nutrition on clinical outcome in mechanically ventilated patients suffering head injury. Crit Care Med. 1999;27(11):2525–31.
125. Wong CS, Aly EH. The effects of enteral immunonutrition in upper gastrointestinal surgery: a systematic review and meta-analysis. Int J Surg. 2016;29:137–50.
126. Marimuthu K, Varadhan KK, Ljungqvist O, Lobo DN. A meta-analysis of the effect of combinations of

immune modulating nutrients on outcome in patients undergoing major open gastrointestinal surgery. Ann Surg. 2012;255(6):1060–8.

127. Liu K, Ji S, Xu Y, Diao Q, Shao C, Luo J, et al. Safety, feasibility, and effect of an enhanced nutritional support pathway including extended preoperative and home enteral nutrition in patients undergoing enhanced recovery after esophagectomy: a pilot randomized clinical trial. Dis Esophagus. 2020;33(2):doz030.
128. Soop M, Carlson GL, Hopkinson J, Clarke S, Thorell A, Nygren J, et al. Randomized clinical trial of the effects of immediate enteral nutrition on metabolic responses to major colorectal surgery in an enhanced recovery protocol. Br J Surg. 2004;91(9):1138–45.
129. Xiang Q, Yuan H, Cai W, Qie S. Effect of early enteral nutrition on laparoscopic common bile duct exploration with enhanced recovery after surgery protocols. Eur J Clin Nutr. 2019;73(9):1244–9.
130. Gillis C, Wischmeyer PE. Pre-operative nutrition and the elective surgical patient: why, how and what? Anaesthesia. 2019;74(Suppl 1):27–35.
131. Singh PM, Panwar R, Borle A, Goudra B, Trikha A, van Wagensveld BA, et al. Efficiency and safety effects of applying ERAS protocols to bariatric surgery: a systematic review with meta-analysis and trial sequential analysis of evidence. Obes Surg. 2017;27(2):489–501.
132. Mazaki T, Ishii Y, Murai I. Immunoenhancing enteral and parenteral nutrition for gastrointestinal surgery: a multiple-treatments meta-analysis. Ann Surg. 2015;261(4):662–9.

Food Allergies and Sensitivities

10

Neil Nadpara, Arnon Matan,
and Keerthana Kesavarapu

Introduction

A food allergy is defined as an adverse immune response after ingestion of a specific food. Food allergies are usually characterized as IgE-mediated or non-IgE mediated immune reactions. This is distinct from food intolerance, which refers to a non-immune reaction. Intolerances are categorized as metabolic, toxic, pharmacologic, or other mechanisms (Fig. 10.1) [1].

Extensive published literature estimates the prevalence of food allergies in the United States to be 8% and 10% in children and adults, respectively [3]. The prevalence of food allergies along with hospitalizations related to allergies has continued to rise over the past decade. These allergies are common in the early years of life and decrease over the first decade. There seems to be a geographic predisposition with more people affected in industrialized and western regions. Eight food categories, including peanuts (1.4%); tree nuts (1%); fish, shellfish, and eggs (1.5%); milk (2.5%); wheat (~0.4%); and soy (~0.4%), comprise a vast majority of allergic disease burden and account for over 90% of food allergens [3].

N. Nadpara
Temple University Hospital, Department of Internal Medicine, Philadelphia, PA, USA

A. Matan · K. Kesavarapu (✉)
Robert Wood Johnson, Department of Gastroenterology, New Brunswick, NJ, USA
e-mail: matan.arnon@tuhs.temple.edu; Keerthana.kesavarapu@tuhs.temple.edu

Food Allergies and Sensitivities

Individual physiologic and immunologic tolerance to ingested foods forms the foundation of food allergies and sensitivities that can be grouped into four categories: IgE-mediated, non-IgE-mediated, mixed, and non-immune. The mucosal immune system interacts with food antigens and is responsible for alterations and modulation of this immune reactivity. The gastrointestinal tract is composed of a single cell layer of the columnar epithelium joined by tight junctions and protected by trefoil factors (protease-resistant proteins that restore barrier), brush border enzymes, bile salts, and mucus. These factors work in combination to destroy pathogens and render antigens non-immunogenic. However, 2% of ingested food antigens are absorbed and transported into the body. These immunologically intact proteins do not usually provoke an immune response because of oral tolerance [4].

Oral tolerance normally occurs when a food antigen crosses an intact mucosal barrier and is delivered to antigen presenting cells (APCs), especially dendritic cells (DCs). Antigen-bound DCs in combination with suppressive cytokines, like interleukin 10, differentiate naïve T cells into

C. Newberry et al. (eds.), *Nutrition, Weight, and Digestive Health*,
https://doi.org/10.1007/978-3-030-94953-2_10

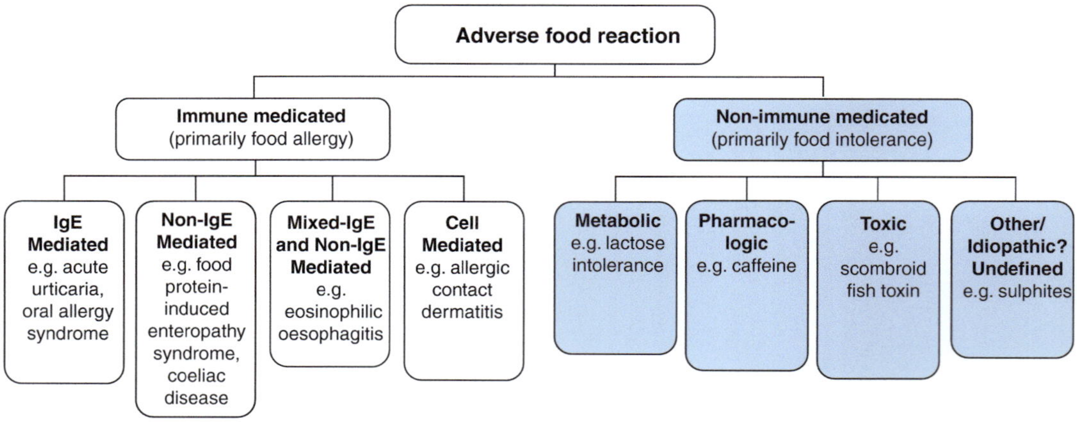

Fig. 10.1 Classification of adverse reactions to food (Reproduced from the Australasian Society of Clinical Immunology and Allergy [2]). Food allergies are characterized into immune-mediated and non-immune-mediated reactions. Immune-mediated food reactions are further categorized based on the pathophysiology into IgE-mediated, non-IgE-mediated, and mixed IgE- and non-IgE mediated etiologies

regulatory T cells rather than food antigen-specific T-helper type 2 (TH_2) cells. Upregulation of food-specific IgA and IgG antibodies with a compensatory decrease of IgE antibodies coupled with immune suppression of effector cells (mast cells and basophils) maintains tolerance and prevents these antigens from causing allergies (Fig. 10.2) [5].

IgE-Mediated Reactions

Pathophysiology

Food allergies occur because of dysfunction of the immune system that normally maintains oral tolerance. An allergic response occurs in two steps: sensitization, which is defined as the development of food-specific IgE, and subsequent exposure. Sensitization occurs when food antigens cross a disrupted intestinal epithelial barrier in genetically predisposed individuals. This compromise in the integrity of the gut membrane results in the release of inflammatory cytokines, such as interleukin 25 (IL-25), IL-33, and thymic stromal lymphopoietin (TSLP), and allows antigens to freely pass through the barrier. When antigens are taken up by DCs in the presence of these inflammatory cytokines, the benign antigen is seen as a "threat."

The activated DCs convert naïve T cells into food antigen-specific Th_2 cells, which results in the release of proinflammatory cytokines such as IL-4. This induces class switching of food antigen-specific B cells from IgA and IgG antibody production to IgE antibody production pro-

Fig. 10.2 Immunopathogenesis of food allergies (Reproduced from Anvari et al. 2018). *Tolerance* (left): Food allergens are exposed to macrophages in the intestinal lumen, which transfer antigens to dendritic cells in the gut lamina propria, which in turn present food peptides to T-cell receptors on naïve T cells. These T cells differentiate into T regulatory cells. Food-specific T cells with the help of cytokines TGF-beta and IL-10 encourage tolerance by suppressing mediator cells. *Allergy* (right): In the setting of immune barrier dysfunction, proinflammatory cytokines IL-25, IL-33, and thymic stromal lymphopoietin (TSLP) are released and activate dendritic cells, which in turn present food peptides to T-cell receptors on naïve T cells to T-helper type 2 (Th2) cells. Food-specific Th2 cells secrete inflammatory cytokines such as IL-4, IL-5, and IL-13, promoting effector cell (eosinophils and basophils) recruitment. IL-4 also allows for B cells to produce food-specific IgE production

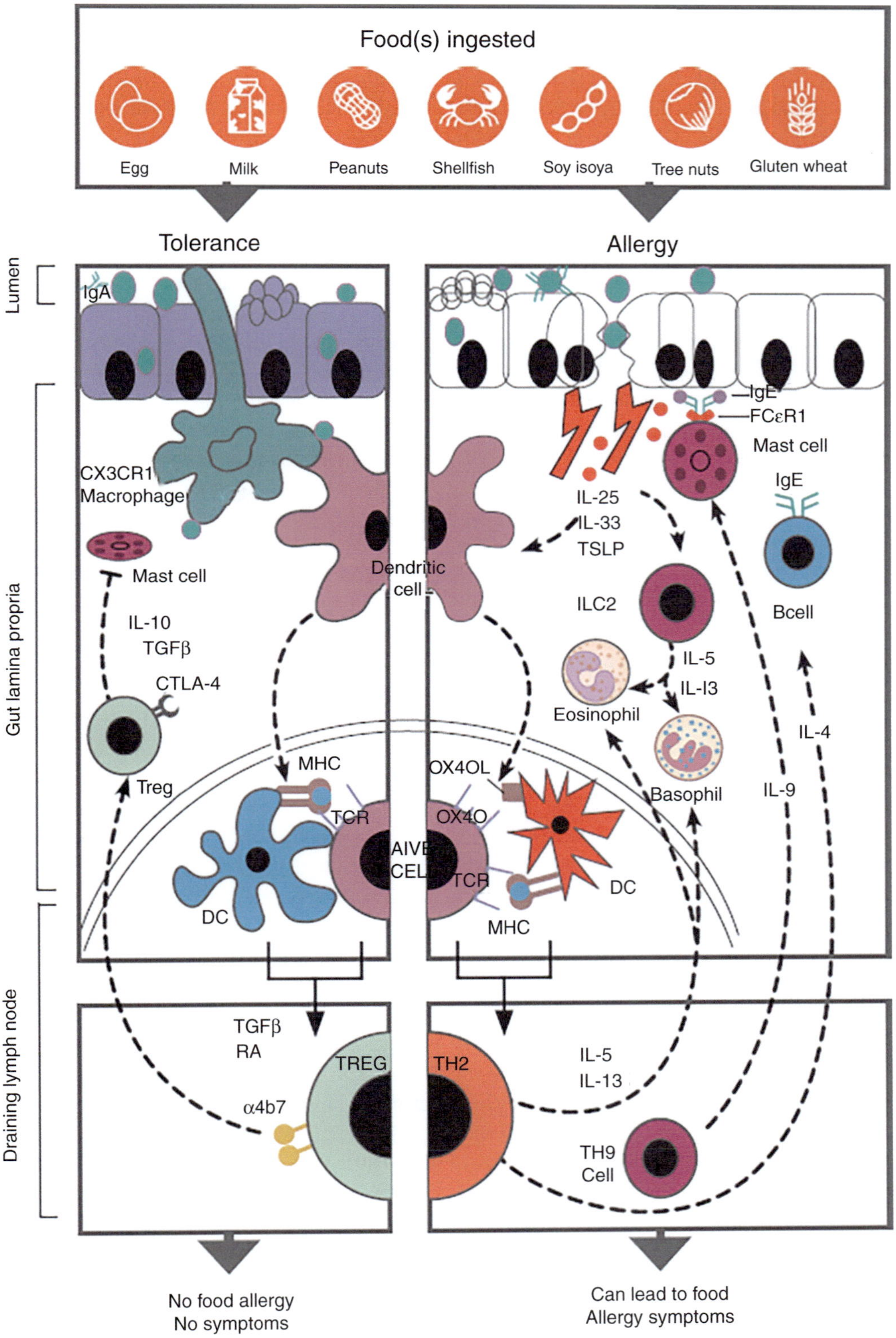
Food(s) ingested
Egg
Milk
Peanuts
Shellfish
Soy isoya
Tree nuts
Gluten wheat
Tolerance
Allergy
Lumen
Gut lamina propria
Draining lymph node
IgA
CX3CR1
Macrophage
Mast cell
IL-10
TGFβ
CTLA-4
Treg
Dendritic cell
MHC
TCR
DC
AIVE
CEL
IgE
FCεR1
Mast cell
IgE
Bcell
IL-25
IL-33
TSLP
ILC2
IL-5
IL-I3
Eosinophil
Basophil
IL-9
IL-4
OX4OL
OX4O
TCR
DC
MHC
TGFβ
RA
TREG
α4b7
TH2
IL-5
IL-13
TH9
Cell
No food allergy
No symptoms
Can lead to food
Allergy symptoms

moting a state of sensitization and allergy. Antibodies remain bound on effector cells (e.g., mast cells and basophils). Upon repeat exposure to the food antigen, cross-linking of IgE and the IgE receptors occurs on the surface of the effector cells resulting in the release of preformed mediators involved in anaphylaxis including histamine, tryptase, platelet-activating factor, prostaglandins, and leukotrienes (Fig. 10.2) [5].

Clinical Manifestations

Typical symptoms occur rapidly within minutes to hours after ingestion of causative food and can involve almost every organ system including the following: cutaneous (i.e., erythema, pruritis), ocular (i.e., tearing, conjunctival erythema), airway (i.e., cough, chest tightness, wheezing), gastrointestinal (i.e., nausea, emesis, diarrhea), and cardiac (i.e., tachycardia, hypotension) [5]. Clinical presentation and organ systems involved depend on certain factors such as underlying comorbidities (e.g., asthma), health status, activities performed during ingestion (e.g., exercise or alcohol consumption), dose ingested, route of exposure, and method of preparation of causative food [6]. Additionally, risk factors for reported fatal and near-fatal reactions include age, underlying respiratory diseases (e.g., asthma), concomitant use of β-blocker medications, reactions that do not involve the skin, and delay in treatment [6].

Most food reactions involve cutaneous manifestations, such as pruritic rash, urticaria, and angioedema. IgE-mediated respiratory symptoms can involve the upper and lower airway. Upper airway symptoms present with nasal congestion, rhinorrhea, and nasal pruritus, and lower airway symptoms include wheezing, shortness of breath, cough, and use of accessory muscles. The most severe airway symptom is stridor resulting from airway obstruction.

Gastrointestinal manifestations include itching of the mouth or throat, nausea, vomiting, abdominal pain, and diarrhea. Bloody diarrhea, delayed diarrhea (>4 hours after ingestion of allergen), constipation, weight loss, and/or malabsorption are not typically the result of IgE-mediated disease, and other etiologies should be investigated [5]. The cardiovascular system can be affected resulting in dizziness, lightheadedness, and syncope with resultant tachycardia, hypotension, cardiovascular collapse, or even death [5].

Diagnostic Evaluation

A detailed food diary can supplement a medical history in unveiling the responsible food as well as in describing the interval between ingestion and symptom presentation. Immediate food-induced allergic reactions begin within minutes to a few hours following ingestion of a causative food and typically are IgE-mediated. Delayed food reactions typically occur several hours to days following ingestion and involve cellular mechanisms.

When the history and food diary are unrevealing, allergy testing with IgE skin or blood tests can be performed. A skin test, performed by either prinking or intradermal injection of allergens, is positive if local pruritis, erythema, and swelling occurs, a manifestation of activated mast cells primed by allergen-specific IgE.

IgE-specific skin or serum tests alone cannot be used for diagnosis given high rates of false positives; however, they can support the patient's clinical history. Specifically, patients can show evidence of sensitization to an allergen in both tests without having a clinical allergic reaction to that allergen. High titer-specific IgE measurements and strongly positive wheal diameters (greater than 8 mm) on skin prick testing, however, are highly predictive of clinical allergy.

Total IgE measurement has been found to have little clinical utility, low positive predictive values, and inability to exclude culprit food allergens [5, 6]. IgG food-specific antibodies, total IgG antibodies, basophil activation, leukotriene release assays, and atopy patch test are similarly not recommended [1, 6].

The gold standard for determining and confirming the responsible antigen is a double-blind, placebo-controlled food challenge. In this setting, the patient receives doses of suspected food allergen or placebo that neither the patient nor allergist is aware of. However, given the expense and inconvenience of this test, single-blind food challenge and open-food challenge are more commonly in clinical settings [1].

Management

The mainstay of therapy is to identify and avoid specific food allergens that incite symptoms. Severe IgE-mediated reactions, such as anaphylaxis, require emergent management. After identifying symptoms as part of an anaphylactic reaction, intramuscular (IM) epinephrine remains the first-line treatment. Delay in epinephrine injection is associated with increased mortality. Epinephrine acts by vasoconstricting blood vessels to maintain blood pressure and dilating airways to decrease airway edema and improve respiration.

Intramuscular epinephrine can be administered via an autoinjector placed into the mid-outer thigh (vastus lateralis muscle). IM route is preferred over intravenous and subcutaneous routes, and autoinjectors can be used in many individuals, except infants weighing under 10 kg and adults weighing over 50 kg (who require weight-based dosing of 0.01 mg/kg).

In the case of anaphylaxis, massive fluid shifts can occur. These patients should receive large volume of fluid resuscitation with normal saline. Following epinephrine and hydration, adjunctive therapies can be used in the treatment of continued reactions including antihistamines, bronchodilators, and glucocorticoids. These medications should not be first-line therapies in anaphylaxis as they do not improve respiratory obstruction or cardiovascular compromise. However, they are the mainstay in managing symptoms of less severe food-induced IgE-mediated allergic reactions.

First- and second-generation antihistamines relive pruritis and hives but can produce side effects (e.g., sedation). In the case of anaphylaxis, IV formulations are preferred, whereas less severe allergic reactions can be treated with oral formulations. H1 antihistamines like diphenhydramine, given with an H2 antihistamine, like ranitidine and famotidine, provide additional relief of hives. Inhaled bronchodilators administered by a mouthpiece and nebulizer can improve bronchospasm not responsive to epinephrine. Glucocorticoids have an onset of action over several hours and are thought to prevent biphasic or protracted reactions. There is an overall lack of evidence supporting the benefit of glucocorticoids, though they are commonly used.

The main long-term management strategy of IgE-mediated food allergies is strict food allergen avoidance. To reduce the risk of recurrence, patients should follow up with an allergist, who may aid in allergen identification, and a registered dietitian, who may counsel on recipes, meal plans, and analysis of food labels. Patients should also be given a prescription for epinephrine with instructions outlining proper use.

Oral immunotherapy, an emerging modality, is accomplished by using a small, increasing amount of culprit allergens or cross-reactive allergens to desensitize the patient and possibly induce tolerance. Allergen-specific immunotherapy improves clinical symptoms of FA while on therapy; however, long-term clinical benefit and safety data of immunotherapy is unknown. Other modes of immunotherapy including epicutaneous and sublingual are also being studied and may become useful in the future.

Non-IgE-Mediated Reactions

Non-IgE-mediated food allergies encompass a wide spectrum of disorders including food protein-induced enterocolitis syndrome (FPIES), allergic proctocolitis (AP), food protein-induced enteropathy (FPE), and gluten-related disorders (Fig. 10.1). The pathophysiology of non-IgE-mediated food allergies is poorly defined but likely T-cell-mediated. Unlike IgE-mediated FA, symptom onset is delayed from hours to weeks after ingestion of causative food. Given the lack of temporal association between ingestion and symptoms as well as paucity of noninvasive confirmatory testing, diagnosis of non-IgE-mediated food hypersensitivity can be challenging.

Food Protein-Induced Enterocolitis Syndrome (FPIES)

FPIES represents the more severe end of the non-IgE-mediated food hypersensitivity spectrum that occurs almost exclusively in infants and young children. Although the pathophysiology is not well understood, it is thought to be a T-cell-mediated disorder. It is hypothesized food allergens promote T-cell activation and release of proinflammatory cytokines resulting in local intestinal inflammation and subsequent increased intestinal permeability and fluid shifts. The local inflammation may be mediated by activated peripheral mononuclear cells, increased TNF-α, and decreased expression of TGF-β receptors in the intestinal mucosa. Humoral responses are also poorly understood, but studies reveal an increased number of IgM- and IgA-containing plasma cells [7]. More studies are required to understand the underlying mechanism of FPIES.

The most common inciting allergens are cow's milk and soy proteins, but proteins in rice, oat, egg, wheat, and fish have also been implicated. The suggested incidence of cow's milk-induced FPIES is 0.34% [8]. Age of onset is generally within the first year of life, and the inciting allergen correlates with early introduction of this food. FPIES to cow's milk and soy usually starts within the first 3–6 months of life, while FPIES to solid foods starts later at 4–8 months of age.

Acute FPIES presents with severe, projectile emesis, diarrhea, dehydration, and possibly shock within 1–6 hours after ingestion of causative food protein. Stools contain occult blood and inflammatory cells including neutrophils and eosinophils. Chronic FPIES is less prevalent and characterized by intermittent but progressive emesis, watery diarrhea, and failure to thrive. Unlike acute FPIES, there does not appear to be a clear temporal association between trigger food antigen and onset of symptoms.

Allergic Proctocolitis (AP)

Allergic proctocolitis (AP) represents a milder end of the non-IgE-mediated food hypersensitivity spectrum. The pathophysiology is not well identified but also thought to be a T-cell-mediated.

This disease is exclusively identified in young infants within months after birth, with a prevalence of 1–2% [9]. Cow's milk, found in either formula or breast milk, remains the most common offending antigen with an incidence of 76% [9]. Other dietary triggers include egg, soy, and corn, with some infants having multiple offenders.

Symptoms can begin as early as the first week of life. While some infants can be fussy and irritable, others can develop altered stool patterns varying from multiple daily stools with visible blood and mucus streaks to infrequent stools with occasional bleeding. Most infants are healthy appearing and thriving. This can result in delayed diagnosis.

Food Protein-Induced Enteropathy (FPE)

Food protein-induced enteropathy (FPE) is rare with unknown prevalence. Cow's milk is the most common food allergen causing FPE; however, it has also been associated with soy, egg, wheat, rice, chicken, and fish protein allergens. Eosinophils, cow's milk-specific TH2 lymphocytes, and localized production of IgE in mucosa of the small intestine have been implicated in the pathophysiology of FPE.

FPE manifests in infancy with the most prominent symptoms being watery diarrhea and failure to thrive accompanied by vomiting and abdominal distention and fullness. Malabsorption and steatorrhea distinguish this entity from FPIES and AP.

Laboratory work-up and endoscopy with biopsies are necessary to confirm the diagnosis and to differentiate this condition from other disorders that cause failure to thrive and diarrhea. Laboratory findings may suggest malabsorption with anemia (20–70%), hypoalbuminemia, and fat-soluble vitamin deficiency. Serologically, milk IgA and IgG antibodies are present. Endoscopic assessment can show villous effacement with histology showing elevation and predominance of intraepithelial lymphocytes, mast cells, and eosinophils. Despite cessation, endoscopic remission may require 6 to 18 months of allergen avoidance.

Gluten-Related Disorders

Gluten is the main structural protein complex found in wheat, rye, and barley. The immunogenic protein fractions of gluten include prolamins (gliadin) and glutenins. Three main forms of gluten reactions exist: (1) allergic (wheat allergy), (2) autoimmune (celiac disease, gluten ataxia, and dermatitis herpetiformis), and (3) possible immune-mediated (gluten sensitivity). Wheat allergy occurs via an IgE-mediated immune response with gluten peptides triggering a classic food allergy affecting the skin, gastrointestinal tract, and/or respiratory tract as described above in the IgE-mediated section.

Celiac Disease (CD)

CD is an immune-mediated enteropathy triggered by ingestion of gluten in genetically susceptible individuals that occurs in up to 1% of the population (see details in Chap. 6). Here we will discuss the immunogenic process of CD. Genetic predisposition plays a role in CD with all patients expressing a gene that encodes for the major histocompatibility complex (MHC) human leukocyte antigen (HLA) class II proteins HLA DQ2 (approximately 95%) and HLD-DQ8, located on chromosome 6p21. While the presence of these HLA class II proteins alone does not ensure CD, their presence is necessary for disease development.

The development of CD relies on exposure to gliadin, one of the soluble protein components of gluten. Gliadin fragments gain entry through the epithelial barrier into the lamina propria and are deaminated by tissue transglutaminase (TTG). Gliadin is then deaminated by TTG activating both the adaptive and innate immune systems. In the adaptive immune response, APCs, including macrophages, DCs, and B cells, express HLA class II DQ2 and/or DQ8 molecules on their surface which then uptake and display gliadin peptides. These APCs bind with gliadin-specific CD4 Th1 cells, producing proinflammatory cytokines. The resultant effect is crypt hyperplasia and villous blunting in the small intestine. Similarly, the innate immune response increases inflammatory mediators like IL-15 and interferon alpha with subsequent recruitment of intraepithelial lymphocytes to the intestinal epithelium.

Classic CD is characterized by diarrhea or signs and symptoms of malabsorption with steatorrhea, weight loss, or vitamin deficiency; however, patients often present with minor gastrointestinal complaints with extraintestinal manifestations including anemia, osteoporosis, arthritis, increased transaminases, neurological symptoms, and/or infertility.

Non-celiac Gluten Sensitivity

Non-celiac gluten sensitivity (NCGS) is a term used to describe individuals who do not have CD or wheat allergy but develop intestinal and/or extraintestinal signs and symptoms induced by gluten ingestion that improve when gluten-containing grains are removed from the diet [10]. The true prevalence is unknown due to the lack of definitive diagnostic testing. It is thought, however, to be more prevalent than celiac disease.

The pathophysiology of NCGS remains largely undetermined. While gliadin plays a prominent role in the pathogenesis of gluten sensitivity, it is hypothesized that other components, like α-amylase/trypsin inhibitors, may also contribute. Gliadin fragments bind the CXCR3 chemokine receptor allowing the release of zonulin, a modulator of intracellular tight junctions which regulates gut permeability. This reaction occurs in all individuals who ingest gluten, usually without any consequences [11]. However, these events can cause an inflammatory process in genetically predisposed individuals when gluten is mistaken as a pathogen by the immunologic surveillance system. Increased permeability of the epithelial barrier facilitates gliadin fragments trafficking from the gut lumen to lamina propria resulting in the activation of the intestinal innate immune system. Unlike in celiac disease, there is no subsequent activation in the adaptive immune system which explains the lack of enteropathy and villous blunting in this condition [11].

Clinical symptoms are like CD and include abdominal pain, bloating, and altered bowel habits (diarrhea, constipation, or both). Extraintestinal manifestations include mental fog, defined as slowed thinking, headache, joint and muscle pain, fatigue, depression, leg or arm numbness, dermatitis, and anemia.

Unlike CD, NCGS has no validated serum biomarkers for diagnosis. Given the overlap in symptoms between CD, NCGS, and wheat allergy, it becomes important to diagnose an underlying disease with serologic and histologic evaluation.

Management

The cornerstone of the management of FPIES, FPE, AP, and gluten-related disorders is the avoidance of offending foods. For acute management of FPIES, intravenous or oral rehydration may be required based on the ability to tolerate oral intake. Anti-emetics, such as ondansetron, may be considered to control emesis. With rehydration and food avoidance, acute FPIES resolves in a few hours, and chronic FPIES resolves in days to weeks. Similarly, FPE symptoms resolve within 1–4 weeks with avoidance; however, resolution of biopsy findings can take up to 18 months.

In breast-fed infants with AP, eliminating the offending agent in mom's diet, usually cow's milk, is key to resolution, with bleeding improving in 72 to 96 hours. Unremitting symptoms can require change from breastfeeding to a casein hydrolysate formula or amino acid-based formula. In formula-fed infants with AP, transition to extensively hydrolyzed formula is considered first-line therapy especially in infants less than 6 months with failure to thrive.

For both AP and FPE, food avoidance is not permanent. Foods can be reintroduced gradually if skin prick test and food-specific IgE antibody levels are negative. In FPIES, food can be reintroduced under medical supervision given the risk of hypotension.

In gluten-related disorders, the mainstay of management is avoidance of gluten-containing foods. Unlike CD and wheat allergy, NCGS may be transient. Current recommendations are to follow a gluten-free diet (GFD). In instances of NCGS, gluten may be introduced after a finite amount of time to determine tolerance. Based on severity of symptoms, some patients with NCGS may choose to follow a GFD indefinitely. These patients, along with patients diagnosed with CD and wheat allergy, should be monitored closely by a gastroenterologist and registered dietician to confirm they are avoiding inadvertent exposures and meeting daily fiber and micronutrient goals.

Mixed IgE- and Non-IgE-Mediated Food Allergy

Eosinophilic Gastrointestinal Disorders

Some food allergy disorders result from both IgE- and non-IgE-mediated immune processes. A common example is allergic eosinophilic gastrointestinal disorders (EGIDs), which are characterized by pathologic eosinophilic infiltration of the esophagus, stomach, small intestine, and/or colon leading to organ dysfunction and clinical symptoms. EGIDs include eosinophilic esophagitis (EoE), eosinophilic gastritis (EG), eosinophilic enteritis (EE), eosinophilic colitis (EC), and eosinophilic gastroenteritis (EGE). The most common of the disorders is eosinophilic esophagitis (EoE), with an estimated prevalence of 1/1000. (refer to Chap. 5 for an in-depth discussion of EoE). For this chapter, we will focus on the other subtypes of EGIDs.

The estimated prevalence of EG, EGE, and EC are 6.3/100,000, 8.4/100,000, and 3.3/100,000, respectively [12]. Overall, the prevalence of non-EoE EGIDs remains rare in the United States with less than 50,000 total people affected [12]. Genetic predisposition in combination with environmental factors and host's immune system plays a role in pathogenesis. Familial clustering has been reported with 10% of patients having an immediate family member with an eosinophilic gastrointestinal disorder [12].

Pathophysiology

Eosinophils are normally present in all regions of the gastrointestinal tract except for the esophagus and participate in immune homeostasis. However, a large number of mucosal eosinophils reflect a pathologic process driven by exposure to food antigen. A T-helper type 2 (Th_2) cell immune response and increased levels of mucosal permeability are the primary abnormalities found in EGIDs. TH2 immune response increases production of cytokines, such as IL-5, which promotes eosinophil development, activation, survival, and recruitment to sites of inflammation, and IL-13, which induces gene expression necessary to accumulate eosinophils in the mucosa [13].

Once densely infiltrated, eosinophils become activated, releasing granules of proinflammatory mediators, leukotrienes, and prostaglandins. The resultant effect is increased epithelial infiltration and alteration of sensory and motor activities of the mucosa. Augmented intestinal permeability makes entry of food and environmental allergens into subepithelial tissues easier. This stimulates a Th_2 cell-mediated immune response which leads to eosinophilic inflammation and eventual tissue remodeling and fibrosis [14].

Clinical Manifestations

The clinical presentation depends on the location, extent, and layer(s) of the gastrointestinal tract involved. The most common symptoms are abdominal pain, nausea, vomiting, early satiety, and diarrhea with only 33% of patients developing weight loss. Those diagnosed with EG primarily present with nausea, vomiting, abdominal pain, and early satiety. Diffuse small bowel involvement in EE and EGE disrupts the intestinal barrier resulting in malabsorption, protein-losing enteropathy, and failure to thrive. Those with EC can present with diarrhea, abdominal pain, and hematochezia.

EGIDs can affect the mucosal, muscular, and serosal layers, with mucosal involvement most common. Involvement of the muscular layer results in wall thickening and impaired motility. Patients may present with gastric or intestinal obstruction reporting nausea, vomiting, abdominal distention, and rarely perforation. Sub-serosal disease is the rarest form and can present with isolated ascites or ascites in combination with symptoms seen in the other subtypes.

Diagnosis

EGIDs are suspected in patients with concerning clinical manifestations associated with peripheral eosinophilia, which is seen in 80% of patients. Eosinophil counts can range from 5% to 35% of total white blood cells with an average absolute eosinophil count of greater than 500 cells/μL. Mucosal and sub-serosal diseases are characterized by higher eosinophil count compared with the disease that involves the muscular layer. Those with malabsorption can have hypoalbuminemia, iron deficiency anemia from occult bleeding and erosions/ulcerations, increased fecal fat excretion, and prolonged prothrombin time due to vitamin deficiencies. Serum IgE levels are markedly elevated. In 25% of the cases, elevated ESR is seen. Evaluation of patients suspected to have an EGID should exclude alternate causes of eosinophilia.

Imaging is not necessary for diagnosis; however, barium studies and cross-sectional imaging may reveal thickening or nodularity in the antrum and thickening or "saw-tooth" mucosa in the small intestine. Despite abnormalities being present, these findings are not sensitive or specific for diagnosis.

Diagnosis is made during upper endoscopy with biopsies. Because eosinophilia can be patchy in patients, multiple biopsies of both normal and abnormal mucosa must be taken to increase sensitivity. It is important to remember that biopsies are normal in sub-serosal and muscular disease. It is important to notify the pathologist for clinical suspicion of this diagnosis. Because the stomach and duodenum are the most affected sites, initial endoscopic evaluation is limited to the upper gastrointestinal tract. Diarrhea-prominent disease should be investigated with a colonoscopy and subsequent examination of the terminal ileum, which can show erythema, nodularity, and thickened folds.

Management

Like EOE, elimination diet and corticosteroids are the mainstay of therapy of EGIDs. Administration of prednisone, a systemic glucocorticoid, at 30–40 mg/day is the most widely used treatment for EGE. The use of swallowed topical administration is also an option; however, effectiveness of this approach has not been elucidated in the literature. Histamine H1 receptor antagonists, leukotriene receptor antagonists, mast cell stabilizers, and immunosuppressive agents have been reported for use in both patients who respond to steroids and those who do not. The effectiveness of these drugs is unknown because randomized controlled trials are limited. A six-food elimination diet, cutting out wheat, milk, egg, soy, nuts and tree nuts, and seafood and reintroducing eliminated components, may allow for improvement in symptoms.

Non-immune-Mediated GI Adverse Reactions to Food

Food intolerance or sensitivity refers to a non-immunologic reaction to food and can result from a wide range of etiologies. It affects up to 15–20% of the population [15]. Intolerances are categorized into metabolic, pharmacologic, and other etiologies based on their pathophysiology. In this section, we will focus on enzymatic defects (e.g., disaccharidase deficiencies), pharmacologic food intolerances, toxic reactions to food, and other food intolerances including those related to specific ingestions (i.e., fermentable oligo-, di-, and monosaccharides and polyols (FODMAPs), food additives, and food pathogens).

Enzymatic Defects: Disaccharide Intolerance

Disaccharides are sugar molecules composed of a combination of two monosaccharides (glucose, fructose, galactose) and include lactose (glucose-galactose), sucrose (glucose-fructose), maltose (glucose-glucose), and trehalose (glucose-glucose). Disaccharides are broken down into their single sugar components by enzymes found in the intestinal brush border known as disaccharidases. Disaccharide intolerance occurs in the setting of disaccharidase ingestion out of proportion of available enzyme and/or activity. Adult-onset lactose intolerance is by far the most common type, affecting up to 67% of the global population [16].

Lactose intolerance is especially prevalent among Asian, African, Native-American, and Mediterranean populations. Lactase activity peaks at birth and is reduced during childhood to facilitate breastfeeding weaning. Lactose intolerance is less common in Caucasians due to a gain of function mutation leading to lactase persistence [17]. Lactose intolerance occurs when there is inadequate lactase activity resulting in unabsorbed lactose after ingestion. Gut bacteria metabolize unabsorbed sugars resulting in the production of hydrogen, methane, and short-chain fatty acids, which lead to the GI symptoms of abdominal pain and cramping, bloating, diarrhea, and borborygmi. Symptom development depends on the mismatch of lactose ingestion with enzyme activity and can be worsened by visceral hypersensitivity associated with anxiety or IBS [17]. Lactose content is higher in milk, ice cream, and butter products compared to yogurt and cheese because bacteria used to produce the latter break-down lactose resulting in lower total lactose levels.

Sucrose intolerance occurs due to inadequate sucrase-isomaltase and can be congenital or acquired. New evidence estimates that 2–9% of Americans of European descent may be affected by sucrose intolerance [18]. Maltase and trehalase deficiencies are rarer types of disaccharidase deficiencies with unknown prevalence. Maltose is a disaccharide formed from two units of glucose with an alpha (1–4) bond, compared to the alpha (1–6) bond of isomaltose. The pathophysiology of these disaccharide intolerances is similar to lactose intolerance in that undigested sugars accumulate in the intestinal lumen leading to osmotic diarrhea and bacterial fermentation that induces additional changes in bowel habits, bloating, and abdominal pain.

Disaccharidase intolerances, such as lactose deficiency, can be assessed by disaccharide breath tests, but clinical aptitude of these tests is questionable, and an elimination diet may be more effective in diagnosing the condition and recommending sugar avoidance. Additionally, saliva tests are available for evaluation of sucrase activity, though these have similar clinical limitations.

Pharmacologic Food Intolerance

Pharmacologic food intolerance results from ingestion of vasoactive amines including dopamine, histamine, norepinephrine, phenylethylamine, serotonin, and tyramine. A common example is ingestion of histamine in the form of matured cheeses, alcoholic beverages, and fermented foods, which leads to systemic and gastrointestinal complaints. Histamine is metabolized extracellularly by diamine oxidase and intracellularly by histamine-N-methyltransferase [19]. Reduced activity of these enzymes leads to histamine toxicity and symptoms. Overall, histamine-rich food avoidance is crucial for diagnosis and management because there is limited utility in checking serum histamine levels.

Tyramine toxicity most frequently occurs in patients taking MAO inhibitors who ingest tyramine-rich foods such as cheese and wine but can also occur due to increased bacterial decarboxylation activity in poorly preserved foods [20]. Excess tyramine results in sympathetic stimulation with hypertensive crisis, headache, and flushing. Management of hypertensive crisis includes administration of phentolamine or nitroprusside. Beta-blockers should be avoided to prevent unopposed alpha receptor activation, which worsens elevated blood pressures.

Toxic Food Intolerance

Ingestion of toxic food components can also induce systemic and gastrointestinal complaints. Scombroid poisoning is the most common presentation, representing a histamine toxicity that occurs due to ingestion of spoiled dark meat fish such as tuna, mahi-mahi, or mackerel. During the spoilage period, bacterial histidine decarboxylase converts histidine to histamine. Symptoms occur 20–30 minutes after ingestion and are usually mild and self-limiting. These include facial flushing, burning sensation of the mouth, abdominal pain, diarrhea, headache, and palpitations [21]. Scombroid poisoning is frequently misdiagnosed as fish allergy, so history-taking and nuanced assessment of symptoms are critical. First-line immediate treatment is antihistamines. Epinephrine is rarely used, though may be necessary if the patient develops anaphylaxis with hypotension, angioedema, and bronchospasm.

Specific Food Component Intolerances

Fermentable Carbohydrates

Fermentable oligo-, di-, and monosaccharides and polyols (FODMAPs) are short-chain carbohydrates and sugar alcohols such as fructose, lactose, sorbitol, and mannitol that are fermented by intestinal bacteria. Examples of high-FODMAP foods include beans, wheat and rye, dairy products, dried fruit, artificial sweeteners, and alcohol.

These foods cause GI symptoms such as bloating, abdominal pain, nausea, and altered bowel habits (diarrhea and/or constipation) due to poor intestinal absorption, high osmotic activity, rapid fermentation, and increased gas production by intestinal bacteria. The combined effects of increased water delivery and gas in the lumen cause distention and lead to pain and discomfort in susceptible patients. Because IBS patients have increased visceral hypersensitivity, they are also more likely to experience functional GI symptoms from FODMAP ingestion.

Studies show that a low-FODMAP diet leads to clinical response and improvement in symptoms for 50–80% of patients with IBS [22]. Low-FODMAP diets have also helped mitigate IBS-like symptoms in IBD patients, but recommendations are still controversial due to the risk of undernutrition with dietary restriction in this population [23]. Low-FODMAP dietary education should be provided to avoid dietary over-restriction and nutritionally replete diet. This education consists of initially eliminating FODMAPs from the diet for 2 to 8 weeks and then, if symptom resolution occurs and patient is considered a responder, sequentially reintroducing foods high in fermentable carbohydrates to determine individual tolerance and define personalized dietary approach.

Food Additives

Food additives, such as preservatives, nutritional additives, coloring, flavoring, and texturing agents, are used during food production at allowed doses. However, these bioactive chemicals can cause physiological changes and have potentially harmful health effects. Specifically, sulphites, nitrites, nitrates, and monosodium glutamate have been implicated as causing asthma, rhinitis, urticaria, pruritus, and migraines. An ongoing area of research is the effect of food additives on the human gut microbiota, which can have pervasive effects on various metabolic processes and diseases such as obesity, diabetes, and cardiovascular disease. Future studies in humans will be critical to define safety.

Food Poisoning

Food poisoning is the ingestion of foods contaminated with bacteria, toxins, viruses, parasites, or chemicals. Common pathogens include staphylococcal enterotoxins, *Bacillus cereus* toxins, gram-negative enteric pathogens, and hepatitis A virus. The time course of developing symptoms varies depending on the pathogen ingested, within hours for toxins and days for bacteria or viruses. Treatment is supportive, and resolution of symptoms is also variable, ranging from hours to weeks depending on the offending agent. Bacterial and protozoal infections are more likely than viral infections to lead to prolonged post-infective irritable bowel syndrome (PI-IBS) [24].

References

1. Boyce JA, Assa'ad A, Burks AW, Jones SM, Sampson HA, Wood RA, et al. Guidelines for the diagnosis and management of food allergy in the United States: report of the NIAID-sponsored expert panel. J Allergy Clin Immunol. 2010;126(6 Suppl):S1–58. https://doi.org/10.1016/j.jaci.2010.10.007.
2. Food Intolerance. In: Information for patients, consumers and carers. Australian society of clinical immunology and allergy. 2019.
3. Gupta RS, Warren CM, Smith BM, Jiang J, Blumenstock JA, Davis MM, et al. Prevalence and severity of food allergies among US adults. JAMA Netw Open. 2019;2(1):e185630. https://doi.org/10.1001/jamanetworkopen.2018.5630.
4. Berin MC, Sampson HA. Mucosal immunology of food allergy. Curr Biol. 2013;23(9):R389–400. https://doi.org/10.1016/j.cub.2013.02.043.
5. Anvari S, Miller J, Yeh CY, Davis CM. IgE-mediated food allergy. Clin Rev Allergy Immunol. 2019;57(2):244–60. https://doi.org/10.1007/s12016-018-8710-3.
6. Atkins D, Bock SA. Fatal anaphylaxis to foods: epidemiology, recognition, and prevention. Curr Allergy Asthma Rep. 2009;9(3):179–85. https://doi.org/10.1007/s11882-009-0027-0.
7. Feuille E, Nowak-Węgrzyn A. Definition, etiology, and diagnosis of food protein-induced enterocolitis syndrome. Curr Opin Allergy Clin Immunol. 2014;14(3):222–8. https://doi.org/10.1097/ACI.0000000000000055.
8. Katz Y, Goldberg MR, Rajuan N, Cohen A, Leshno M. The prevalence and natural course of food protein-induced enterocolitis syndrome to cow's milk: a large-scale, prospective population-based study. J Allergy Clin Immunol. 2011;127(3):647–53.e1-3. https://doi.org/10.1016/j.jaci.2010.12.1105.
9. Lake AM. Food-induced eosinophilic proctocolitis. J Pediatr Gastroenterol Nutr. 2000;30(Suppl):S58–60. https://doi.org/10.1097/00005176-200001001-00009.
10. Fasano A, Sapone A, Zevallos V, Schuppan D. Nonceliac gluten sensitivity. Gastroenterology. 2015;148(6):1195–204. https://doi.org/10.1053/j.gastro.2014.12.049.
11. Leonard MM, Sapone A, Catassi C, Fasano A. Celiac disease and nonceliac gluten sensitivity: a review. JAMA. 2017;318(7):647–56. https://doi.org/10.1001/jama.2017.9730.
12. Jensen ET, Martin CF, Kappelman MD, Dellon ES. Prevalence of eosinophilic gastritis, gastroenteritis, and colitis: estimates from a National Administrative Database. J Pediatr Gastroenterol Nutr. 2016;62(1):36–42. https://doi.org/10.1097/MPG.0000000000000865.
13. Hill DA, Spergel JM. The immunologic mechanisms of eosinophilic esophagitis. Curr Allergy Asthma Rep. 2016;16(2):9. https://doi.org/10.1007/s11882-015-0592-3.

14. Kinoshita Y, Oouchi S, Fujisawa T. Eosinophilic gastrointestinal diseases – pathogenesis, diagnosis, and treatment. Allergol Int. 2019;68(4):420–9. https://doi.org/10.1016/j.alit.2019.03.003.
15. Zopf Y, Baenkler HW, Silbermann A, Hahn EG, Raithel M. The differential diagnosis of food intolerance. Dtsch Arztebl Int. 2009;106(21):359–69; quiz 69–70; 4 p following 70. https://doi.org/10.3238/arztebl.2009.0359.
16. Storhaug CL, Fosse SK, Fadnes LT. Country, regional, and global estimates for lactose malabsorption in adults: a systematic review and meta-analysis. Lancet Gastroenterol Hepatol. 2017;2(10):738–46. https://doi.org/10.1016/S2468-1253(17)30154-1.
17. Misselwitz B, Butter M, Verbeke K, Fox MR. Update on lactose malabsorption and intolerance: pathogenesis, diagnosis and clinical management. Gut. 2019;68(11):2080–91. https://doi.org/10.1136/gutjnl-2019-318404.
18. Cohen SA. The clinical consequences of sucrase-isomaltase deficiency. Mol Cell Pediatr. 2016;3(1):5. https://doi.org/10.1186/s40348-015-0028-0.
19. Maintz L, Novak N. Histamine and histamine intolerance. Am J Clin Nutr. 2007;85(5):1185–96. https://doi.org/10.1093/ajcn/85.5.1185.
20. Marcobal A, De las Rivas B, Landete JM, Tabera L, Munoz R. Tyramine and phenylethylamine biosynthesis by food bacteria. Crit Rev Food Sci Nutr. 2012;52(5):448–67. https://doi.org/10.1080/10408398.2010.500545.
21. Feng C, Teuber S, Gershwin ME. Histamine (Scombroid) fish poisoning: a comprehensive review. Clin Rev Allergy Immunol. 2016;50(1):64–9. https://doi.org/10.1007/s12016-015-8467-x.
22. Staudacher HM, Whelan K. The low FODMAP diet: recent advances in understanding its mechanisms and efficacy in IBS. Gut. 2017;66(8):1517–27. https://doi.org/10.1136/gutjnl-2017-313750.
23. Gibson PR. Use of the low-FODMAP diet in inflammatory bowel disease. J Gastroenterol Hepatol. 2017;32(Suppl 1):40–2. https://doi.org/10.1111/jgh.13695.
24. Spiller R, Garsed K. Postinfectious irritable bowel syndrome. Gastroenterology. 2009;136(6):1979–88. https://doi.org/10.1053/j.gastro.2009.02.074.

Prebiotics, Probiotics, and Dietary Supplements

11

Pratima Dibba, Megha Kothari, and Irwin Grosman

Introduction to the Gut Microbiome

The human gut is inoculated at birth and develops a microbiome resembling that of an adult by age 3–5 [1]. The fermentation of dietary carbohydrates, lipids, proteins, and secretions such as mucin by anaerobic gut bacteria contributes to homeostasis and energy balance as well as physiologic resistance [1]. Dysbiosis, or disruption of the microbiota, can occur secondary to medications, infections, aging, lifestyle, poor nutrition, and chronic gastrointestinal diseases [1]. It is hypothesized that alteration of the colonic bacteria may be a contributing etiology for irritable bowel syndrome (IBS) and that IBS symptoms such as bloating, slowed intestinal transit, and early satiety may be associated with specific gut microbiota profiles, indicating a potential therapeutic role for prebiotics and probiotics [2].

Prebiotics

Prebiotics, which include non-digestible oligosaccharides or short-chain polysaccharides, are defined as selectively fermented ingredients or substrates that are utilized by host microorganisms. These compounds promote specific changes, both in the composition and activity of the gastrointestinal microbiota that may confer health benefits [3, 4]. By increasing specific bacteria within the colonic flora, for example, *lactobacilli* and *bifidobacteria*, there is alteration and modification of the microbiome resulting in the replacement of potentially pathogenic species with beneficial microorganisms which may have therapeutic benefit in gastrointestinal disease [5–7]. Prebiotics are resistant to gastric acid, hydrolysis, and gastrointestinal absorption. They are fermented by intestinal microorganisms and selectively stimulate growth of intestinal bacteria associated with health and well-being [8, 9]. Byproducts of the fermentation of prebiotics may also play a role in immune modulation, defense against pathogens, increasing satiety, increasing calcium absorption, increasing fecal weight, and shortening gastrointestinal transit time, among other metabolic effects [2, 6]. Examples of prebiotics include inulin, fructo-oligosaccharides, galacto-oligosaccharides, soybean oligosaccharides, breast milk oligosaccharides, lactulose, and complex polysaccharides that constitute fiber [6, 10]. Prebiotics have been proposed to have therapeutic benefit in IBS, chronic idiopathic constipation, inflammatory bowel disease (IBD), and nonalcoholic fatty liver disease (NAFLD) [11]. Animal studies reveal that prebiotics may play a role in colorectal cancer (CRC) although no human trials have been conducted to date [12].

P. Dibba (✉) · M. Kothari · I. Grosman
Department of Gastroenterology and Liver Disease, New York Presbyterian Brooklyn Methodist Hospital, Brooklyn, NY, USA
e-mail: mek9037@nyp.org; img9004@nyp.org

C. Newberry et al. (eds.), *Nutrition, Weight, and Digestive Health*,
https://doi.org/10.1007/978-3-030-94953-2_11

Use in Digestive Disease Management

The use of prebiotics in IBS is weakly recommended due to low-quality evidence [2]. In a double-blind randomized placebo-controlled trial including 128 patients with IBS treated with prebiotics derived from chicory, abdominal pain relief scores and flatulence scores were significantly improved with prebiotic therapy [2, 13]. Another double-blind randomized controlled trial in patients with IBS compared prebiotic supplements with a low-FODMAP diet and placebo; results demonstrated that although both active treatments improved daily symptom scores and flatulence, symptoms relapsed more quickly after discontinuation of the low-FODMAP diet versus prebiotics [14]. A recent systematic review and meta-analysis of 11 randomized controlled trials with notable limitations including lack of standardization in prebiotic formulas failed to find significant improvement of symptoms or quality of life in patients with IBS or functional gastrointestinal disorders treated with prebiotic supplements [15]. While prebiotics were hypothesized to play a role in chronic idiopathic constipation based on an early study, a subsequent randomized controlled trial revealed no significant relief in constipation in patients treated with prebiotics versus placebo [16–18].

Prebiotics have been studied minimally in IBD. Although animal studies suggest that prebiotics may be effective in treating Crohn's disease (CD), these findings have not been corroborated in human studies [19]. A small pilot study of ten patients with CD showed that prebiotics increased colonic bifidobacteria and reduced disease activity; however, two larger randomized controlled trials showed no benefit [20–22]. Prebiotics were studied in comparison to mesalamine in one randomized controlled trial of 102 patients with ulcerative colitis (UC) [23]. Results indicated that both agents were similarly effective in sustaining clinical and endoscopic remission [23]. When investigated in combination with probiotics as a symbiotic, a small pilot study demonstrated reduced endoscopic disease activity and mucosal inflammatory cytokines in nine treated patients, although clinical disease activity was not significantly decreased in comparison to placebo [24]. The role of prebiotics in treatment of inflammatory bowel disease therefore remains unclear.

Probiotics

Probiotics were first defined in 1965 as substances secreted by one microorganism which stimulate the growth of another [25]. Currently, probiotics are defined as live organisms which, when administered in adequate amounts, confer a health benefit to the host. They are divided into four categories: (1) live or active cultures, (2) probiotics in food or supplements without a health claim, (3) probiotics in food or supplements with a specific health claim, and (4) probiotic drugs [26, 27]. Probiotics exert their effects on the digestive tract by increasing beneficial anaerobic bacteria, decreasing potentially pathogenic organisms, and modifying the microbiota and luminal milieu, gut barrier, intestinal immune response, neuromuscular function of the gastrointestinal tract, and microbiota of the gut-brain axis [27, 28]. Probiotics inhibit epithelial apoptosis, promote integrity of the mucus layer, increase production of tight junction proteins, and stimulate IgA secretion, thereby strengthening the gut barrier [28]. Probiotics also reduce visceral hypersensitivity, enhance gut transit, and enhance neurotransmitter production [28]. They interact with the gut microbiota, compete for nutrients, and produce organic acids and enzymes such as beta-galactosidase, bile salt hydrolase, and lactase [2].

Probiotics are generally identified by the genus, species, subspecies, and strain [28]. The most common probiotics are *Lactobacillus* and *Bifidobacterium* species, but others utilized include *Bacillus*, *Saccharomyces*, *E. coli*, *Clostridium*, *Enterococcus*, *Lactococcus*, *Leuconostoc*, *Pediococcus*, *Propionibacterium*, and *Streptococcus* [28, 29]. Combinations of probiotics that have been well studied include Align®, which is composed of *Bifidobacterium longum;* VSL#3, which is composed of *Bifidobacterium breve*, *longum*, *and infantis*;

Lactobacillus acidophilus, *Lactobacillus delbrueckii*, *Lactobacillus plantarum*, *Lactobacillus paracasei*, and *Lactobacillus bulgaricus*; and *Streptococcus thermophilus* [29, 30]. The potential application of probiotics has been studied for the treatment of antibiotic-associated diarrhea (AAD), *Clostridioides difficile* infection (CDI), radiation-induced diarrhea, small intestinal bacterial overgrowth, infectious diarrhea, traveler's diarrhea, *H. pylori* gastritis, IBD, IBS, colic, necrotizing enterocolitis, NAFLD, and hepatic encephalopathy [28, 29]. Several systemic reviews and meta-analyses regarding the use of probiotics in gastrointestinal disorders have been published. Limitations of published data, however, include the heterogeneity of studies in terms of the types and formulations of probiotics used, dosage administered, duration of therapy, outcome measures, sample size, and patient population studied [26].

Use in Digestive Disease Management

Probiotics have been considered as possibly beneficial in IBD based on the hypothesis that dysbiosis may be a pathogenic mechanism for CD and UC [31]. In a systematic review of case-control studies evaluating the microbiota of patients with IBD compared with healthy controls, patients with CD had decreased amounts of *Christensenellaceae*, *Coriobacteriaceae*, and *Faecalibacterium prausnitzii* and increased *Actinomyces*, *Veillonella*, and *Escherichia coli* [31]. *Eubacterium rectale* and *Akkermansia* were decreased in patients with UC, whereas *E. coli* was increased [31]. Given the variation of the gut microbiome between patients with IBD and healthy controls and the aforementioned immunomodulatory, anti-inflammatory, and gut barrier protective mechanisms of probiotics, probiotics have been considered a potential complementary/alternative therapy in this population [32, 33]. In a systematic review of seven small randomized controlled trials comparing probiotics to placebo in patients with mild to moderately active UC, probiotics had potential remission-inducing effects [34]. Three of the seven trials demonstrated that specifically the product VSL#3 demonstrated significant increase in response and remission rates [34]. Although another study found no difference in remission rates based a global assessment scale, VSL#3-treated patients showed improvement in rectal bleeding and stool frequency scores [35]. A small study included 29 pediatric patients with UC who received steroid induction and mesalamine maintenance therapy and were treated with VSL#3 or placebo; remission was achieved in a greater number of patients receiving VSL#3 as compared to placebo [36]. In the review by Koretz, two of five low-quality randomized controlled trials analyzed showed that *Bifidobacterium* may be effective for maintenance of remission in patients with UC [34]. Other probiotics that have been evaluated in the management of UC include *E. coli* (Nissle), *Lactobacillus*, and *Streptococcus* [29, 32–34]. A more recent technical review of the seven aforementioned randomized controlled trials in UC analyzed by Koretz found that probiotics were no more effective than placebo in the induction of remission and probiotic-treated patients had lower rates of relapse compared to placebo, though the results were not statistically significant [37]. Evidence was considered low quality due to imprecision, inconsistency, and risk of bias [37]. Additionally, studies comparing probiotic *E. coli* to mesalamine showed no significant difference in induction or maintenance of remission in patients with UC [37]. Probiotics have also been studied in post-surgical UC patients with ileal pouch anal anastomoses complicated by pouchitis. In a Cochrane systematic review of six randomized controlled trials, *Lactobacillus* had no effect on active pouchitis, but VSL#3 was effective as prophylaxis and induced maintenance of remission [37–40]. Although a small randomized controlled trial of *Saccharomyces boulardii* showed some benefit in CD, four other trials demonstrated either no effect or adverse effects associated with the use of probiotics in CD [34]. Probiotics have also been found to be ineffective in maintaining clinical remission in patients with CD who have undergone surgical resection [33, 41–45].

Data supporting the use of probiotics in microscopic colitis, traveler's diarrhea, and infectious colitis is limited [34]. Studies showed no benefit conferred by probiotics in microscopic colitis or traveler's diarrhea [34]. Low-quality studies demonstrate that probiotics may improve clearance of *Giardia* cysts and may result in more rapid recovery from amebiasis [34]. One systematic review and meta-analysis revealed that probiotic use may play a role in the prevention and treatment of SIBO, although the heterogeneity of the studies limited the validity of these findings [46]. In patients with diverticular disease who had symptoms of chronic abdominal pain and altered bowel habits not necessarily associated with acute diverticulitis, probiotics improved pain independently or in combination with mesalamine when compared to placebo [34].

A systematic review was unable to assess the utility of probiotics in IBS given the heterogeneity and limitations of the studies evaluated, although several studies suggested benefit for *Bifidobacterium infantis* [47–50]. To date, there are more than 50 randomized controlled trials studying the effects of probiotics in IBS [51–53]. Although there is significant heterogeneity among studies comparing probiotics to placebo, probiotics have demonstrated statistically significant superiority to placebo in regard to global IBS symptoms scores, flatulence scores, bloating scores, and abdominal pain scores [2, 17]. It is important to note that benefits are strain and dose-specific and that high-quality studies regarding the role of probiotics in IBS are warranted [54].

Studies regarding the use of probiotics in antibiotic-associated diarrhea (AAD) and *C. difficile* infection (CDI) have had varying conclusions but have trended toward efficacy. The etiology of AAD and CDI is presumed to be an alteration in the intestinal microbiome secondary to the use of antibiotics [34]. An early meta-analysis of 25 randomized controlled trials found that probiotics (specifically *Saccharomyces boulardii*, *Lactobacillus rhamnosus GG*, and probiotic mixtures) reduced the development of AAD, with *S. boulardii* being the only probiotic effective for the prevention of CDI [55]. Similar conclusions about the efficacy of probiotics in AAD in the pediatric population were reported in a systematic review of 16 studies. A systematic review and meta-analysis of 31 randomized controlled trials studying the prevention of CDI by probiotics in all age groups and a large systematic review and meta-analysis of 82 randomized controlled trials studying the evidence for probiotics in the prevention and treatment of AAD in all age groups also reported benefit [56–58]. A large multicenter double-blind randomized controlled trial, known as the PLACIDE trial, in approximately 3,000 patients exposed to antibiotics randomized subjects to a multi-strain preparation of *Lactobacilli* and *Bifidobacteria* or placebo to assess the occurrence of ADD and CDI [59]. Findings did not support the use of probiotics in the prevention of ADD or CDI [59]. While this study failed to support the use of this probiotic combination, a recent systematic review with meta-regression analysis of 19 studies reintroduced the potential benefit of probiotics in this clinical setting [60]. The study found that the administration of probiotics closer to the first dose of antibiotics reduces the risk of CDI by more than 50% in hospitalized adults and found that the PLACIDE trial may not have been adequately powered to demonstrate benefit [60]. Although heterogeneity in probiotic dose and species was acknowledged, pooled estimates did not demonstrate significant statistical heterogeneity [60].

Although one systematic review was unable to draw conclusions about the potential benefit of probiotics in patients with hepatic encephalopathy (HE) due to the high risk of bias and high risk of random errors among the existing trials, there are some data supporting their use in this setting [61]. In one small unblinded randomized controlled trial of nonalcoholic cirrhotic patients with minimal hepatic encephalopathy (MHE), probiotic yogurt supplementation demonstrated MHE reversal [62]. A randomized controlled trial comparing probiotics, lactulose, and

Table 11.1 The role of probiotics in specific digestive diseases

Digestive condition	Role of probiotics
Traveler's diarrhea	None
IBD	None
Microscopic colitis	None
Clearance of *Giardia* cysts	Possible
SIBO	Possible
Diverticular disease	Possible
Antibiotic-associated diarrhea	Possible
C. difficile	Possible
Hepatic encephalopathy	Possible
NAFLD	Possible
CRC	Possible
IBS	Possible

placebo for overt HE concluded that probiotics and lactulose reduced HE re-admission rates [63]. These findings were supported by a double-blind, randomized, controlled trial that also noted reduced hospitalizations for HE, in addition to improved Child-Turcotte-Pugh scores and model for end-stage liver disease scores [64]. Two low-quality randomized controlled trials that studied the role of probiotics in NAFLD showed some reduction of hepatic steatosis, but studies were limited by lack of assessment of clinical outcomes [34].

Studies regarding the association between the gut microbiome and CRC have primarily been conducted in in vitro models [65]. Studies have demonstrated that there is increased microbial diversity and reduced temporal stability in the fecal microbiota as well as overexpression of certain strains in subjects with colonic polyposis syndromes and CRC [63]. The interaction of the diet with the gut microbiome and the resulting byproducts of metabolism by gut microbes may also play a role in the development of CRC [63]. The limited number of clinical studies of probiotics and CRC vary in design and methodology. One prospective study suggested that the intake of probiotics in the form of yogurt was associated with a decreased risk of CRC [66]. There are insufficient data from other clinical studies to draw conclusive recommendations [12]. Table 11.1 summarizes whether existing data supports, refutes, or suggests a possible therapeutic role for probiotics in the aforementioned digestive diseases.

Safety Profile

The majority of clinical trials have found probiotic use to be safe with a low risk of significant adverse events [67]. There have been reports of bacterial sepsis (specifically associated with probiotics containing lactobacilli), pancreatitis, and death from gastrointestinal mucormycosis in a preterm infant (although the latter was associated with mold contamination of the supplement) [66]. Cases of bacteremia have typically been reported in patients with underlying immunosuppression or disruption in the integrity of the gastrointestinal tract [34, 66]. Nonetheless, serious adverse events have been reported rarely, and probiotics have been generally deemed as safe [26].

Dietary Supplements

Dietary supplements are defined as over-the-counter products taken orally (as pills, capsules, tablets, powders, or liquids) that contain dietary ingredients such as vitamins, minerals, amino acids, herbs, botanicals, or other substances whose use, often to supplement diet, does not require medical or physician supervision [68, 69]. According to data collected from the National Health and Nutrition Examination Survey in 2011, 52% of US adults reported the use of supplements due to their perceived medicinal and health benefits [70, 71]. Consumers use dietary supplements to address ailments and to maintain and improve overall health [72]. The true impact of dietary supplements on disease prevention and health promotion has been limited by the inability to isolate supplement use from health-seeking behaviors, the difficulty of assessing the impact of a supplement over a short duration of use, and variability in supplement composition due to lack of standardization and government oversight [72].

Dietary Supplement Regulation

The Bureau of Chemistry was the first US federal agency to attempt to regulate dietary supplements through the Federal Food and Drugs Act of 1906, which required transparent labeling [73, 74]. With the emergence of vitamins as dietary supplements in the 1920s, the concern over their indiscriminate use prompted further regulation by the Bureau of Chemistry. Several subsequent efforts to tighten the regulation of dietary supplements were made by the successor to the Bureau of Chemistry, the US Food and Drug Administration (FDA), from 1938 to 1960 [74].

After 38 people died and 1,500 others were sickened by the consumption of L-tryptophan, the FDA began to more aggressively regulate dietary supplements [75]. The Dietary Supplement Health and Education Act of 1994 (DSHEA) was passed by Congress with the intention of balancing consumer access and product safety [73, 76, 77]. Unlike pharmaceutical drugs, which require proof of safety and efficacy prior to approval by the FDA, dietary supplements may be marketed to consumers if the manufacturer determines that the product is generally recognized as safe [74, 75]. The safety of dietary supplements is subsequently monitored through post-market surveillance for serious adverse events resulting in hospitalization, disability, or death which must be reported to the FDA [78, 79]. Additional avenues for product recall include spot inspection of manufacturer facilities by the FDA, reports by physicians or consumers of adverse events, and tips from retailers of potentially adulterated products [80]. Still, lack of formal assessments, scientific research, and government oversight has led to variable composition of supplements and lack of adequate objective data to support or refute their use.

The Role of Dietary Supplements in Gastrointestinal Disease

Many dietary supplements have been proposed as potential treatments for gastrointestinal illnesses. Studies regarding the use of supplements for gastrointestinal health in people who prefer nonpharmaceutical therapy have been published with mixed evidence of benefit. Table 11.2 summarizes the proposed gastrointestinal effects of dietary supplements, excluding weight loss supplements and medical foods.

Peppermint

Peppermint oil, composed of menthol and menthone, is derived from the plant *Mentha* x *piperita* L. [81]. The proposed benefit of peppermint oil in gastrointestinal conditions, such as IBS, functional dyspepsia, gastroduodenal dysmotility, and spasm during endoscopy, has been attributed to its antispasmodic effects on gastrointestinal smooth muscle. A meta-analysis of five double-blind, randomized controlled trials suggested statistically significant global improvement of IBS symptoms in patients treated with peppermint oil compared to placebo, although strong limitations were noted due to the variability of parameters across studies [82]. A later double-blind randomized controlled trial of 110 patients evaluating the efficacy of enteric-coated peppermint oil as a treatment in IBS concluded that patients receiving the peppermint oil experienced improvement in IBS symptoms compared to those on placebo, although this study included patients whose IBS diagnosis was not based on established criteria [83]. A double-blind randomized trial of 74 patients similarly concluded that peppermint oil transiently improved abdominal pain but only in patients with diarrhea-predominant IBS [84]. In a limited meta-analysis of over 1,000 treated IBS patients, peppermint oil was found to alleviate abdominal pain, abdominal distention, bowel frequency, borborygmi, and flatulence [85]. In another meta-analysis, four studies of 392 patients with IBS (diagnosed according to established Rome criteria) comparing peppermint oil versus placebo found improvement of symptoms with no statistically significant heterogeneity. The authors concluded that the number needed to treat to prevent one patient from having persistent symptoms was 2.5 [86]. A later meta-analysis evaluated nine studies that included 726 patients; results demon-

Table 11.2 Proposed gastrointestinal effects of dietary supplements and support for use

Supplement	Proposed gastrointestinal effect	Evidence supporting use
Peppermint oil	1. Antispasmodic effects on smooth muscles 2. Improvement in IBS symptoms (most improvement in abdominal pain) 3. Improvement in functional dyspepsia	Literature supports use in IBS and dyspepsia
Ginger	1. Alleviation of nausea/vomiting of pregnancy 2. Alleviation of chemotherapy-induced nausea 3. Alleviation of postoperative nausea 4. Reduction in hepatic steatosis score in NAFLD patients 5. Role in improvement in dysphagia and prevention of aspiration 6. Bactericidal against *H. pylori* 7. Chemo-preventative and chemotherapeutic benefits 8. Preventative role in patients with an increased risk of colon cancer 9. Alleviation of IBS symptoms 10. Improvement in dyspepsia	Literature supports use in nausea
STW 5 (Iberogast)	1. Improvement in functional dyspepsia 2. Improvement in IBS symptoms 3. Affects gastric motility 4. Alleviation of gastrointestinal hypersensitivity 5. Inhibition of inflammation 6. Suppression of gastric hypersecretion 7. Modulation of the microbiota 8. Binding of 5-HT3, 5-HT4, muscarinic M3, and opioid receptors 9. Reduction in oxidative stress 10. Protection against irritant-induced inflammation 11. Provides stimulatory and protective effects on mucosal integrity and secretion	More studies required to support its use
Licorice	1. Healing of gastric ulcers 2. Improves histologic inflammation associated with *H. pylori* 3. Anti-viral activity 4. Influences gut bacteria 5. Spasmogenic and spasmolytic effects 6. Gastroprotective and anti-inflammatory properties 7. Reduces body weight, hepatic steatosis, and hepatic inflammation in NAFLD patients	More studies required to support its use

(continued)

Table 11.2 (continued)

Supplement	Proposed gastrointestinal effect	Evidence supporting use
Curcumin	1. Reduction of inflammation and tumorigenesis by suppression of nuclear factor kappa B (NF-κB), resulting in a secondary suppression of cyclooxygenase-2 (COX-2) and inducible nitric oxide synthase (iNOS) 2. Protection against intestinal permeability 3. Antibacterial, antifungal, and antiparasitic properties against gastrointestinal infections such as *H. pylori*, *Candida*, *Giardia*, *E. coli*, and *Toxoplasma gondii* 4. Protects normal tissue from chemotherapy-induced toxicity by clearing intracellular radical oxygen species 5. Improvement hematologically, biochemically, and endoscopically in patients with UC 6. Improvement in Crohn's disease activity index (CDAI) score in patients with CD 7. Improvement in clinical activity index and endoscopic index in patients with UC 8. Prevention of carcinogenesis and tumor initiation 9. Reduction of tumor proliferation and progression 10. Decrease in prostaglandin E2, which has been found to enhance the growth of human CRC cells 11. Regression in both number and size of polyps in patients with FAP 12. Reductions in transaminase elevations in patients with NAFLD 13. Antifibrotic and hepatoprotective effects in patients with cirrhosis 14. Improved quality of life in patients with cirrhosis	More studies required to support its use
Chamomile	1. Anti-diarrheal properties in acute inflammatory disorders, IBD, or IBS 2. Hepatoprotective properties 3. Anti-inflammatory properties	More studies required to support its use
Glutamine	1. Energy source in intestinal enterocytes 2. Substrate in hepatic gluconeogenesis 3. Decreased gut mucosal atrophy in animals fed with parenteral nutrition 4. Decreased intestinal permeability 5. Decreased mucosal damage in animals subjected to gram-negative sepsis 6. Preservation of glutathione concentrations in intestinal tracts subject to ischemia and reperfusion 7. Improvement in mucosal and plasma glutathione concentrations 8. Protection against bacterial translocation from the gut with parenteral nutrition 9. Mediation of intestinal adaptation in animals with short bowel syndrome 10. Improve absorption of protein and reduce parenteral nutrition requirements in parenteral nutrition-dependent patients with short bowel syndrome 11. Protective effect of glutamine from radiation and chemotherapy-induced gastrointestinal mucosal injury 12. Mucosal regeneration and immune enhancement in patients with CD 13. Reduction in intestinal hyperpermeability and decreasing visceral hypersensitivity in patients with IBS	More studies required to support its use

strated evidence for global improvement in IBS symptoms, with improvement in abdominal pain being most significant [87].

Peppermint has been evaluated for other gastrointestinal conditions, including functional dyspepsia, postoperative nausea, gastroduodenal motility disorders, and gastrointestinal spasm during endoscopic procedures [88–95]. A double-blind randomized controlled trial of 97 patients determined that peppermint oil decreased the intensity of abdominal pain and offered global improvement in symptoms of functional dyspepsia [88]. A double-blind randomized controlled trial of 100 patients undergoing upper endoscopy who received intramuscular hyoscyamine or intraluminal peppermint oil demonstrated that peppermint oil exhibited greater antispasmodic properties as evidenced by more dramatic opening of the pyloric ring, smaller contraction ratios, and disappearance of the contraction ring in the gastric antrum [91]. Peppermint oil demonstrated similar antispasmodic properties in the duodenum as observed by reduction of duodenal motility in 39 patients undergoing ERCP who received peppermint oil in a prospective fashion [92]. The use of peppermint oil, however, is limited in patients with GERD as it may exacerbate esophageal reflux and heartburn, although reflux may be minimized with the use of enteric coated capsules [83].

Ginger

Ginger, also known as *Zingiber officinale*, is used commonly in Asian countries as a complementary treatment for a wide array of medical problems including dental, rheumatological, respiratory, and gastrointestinal illness [96]. The use of ginger in gastrointestinal health has been studied primarily in nausea and vomiting. It has also been assessed in the management of nonalcoholic fatty liver disease (NAFLD), dysphagia, gastrointestinal malignancies, IBS, and other functional disorders with less conclusive findings [96].

Ginger has demonstrated therapeutic benefits in nausea and vomiting of pregnancy, postoperative nausea and vomiting, motion sickness, and nausea and vomiting of chemotherapy. In a systematic review of six double-blind randomized controlled trials of patients receiving ginger as a monotherapy compared to placebo for nausea and vomiting, five out of six studies found that ginger alleviated nausea [97, 98]. In a more recent systematic review and meta-analysis, 12 randomized controlled trials were included in the analysis, and the authors concluded that ginger was effective for the alleviation of nausea though there was less evidence for reduction in the number of episodes of emesis [99]. Another meta-analysis of six studies including 256 patients concluded that ginger was better than placebo in improving nausea and vomiting of pregnancy [100]. When ginger was compared to other antiemetics given in pregnancy, it had similar efficacy to vitamin B6 and metoclopramide. [99].

A randomized controlled trial of 41 patients with leukemia suffering from chemotherapy-induced nausea showed that ginger was more effective in alleviating symptoms than placebo, although no p-value was reported [97, 101]. The largest double-blind multicenter trial of 576 cancer patients receiving either placebo or different concentrations of ginger in addition to a 5-HT3 receptor antagonist antiemetic revealed that ginger supplementation significantly reduced chemotherapy-induced nausea [102]. Later studies demonstrated conflicting results regarding the efficacy of ginger in the management of this condition. [103].

Studies regarding the use of ginger to treat postoperative nausea have yielded mixed results. Although some studies found ginger comparable in efficacy to metoclopramide, others have found ginger is no more effective than placebo and ineffective as a single agent or in combination with diazepam [97, 104–108]. Similar findings have been reported when used intraoperatively [96, 109–113].

Ginger has also been studied in NAFLD, dysphagia, *H. pylori*, and gastrointestinal malignancy in limited studies [96]. In a double-blind, randomized controlled trial of 44 patients with NAFLD, ginger demonstrated reduction in hepatic steatosis score, which is an estimate of hepatic liver accumulation as determined by ultrasound elastography, compared to placebo, although the results were not verified by histology [114]. A small, limited study demonstrated lack of aspiration and improvement in the swallowing function score in patients above age 63 with dysphagia after using ginger [115]. Ginger may also be bactericidal against *H. pylori* according to preclinical investigation [116]. Preclinical investigation in in vivo and in vitro gastrointestinal cancer models (hepatocellular, gastric, colon, and gallbladder) has yielded multiple mechanisms by which ginger may have potential chemo-preventative and chemotherapeutic benefits [117]. There is some limited data to suggest that ginger may provide some benefit in patients at increased risk of colorectal cancer (CRC) through the reduction in prostaglandin E2 and 5-hydroxyeicosatetraenoic acid, both of which have been implicated in the development of CRC and the proliferation of CRC cells [118].

Although the efficacy of ginger has not been well-proven in functional disorders such as IBS, functional diarrhea, functional constipation, and functional dyspepsia, it remains one of the most frequently used complementary medicines for these conditions [119, 120]. In a double-blind randomized controlled trial of 45 patients with IBS, ginger was well-tolerated but not more effective than the placebo in alleviating IBS symptoms [121]. Although one small pilot study of patients with functional dyspepsia demonstrated improvement in symptoms with the use of ginger, other studies have demonstrated improved gastric emptying and antral contractions without associated symptom improvement [122–125]. Additional, larger-scale, well-designed trials will be necessary to elicit the true effect of ginger on these digestive conditions.

Herbal Combinations (STW 5, Iberogast®)

STW 5, also known as the commercial preparation, Iberogast®, is an herbal formulation composed of nine medicinal herbs, including *Iberis amara*, *Melissa officinalis*, *Matricaria recutita*, *Carum carvi*, *Mentha piperita*, *Angelica archangelica*, *Silybum marianum*, *Chelidonium majus*, and *Glycyrrhiza glabra* [126]. Its use has been studied in patients with functional dyspepsia and IBS. In a prospective double-blind, placebo-controlled study of 243 patients with functional dyspepsia, STW 5 was found to be effective in improving symptoms [127]. A larger study of more than 300 patients, including those with functional dyspepsia as defined by Rome II criteria, found that treatment with STW 5 over an 8-week period resulted in immediate and sustained symptom improvement [128, 129]. SWT 5 was comparable to the prokinetic drug cisapride in patients with functional dyspepsia of the dysmotility subtype with symptoms of bloating, abdominal fullness, nausea, vomiting, belching, and early satiety [130, 131].

Studies in IBS have been equally positive. In one observational study of over 2,500 patients with IBS, treatment with STW 5 resulted in significant improvement in symptoms as determined by both physician and patient assessment [127]. Similar results were reported in a study of more than 900 pediatric patients with functional gastrointestinal disorders, including IBS, who were treated with STW 5 [132].

In a double-blind randomized controlled trial, the effect of SWT 5 was compared to that of placebo on gastric volume, antropyloroduodenal motility, gastric emptying, and intragastric distribution of a solid/liquid meal [133]. SWT 5 was found to increase gastric volume, increase the motility index of antral pressure waves, and increase retention of liquid, suggesting that it affects gastric motility [66]. Other potential mechanisms for the gastrointestinal effects of STW 5 include the alleviation of gastrointestinal hypersensitivity, inhibition of inflammation, suppression of gastric hypersecretion, modulation of the microbiota, and binding of 5-HT3, 5-HT4, muscarinic M3, and opioid receptors [134, 135]. STW 5 has been shown to reduce oxidative stress, protect against irritant-induced inflammation, and provide stimulatory and protective effects on mucosal integrity and secretion [135]. It therefore may have a role in treating a variety of functional disorders in the upper and lower GI tracts.

Licorice

Licorice, also known as *Glycyrrhiza* spp., has been used as a laxative, demulcent, and anti-inflammatory agent in Ayurvedic medicine practices singly and as a component of Iberogast® [136]. There are very few randomized controlled trials that have been conducted to support the use of licorice alone in the treatment of gastrointestinal disease; its use has primarily been studied in in vitro and in vivo models. One randomized placebo-controlled trial of 38 patients with gastric ulcers who were treated with licorice refuted the previously reported healing effect of licorice on ulcers [137, 138]. Another randomized controlled trial studying *Glycyrrhiza glabra* in combination with *Lactobacillus paracasei* in *H. pylori* gastritis demonstrated that the combination of agents decreased *H. pylori* density and improved histologic inflammation when compared with placebo [139]. In vivo and in vitro studies suggest that different species of *Glycyrrhiza* possess antiviral activity, influence gut bacteria, have spasmogenic and spasmolytic effects, and exhibit gastroprotective and anti-inflammatory properties [68, 140–144]. In a murine model, diammonium glycyrrhizinate, a component of licorice root extract, reduced body weight, hepatic steatosis, and hepatic inflammation in mice with high-fat diet-induced NAFLD, possibly mediated by modulation of gut microbiota and restoration of the intestinal barrier [145].

Curcumin

Curcumin is a constituent of the herb *Curcuma Longa*, commonly known as turmeric [146]. Its anti-inflammatory and anti-neoplastic properties have supported the investigation of its therapeutic potential in various gastrointestinal disorders IBD, NAFLD, CRC, cirrhosis, and *H. pylori*. A meta-analysis of five clinical trials proposed that curcumin may be beneficial in IBS; however, only three studies demonstrated positive and statistically significant effects [147]. In vivo and in vitro models have been useful in identifying the effects of curcumin that may be beneficial in gastrointestinal disease, including reduction of inflammation and tumorigenesis by suppression of nuclear factor kappa B (NF-κB), resulting in a secondary suppression of cyclooxygenase-2 (COX-2) and inducible nitric oxide synthase (iNOS) [146]. In vivo and in vitro studies have also confirmed the role of curcumin in protecting against intestinal permeability and as an antibacterial, antifungal, and antiparasitic agent against gastrointestinal infections such as *H. pylori*, *Candida*, *Giardia*, *E. coli*, and *Toxoplasma gondii* [148–150]. Other in vivo and in vitro studies suggest that curcumin can protect normal tissue from chemotherapy-induced toxicity by clearing intracellular radical oxygen species [151].

Because curcumin has been hypothesized to suppress NF-κB and other inflammatory cytokines, it has been studied as a potential IBD therapy [152]. In a small pilot study, all five patients with UC treated with curcumin demonstrated improvement hematologically, biochemically, and endoscopically although these patients were on concomitant standard maintenance therapy [146, 153]. Four out of five patients with Crohn's disease (CD) showed improvement in Crohn's disease activity index (CDAI) score [153]. In a multicenter double-blind randomized controlled trial of 89 UC patients, curcumin was studied in comparison to placebo, given in combination with either sulfasalazine or mesalamine [154]. Of the final 43 patients in the curcumin group, two patients demonstrated relapse at 6 months versus eight out of 39 patients in the placebo group [154]. Curcumin also improved the clinical activity index and endoscopic index in patients with UC [154]. A recent review of three randomized placebo-controlled trials totaling 169 patients with mild-to-moderate UC found a trend toward the benefit in maintaining clinical remission with the addition of curcumin to standard maintenance therapy, although the results were not statistically significant [37]. Other meta-analyses and systematic reviews demonstrated conflicting results regarding the use of curcumin as adjunctive therapy in the induction and/or maintenance of remission in patients with mild-to-moderate UC [155, 156]. As a result, support for the use of curcumin for induction or maintenance of remission in UC is currently not recommended as only low-quality evidence exists [37]. The role of curcumin in CD has been less frequently studied. In one double-blind randomized controlled trial of 62 patients with CD who underwent surgery and received postoperative thiopurine treatment, patients additionally treated with curcumin experienced more severe recurrence compared to those treated with placebo; quality of life scores did not differ between the two groups [157].

Curcumin is hypothesized to play a beneficial role in the prevention of carcinogenesis and tumor initiation as well as the reduction of tumor proliferation and progression [158]. One clinical trial of 15 patients with CRC treated with curcumin demonstrated a decrease in prostaglandin E2, which has been found to enhance the growth of human CRC cells [146]. While earlier studies in patients with familial adenomatous polyposis (FAP) treated with a combination of curcumin and quercetin showed regression in both number and size of polyps, a recent double-blind randomized controlled trial of 44 patients with FAP treated with curcumin did not demonstrate adenoma regression indicating an overall effect on polyposis is still unknown [159, 160].

A meta-analysis of four randomized controlled trials comprised of 228 patients with NAFLD treated with curcumin found significant reductions in transaminase elevations though effects on liver histology were not studied [161]. Curcumin may also have antifibrotic and hepatoprotective properties, suggesting that it may be beneficial in patients with cirrhosis [146, 162]. Indeed, one study showed improved quality of life in cirrhotic patients treated with curcumin as compared with placebo [163].

Chamomile

Understanding the benefits unique to chamomile, a member of the Asteraceae family, has been limited by its frequent use in combination with other supplements [164]. Potential antidiarrheal and hepatoprotective properties of chamomile have been inferred from observations in murine models [162]. Chamomile has been studied as a component of Iberogast® (vide supra) and Gastritol® Liquid (which is composed of chamomile, silverweed, licorice, angelica, blessed thistle, and wormwood) and in combination with myrrh and coffee charcoal [165–167]. A non-interventional open-label study of Gastritol® Liquid determined that this formulation may be effective in the treatment of mild gastrointestinal disorders [167]. The combination of chamomile, myrrh, and coffee charcoal has been proposed to have anti-inflammatory properties, possibly by influencing the activity of macrophages in the setting of intestinal inflammation [168]. In a post-marketing open-label observational study, this formulation was reported to be effective in treating diarrhea secondary to acute inflammatory disorders, IBD, or IBS [169]. The same formulation was studied against mesalamine in a double-blind randomized controlled trial of 96 patients with inactive UC [170]. The aforementioned formulation was non-inferior to mesalamine with regard to relapse rates, relapse-free time intervals, endoscopy findings, and fecal biomarkers, though these results could not be attributed to chamomile alone [170].

Glutamine

Glutamine is a non-essential amino acid that has been postulated to be crucial to metabolism in a catabolic state [171, 172]. It is utilized as a substrate in hepatic gluconeogenesis and as an important source of energy by small intestinal enterocytes [169, 170]. Other functions of glutamine include decreased gut mucosal atrophy in animals fed with parenteral nutrition, decreased intestinal permeability, decreased mucosal damage in animals subjected to gram-negative sepsis, preservation of glutathione concentrations in animals whose intestinal tracts were subject to ischemia and reperfusion, improvement in mucosal and plasma glutathione concentrations, protection against bacterial translocation from the gut with parenteral nutrition, and mediation of intestinal adaptation in animals with short bowel syndrome [169, 170, 173]. Glutamine supplementation was found to improve absorption of protein and reduce parenteral nutrition requirements in parenteral nutrition-dependent patients with short bowel syndrome although most studies have demonstrated no significant effect, deterring its use as standard of care [174]. It is also important to note that glutamine has been studied in combination with other interventions (such as growth hormone supplementation and a high carbohydrate, low-fat diet) that may have contributed to the observed effects of weight gain and favorable changes to body composition; however, these benefits are not sustained, and absorption is generally not improved.

Glutamine has been studied in chemotherapy and radiation-induced gastrointestinal disease and in IBD. Animal studies have demonstrated a protective effect of glutamine from radiation and chemotherapy-induced gastrointestinal mucosal injury, although results from human trials are inconclusive [175, 176]. One double-blind randomized controlled trial of 69 patients with pelvic or abdominal solid tumors failed to demonstrate a protective benefit from glutamine in patients receiving radiation therapy; in fact, more patients developed enteritis with glutamine than those given placebo [177]. Its use in CD is therefore controversial. While some studies indicated no improvement in CDAI and intestinal permeability in patients with CD supplemented with glutamine, other studies revealed that it may be beneficial in small bowel CD via mucosal regeneration and immune enhancement [178, 179]. Some data suggest that glutamine may worsen colonic injury in CD involving the colon [176].

Glutamine has had limited study in IBS. Glutamine may function in this patient population by reducing intestinal hyperpermeability and decreasing visceral hypersensitivity [180, 181]. One double-blind randomized controlled trial in patients with diarrhea-predominant IBS, although underpowered, demonstrated improvement in bowel movement frequency [182, 183].

Weight Loss Supplements

Garcinia

Hydroxycitric acid is the main active component of the tropical fruit *Garcinia cambogia*, which is used in commercial weight loss products [184]. In vivo and in vitro studies show that it competitively inhibits citrate cleavage enzyme, suppresses de novo fatty acid synthesis, increases the rate of hepatic glycogen synthesis, suppresses food intake, and decreases weight gain [182]. Although initial studies and unpublished data in humans yielded positive results, a double-blind randomized controlled trial of 135 patients, as well as other smaller randomized controlled trials, demonstrated that *Garcinia* did not produce weight loss or fat mobilization beyond that of placebo [182, 185]. Other studies suggest that *Garcinia* decreases gastric acidity and has gastroprotective, anti-diarrheal, and antispasmodic properties [186–188]. The clinical use of *Garcinia cambogia*, however, has been limited by multiple reports of hepatic injury, including hepatitis and acute liver failure [189–192].

Chitosan

Chitosan is a deacetylated polymer derived from the polysaccharide chitin found in the exoskeleton of crustaceans [193]. It has been proposed to aid in weight loss and in the lowering of blood lipids, glucose, and blood pressure [194]. Multiple clinical studies have been published to date regarding the effects of chitosan on weight loss and cholesterol levels, albeit with conflicting results [194]. An early systematic review of clinical trials studying the benefits of chitosan in overweight and obese patients included 14 potential randomized controlled studies [194]. The authors concluded that participants taking chitosan demonstrated limited weight loss and decrease in total cholesterol levels compared to those taking placebo, although the validity of their conclusions is limited by the exclusion of potentially informative trials and other methodological concerns [194]. A recent meta-analysis of 14 randomized controlled trials concluded that compared to patients taking placebo, patients taking oral chitosan achieved greater weight loss, better control of blood pressure and lower total cholesterol, low-density lipoprotein (LDL) cholesterol, triglycerides, along with an increase in high-density lipoprotein cholesterol [194]. The analysis was limited by the inclusion of studies which were of limited size and duration and studies in which chitosan was administered in addition to other active substances [194]. Given the therapeutic potential of chitosan in obesity and secondary cardiovascular processes, it may also be potentially beneficial in NAFLD as suggested by in vivo studies, though this needs to be further studied [195].

Glucomannan

Glucomannan is a fermentable fiber gel polysaccharide derived from the *Amorphophallus konjac* plant [196]. It has been studied as a possible therapeutic intervention for obesity, functional gastrointestinal disorders, and constipation. In one systematic review and meta-analysis of 14 studies, although limited by the inclusion of crossover and parallel studies and possible publication bias, glucomannan demonstrated benefits in reducing total cholesterol, LDL cholesterol, triglycerides, body weight, and fasting blood glucose levels [197]. Short-term studies demonstrate that glucomannan is well tolerated with mild adverse gastrointestinal effects, although reports of esophageal obstruction secondary to swelling of glucomannan tablets have been published [195, 198]. Two later studies failed to demonstrate statistically significant weight loss with glucomannan [196, 199]. In randomized controlled trials conducted in children, glucomannan was not effective in treating obesity or functional gastrointestinal disorders, although some data support glucomannan as a therapeutic intervention for constipation in children [194, 200–203]. Overall, like other weight loss supplements, data is lacking to support routine use.

Green Tea Extract

Green tea extracts (GTE) are concentrated forms of green tea made from the plant, *Camellia sinensis* [204]. The major active compounds of this plant, known as catechins, include *epicatechin* (EC), *epicatechin gallate* (ECG), *epigallocatechin* (EGC), and *epigallocatechin-3-gallate* (EGCG) [205]. EGCG is the most abundant catechin, and, in combination with caffeine, it is believed to be responsible for the pharmacologic activity of GTE [202, 203]. In one systematic review of 18 randomized controlled trials, meta-analysis of six studies revealed that GTE produced a small, statistically non-significant effect on weight loss, body mass index, and waist circumference [202]. A double-blind randomized controlled trial conducted in 102 women with central obesity designed to examine the efficacy and safety of high-dose EGCG revealed significant weight loss, reduction in waist circumference, and decrease in total cholesterol and LDL levels [206]. However, the results were not superior to placebo, and the dose of EGCG administered was in the potentially toxic range [207]. Another randomized controlled trial suggested that GTE may promote maintenance of body weight after intentional weight loss [208]. In vitro and in vivo studies suggest that GTE may also play a role in the reduction of steatosis in patients with NAFLD by modifying lipid metabolism and improving insulin sensitivity [203].

Adverse events reported with the use of GTE include the following: hepatotoxicity; gastrointestinal, central nervous system, and cardiovascular effects; renal tubular necrosis; nasal and olfactory toxicity; and thyroid dysfunction [202, 209]. Hepatotoxicity has been widely reported with liver damage ranging from acute hepatitis to fulminant hepatic failure requiring liver transplantation [210–212].

Medical Foods

Medical foods, as defined in the Orphan Drug Act, are foods formulated to be consumed or administered enterally under the supervision of a physician, intended for the dietary management of a disease or condition for which distinctive nutritional requirements, based on recognized scientific principles, are established by medical evaluation [213]. Medical foods are formulated in a manner whereby they cannot be purchased over the counter or obtained by modification of a normal diet; they cannot be used for a condition that can be managed with adjustment of a normal diet [214]. Unlike dietary supplements, medical foods require clinical trials to substantiate their use and must be recognized as safe by expert panel review (though they do not require proof of safety through clinical phase trials as do FDA-approved drugs) [67]. Medical foods currently available for gastrointestinal disorders include EnteraGam, Modulen IBD, Vivonex, and VSL#3 [67].

EnteraGam is a combination of serum-derived bovine immunoglobulin/protein isolate (SBI) from edible plasma, dextrose, and trace amounts of sunflower lecithin [67]. This formulation functions by maintaining the integrity of the microbiologic, physical (via tight junctions), and immune barriers of the gastrointestinal system [67]. It is intended for the management of chronic diarrhea and loose stools but has been studied in IBS-D, HIV-associated enteropathy, and IBD [67]. Results from retrospective case studies and a double-blind randomized controlled trial of 66 patients with IBS-D demonstrated improvement in symptoms in patients treated with SBI [67]. An open-label study and a follow-up multicenter randomized controlled trial of 103 patients with HIV-associated enteropathy found that SBI led to improvement in symptoms and quality of life and increased CD4+ counts in the duodenum [67]. Retrospective case series of patients with UC and CD have demonstrated that addition of EnteraGam to standard therapies has led to clinical improvement in patients with refractory disease with evidence of mucosal healing in two case studies [67]. Adverse events that have been reported have been mild [67].

Modulen IBD is a powdered, whole-protein, calorie-dense formula, rich in TGF beta, used singly in patients with active CD and as a supplementary formula in CD patients in remission [67]. In two studies of pediatric patients with CD, Modulen IBD was found to induce mucosal healing and clinical improvement; additionally, decreased proinflammatory markers and increased anti-inflammatory markers were noted as well as changes in the fecal microbiome [67]. In a recent study comparing exclusive enteral nutrition to partial enteral nutrition combined with a whole-food diet in 74 children with mild to moderate CD, Modulen was utilized to assess the effects of dietary components on the microbiome, intestinal barrier, and intestinal immunity in pediatric CD patients [215]. Although both diets were associated with higher and comparable rates of clinical remission and decreased inflammation, subjects who received a combined whole-food diet and partial enteral nutrition with Modulen demonstrated sustained remission in higher proportions [215]. The only potential adverse effect associated with Modulen IBD is milk allergy [67].

Vivonex is an elemental formula of free amino acids with low levels of fat that has been studied in the management of CD, gastrointestinal dysfunction in burn victims, bile acid-induced diarrhea, and pancreatic insufficiency [67]. Although several small historic studies suggest that Vivonex may induce remission in patients with CD at similar rate as corticosteroids, when analyzed in comparison with other enteral formulas, Vivonex did not demonstrate similar or superior efficacy to corticosteroid therapy in inducing remission of active CD [67, 216]. In animal models of burn victims, Vivonex was not effective in altering intestinal motility [67]. However, other clinical studies suggest that Vivonex may decrease length of stay, rate of sepsis, hepatic steatosis, and organomegaly in burn victims, although no decrease in overall mortality rate was seen [67]. The high cost of elemental formulas is a barrier to their widespread use as polymeric formulas have demonstrated equal efficacy and are available at lesser expense.

Conclusion

Prebiotics, probiotics, and dietary supplements are widely consumed products despite the absence of federal regulation and consistent, compelling evidence of benefit. Some of these products have shown promising benefits in certain digestive disorders, and the role of these products continues to evolve with additional data from ongoing clinical trials. Further high-quality studies and thoughtful federal regulation may allow for a broader understanding of the potential role of prebiotics, probiotics, and dietary supplements in a spectrum of digestive diseases.

References

1. Sanders ME, Merenstein DJ, Reid G, Gibson GR, Rastall RA. Probiotics and prebiotics in intestinal health and disease: from biology to the clinic. Nat Rev Gastroenterol Hepatol. 2019:1–12.
2. Ford AC, Moayyedi P, Chey WD, Harris LA, Lacy BE, Saito YA, Quigley EM. American College of Gastroenterology monograph on management of irritable bowel syndrome. Am J Gastroenterol. 2018;113:1–18.
3. Gibson GR, Roberfroid MB. Dietary modulation of the human colonic microbiota: introducing the concept of prebiotics. J Nutr. 1995;125(6):1401–12.
4. Gibson GR, Scott KP, Rastall RA, Tuohy KM, Hotchkiss A, Dubert-Ferrandon A, Gareau M, Murphy EF, Saulnier D, Loh G, Macfarlane S. Dietary prebiotics: current status and new definition. Food Sci Technol Bull Funct Foods. 2010;7(1):1–19.
5. Gibson GR, Hutkins R, Sanders ME, Prescott SL, Reimer RA, Salminen SJ, Scott K, Stanton C, Swanson KS, Cani PD, Verbeke K. Expert consensus document: The International Scientific Association for Probiotics and Prebiotics (ISAPP) consensus statement on the definition and scope of prebiotics. Nat Rev Gastroenterol Hepatol. 2017;14(8):491.
6. Guarner F, Khan AG, Garisch J, Eliakim R, Gangl A, Thomson A, Krabshuis J, Lemair T, Kaufmann P, De Paula JA, Fedorak R. World gastroenterology organisation global guidelines: probiotics and prebiotics october 2011. J Clin Gastroenterol. 2012;46(6):468–81.
7. Quigley EM. Prebiotics and probiotics: their role in the management of gastrointestinal disorders in adults. Nutr Clin Pract. 2012;27(2):195–200.
8. Holscher HD. Dietary fiber and prebiotics and the gastrointestinal microbiota. Gut Microbes. 2017;8(2):172–84.
9. Bindels LB, Delzenne NM, Cani PD, Walter J. Towards a more comprehensive concept for prebiotics. Nat Rev Gastroenterol Hepatol. 2015;12(5):303.
10. Trop TK. Intestinal microbiota, probiotics and prebiotics in inflammatory bowel disease. World J Gastroenterol: WJG. 2014;20(33):11505.
11. Lambert JE, Parnell JA, Eksteen B, Raman M, Bomhof MR, Rioux KP, Madsen KL, Reimer RA. Gut microbiota manipulation with prebiotics in patients with non-alcoholic fatty liver disease: a randomized controlled trial protocol. BMC Gastroenterol. 2015;15(1):169.
12. Serban DE. Gastrointestinal cancers: influence of gut microbiota, probiotics and prebiotics. Cancer Lett. 2014;345(2):258–70.
13. Alexea O, Bacarea V, Piqué N. The combination of oligo-and polysaccharides and reticulated protein for the control of symptoms in patients with irritable bowel syndrome: Results of a randomised, placebo-controlled, double-blind, parallel group, multicentre clinical trial. United European Gastroenterol J. 2016;4(3):455–65.
14. Huaman JW, Mego M, Manichanh C, Cañellas N, Cañueto D, Segurola H, Jansana M, Malagelada C, Accarino A, Vulevic J, Tzortzis G. Effects of prebiotics vs a diet low in FODMAPs in patients with functional gut disorders. Gastroenterology. 2018;155(4):1004–7.
15. Wilson B, Rossi M, Dimidi E, Whelan K. Prebiotics in irritable bowel syndrome and other functional bowel disorders in adults: a systematic review and meta-analysis of randomized controlled trials. Am J Clin Nutr. 2019;109(4):1098–111.
16. Cummings JH, Branch W, Jenkins DJA, Southgate DAT, Houston H, James WPT. Colonic response to dietary fibre from carrot, cabbage, apple, bran, and guar gum. The Lancet. 1978;311(8054):5–9.
17. Ford AC, Quigley EM, Lacy BE, Lembo AJ, Saito YA, Schiller LR, Soffer EE, Spiegel BM, Moayyedi P. Efficacy of prebiotics, probiotics, and synbiotics in irritable bowel syndrome and chronic idiopathic constipation: systematic review and meta-analysis. Am J Gastroenterol. 2014;109(10):1547–61.
18. Waitzberg DL, Pereira CC, Logullo L, Jacintho TM, Almeida D. Microbiota benefits after inulin and partially hydrolyzed guar gum supplementation-a randomized clinical trial in constipated women. Nutr Hosp. 2012;27(1):123–9.
19. Wilson B, Whelan K. Prebiotic inulin-type fructans and galacto-oligosaccharides: definition, specificity, function, and application in gastrointestinal disorders. J Gastroenterol Hepatol. 2017;32:64–8.
20. Lindsay JO, Whelan K, Stagg AJ, Gobin P, Al-Hassi HO, Rayment N, Kamm MA, Knight SC, Forbes A. Clinical, microbiological, and immunological effects of fructo-oligosaccharide in patients with Crohn's disease. Gut. 2006;55(3):348–55.
21. Benjamin JL, Hedin CR, Koutsoumpas A, Ng SC, McCarthy NE, Hart AL, Kamm MA, Sanderson

JD, Knight SC, Forbes A, Stagg AJ. Randomised, double-blind, placebo-controlled trial of fructo-oligosaccharides in active Crohn's disease. Gut. 2011;60(7):923–9.
22. Joossens M, De Preter V, Ballet V, Verbeke K, Rutgeerts P, Vermeire S. Effect of oligofructose-enriched inulin (OF-IN) on bacterial composition and disease activity of patients with Crohn's disease: results from a double-blinded randomised controlled trial. Gut. 2012;61(6):958.
23. Fernandez-Banares F, Hinojosa J, Sanchez-Lombrana JL, Navarro E, Martınez-Salmerón JF, Garcıa-Pugés A, Gonzalez-Huix F, Riera J, Gonzalez-Lara V, Domınguez-Abascal F, Gine JJ. Randomized clinical trial of Plantago ovata seeds (dietary fiber) as compared with mesalamine in maintaining remission in ulcerative colitis. Am J Gastroenterol. 1999;94(2):427–33.
24. Furrie E, Macfarlane S, Kennedy A, Cummings JH, Walsh SV, O'neil DA, Macfarlane GT. Synbiotic therapy (Bifidobacterium longum/Synergy 1) initiates resolution of inflammation in patients with active ulcerative colitis: a randomised controlled pilot trial. Gut. 2005;54(2):242–9.
25. Lilly DM, Stillwell RH. Probiotics: growth-promoting factors produced by microorganisms. Science. 1965;147(3659):747–8.
26. Quigley EM. Prebiotics and probiotics in digestive health. Clin Gastroenterol Hepatol. 2019;17(2):333–44.
27. Hill C, Guarner F, Reid G, Gibson GR, Merenstein DJ, Pot B, Morelli L, Canani RB, Flint HJ, Salminen S, Calder PC. Expert consensus document: The International Scientific Association for Probiotics and Prebiotics consensus statement on the scope and appropriate use of the term probiotic. Nat Rev Gastroenterol Hepatosl. 2014;11(8):506–14.
28. Guarner, F., Sanders, M.E. and Eliakim, R., World Gastroenterology Organization. World gastroenterology organisation global guidelines: probiotics and prebiotics. February 2017.
29. Wilkins T, Sequoia J. Probiotics for gastrointestinal conditions: a summary of the evidence. Am Fam Physician. 2017;96(3):170–8.
30. Park J, Floch MH. Prebiotics, probiotics, and dietary fiber in gastrointestinal disease. Gastroenterol Clin North Am. 2007;36(1):47–63.
31. Pittayanon R, Lau JT, Leontiadis GI, Tse F, Yuan Y, Surette M, Moayyedi P. Differences in gut microbiota in patients with vs without inflammatory bowel diseases: a systematic review. Gastroenterology. 2020;158(4):930–46.
32. Cheifetz AS, Gianotti R, Luber R, Gibson PR. Complementary and alternative medicines used by patients with inflammatory bowel. Gastroenterology. 2017;152(2):415–429.e15.
33. Abraham BP, Quigley EM. Probiotics in inflammatory bowel disease. Gastroenterology Clin. 2017;46(4):769–82.
34. Koretz RL. Probiotics in gastroenterology: how pro is the evidence in adults? Am J Gastroenterol. 2018;113(7):1125–36.
35. Tursi A, Brandimarte G, Papa A, Giglio A, Elisei W, Giorgetti GM, Forti G, Morini S, Hassan C, Pistoia MA, Modeo ME. Treatment of relapsing mild-to-moderate ulcerative colitis with the probiotic VSL# 3 as adjunctive to a standard pharmaceutical treatment: a double-blind, randomized, placebo-controlled study. Am J Gastroenterol. 2010;105(10):2218.
36. Miele E, Pascarella F, Giannetti E, Quaglietta L, Baldassano RN, Staiano A. Effect of a probiotic preparation (VSL# 3) on induction and maintenance of remission in children with ulcerative colitis. Am J Gastroenterol. 2009;104(2):437–43.
37. Singh S, Feuerstein JD, Binion DG, Tremaine WJ. AGA technical review on the management of mild-to-moderate ulcerative colitis. Gastroenterology. 2019;156(3):769–808.
38. Gionchetti P, Rizzello F, Helwig U, Venturi A, Lammers KM, Brigidi P, Vitali B, Poggioli G, Miglioli M, Campieri M. Prophylaxis of pouchitis onset with probiotic therapy: a double-blind, placebo-controlled trial. Gastroenterology. 2003;124(5):1202–9.
39. Mimura T, Rizzello F, Helwig U, Poggioli G, Schreiber S, Talbot IC, Nicholls RJ, Gionchetti P, Campieri M, Kamm MA. Once daily high dose probiotic therapy (VSL# 3) for maintaining remission in recurrent or refractory pouchitis. Gut. 2004;53(1):108–14.
40. Gionchetti P, Rizzello F, Venturi A, Brigidi P, Matteuzzi D, Bazzocchi G, Poggioli G, Miglioli M, Campieri M. Oral bacteriotherapy as maintenance treatment in patients with chronic pouchitis: a double-blind, placebo-controlled trial. Gastroenterology. 2000;119(2):305–9.
41. Prantera C, Scribano ML, Falasco G, Andreoli A, Luzi C. Ineffectiveness of probiotics in preventing recurrence after curative resection for Crohn's disease: a randomised controlled trial with Lactobacillus GG. Gut. 2002;51(3):405–9.
42. Regueiro M, Velayos F, Greer JB, Bougatsos C, Chou R, Sultan S, Singh S. American Gastroenterological Association Institute technical review on the management of Crohn's disease after surgical resection. Gastroenterology. 2017;152(1):277–95.
43. Marteau P, Lémann M, Seksik P, Laharie D, Colombel JF, Bouhnik Y, Cadiot G, Soulé JC, Bourreille A, Metman E, Lerebours E. Ineffectiveness of Lactobacillus johnsonii LA1 for prophylaxis of postoperative recurrence in Crohn's disease: a randomised, double blind, placebo controlled GETAID trial. Gut. 2006;55(6):842–7.
44. Fedorak RN, Feagan BG, Hotte N, Leddin D, Dieleman LA, Petrunia DM, Enns R, Bitton A, Chiba N, Paré P, Rostom A. The probiotic VSL# 3 has anti-inflammatory effects and could reduce endoscopic recurrence after surgery for Crohn's disease. Clin Gastroenterol Hepatol. 2015;13(5):928–35.

45. Van Gossum A, Dewit O, Louis E, de Hertogh G, Baert F, Fontaine F, DeVos M, Enslen M, Paintin M, Franchimont D. Multicenter randomized-controlled clinical trial of probiotics (Lactobacillus johnsonii, LA1) on early endoscopic recurrence of Crohn's disease after ileo-caecal resection. Inflamm Bowel Dis. 2007;13(2):135–42.
46. Zhong C, Qu C, Wang B, Liang S, Zeng B. Probiotics for preventing and treating small intestinal bacterial overgrowth. J Clin Gastroenterol. 2017;51(4):300–11.
47. Brenner DM, Moeller MJ, Chey WD, Schoenfeld PS. The utility of probiotics in the treatment of irritable bowel syndrome: a systematic review. Am J Gastroenterol. 2009;104(4):1033–49.
48. O'Mahony L, McCarthy J, Kelly P, Hurley G, Luo F, Chen K, O'Sullivan GC, Kiely B, Collins JK, Shanahan F, Quigley EM. Lactobacillus and bifidobacterium in irritable bowel syndrome: symptom responses and relationship to cytokine profiles. Gastroenterology. 2005;128(3):541–51.
49. Whorwell PJ, Altringer L, Morel J, Bond Y, Charbonneau D, O'mahony, L., Kiely, B., Shanahan, F. and Quigley, E.M. Efficacy of an encapsulated probiotic Bifidobacterium infantis 35624 in women with irritable bowel syndrome. Am J Gastroenterol. 2006;101(7):1581–90.
50. Ringel-Kulka T, McRorie J, Ringel Y. Multi-center, double-blind, randomized, placebo-controlled, parallel-group study to evaluate the benefit of the probiotic Bifidobacterium infantis 35624 in non-patients with symptoms of abdominal discomfort and bloating. Am J Gastroenterol. 2017;112(1):145–51.
51. Moayyedi P, Ford AC, Talley NJ, Cremonini F, Foxx-Orenstein AE, Brandt LJ, Quigley EM. The efficacy of probiotics in the treatment of irritable bowel syndrome: a systematic review. Gut. 2010;59(3):325–32.
52. McFarland LV, Dublin S. Meta-analysis of probiotics for the treatment of irritable bowel syndrome. World J Gastroenterol: WJG. 2008;14(17):2650.
53. Hoveyda N, Heneghan C, Mahtani KR, Perera R, Roberts N, Glasziou P. A systematic review and meta-analysis: probiotics in the treatment of irritable bowel syndrome. BMC Gastroenterol. 2009;9(1):15.
54. Whelan K, Quigley EM. Probiotics in the management of irritable bowel syndrome and inflammatory bowel disease. Curr Opin Gastroenterol. 2013;29(2):184–9.
55. McFarland LV. Meta-analysis of probiotics for the prevention of antibiotic associated diarrhea and the treatment of Clostridium difficile disease. Am J Gastroenterol. 2006;101(4):812–22.
56. Johnston BC, Goldenberg JZ, Vandvik PO, Sun X, Guyatt GH. Probiotics for the prevention of pediatric antibiotic-associated diarrhea. Cochrane Database Syst Rev. 2011;9(11):CD004827.
57. Goldenberg JZ, Yap C, Lytvyn L, Lo CKF, Beardsley J, Mertz D, Johnston BC. Probiotics for the prevention of Clostridium difficile-associated diarrhea in adults and children. Cochrane Database Syst Rev. 2017;12(12):CD006095.
58. Hempel S, Newberry SJ, Maher AR, Wang Z, Miles JN, Shanman R, Johnsen B, Shekelle PG. Probiotics for the prevention and treatment of antibiotic-associated diarrhea: a systematic review and meta-analysis. JAMA. 2012;307(18):1959–69.
59. Allen SJ, Wareham K, Wang D, Bradley C, Hutchings H, Harris W, Dhar A, Brown H, Foden A, Gravenor MB, Mack D. Lactobacilli and bifidobacteria in the prevention of antibiotic-associated diarrhoea and Clostridium difficile diarrhoea in older inpatients (PLACIDE): a randomised, double-blind, placebo-controlled, multicentre trial. The Lancet. 2013;382(9900):1249–57.
60. Shen NT, Maw A, Tmanova LL, Pino A, Ancy K, Crawford CV, Simon MS, Evans AT. Timely use of probiotics in hospitalized adults prevents Clostridium difficile infection: a systematic review with meta-regression analysis. Gastroenterology. 2017;152(8):1889–900.
61. McGee RG, Bakens A, Wiley K, Riordan SM, Webster AC. Probiotics for patients with hepatic encephalopathy. Cochrane Database Syst Rev. 2011;9(11):CD008716.
62. Bajaj JS, Saeian K, Christensen KM, Hafeezullah M, Varma RR, Franco J, Pleuss JA, Krakower G, Hoffmann RG, Binion DG. Probiotic yogurt for the treatment of minimal hepatic encephalopathy. Am J Gastroenterol. 2008;103(7):1707–15.
63. Agrawal A, Sharma BC, Sharma P, Sarin SK. Secondary prophylaxis of hepatic encephalopathy in cirrhosis: an open-label, randomized controlled trial of lactulose, probiotics, and no therapy. Am J Gastroenterol. 2012;107(7):1043–50.
64. Dhiman RK, Rana B, Agrawal S, Garg A, Chopra M, Thumburu KK, Khattri A, Malhotra S, Duseja A, Chawla YK. Probiotic VSL# 3 reduces liver disease severity and hospitalization in patients with cirrhosis: a randomized, controlled trial. Gastroenterology. 2014;147(6):1327–37.
65. Marchesi JR, Adams DH, Fava F, Hermes GD, Hirschfield GM, Hold G, Quraishi MN, Kinross J, Smidt H, Tuohy KM, Thomas LV. The gut microbiota and host health: a new clinical frontier. Gut. 2016;65(2):330–9.
66. Pala V, Sieri S, Berrino F, Vineis P, Sacerdote C, Palli D, Masala G, Panico S, Mattiello A, Tumino R, Giurdanella MC. Yogurt consumption and risk of colorectal cancer in the Italian European prospective investigation into cancer and nutrition cohort. Int J Cancer. 2011;129(11):2712–9.
67. De Simone C. The unregulated probiotic market. Clin Gastroenterol Hepatol. 2019;17(5):809–17.
68. US Food and Drug Administration. FDA 101: dietary supplements. FDA Consumer Health. Inf Dent. 4. 2008. https://www.fda.gov/consumers/consumer-updates/fda-101-dietary-supplements.
69. Ciampa BP, Ramos ER, Borum M, Doman DB. The emerging therapeutic role of medical foods for

gastrointestinal disorders. Gastroenterol Hepatol. 2017;13(2):104. https://www.ncbi.nlm.nih.gov/pmc/articles/PMC5402682/
70. Kantor ED, Rehm CD, Du M, White E, Giovannucci EL. Trends in dietary supplement use among US adults from 1999-2012. JAMA. 2016;316(14):1464–74. https://jamanetwork.com/journals/jama/article-abstract/2565748
71. Bloomberg: https://www.bloomberg.com/press-releases/2019-12-04/dietary-supplements-market-to-reach-usd-216-3-billion-by-2026-reports-and-data
72. Bailey RL, Gahche JJ, Miller PE, Thomas PR, Dwyer JT. Why US adults use dietary supplements. JAMA Intern Med. 2013;173(5):355–61. https://jamanetwork.com/journals/jamainternalmedicine/article-abstract/1568520
73. Swann JP. The history of efforts to regulate dietary supplements in the USA. Drug Test Anal. 2016;8(3-4):271–82. https://onlinelibrary.wiley.com/doi/full/10.1002/dta.1919
74. Hutt PB. FDA statutory authority to regulate the safety of dietary supplements. Am J Law Med. 2005;31(2-3):155–74. https://journals.sagepub.com/doi/abs/10.1177/009885880503100202?journalCode=jlma
75. Denham BE. Dietary supplements—regulatory issues and implications for public health. JAMA. 2011;306(4):428–9. https://jamanetwork.com/journals/jama/article-abstract/1104131
76. Cohen PA. Assessing supplement safety—the FDA's controversial proposal. N Engl J Med. 2012;366(5):389–91. https://www.nejm.org/doi/full/10.1056/NEJMp1113325
77. Ziker D. What lies beneath: an examination of the underpinnings of dietary supplement safety regulation. Am J Law Med. 2005;31(2-3):269–84. https://journals.sagepub.com/doi/abs/10.1177/009885880503100205?journalCode=jlma
78. Ashar BH, Rice TN, Sisson SD. Physicians' understanding of the regulation of dietary supplements. Arch Intern Med. 2007;167(9):966–9. https://jamanetwork.com/journals/jamainternalmedicine/article-abstract/412433
79. Geller AI, Shehab N, Weidle NJ, Lovegrove MC, Wolpert BJ, Timbo BB, Mozersky RP, Budnitz DS. Emergency department visits for adverse events related to dietary supplements. N Engl J Med. 2015;373(16):1531–40. https://www.nejm.org/doi/full/10.1056/nejmsa1504267
80. Harel Z, Harel S, Wald R, Mamdani M, Bell CM. The frequency and characteristics of dietary supplement recalls in the United States. JAMA Intern Med. 2013;173(10):929–30. https://jamanetwork.com/journals/jamainternalmedicine/article-abstract/1678813
81. Hills JM, Aaronson PI. The mechanism of action of peppermint oil on gastrointestinal smooth muscle: an analysis using patch clamp electrophysiology and isolated tissue pharmacology in rabbit and guinea pig. Gastroenterology. 1991;101(1):55–65.
82. Pittler MH, Ernst E. Peppermint oil for irritable bowel syndrome: a critical review and metaanalysis. Am J Gastroenterol. 1998;93(7):1131–5.
83. Liu JH, Chen GH, Yeh HZ, Huang CK, Poon SK. Enteric-coated peppermint-oil capsules in the treatment of irritable bowel syndrome: a prospective, randomized trial. J Gastroenterol. 1997;32(6):765.
84. Alam MS, Roy PK, Miah AR, Mollick SH, Khan MR, Mahmud MC, Khatun S. Efficacy of Peppermint oil in diarrhea predominant IBS-a double blind randomized placebo-controlled study. Mymensingh Med J. 2013;22(1):27–30.
85. Mann NS, Sandhu KS. Peppermint oil in irritable bowel syndrome: systematic evaluation of 1634 cases with meta-analysis. Intern Med J. 2012;19(1):5–6.
86. Ford AC, Talley NJ, Spiegel BM, Foxx-Orenstein AE, Schiller L, Quigley EM, Moayyedi P. Effect of fibre, antispasmodics, and peppermint oil in the treatment of irritable bowel syndrome: systematic review and meta-analysis. BMJ. 2008;337:a2313.
87. Khanna R, MacDonald JK, Levesque BG. Peppermint oil for the treatment of irritable bowel syndrome: a systematic review and meta-analysis. J Clin Gastroenterol. 2014;48(6):505–12.
88. May B, Köhler S, Schneider B. Efficacy and tolerability of a fixed combination of peppermint oil and caraway oil in patients suffering from functional dyspepsia. Aliment Pharmacol Ther. 2000;14(12):1671–7.
89. Tate S. Peppermint oil: a treatment for postoperative nausea. J Adv Nurs. 1997;26(3):543–9.
90. Micklefield GH, Greving I, May B. Effects of peppermint oil and caraway oil on gastroduodenal motility. Phytother Res. 2000;14(1):20–3.
91. Hiki N, Kurosaka H, Tatsutomi Y, Shimoyama S, Tsuji E, Kojima J, Shimizu N, Ono H, Hirooka T, Noguchi C, Mafune KI. Peppermint oil reduces gastric spasm during upper endoscopy: a randomized, double-blind, double-dummy controlled trial. Gastrointest Endosc. 2003;57(4):475–82.
92. Yamamoto N, Nakai Y, Sasahira N, Hirano K, Tsujino T, Isayama H, Komatsu Y, Tada M, Yoshida H, Kawabe T, Hiki N. Efficacy of peppermint oil as an antispasmodic during endoscopic retrograde cholangiopancreatography. J Gastroenterol Hepatol. 2006;21(9):1394–8.
93. Asao T, Kuwano H, Ide M, Hirayama I, Nakamura JI, Fujita KI, Horiuti R. Spasmolytic effect of peppermint oil in barium during double-contrast barium enema compared with Buscopan. Clin Radiol. 2003;58(4):301–5.
94. Sparks MJW, O'sullivan P, Herrington AA, Morcos SK. Does peppermint oil relieve spasm during barium enema? Br J Radiol. 1995;68(812):841–3.
95. Kligler B, Chaudary S. Peppermint oil. Am Fam Physician. 2007;75(7):1027–30.
96. Nikkhah Bodagh M, Maleki I, Hekmatdoost A. Ginger in gastrointestinal disorders: a systematic review of clinical trials. Food Sci Nutr. 2019;7(1):96–108.

97. Ernst E, Pittler MH. Efficacy of ginger for nausea and vomiting: a systematic review of randomized clinical trials. Br J Anaesth. 2000;84(3):367–71.
98. Koretz RL, Rotblatt M. Complementary and alternative medicine in gastroenterology: the good, the bad, and the ugly. Clin Gastroenterol Hepatol. 2004;2(11):957–67.
99. Viljoen E, Visser J, Koen N, Musekiwa A. A systematic review and meta-analysis of the effect and safety of ginger in the treatment of pregnancy-associated nausea and vomiting. Nutr J. 2014;13(1):20.
100. Thomson M, Corbin R, Leung L. Effects of ginger for nausea and vomiting in early pregnancy: a meta-analysis. J Am Board Fam Med. 2014;27(1):115–22.
101. Pace, J.C. Oral ingestion of encapsulated ginger and reported self-care actions for the relief of chemotherapy-associated nausea and vomiting. 1987.
102. Ryan JL, Heckler CE, Roscoe JA, Dakhil SR, Kirshner J, Flynn PJ, Hickok JT, Morrow GR. Ginger (Zingiber officinale) reduces acute chemotherapy-induced nausea: a URCC CCOP study of 576 patients. Support Care Cancer. 2012;20(7):1479–89.
103. Marx WM, Teleni L, McCarthy AL, Vitetta L, McKavanagh D, Thomson D, Isenring E. Ginger (Zingiber officinale) and chemotherapy-induced nausea and vomiting: a systematic literature review. Nutr Rev. 2013;71(4):245–54.
104. Bone ME, Wilkinson DJ, Young JR, McNeil J, Charlton S. Ginger root—a new antiemetic. The effect of ginger root on postoperative nausea and vomiting after major gynaecological surgery. Anaesthesia. 1990;45(8):669–71.
105. Phillips S, Ruggier R, Hutchinson SE. Zingiber officinale (ginger)–an antiemetic for day case surgery. Anaesthesia. 1993;48(8):715–7.
106. Arfeen Z, Owen H, Plummer JL, Ilsley AH, Sorby-Adams RAC, Doecke CJ. A double-blind randomized controlled trial of ginger for the prevention of postoperative nausea and vomiting. Anaesth Intensive Care. 1995;23(4):449–52.
107. Visalyaputra S, Petchpaisit N, Somcharoen K, Choavaratana R. The efficacy of ginger root in the prevention of postoperative nausea and vomiting after outpatient gynaecological laparoscopy. Anaesthesia. 1998;53(5):506–10.
108. Eberhart LH, Mayer R, Betz O, Tsolakidis S, Hilpert W, Morin AM, Geldner G, Wulf H, Seeling W. Ginger does not prevent postoperative nausea and vomiting after laparoscopic surgery. Anesth Anal. 2003;96(4):995–8.
109. Kalava A, Darji SJ, Kalstein A, Yarmush JM, SchianodiCola J, Weinberg J. Efficacy of ginger on intraoperative and postoperative nausea and vomiting in elective cesarean section patients. Eur J Obstet Gynecol Reprod Biol. 2013;169(2):184–8.
110. Mandal P, Das A, Majumdar S, Bhattacharyya T, Mitra T, Kundu R. The efficacy of ginger added to ondansetron for preventing postoperative nausea and vomiting in ambulatory surgery. Pharm Res. 2014;6(1):52.
111. Montazeri AS, Hamidzadeh A, Raei M, Mohammadiun M, Montazeri AS, Mirshahi R, Rohani H. Evaluation of oral ginger efficacy against postoperative nausea and vomiting: a randomized, double-blinded clinical trial. Iran Red Crescent Med J. 2013;15(12):e12268.
112. Zeraati H, Shahinfar J, Hesari SI, Masrorniya M, Nasimi F. The effect of ginger extract on the incidence and severity of nausea and vomiting after cesarean section under spinal anesthesia. Anesthesiol Pain Med. 2016;6(5):e38943.
113. Seidi J, Ebnerasooli S, Shahsawari S, Nzarian S. The influence of oral ginger before operation on nausea and vomiting after cataract surgery under general anesthesia: a double-blind placebo-controlled randomized clinical trial. Electron Physician. 2017;9(1):3508.
114. Rahimlou M, Yari Z, Hekmatdoost A, Alavian SM, Keshavarz SA. Ginger supplementation in nonalcoholic fatty liver disease: a randomized, double-blind, placebo-controlled pilot study. Hepat Mon. 2016;16(1):e34897.
115. Hirata A, Funato H, Nakai M, Iizuka M, Abe N, Yagi Y, Shiraishi H, Jobu K, Yokota J, Hirose K, Hyodo M. Ginger orally disintegrating tablets to improve swallowing in older people. Biol Pharm Bull. 2016;39(7):1107–11.
116. Ali BH, Blunden G, Tanira MO, Nemmar A. Some phytochemical, pharmacological and toxicological properties of ginger (Zingiber officinale Roscoe): a review of recent research. Food Chem Toxicol. 2008;46(2):409–20.
117. Prasad S, Tyagi AK. Ginger and its constituents: role in prevention and treatment of gastrointestinal cancer. Gastroenterol Res Pract. 2015;2015:142979.
118. Zick SM, Turgeon DK, Vareed SK, Ruffin MT, Litzinger AJ, Wright BD, Alrawi S, Normolle DP, Djuric Z, Brenner DE. Phase II study of the effects of ginger root extract on eicosanoids in colon mucosa in people at normal risk for colorectal cancer. Cancer Prev Res. 2011;4(11):1929–37.
119. van Tilburg MA, Palsson OS, Levy RL, Feld AD, Turner MJ, Drossman DA, Whitehead WE. Complementary and alternative medicine use and cost in functional bowel disorders: a six month prospective study in a large HMO. BMC Complement Altern Med. 2008;8(1):1–7.
120. Esmaillzadeh A, Keshteli AH, Hajishafiee M, Feizi A, Feinle-Bisset C, Adibi P. Consumption of spicy foods and the prevalence of irritable bowel syndrome. World J Gastroenterol: WJG. 2013;19(38):6465.
121. van Tilburg MA, Palsson OS, Ringel Y, Whitehead WE. Is ginger effective for the treatment of irritable bowel syndrome? A double blind randomized controlled pilot trial. Complement Ther Med. 2014;22(1):17–20.
122. Attari VE, Somi MH, Jafarabadi MA, Ostadrahimi A, Moaddab SY, Lotfi N. The gastro-protective

effect of ginger (Zingiber officinale Roscoe) in helicobacter pylori positive functional dyspepsia. Adv Pharm Bull. 2019;9(2):321.

123. Micklefield GH, Redeker Y, Meister V, Jung O, Greving I, May B. Effects of ginger on gastroduodenal motility. Int J Clin Pharmacol Ther. 1999;37(7):341–6.
124. Hu ML, Rayner CK, Wu KL, Chuah SK, Tai WC, Chou YP, Chiu YC, Chiu KW, Hu TH. Effect of ginger on gastric motility and symptoms of functional dyspepsia. World J Gastroenterol: WJG. 2011;17(1):105.
125. Wu KL, Rayner CK, Chuah SK, Changchien CS, Lu SN, Chiu YC, Chiu KW, Lee CM. Effects of ginger on gastric emptying and motility in healthy humans. Eur J Gastroenterol Hepatol. 2008;20(5):436–40.
126. Khayyal MT, Wadie W, El-Haleim EAA, Ahmed KA, Kelber O, Ammar RM, Abdel-Aziz H. STW 5 is effective against nonsteroidal anti-inflammatory drugs induced gastro-duodenal lesions in rats. World J Gastroenterol. 2019;25(39):5926.
127. Malfertheiner P. STW 5 (Iberogast) therapy in gastrointestinal functional disorders. Dig Dis. 2017;35(S1):25–9.
128. Von Arnim U, Peitz U, Vinson B, Gundermann KJ, Malfertheiner P. STW 5, a phytopharmacon for patients with functional dyspepsia: results of a multicenter, placebo-controlled double-blind study. Am J Gastroenterol. 2007;102(6):1268–75.
129. Grundmann O, Yoon SL. Complementary and alternative medicines in irritable bowel syndrome: an integrative view. World J Gastroenterol: WJG. 2014;20(2):346.
130. Rösch W, Vinson B, Sassin I. A randomised clinical trial comparing the efficacy of a herbal preparation STW 5 with the prokinetic drug cisapride in patients with dysmotility type of functional dyspepsia. Z Gastroenterol. 2002;40(06):401–8.
131. Gundermann KJ, Godehardt E, Ulbrich M. Efficacy of a herbal preparation in patients with functional dyspepsia: a meta-analysis of double-blind, randomized, clinical trials. Adv Ther. 2003;20(1):43–9.
132. Vinson BR, Radke M. The herbal preparation STW 5 for the treatment of functional gastrointestinal diseases in children aged 3-14 years–a prospective non interventional study. Gastroenterology. 2011;140(5):S-102.
133. Pilichiewicz AN, Horowitz M, Russo A, Maddox AF, Jones KL, Schemann M, Holtmann G, Feinle-Bisset C. Effects of Iberogast® on proximal gastric volume, antropyloroduodenal motility and gastric emptying in healthy men. Am J Gastroenterol. 2007;102(6):1276–83.
134. Lapina TL, Trukhmanov AS. Herbal preparation STW 5 for functional gastrointestinal disorders: clinical experience in everyday practice. Dig Dis. 2017;35(S1):30–5.
135. Allescher HD, Abdel-Aziz H. Mechanism of action of STW 5 in functional dyspepsia and IBS: the origin of multi-target. Dig Dis. 2017;35(S1):18–24.
136. Peterson CT, Sharma V, Uchitel S, Denniston K, Chopra D, Mills PJ, Peterson SN. Prebiotic potential of herbal medicines used in digestive health and disease. J Altern Complement Med. 2018;24(7):656–65.
137. Cooke WM, Baron JH. Metabolic studies of deglycyrrhizinised liquorice in two patients with gastric ulcer. Digestion. 1971;4(5):264–8.
138. Isbrucker RA, Burdock GA. Risk and safety assessment on the consumption of Licorice root (Glycyrrhiza sp.), its extract and powder as a food ingredient, with emphasis on the pharmacology and toxicology of glycyrrhizin. Regul Toxicol Pharmacol. 2006;46(3):167–92.
139. Yoon JY, Cha JM, Hong SS, Kim HK, Kwak MS, Jeon JW, Shin HP. Fermented milk containing Lactobacillus paracasei and Glycyrrhiza glabra has a beneficial effect in patients with Helicobacter pylori infection: A randomized, double-blind, placebo-controlled study. Medicine. 2019;98(35):e16601.
140. Kwon HJ, Kim HH, Ryu YB, Kim JH, Jeong HJ, Lee SW, Chang JS, Cho KO, Rho MC, Park SJ, Lee WS. In vitro anti-rotavirus activity of polyphenol compounds isolated from the roots of Glycyrrhiza uralensis. Bioorg Med Chem. 2010;18(21):7668–74.
141. Knipping K, Garssen J, van't Land, B. An evaluation of the inhibitory effects against rotavirus infection of edible plant extracts. Virol J. 2012;9(1):137.
142. Nugroho AE, Wijayanti A, Mutmainah M, Susilowati R, Rahmawati N. Gastroprotective effect of combination of hot water extracts of Licorice (Glycyrrhiza glabra), Pulasari Stem Bark (Alyxia reinwardtii), and Sembung Leaf (Blumea balsamifera) against aspirin-induced gastric ulcer model rats. J Evid Based Complementary Altern Med. 2016;21(4):NP77-NP84.
143. Aly AM, Al-Alousi L, Salem HA. Licorice: a possible anti-inflammatory and anti-ulcer drug. AAPS PharmSciTech. 2005;6(1):E74–82.
144. Sadra A, Kweon HS, Huh SO, Cho J. Gastroprotective and gastric motility benefits of AD-lico/Healthy Gut™ Glycyrrhiza inflata extract. Animal Cells Syst. 2017;21(4):255–62.
145. Li Y, Liu T, Yan C, Xie R, Guo Z, Wang S, Zhang Y, Li Z, Wang B, Cao H. Diammonium glycyrrhizinate protects against nonalcoholic fatty liver disease in mice through modulation of gut microbiota and restoration of intestinal barrier. Mol Pharm. 2018;15(9):3860–70.
146. Dulbecco P, Savarino V. Therapeutic potential of curcumin in digestive diseases. World J Gastroenterol: WJG. 2013;19(48):9256.
147. Ng QX, Soh AYS, Loke W, Venkatanarayanan N, Lim DY, Yeo WS. A meta-analysis of the clinical use of curcumin for irritable bowel syndrome (IBS). J Clin Med. 2018;7(10):298.
148. Lopresti AL. The problem of curcumin and its bioavailability: could its gastrointestinal influence contribute to its overall health-enhancing effects? Adv Nutr. 2018;9(1):41–50.

149. Sarkar A, De R, Mukhopadhyay AK. Curcumin as a potential therapeutic candidate for Helicobacter pylori associated diseases. World J Gastroenterol. 2016;22(9):2736.
150. Burge K, Gunasekaran A, Eckert J, Chaaban H. Curcumin and intestinal inflammatory diseases: molecular mechanisms of protection. Int J Mol Sci. 2019;20(8):1912.
151. Liu Z, Huang P, Law S, Tian H, Leung W, Xu C. Preventive effect of curcumin against chemotherapy-induced side-effects. Front Pharmacol. 2018;9:1374.
152. Kozuch PL, Hanauer SB. Treatment of inflammatory bowel disease: a review of medical therapy. World J Gastroenterol: WJG. 2008;14(3):354.
153. Holt PR, Katz S, Kirshoff R. Curcumin therapy in inflammatory bowel disease: a pilot study. Dig Dis Sci. 2005;50(11):2191–3.
154. Hanai H, Iida T, Takeuchi K, Watanabe F, Maruyama Y, Andoh A, Tsujikawa T, Fujiyama Y, Mitsuyama K, Sata M, Yamada M. Curcumin maintenance therapy for ulcerative colitis: randomized, multicenter, double-blind, placebo-controlled trial. Clin Gastroenterol Hepatol. 2006;4(12):1502–6.
155. Grammatikopoulou MG, Gkiouras K, Theodoridis X, Asteriou E, Forbes A, Bogdanos DP. Oral adjuvant curcumin therapy for attaining clinical remission in ulcerative colitis: a systematic review and meta-analysis of randomized controlled trials. Nutrients. 2018;10(11):1737.
156. Zheng T, Wang X, Chen Z, He A, Zheng Z, Liu G. Efficacy of adjuvant curcumin therapy in ulcerative colitis: A metaanalysis of randomized controlled trials. Journal of gastroenterology and hepatology. 2020;35(5):722–9.
157. Bommelaer G, Laharie D, Nancey S, Hebuterne X, Roblin X, Nachury M, Peyrin-Biroulet L, Fumery M, Richard D, Pereira B, Goutte M. Oral curcumin no more effective than placebo in preventing recurrence of crohn's disease after surgery in a randomized controlled trial. Clin Gastroenterol Hepatol. 2019;18(7):1553–60.
158. Park J, Conteas CN. Anti-carcinogenic properties of curcumin on colorectal cancer. World J Gastrointest Oncol. 2010;2(4):169.
159. CruzCorrea M, Hylind LM, Marrero JH, Zahurak ML, Murray-Stewart T, Casero RA Jr, Montgomery EA, Iacobuzio-Donahue C, Brosens LA, Offerhaus GJ, Umar A. Efficacy and safety of curcumin in treatment of intestinal adenomas in patients with familial adenomatous polyposis. Gastroenterology. 2018;155(3):668–73.
160. Cruz-Correa M, Shoskes DA, Sanchez P, Zhao R, Hylind LM, Wexner SD, Giardiello FM. Combination treatment with curcumin and quercetin of adenomas in familial adenomatous polyposis. Clin Gastroenterol Hepatol. 2006;4(8):1035–8.
161. Mansour-Ghanaei F, Pourmasoumi M, Hadi A, Joukar F. Efficacy of curcumin/turmeric on liver enzymes in patients with non-alcoholic fatty liver disease: a systematic review of randomized controlled trials. Integr Med Res. 2019;8(1):57–61.
162. Rajasekaran SA. Therapeutic potential of curcumin in gastrointestinal diseases. World J Gastrointest Pathophysiol. 2011;2(1):1.
163. Nouri-Vaskeh M, Afshan H, Mahdavi AM, Alizadeh L, Fan X, Zarei M. Curcumin ameliorates health-related quality of life in patients with liver cirrhosis: A randomized, double-blind placebo-controlled trial. Complement Ther Med. 2020;49:102351.
164. Miraj S, Alesaeidi S. A systematic review study of therapeutic effects of Matricaria recuitta chamomile (chamomile). Electron Physician. 2016;8(9):3024.
165. Madisch A, Holtmann G, Plein K, Hotz J. Treatment of irritable bowel syndrome with herbal preparations: results of a double-blind, randomized, placebo-controlled, multi-centre trial. Aliment Pharmacol Ther. 2004;19(3):271–9.
166. Khan I, Samson SE, Grover AK. Antioxidant supplements and gastrointestinal diseases: a critical appraisal. Med Princ Pract. 2017;26(3):201–17.
167. Wegener T, Heimueller E. Treatment of mild gastrointestinal disorders with a herbal combination: results of a non-interventional study with gastritol® liquid. Phytother Res. 2016;30(1):72–7.
168. Vissiennon C, Hammoud D, Rodewald S, Fester K, Goos KH, Nieber K, Arnhold J. Chamomile flower, myrrh, and coffee charcoal, components of a traditional herbal medicinal product, diminish proinflammatory activation in human macrophages. Planta Med. 2017;83(10):846–54.
169. Albrecht U, Müller V, Schneider B, Stange R. Efficacy and safety of a herbal medicinal product containing myrrh, chamomile and coffee charcoal for the treatment of gastrointestinal disorders: a non-interventional study. BMJ Open Gastroenterol. 2014;1(1):e000015.
170. Langhorst J, Varnhagen I, Schneider SB, Albrecht U, Rueffer A, Stange R, Michalsen A, Dobos GJ. Randomised clinical trial: a herbal preparation of myrrh, chamomile and coffee charcoal compared with mesalazine in maintaining remission in ulcerative colitis–a double-blind, double-dummy study. Aliment Pharmacol Ther. 2013;38(5):490–500.
171. Duggan C, Gannon J, Walker WA. Protective nutrients and functional foods for the gastrointestinal tract. Am J Clin Nutr. 2002;75(5):789–808.
172. Limketkai BN, Wolf A, Parian AM. Nutritional interventions in the patient with inflammatory bowel disease. Gastroenterol Clin North Am. 2018;47(1):155–77.
173. Burke DJ, Alverdy JC, Aoys E, Moss GS. Glutamine-supplemented total parenteral nutrition improves gut immune function. Arch Surg. 1989;124(12):1396–9.
174. Byrne TA, Persinger RL, Young LS, Ziegler TR, Wilmore DW. A new treatment for patients with short-bowel syndrome. Growth hormone, glutamine, and a modified diet. Ann Surg. 1995;222(3):243.

175. Klimberg VS, Souba WW, Dolson DJ, Salloum RM, Hautamaki RD, Plumley DA, Mendenhall WM, Bova FJ, Khan SR, Hackett RL, Bland KI. Prophylactic glutamine protects the intestinal mucosa from radiation injury. Cancer. 1990;66(1):62–8.
176. Takechi H, Mawatari K, Harada N, Nakaya Y, Asakura M, Aihara M, Takizawa H, Goto M, Nishino T, Minato T, Furukita Y. Glutamine protects the small intestinal mucosa in anticancer drug-induced rat enteritis model. J Med Invest. 2014;61(1.2):59–64.
177. Vidal-Casariego A, Calleja-Fernández A, de Urbina-González JJO, Cano-Rodríguez I, Cordido F, Ballesteros-Pomar MD. Efficacy of glutamine in the prevention of acute radiation enteritis: a randomized controlled trial. J Parenter Enteral Nutr. 2014;38(2):205–13.
178. Goh J, O'morain, C.A. Nutrition and adult inflammatory bowel disease. Aliment Pharmacol Ther. 2003;17(3):307–20.
179. Sido B, Seel C, Hochlehnert A, Breitkreutz R, Dröge W. Low intestinal glutamine level and low glutaminase activity in Crohn's disease: a rational for glutamine supplementation? Dig Dis Sci. 2006;51(12):2170–9.
180. Zhou Q, Souba WW, Croce CM, Verne GN. MicroRNA-29a regulates intestinal membrane permeability in patients with irritable bowel syndrome. Gut. 2010;59(6):775–84.
181. Coëffier M, Déchelotte P, Ducrotté P. Intestinal permeability in patients with diarrhea-predominant irritable bowel syndrome: is there a place for glutamine supplementation? Gastroenterology. 2015;148(5):1079–80.
182. Zhou Q, Verne ML, Fields JZ, Lefante JJ, Basra S, Salameh H, Verne GN. Randomised placebo-controlled trial of dietary glutamine supplements for postinfectious irritable bowel syndrome. Gut. 2019;68(6):996–1002.
183. Ford AC, Gibson PR. Efficacy of glutamine in postinfection IBS. Gut. 2019;68(10):1905–6.
184. Heymsfield SB, Allison DB, Vasselli JR, Pietrobelli A, Greenfield D, Nunez C. Garcinia cambogia (hydroxycitric acid) as a potential antiobesity agent: a randomized controlled trial. JAMA. 1998;280(18):1596–600.
185. Pittler MH, Ernst E. Dietary supplements for body-weight reduction: a systematic review. Am J Clin Nutr. 2004;79(4):529–36.
186. Mahendran P, Vanisree AJ, Shyamala Devi CS. The antiulcer activity of Garcinia cambogia extract against indomethacin-induced gastric ulcer in rats. Phytother Res. 2002;16(1):80–3.
187. Boakye PA, Stenkamp-Strahm C, Bhattarai Y, Heckman MD, Brierley SM, Pasilis SP, Balemba OB. 5-HT3 and 5-HT4 receptors contribute to the antimotility effects of Garcinia buchananii bark extract in the guinea-pig distal colon. Neurogastroenterol Motil. 2012;24(1):e27–40.
188. Udia PM, Braide VB, Owu DU. Antispasmodic and spasmolytic effects of methanolic extract from seeds of Garcinia kola on isolated rat small intestine. Niger J Physiol Sci. 2009;24(2):111.
189. Lunsford KE, Bodzin AS, Reino DC, Wang HL, Busuttil RW. Dangerous dietary supplements: Garcinia cambogia-associated hepatic failure requiring transplantation. World J Gastroenterol. 2016;22(45):10071.
190. Sharma A, Akagi E, Njie A, Goyal S, Arsene C, Krishnamoorthy G, Ehrinpreis M. Acute hepatitis due to Garcinia cambogia extract, an herbal weight loss supplement. Case Rep Gastrointest Med. 2018;2018:9606171.
191. Yousaf MN, Chaudhary FS, Hodanazari SM, Sittambalam CD. Hepatotoxicity associated with Garcinia cambogia: A case report. World J Hepatol. 2019;11(11):735.
192. Kothadia JP, Kaminski M, Samant H, Olivera-Martinez M. Hepatotoxicity associated with use of the weight loss supplement Garcinia cambogia: a case report and review of the literature. Case Reports Hepatol. 2018;2018:6483605.
193. Mhurchu CCN, Dunshea-Mooij CA, Bennett DA, Rodgers AA. Chitosan for overweight or obesity. Cochrane Database Syst Rev. 2005;3:CD003892.
194. Moraru C, Mincea MM, Frandes M, Timar B, Ostafe V. A meta-analysis on randomised controlled clinical trials evaluating the effect of the dietary supplement chitosan on weight loss, lipid parameters and blood pressure. Medicina. 2018;54(6):109.
195. Qian M, Lyu Q, Liu Y, Hu H, Wang S, Pan C, Duan X, Gao Y, Qi LW, Liu W, Wang L. Chitosan Oligosaccharide Ameliorates Nonalcoholic Fatty Liver Disease (NAFLD) in Diet-Induced Obese Mice. Mar Drugs. 2019;17(7):391.
196. Loening-Baucke V, Miele E, Staiano A. Fiber (glucomannan) is beneficial in the treatment of childhood constipation. Pediatrics. 2004;113(3):e259–64.
197. Sood N, Baker WL, Coleman CI. Effect of glucomannan on plasma lipid and glucose concentrations, body weight, and blood pressure: systematic review and meta-analysis. Am J Clin Nutr. 2008;88(4):1167–75.
198. Onakpoya I, Posadzki P, Ernst E. The efficacy of glucomannan supplementation in overweight and obesity: a systematic review and meta-analysis of randomized clinical trials. J Am Coll Nutr. 2014;33(1):70–8.
199. Keithley JK, Swanson B, Mikolaitis SL, DeMeo M, Zeller JM, Fogg L, Adamji J. Safety and efficacy of glucomannan for weight loss in overweight and moderately obese adults. J Obes. 2013;2013:610908.
200. Zalewski BM, Szajewska H. No effect of glucomannan on body weight reduction in children and adolescents with overweight and obesity: a randomized controlled trial. J Pediatr. 2019;211:85–91.
201. Horvath A, Dziechciarz P, Szajewska H. Glucomannan for abdominal pain-related functional gastrointestinal disorders in children: a

randomized trial. World J Gastroenterol: WJG. 2013;19(20):3062.
202. Chmielewska A, Horvath A, Dziechciarz P, Szajewska H. Glucomannan is not effective for the treatment of functional constipation in children: a double-blind, placebo-controlled, randomized trial. Clin Nutr. 2011;30(4):462–8.
203. Han Y, Zhang L, Liu XQ, Zhao ZJ, Lv LX. Effect of glucomannan on functional constipation in children: a systematic review and meta-analysis of randomised controlled trials. Asia Pac J Clin Nutr. 2017;26(3):471.
204. Jurgens TM, Whelan AM, Killian L, Doucette S, Kirk S, Foy E. Green tea for weight loss and weight maintenance in overweight or obese adults. Cochrane Database Syst Rev. 2012;12(12):CD008650.
205. Masterjohn C, Bruno RS. Therapeutic potential of green tea in nonalcoholic fatty liver disease. Nutr Rev. 2012;70(1):41–56.
206. Chen IJ, Liu CY, Chiu JP, Hsu CH. Therapeutic effect of high-dose green tea extract on weight reduction: A randomized, double-blind, placebo-controlled clinical trial. Clin Nutr. 2016;35(3):592–9.
207. Hoofnagle JH, Wright EC. Weight loss from green tea extracts. Clin Nutr. 2016;35(1):238.
208. Gilardini L, Pasqualinotto L, Di Pierro F, Risso P, Invitti C. Effects of Greenselect Phytosome® on weight maintenance after weight loss in obese women: a randomized placebo-controlled study. BMC Complement Altern Med. 2016;16(1):233.
209. Hu J, Webster D, Cao J, Shao A. The safety of green tea and green tea extract consumption in adults–results of a systematic review. Regul Toxicol Pharmacol. 2018;95:412–33.
210. Patel SS, Beer S, Kearney DL, Phillips G, Carter BA. Green tea extract: a potential cause of acute liver failure. World J Gastroenterol: WJG. 2013;19(31):5174.
211. Molinari M, Watt KD, Kruszyna T, Nelson R, Walsh M, Huang WY, Nashan B, Peltekian K. Acute liver failure induced by green tea extracts: case report and review of the literature. Liver Transpl. 2006;12(12):1892–5.
212. Sarma DN, Barrett ML, Chavez ML, Gardiner P, Ko R, Mahady GB, Marles RJ, Pellicore LS, Giancaspro GI, Dog TL. Safety of green tea extracts. Drug Saf. 2008;31(6):469–84.
213. Food and Drug Administration (FDA). Food composition, standards, labeling and economics: Chapter 21, Compliance Program 7321.002. Compliance Program Guidance Manual. 2008.
214. US Food and Drug Administration (FDA). Guidance for industry: frequently asked questions about medical foods; second edition. 2007. Retrieved from https://www.fda.gov/regulatory-information/search-fda-guidance-documents/guidance-industry-frequently-asked-questions-about-medical-foods-second-edition. Updated 12 Dec 2016.
215. Levine A, Wine E, Assa A, Boneh RS, Shaoul R, Kor i M, Cohen S, Peleg S, Shamaly H, On A, Millman P. Crohn's disease exclusion diet plus partial enteral nutrition induces sustained remission in a randomized controlled trial. Gastroenterology. 2019;157(2):440–50.
216. Narula N, Dhillon A, Zhang D, Sherlock ME, Tondeur M, Zachos M. Enteral nutritional therapy for induction of remission in Crohn's disease. Cochrane Database of Systematic Reviews. 2018(4).

Part III

Obesity and Weight Management

12 Obesity Diagnosis and Pathophysiology

Amit Mehta, Shawn L. Shah, Katherine H. Saunders, and Reem Z. Sharaiha

Epidemiology of Obesity

The global obesity pandemic is among the most significant public health crises today. The national prevalence of obesity in the United States is greater than 40%, and rates have continued to increase in all ages and both sexes, independent of geography, ethnicity, or socioeconomic status (SES) [1–3]. The prevalence of obesity is varied, with women of limited education (less than a high school level education) and lower incomes in Western countries having the greatest risk [4]. Similarly, obesity disproportionately affects certain racial and ethnic groups more than others. In the United States, non-Hispanic blacks have the highest age-adjusted rates of obesity (49.5%), compared with Hispanics (39.1%), and non-Hispanic whites (34.3%) [1]. Within the pediatric population, the prevalence of obesity in the United States has also increased. Approximately 18% of children and adolescents are obese [1]. Given its broad prevalence, it is not surprising that obesity has a large impact on total health-care expenditure. In the United States, it has been estimated that the annual medical cost of obesity is $149.4 billion annually, with the medical cost for people who have obesity being $1429 higher than those of normal weight [1, 5].

Many of the leading causes of preventable death among adults are obesity-related comorbidities; most notably, these include type 2 diabetes, coronary heart disease, chronic renal disease, and some types of cancer (e.g., endometrial, breast, and colon) [1, 6, 7]. Moreover, it is well established that obesity is associated with an increase in all-cause mortality independent of age, race, and sex [8]. The psychosocial complications of obesity are also significant. Adults with obesity are more likely to face discrimination at work, and studies show that they have higher rates of depression and anxiety [9]. However, a causal relationship between obesity and mental illness remains unclear, and further study in this area is needed.

A. Mehta (✉)
Divison of Gastroenterology, The Johns Hopkins Hospital, Baltimore, MD, USA
e-mail: amm9102@nyp.org

S. L. Shah
Division of Digestive and Liver Diseases, UT Southwestern Medical Center, Dallas, TX, USA

K. H. Saunders
Division of Endocrinology, Diabetes and Metabolism, New York-Presbyterian Hospital and Weill Cornell Medical Center, New York, NY, USA
e-mail: kph2001@med.cornell.edu

R. Z. Sharaiha
Division of Gastroenterology and Hepatology, New York-Presbyterian Hospital and Weill Cornell Medical Center, New York, NY, USA

C. Newberry et al. (eds.), *Nutrition, Weight, and Digestive Health*,
https://doi.org/10.1007/978-3-030-94953-2_12

Diagnosis of Obesity

Body Mass Index (BMI)

According to the Obesity Medicine Association (OMA), obesity is defined as a "chronic, relapsing, multi-factorial, neurobehavioral disease, wherein an increase in body fat promotes adipose tissue dysfunction and abnormal fat mass physical forces, resulting in adverse metabolic, biomechanical, and psychosocial health consequences" [10]. In the clinical setting, obesity has been most commonly characterized by use of body mass index (BMI), calculated as weight in kilograms divided by height squared in meters. According to the National Institutes of Health (NIH) and WHO, obesity for white, black, and Hispanic individuals is defined as a BMI $\geq$30 kg/m^2 [11, 12]. This classification is based on the greater risk of mortality associated with a BMI of 30 kg/m^2 or higher [8, 11, 12]. Overweight is classified as a BMI between 25.0 and 29.9 kg/m^2, normal weight between 18.5 and 24.9 kg/m^2, and underweight below 18.5 kg/m^2. The degree of obesity can be further subcategorized into class 1 (BMI of 30 to <35 kg/m^2), class 2 (BMI of 35 to <40 kg/m^2), and class 3 (BMI $\geq$ 40 kg/m^2).

The chief advantage of BMI is that it serves as an easily calculated, reliable, and noninvasive surrogate measure of fat mass. Furthermore, multiple epidemiological studies have established its association with morbidity and mortality [8, 13]. However, BMI also has a number of important limitations in diagnosing obesity. While BMI does correlate with body fat mass, it does not distinguish between fat and lean muscle mass. Consequently, BMI can be confounded in individuals who have significant muscle mass, resulting in a high BMI despite having only little body fat. As well, in older adults with a loss of muscle mass, BMI may underestimate the degree of adiposity. BMI has also been found to vary based upon ethnicity and age. Ethnicity-specific BMI cutoffs to better capture body fat and risk associated with obesity have been proposed. For example, the current Asian-Pacific guidelines define obesity among Asian individuals as a BMI $\geq$ 25 [14]. Finally, BMI is also a limited tool in that it does not reflect body fat distribution.

There is a wide range of body fat distribution. Abdominal fat is described as having three compartments: visceral, retroperitoneal, and subcutaneous. Subcutaneous adipose tissue (i.e., fat tissue beneath the skin) is the largest of these compartments. Visceral fat, however, is the more hormonally active and known to promote insulin resistance and low-grade inflammatory changes [15]. Moreover, visceral fat is an important independent risk factor for a number of obesity-related metabolic complications, including cardiovascular disease, type 2 diabetes, and hypertension [16].

Ultimately, clinicians should regularly assess obesity with BMI as it remains a practical way to identify individuals who are overweight or obese. Furthermore, calculating BMI is still a good way to evaluate changes over time, as incremental increases most likely represent gains in body fat.

Weight Circumference (WC) and Waist-to-Hip Ratio (WHR)

As stated earlier, BMI serves as an effective surrogate measure of fat mass; however, it does not reflect body fat composition or distribution. In contrast, waist circumference and waist-to-hip ratio are alternative measurements to assess body fat distribution and are more strongly correlated with visceral fat mass than BMI [17]. The National Heart, Lung, and Blood Institute (NHLBI) recommends that in patients with a BMI between 25.0 and 35, additional measurements to further characterize abdominal obesity be pursued, specifically either waist circumference or waist-to-hip ratio (WHR) measurement [12]. Guidelines for measuring waist circumference typically recommend measuring at the superior border of the iliac crest [12, 18]. The measurement is also usually made at a normal minimal respiration. The NHLBI defines abdominal obesity as a weight circumference greater than 102 cm in men and greater than 88 cm in women. The proposed cutoffs for WHR are 0.95 in men and 0.80 in women. A number of studies have shown that both waist circumference and WHR are associated with a greater risk of cardiometabolic disease and death, even after adjusting for BMI, compared with individuals with waist measurements in the normal range [19, 20].

Body Composition Testing

A number of imaging techniques have been developed to better asses body compartments, including bioimpedance analysis (BIA) instruments, dual-energy X-ray absorptiometry (DEXA), body volume determination techniques, dilution techniques using isotope labeled water, and magnetic resonance imaging (MRI) or magnetic resonance spectroscopy (MRS) scans [21]. These techniques are accurate tools to quantify the volume and mass of different body compartments, including subcutaneous and visceral fat. Furthermore, they can accurately distinguish body fat compartments from fat-free lean compartments, such as bone marrow and skeletal muscle tissue [22–25].

BIA techniques use an electric current to estimate total body water and thereby calculate fat and fat-free mass. These instruments are relatively inexpensive, safe, and convenient to use. However, because of their use of an electric current, this technique is contraindicated in patients with pacemakers [21]. Dilution techniques using isotope labeled water can also measure body composition, again by estimating total body water to calculate fat and fat-free mass. Furthermore, this technique can also be used to calculate free-living energy expenditure [21]. Body volume determination techniques include air displacement plethysmography and 3D photonic scanning and are used to estimate total body volume and therefore body density. Unlike BIA and dilutional techniques, body volume determination can be used in all age groups [21]. Radiographic techniques to measure body composition include DEXA and MRI/MRS. DEXA measures bone mass and fat and fat-free mass and also provides information on regional composition. DEXA can be used across all age groups and disease states [21]. MRI and MRS are the most accurate and reliable tool to asses body composition, allowing quantification of specific fat depots (i.e., visceral, subcutaneous, intramuscular, and epicardial). However, MR-based techniques cannot be used in patients with pacemakers or very high BMIs. Furthermore, they are expensive and complex [22–25].

These imaging modalities have been increasingly adopted in obesity research; however, their clinical utility in better defining and characterizing obesity is complicated. While these modalities are accurate, they are expensive and still not widely available. Moreover, there remain no guidelines or standardized cutoffs as to what amount of measured fat mass is associated with clinical significance or harm. Furthermore, there remains very little data comparing each of the different modalities in measuring or evaluating changes in body fat with weight reduction or weight loss therapy.

Obesity Biomarkers

A growing number of studies have identified and investigated the association between obesity-related biomarkers and chronic obesity-related disease risk. The major pathways studied include the insulin/insulin-like growth factor (IGF) axis, adipokines, and chronic inflammation.

The association between insulin metabolism and obesity has long been established [26, 27]. Insulin metabolism is also tightly linked with the IGF system [28]. Biomarkers of the insulin and IGF axis include IGF-1, fasting insulin, and C-peptide. Fasting insulin and C-peptide have been shown to positively correlate with BMI [26, 29]. Higher fasting insulin concentrations were associated with higher risk of hypertension and coronary heart disease [30]. Similarly, C-peptide has been shown to predict total and cardiovascular mortality [31, 32].

The role of adipokines, such as leptin and adiponectin, in identifying and characterizing obesity has also been explored. Both adiponectin and leptin are primarily expressed by adipose tissue. The main function of leptin is the long-term regulation of appetite and energy balance. Furthermore, leptin is considered a pro-inflammatory adipokine [33]. Individuals with obesity are known to have higher leptin concentrations than normal-weight individuals, suggesting a state of leptin resistance in obesity [34]. Adiponectin helps to regulate energy metabolism and has an anti-inflammatory and insulin-sensitizing effect. In contrast to leptin, adiponectin expression is decreased with obesity compared to individuals with normal weight [35]. However, while these differential patterns of adipokine expression in obesity have been well characterized, no studies have definitively shown a causal role between adipokines and the development of obesity.

Obesity has been clearly associated with chronic inflammation, mediating the increased risk for cardiovascular disease. Studies have shown that in people with obesity, the release of pro-inflammatory cytokines such as tumor necrosis factor α (TNF-α) and interleukin 6 (IL-6) is upregulated [33]. However, the data for these inflammatory biomarkers, or others like C-reactive protein (CRP), and their direct association with both obesity development and related chronic illnesses remains limited [36].

With additional investigation, these biomarkers of obesity may one day be used to better characterize obesity beyond anthropometric measurements, possibly identifying obesity phenotypes more prone to chronic disease development. At this time, however, our understanding of obesity-related biomarkers in disease development is limited and their role in obesity diagnosis is uncertain.

Screening

When physicians encounter patients in the clinical setting, the opportunity exists for the early identification of overweight and obesity, as well as accompanying risk factors. However, the appropriate diagnosis and management of obesity remains limited by the persistent stigma associated with obesity, lack of education regarding obesity management, as well as the diversity of attitudes among both patients and health-care providers regarding the underlying causes and treatments. In the recent past, there were few guidelines regarding the diagnosis and treatment of obesity and few FDA-approved pharmacologic options. In addition, there is insufficient teaching in medical schools and inadequate training in residency programs on the management of patients with obesity [37]. In fact, the 2017 National ACTION Study found that only 55% of patients with obesity carried a formal diagnosis and only 18% had a formal weight loss plan [38].

The United States Preventive Services Task Force (USPTF) recommends that all adults over the age of 18 be screened for obesity with use BMI. Those patients with a BMI $\geq$30 kg/m^2 should be offered or referred to intensive, multicomponent behavioral interventions [39]. The USPTF does not provide guidance regarding the appropriate intervals for screening, though frequent reassessment with routine medical examination is generally recommended by most society guidelines to identify those who are overweight or with obesity [40, 41]. Unsurprisingly, with the global increase in obesity prevalence, "metabolic syndrome," or the co-occurrence of certain metabolic risk factors, is also becoming increasingly common. Metabolic syndrome is defined by a cluster of metabolic risk factors, specifically abdominal obesity, dyslipidemia, hypertension, and hyperglycemia. Health-care providers should include the routine assessment of metabolic syndrome in at-risk individuals with a history, physical exam, and/or laboratory studies. The Endocrine Society clinical practice guidelines suggest screening at 3-year intervals in individuals with one or more risk factors [42]. The assessment should include measurement of blood pressure, waist circumference, fasting lipids, fasting glucose, thyroid-stimulating hormone (TSH), and liver enzymes.

Pathophysiology of Obesity

While there is strong evidence from epidemiological studies on the detrimental effects of obesity defined by classical anthropometric measures on health outcomes, the underlying biological mechanisms are less understood. A growing body of evidence suggests that obesity pathogenesis is governed by a disorder of energy homeostasis: (1) the sustained positive energy balance and (2) the resetting of the body weight set point to an increased value. Furthermore, despite weight loss efforts, studies show that the body still works to defend this higher set point through a mechanism referred to as thermogenesis or metabolic adaptation – promoting increased appetite and slowing the metabolic rate [43, 44]. These processes are in turn further affected and molded by a combination of genetic, epigenetic, developmental, hormonal, and environmental factors.

Genetic Mechanisms of Obesity Pathogenesis

The genetic mechanisms driving the regulation of body weight in humans remains an area of much interest. Studies of twins and adopted children suggest the influential role of genetic factors in humans with obesity. However, concordance rates from twin studies have ranged widely, suggesting that anywhere from 25% to 77% of the risk for obesity is heritable [45–47].

Additional research using genome-wide association studies (GWASs) has identified a number of gene variants associated with weight regulation and obesity [48]. Among the genes identified by GWAS, the fat mass and obesity-associated (*FTO*) gene on chromosome 16 has the strongest genetic association with obesity and may account for up to 15 to 20 percent of the risk for obesity [49, 50]. The mechanisms associated with FTO mutations and obesity have not been fully characterized, but may involve functional "reprogramming" of adipocytes from energy utilization (i.e., beige fat) to energy storage (i.e., white fat) [51]. Furthermore, studies have shown that physical activity and diet influence the impact of obesity risk alleles of the FTO gene [52]. These genetic mechanisms, while an important player in obesity pathogenesis, cannot solely account for the rapid increase in obesity prevalence over the last three decades. Genetic factors, however, may predispose individuals to a positive energy balance and weight gain and are further modulated by environmental and lifestyle factors to promote the obesity phenotype.

Though extremely rare, there are also a number of monogenic obesity disorders that result from a mutation or deficiency of a single gene. The most common monogenic form of obesity results from heterozygous mutations in the gene encoding the melanocortin-4-receptor (MC4R). This mutation is present in 2–3% of obese children and adults. MC4R is expressed in second-order neurons of the hypothalamus and is essential for the homeostatic regulation of food intake and energy expenditure. MC4R mutations are inherited in an autosomal dominant fashion and result in hyperphagia, early-onset obesity, tall stature, rapid growth, and normal mental status. Interestingly, studies have shown that heterozygous patients have the same distribution of weight loss response to bariatric surgery as non-carriers [53].

There are also several syndromic forms of obesity that typically result from mutations in multiple genes rather than one single gene. They present with both severe obesity and characteristic neurodevelopmental abnormalities and other organ/system malformations. The most common form of syndromic obesity is Prader-Willi syndrome (PWS), with an estimated prevalence of 1:10,000–1:30,000 live births. PWS results from the inactivation of the Prader-Willi critical region (PWCR) located on chromosome 15q and typically presents with hyperphagia, early-onset obesity, short stature, developmental delay, and increased serum ghrelin levels at baseline [53].

Environmental and Socioeconomic Factors

A number of studies have identified a clear link between environmental factors (e.g., diet, physical activity, property values and environment, nutrition education, food environments, and income) and obesity risk [54, 55]. Processed food and sugar-sweetened beverage consumption increased rapidly over the second half of the twentieth century, further exacerbated by a decrease in physical activity [56–60]. Together, these changes produced an "obesogenic" environment, promoting increased energy intake and decreased energy expenditure and exacerbating genetic variants on weight [61]. Processed foods in particular have been shown to promote increased appetite and overeating, which may result in pathological eating behavior [62, 63]. Furthermore, Hall and colleagues recently showed that an ultra-processed diet was directly correlated with weight gain and the development of obesity [64].

Obesity rates in the United States have also been linked inversely to socioeconomic status (SES), especially among women [65–69]. Disparities in the types and amounts of food may be one driver of the disparities across different socioeconomic groups [70–72]. Low-cost foods are typically highly processed, have high energy density, and tend to be more widely available and selected in underserved areas [73, 74]. Other environmental variables that influence diet choices and physical activity levels, such as neighborhood crime rates and proximity to parks and grocery stores, have also been identified as independent predictors of obesity risk [75–77]. Environmental and economic variables that act as barriers to healthy diet and physical activity among low-income groups ultimately predispose to positive energy balance and weight gain.

Medications

Drug-induced weight gain is a common problem that can contribute to both the development of obesity and its associated metabolic comorbidities. Classes of medications commonly associated with weight gain include diabetes medications, such as insulin, sulfonylureas, and thiazolidinediones. Treatment with corticosteroids, oral contraceptives, and antineoplastic hormonal therapies (i.e., tamoxifen) are often associated with weight gain in patients. Antidepressants (selective serotonin reuptake inhibitors, tricyclic antidepressants, and trazodone), antipsychotics (olanzapine, clozapine, risperidone, and quetiapine), and anti-seizure medications (valproic acid, gabapentin, and carbamazepine) are all also commonly associated with weight gain [10]. The mechanisms by which these medications induce weight gain vary based on the drug class and include stimulation of food intake and fat storage, decrease in energy expenditure, and impaired exercise tolerance [10].

Circadian Rhythm and Sleep Disruption

A number of studies have demonstrated that the circadian rhythm plays an important role in modulating energy metabolism. Multiple genes and hormones involved in energy regulation and nutrient metabolism (i.e., insulin, leptin, ghrelin, and cortisol) display rhythmic oscillations [78, 79]. Mouse model studies have found that mutations in circadian clock genes result in altered feeding behavior, endocrine signaling, and dietary fat absorption resulting in increased weight gain [79]. Human epidemiological studies have also shown that disruption to the normal sleep pattern and circadian rhythm, such as with shift work, results in higher rates of obesity, hypertension, hyperlipidemia, and insulin resistance [80]. These results suggest that disrupted sleep and circadian misalignments are independent risk factors for the development of obesity and its metabolic complications.

Gut Hormones

Several gut hormones are involved in the regulation of food intake and communication between the gastrointestinal (GI) tract and the regions of the brain regulating energy homeostasis. This interplay between gut endocrine pathways and the brains neural circuits has been referred to as the "gut-brain axis." Increasing evidence suggests these hormones and the gut-brain axis play an important role in development of obesity and the biological defense of body fat mass [81]. Gastric and intestinal hormones involved in the gut-brain axis include ghrelin, glucagon-like peptide (GLP)-1, cholecystokinin, enterostatin, and peptide YY 3–36. All of these circulating hormones, except ghrelin, inhibit food intake (i.e., anorexigenic). Ghrelin, a gastrointestinal peptide produced in the stomach and duodenum, has two major effects: (1) stimulates growth hormone (GH) secretion and (2) increases food intake (i.e., orexigenic) [82–85]. Studies have shown that ghrelin levels increase with diet-induced weight loss, suggesting it plays a role in the compensatory changes in appetite and energy homeostasis that make maintaining weight loss difficult [82]. This effect is further exacerbated by a decrease in anorexigenic mediators following weight loss, again promoting a positive energy balance [81]. Interestingly, bariatric surgery appears to be associated with low serum ghrelin concentrations [82, 86]. Researchers have suggested that this suppression of ghrelin following surgery may be a possible mechanism for why patients are less hungry following these procedures, even in the face of significant weight loss.

Gastrointestinal Microbiome

The GI or "gut" microbiome may be another factor that directly influences both obesity and the response to weight loss interventions. Alterations in diet can profoundly affect the composition of gut microbiota at multiple levels of the GI tract [87]. However, obesity may also directly influence the composition of gut microbiota as well [81, 88, 89]. The bacteria of the microbiome in turn can generate biological signals that impact energy homeostasis [90]. Consequently, changes in the composition of the microbiome likely have an impact on these signals that may influence weight and the development of obesity.

Studies have shown that individuals who have a higher gut *Prevotella*-to-*Bacteroides* (P/B) ratio lost significantly more weight with lifestyle changes and dietary restrictions, compared to those with a lower ratio [91]. In individuals with obesity, the *Firmicutes*-to-*Bacteroidetes* (F/B) ratio is higher than in individuals with normal weight. Furthermore, following weight loss, researchers found that the F/B ratio decreases, and when the same individuals regain weight, the F/B ratio again increases [89]. A number of mouse model studies have also shown that transferring bacteria from mice with obesity into the GI tract of germ-free normal weight mice leads to weight gain and an obese phenotype [88]. It has been postulated that there may be an "obese microbiome" capable of harvesting more calories from ingested food than a "lean" microbiome [88, 90, 92].

While studies have increasingly explored the relationship between specific gut microbiome compositions and weight regulation, a causal relationship to obesity has still not been established in human studies. Ultimately, significant work needs to be done to better understand the impact of the microbiome on obesity pathogenesis and its role in future interventions for obesity prevention or treatment.

Insulin Resistance and Metabolic Syndrome

Obesity, or the presence of excess visceral fat, has long been associated with insulin resistance. However, more recent studies have suggested that obesity itself may first induce hyperinsulinemia, later resulting in insulin resistance via downstream pathways [26, 27]. Insulin resistance then drives hyperglycemia and the production of pro-inflammatory adipocyte cytokines and ultimately leads to vascular endothelial dysfunction and dyslipidemia, resulting in a constellation of metabolic derangements: atherosclerotic cardiovascular disease, hypertension, and type 2 diabetes [93–95]. Studies have shown that the predominant underlying risk factors for metabolic syndrome are abdominal obesity and insulin resistance [93–95].

Conclusion

The global obesity pandemic is still one of the most significant public health crises today. While multifactorial, obesity pathogenesis is governed by a disorder of energy homeostasis that promotes a positive energy balance. The pathways regulating energy homeostasis are in turn affected and molded by a combination of genetic, epigenetic, developmental, hormonal, and environmental factors. Given the widespread prevalence of obesity and numerous associated comorbidities, most medical governing bodies advocate for early and frequent screening of obesity, most commonly using BMI. Still, the appropriate diagnosis and management of obesity remains limited by the persistent stigma, the diversity of attitudes among both patients and health-care providers regarding the underlying causes and treatments for obesity, as well as the lack of formal education and training regarding obesity diagnosis and treatment. Ultimately, further education and research regarding the pathogenesis of obesity and widespread utilization of clinical screening is necessary to address the obesity pandemic.

References

1. Hales CM, Fryar CD, Carroll MD, Freedman DS, Ogden CL. Trends in obesity and severe obesity prevalence in US youth and adults by sex and age, 2007-2008 to 2015-2016. JAMA. 2018;319(16):1723–5.
2. Ward ZJ, Bleich SN, Cradock AL, Barrett JL, Giles CM, Flax C, et al. Projected U.S. state-level prevalence of adult obesity and severe obesity. N Engl J Med. 2019;381(25):2440–50.
3. Collaborators GBDO, Afshin A, Forouzanfar MH, Reitsma MB, Sur P, Estep K, et al. Health effects of overweight and obesity in 195 countries over 25 years. N Engl J Med. 2017;377(1):13–27.
4. Swinburn BA, Sacks G, Hall KD, McPherson K, Finegood DT, Moodie ML, et al. The global obesity pandemic: shaped by global drivers and local environments. Lancet. 2011;378(9793):804–14.
5. Kim DD, Basu A. Estimating the medical care costs of obesity in the United States: systematic review, meta-analysis, and empirical analysis. Value Health. 2016;19(5):602–13.
6. Haslam DW, James WP. Obesity. Lancet. 2005;366(9492):1197–209.
7. Nimptsch K, Pischon T. Body fatness, related biomarkers and cancer risk: an epidemiological perspective. Horm Mol Biol Clin Investig. 2015;22(2):39–51.
8. Prospective Studies C, Whitlock G, Lewington S, Sherliker P, Clarke R, Emberson J, et al. Body-mass index and cause-specific mortality in 900 000 adults: collaborative analyses of 57 prospective studies. Lancet. 2009;373(9669):1083–96.
9. Karasu SR. Of mind and matter: psychological dimensions in obesity. Am J Psychother. 2012;66(2):111–28.
10. Bays HE, McCarthy W, Burridge K, Tondt J, Karjoo S, Christensen S, Ng J, Golden A, Davisson L, Richardson L. Obesity algorithm eBook, presented by the Obesity Medicine Association. 2021.
11. Obesity: preventing and managing the global epidemic. Report of a WHO consultation. World Health Organ Tech Rep Ser. 2000;894:i–xii, 1–253.
12. Clinical guidelines on the identification, evaluation, and treatment of overweight and obesity in adults--the evidence report. Natl Instit Health Obes Res. 1998;6 Suppl 2:51S–209S.
13. Okorodudu DO, Jumean MF, Montori VM, Romero-Corral A, Somers VK, Erwin PJ, et al. Diagnostic performance of body mass index to identify obesity as defined by body adiposity: a systematic review and meta-analysis. Int J Obes. 2010;34(5):791–9.
14. Choo V. WHO reassesses appropriate body-mass index for Asian populations. Lancet. 2002;360(9328):235.
15. Galic S, Oakhill JS, Steinberg GR. Adipose tissue as an endocrine organ. Mol Cell Endocrinol. 2010;316(2):129–39.
16. Karlsson T, Rask-Andersen M, Pan G, Hoglund J, Wadelius C, Ek WE, et al. Contribution of genetics to visceral adiposity and its relation to cardiovascular and metabolic disease. Nat Med. 2019;25(9):1390–5.
17. Ping Z, Pei X, Xia P, Chen Y, Guo R, Hu C, et al. Anthropometric indices as surrogates for estimating abdominal visceral and subcutaneous adipose tissue: a meta-analysis with 16,129 participants. Diabetes Res Clin Pract. 2018;143:310–9.
18. Bosy-Westphal A, Booke CA, Blocker T, Kossel E, Goele K, Later W, et al. Measurement site for waist circumference affects its accuracy as an index of visceral and abdominal subcutaneous fat in a Caucasian population. J Nutr. 2010;140(5):954–61.
19. Feller S, Boeing H, Pischon T. Body mass index, waist circumference, and the risk of type 2 diabetes mellitus: implications for routine clinical practice. Dtsch Arztebl Int. 2010;107(26):470–6.
20. Pischon T, Boeing H, Hoffmann K, Bergmann M, Schulze MB, Overvad K, et al. General and abdominal adiposity and risk of death in Europe. N Engl J Med. 2008;359(20):2105–20.
21. Lee SY, Gallagher D. Assessment methods in human body composition. Curr Opin Clin Nutr Metab Care. 2008;11(5):566–72.
22. Karlsson AK, Kullberg J, Stokland E, Allvin K, Gronowitz E, Svensson PA, et al. Measurements of total and regional body composition in preschool children: a comparison of MRI, DXA, and anthropometric data. Obesity (Silver Spring). 2013;21(5):1018–24.
23. Lee S, Kuk JL. Changes in fat and skeletal muscle with exercise training in obese adolescents: comparison of whole-body MRI and dual energy X-ray absorptiometry. Obesity (Silver Spring). 2013;21(10):2063–71.
24. Ross R. Advances in the application of imaging methods in applied and clinical physiology. Acta Diabetol. 2003;40(Suppl 1):S45–50.
25. Wald D, Teucher B, Dinkel J, Kaaks R, Delorme S, Boeing H, et al. Automatic quantification of subcutaneous and visceral adipose tissue from whole-body magnetic resonance images suitable for large cohort studies. J Magn Reson Imaging. 2012;36(6):1421–34.
26. Reaven GM. Insulin resistance: the link between obesity and cardiovascular disease. Med Clin North Am. 2011;95(5):875–92.

27. Kahn SE, Hull RL, Utzschneider KM. Mechanisms linking obesity to insulin resistance and type 2 diabetes. Nature. 2006;444(7121):840–6.
28. van Heemst D. Insulin, IGF-1 and longevity. Aging Dis. 2010;1(2):147–57.
29. Aleksandrova K, Drogan D, Boeing H, Jenab M, Bas Bueno-de-Mesquita H, Jansen E, et al. Adiposity, mediating biomarkers and risk of colon cancer in the European prospective investigation into cancer and nutrition study. Int J Cancer. 2014;134(3):612–21.
30. Xun P, Wu Y, He Q, He K. Fasting insulin concentrations and incidence of hypertension, stroke, and coronary heart disease: a meta-analysis of prospective cohort studies. Am J Clin Nutr. 2013;98(6):1543–54.
31. Min JY, Min KB. Serum C-peptide levels and risk of death among adults without diabetes mellitus. CMAJ. 2013;185(9):E402–8.
32. Patel N, Taveira TH, Choudhary G, Whitlatch H, Wu WC. Fasting serum C-peptide levels predict cardiovascular and overall death in nondiabetic adults. J Am Heart Assoc. 2012;1(6):e003152.
33. Tilg H, Moschen AR. Adipocytokines: mediators linking adipose tissue, inflammation and immunity. Nat Rev Immunol. 2006;6(10):772–83.
34. Engin A. Diet-induced obesity and the mechanism of leptin resistance. Adv Exp Med Biol. 2017;960:381–97.
35. Chandran M, Phillips SA, Ciaraldi T, Henry RR. Adiponectin: more than just another fat cell hormone? Diabetes Care. 2003;26(8):2442–50.
36. Zhuang Q, Shen C, Chen Y, Zhao X, Wei P, Sun J, et al. Association of high sensitive C-reactive protein with coronary heart disease: a Mendelian randomization study. BMC Med Genet. 2019;20(1):170.
37. Kushner RF. Weight loss strategies for treatment of obesity: lifestyle management and pharmacotherapy. Prog Cardiovasc Dis. 2018;61(2):246–52.
38. Kaplan LM, Golden A, Jinnett K, Kolotkin RL, Kyle TK, Look M, et al. Perceptions of barriers to effective obesity care: results from the national ACTION study. Obesity (Silver Spring). 2018;26(1):61–9.
39. U.S. Preventive Services Task Force. Screening for obesity in adults: recommendations and rationale. Ann Intern Med. 2003;139(11):930–2.
40. Jensen MD, Ryan DH, Apovian CM, Ard JD, Comuzzie AG, Donato KA, et al. 2013 AHA/ACC/TOS guideline for the management of overweight and obesity in adults: a report of the American College of Cardiology/American Heart Association Task Force on Practice Guidelines and the Obesity Society. J Am Coll Cardiol. 2014;63(25 Pt B):2985–3023.
41. Apovian CM, Aronne LJ, Bessesen DH, McDonnell ME, Murad MH, Pagotto U, et al. Pharmacological management of obesity: an endocrine society clinical practice guideline. J Clin Endocrinol Metab. 2015;100(2):342–62.
42. Rosenzweig JL, Bakris GL, Berglund LF, Hivert MF, Horton ES, Kalyani RR, et al. Primary prevention of ASCVD and T2DM in patients at metabolic risk: an Endocrine Society* clinical practice guideline. J Clin Endocrinol Metab. 2019; https://doi.org/10.1210/jc.2019-01338.
43. Rosenbaum M, Leibel RL. Adaptive thermogenesis in humans. Int J Obes. 2010;34(Suppl 1):S47–55.
44. Fothergill E, Guo J, Howard L, Kerns JC, Knuth ND, Brychta R, et al. Persistent metabolic adaptation 6 years after "The Biggest Loser" competition. Obesity (Silver Spring). 2016;24(8):1612–9.
45. O'Rahilly S, Farooqi IS. Human obesity as a heritable disorder of the central control of energy balance. Int J Obes. 2008;32(Suppl 7):S55–61.
46. Wardle J, Carnell S, Haworth CM, Plomin R. Evidence for a strong genetic influence on childhood adiposity despite the force of the obesogenic environment. Am J Clin Nutr. 2008;87(2):398–404.
47. Perusse L, Rankinen T, Zuberi A, Chagnon YC, Weisnagel SJ, Argyropoulos G, et al. The human obesity gene map: the 2004 update. Obes Res. 2005;13(3):381–490.
48. Locke AE, Kahali B, Berndt SI, Justice AE, Pers TH, Day FR, et al. Genetic studies of body mass index yield new insights for obesity biology. Nature. 2015;518(7538):197–206.
49. Frayling TM, Timpson NJ, Weedon MN, Zeggini E, Freathy RM, Lindgren CM, et al. A common variant in the FTO gene is associated with body mass index and predisposes to childhood and adult obesity. Science. 2007;316(5826):889–94.
50. Dina C, Meyre D, Gallina S, Durand E, Korner A, Jacobson P, et al. Variation in FTO contributes to childhood obesity and severe adult obesity. Nat Genet. 2007;39(6):724–6.
51. Claussnitzer M, Dankel SN, Kim KH, Quon G, Meuleman W, Haugen C, et al. FTO obesity variant circuitry and adipocyte browning in humans. N Engl J Med. 2015;373(10):895–907.
52. Kim JY, DeMenna JT, Puppala S, Chittoor G, Schneider J, Duggirala R, et al. Physical activity and FTO genotype by physical activity interactive influences on obesity. BMC Genet. 2016;17:47.
53. Beales PL, Farooqi IS, O'Rahilly S. The genetics of obesity syndromes, vol. x. Oxford; New York: Oxford University Press; 2009. p. 288.
54. Drewnowski A, Rehm CD, Arterburn D. The geographic distribution of obesity by census tract among 59 767 insured adults in King County, WA. Int J Obes (Lond). 2014;38(6):833–9.
55. Drewnowski A, Aggarwal A, Cook A, Stewart O, Moudon AV. Geographic disparities in Healthy Eating Index scores (HEI-2005 and 2010) by residential property values: findings from Seattle Obesity Study (SOS). Prev Med. 2016;83:46–55.
56. Nielsen SJ, Popkin BM. Changes in beverage intake between 1977 and 2001. Am J Prev Med. 2004;27(3):205–10.

57. Nielsen SJ, Popkin BM. Patterns and trends in food portion sizes, 1977-1998. JAMA. 2003;289(4):450–3.
58. Nielsen SJ, Siega-Riz AM, Popkin BM. Trends in energy intake in U.S. between 1977 and 1996: similar shifts seen across age groups. Obes Res. 2002;10(5):370–8.
59. Wright JD, Wang CY. Trends in intake of energy and macronutrients in adults from 1999-2000 through 2007-2008. NCHS Data Brief. 2010;49:1–8.
60. Guo G, Liu H, Wang L, Shen H, Hu W. The genome-wide influence on human BMI depends on physical activity, life course, and historical period. Demography. 2015;52(5):1651–70.
61. Walter S, Mejia-Guevara I, Estrada K, Liu SY, Glymour MM. Association of a genetic risk score with body mass index across different birth cohorts. JAMA. 2016;316(1):63–9.
62. Poti JM, Braga B, Qin B. Ultra-processed food intake and obesity: what really matters for health-processing or nutrient content? Curr Obes Rep. 2017;6(4):420–31.
63. Schulte EM, Smeal JK, Gearhardt AN. Foods are differentially associated with subjective effect report questions of abuse liability. PLoS One. 2017;12(8):e0184220.
64. Hall KD, Ayuketah A, Brychta R, Cai H, Cassimatis T, Chen KY, et al. Ultra-processed diets cause excess calorie intake and weight gain: an inpatient randomized controlled trial of ad libitum food intake. Cell Metab. 2019;30(1):67–77 e3.
65. Sobal J, Stunkard AJ. Socioeconomic status and obesity: a review of the literature. Psychol Bull. 1989;105(2):260–75.
66. McLaren L. Socioeconomic status and obesity. Epidemiol Rev. 2007;29:29–48.
67. Drewnowski A. Obesity, diets, and social inequalities. Nutr Rev. 2009;67(Suppl 1):S36–9.
68. Ogden CL, Lamb MM, Carroll MD, Flegal KM. Obesity and socioeconomic status in adults: United States, 2005-2008. NCHS Data Brief. 2010;50:1–8.
69. Lebel A, Kestens Y, Clary C, Bisset S, Subramanian SV. Geographic variability in the association between socioeconomic status and BMI in the USA and Canada. PLoS One. 2014;9(6):e99158.
70. Gustafson AA, Sharkey J, Samuel-Hodge CD, Jones-Smith J, Folds MC, Cai J, et al. Perceived and objective measures of the food store environment and the association with weight and diet among low-income women in North Carolina. Public Health Nutr. 2011;14(6):1032–8.
71. Jennings A, Welch A, Jones AP, Harrison F, Bentham G, van Sluijs EM, et al. Local food outlets, weight status, and dietary intake: associations in children aged 9-10 years. Am J Prev Med. 2011;40(4):405–10.
72. Caspi CE, Sorensen G, Subramanian SV, Kawachi I. The local food environment and diet: a systematic review. Health Place. 2012;18(5):1172–87.
73. Drewnowski A, Specter SE. Poverty and obesity: the role of energy density and energy costs. Am J Clin Nutr. 2004;79(1):6–16.
74. Darmon N, Drewnowski A. Does social class predict diet quality? Am J Clin Nutr. 2008;87(5):1107–17.
75. Rundle A, Quinn J, Lovasi G, Bader MD, Yousefzadeh P, Weiss C, et al. Associations between body mass index and park proximity, size, cleanliness, and recreational facilities. Am J Health Promot. 2013;27(4):262–9.
76. Duncan MJ, Spence JC, Mummery WK. Perceived environment and physical activity: a meta-analysis of selected environmental characteristics. Int J Behav Nutr Phys Act. 2005;2:11.
77. Boehmer TK, Hoehner CM, Deshpande AD, Brennan Ramirez LK, Brownson RC. Perceived and observed neighborhood indicators of obesity among urban adults. Int J Obes. 2007;31(6):968–77.
78. Froy O, Miskin R. Effect of feeding regimens on circadian rhythms: implications for aging and longevity. Aging (Albany NY). 2010;2(1):7–27.
79. Fonken LK, Nelson RJ. The effects of light at night on circadian clocks and metabolism. Endocr Rev. 2014;35(4):648–70.
80. Antunes LC, Levandovski R, Dantas G, Caumo W, Hidalgo MP. Obesity and shift work: chronobiological aspects. Nutr Res Rev. 2010;23(1):155–68.
81. Torres-Fuentes C, Schellekens H, Dinan TG, Cryan JF. The microbiota-gut-brain axis in obesity. Lancet Gastroenterol Hepatol. 2017;2(10):747–56.
82. Koepp GA, Moore GK, Levine JA. Chair-based fidgeting and energy expenditure. BMJ Open Sport Exerc Med. 2016;2(1):e000152.
83. Cummings DE, Weigle DS, Frayo RS, Breen PA, Ma MK, Dellinger EP, et al. Plasma ghrelin levels after diet-induced weight loss or gastric bypass surgery. N Engl J Med. 2002;346(21):1623–30.
84. Tschop M, Smiley DL, Heiman ML. Ghrelin induces adiposity in rodents. Nature. 2000;407(6806):908–13.
85. Wren AM, Seal LJ, Cohen MA, Brynes AE, Frost GS, Murphy KG, et al. Ghrelin enhances appetite and increases food intake in humans. J Clin Endocrinol Metab. 2001;86(12):5992.
86. Sumithran P, Prendergast LA, Delbridge E, Purcell K, Shulkes A, Kriketos A, et al. Long-term persistence of hormonal adaptations to weight loss. N Engl J Med. 2011;365(17):1597–604.
87. Sommer F, Backhed F. The gut microbiota--masters of host development and physiology. Nat Rev Microbiol. 2013;11(4):227–38.
88. Turnbaugh PJ, Gordon JI. The core gut microbiome, energy balance and obesity. J Physiol. 2009;587(Pt 17):4153–8.
89. Mathur R, Barlow GM. Obesity and the microbiome. Expert Rev Gastroenterol Hepatol. 2015;9(8):1087–99.
90. Rosenbaum M, Knight R, Leibel RL. The gut microbiota in human energy homeostasis and obesity. Trends Endocrinol Metab. 2015;26(9):493–501.

91. Hjorth MF, Blaedel T, Bendtsen LQ, Lorenzen JK, Holm JB, Kiilerich P, et al. Prevotella-to-Bacteroides ratio predicts body weight and fat loss success on 24-week diets varying in macronutrient composition and dietary fiber: results from a post-hoc analysis. Int J Obes. 2019;43(1):149–57.
92. Turnbaugh PJ, Ley RE, Mahowald MA, Magrini V, Mardis ER, Gordon JI. An obesity-associated gut microbiome with increased capacity for energy harvest. Nature. 2006;444(7122):1027–31.
93. Ervin RB. Prevalence of metabolic syndrome among adults 20 years of age and over, by sex, age, race and ethnicity, and body mass index: United States, 2003-2006. Natl Health Stat Rep. 2009;13:1–7.
94. Grundy SM, Cleeman JI, Daniels SR, Donato KA, Eckel RH, Franklin BA, et al. Diagnosis and management of the metabolic syndrome: an American Heart Association/National Heart, Lung, and Blood Institute Scientific Statement. Circulation. 2005;112(17):2735–52.
95. Grundy SM, Cleeman JI, Daniels SR, Donato KA, Eckel RH, Franklin BA, et al. Diagnosis and management of the metabolic syndrome: an American Heart Association/National Heart, Lung, and Blood Institute scientific statement. Curr Opin Cardiol. 2006;21(1):1–6.

Obesity-Related Gastrointestinal Disorders

13

Elissa Lin, Aaron Justin Yeoh, and Violeta Popov

Introduction

Obesity is a complex disease rising from both environmental and genetic etiologies. Broadly defined as excess body weight for a given height, obesity has become a global health concern that affects multiple organ systems. As obesity plays a main role in the development of the metabolic syndrome, it is often associated with cardiovascular disease and diabetes mellitus. There is increasing evidence for the association of obesity with a wide range of gastrointestinal diseases (Fig. 13.1). The prevalence of obesity has risen in parallel with malignancies and organ dysfunction. In this chapter, we discuss key associations between obesity and major gastrointestinal diseases while also considering ways in which obesity affects disease course and management.

E. Lin · A. J. Yeoh
Department of Medicine, NYU Langone Health, New York, NY, USA
e-mail: Elissa.lin@nyulangone.org; ayeoh@stanford.edu

V. Popov (✉)
Department of Medicine, NYU Langone Health, New York, NY, USA

New York VA Harbor Healthcare System (Manhattan), New York, NY, USA
e-mail: Violeta.popov@nyulangone.org

Esophageal Disorders

Obesity is associated with increased esophageal acid exposure that can result in burdensome symptoms. Overtime, increased acid exposure can lead to erosive esophagitis, Barrett's esophagus (BE), and esophageal adenocarcinoma (EAC). As such it is prudent to consider these conditions in patients with obesity [1].

Gastroesophageal Reflux Disease

Gastroesophageal reflux disease (GERD) is characterized by pathologic reflux associated with symptoms of reflux and/or complications of mucosal injury. Epidemiology studies have shown a dose-response relationship between BMI and GERD risk [2]. According to a cross-sectional study of 505 total patients, central obesity independently increased the risk of GERD by 88% [3]. There are several proposed mechanisms of the association between BMI and prolonged acid exposure. Transient relaxations of the lower esophageal sphincter (LES) have been observed to be more common in patients with obesity [4, 5]. A hypotensive LES is a risk factor for GERD. Another mechanism by which obesity predisposes one to GERD is structural. Excess adipose tissue results in an increase in intra-abdominal pressure which increases the pressure gradient between the abdomen and the chest [6, 7].

C. Newberry et al. (eds.), *Nutrition, Weight, and Digestive Health*,
https://doi.org/10.1007/978-3-030-94953-2_13

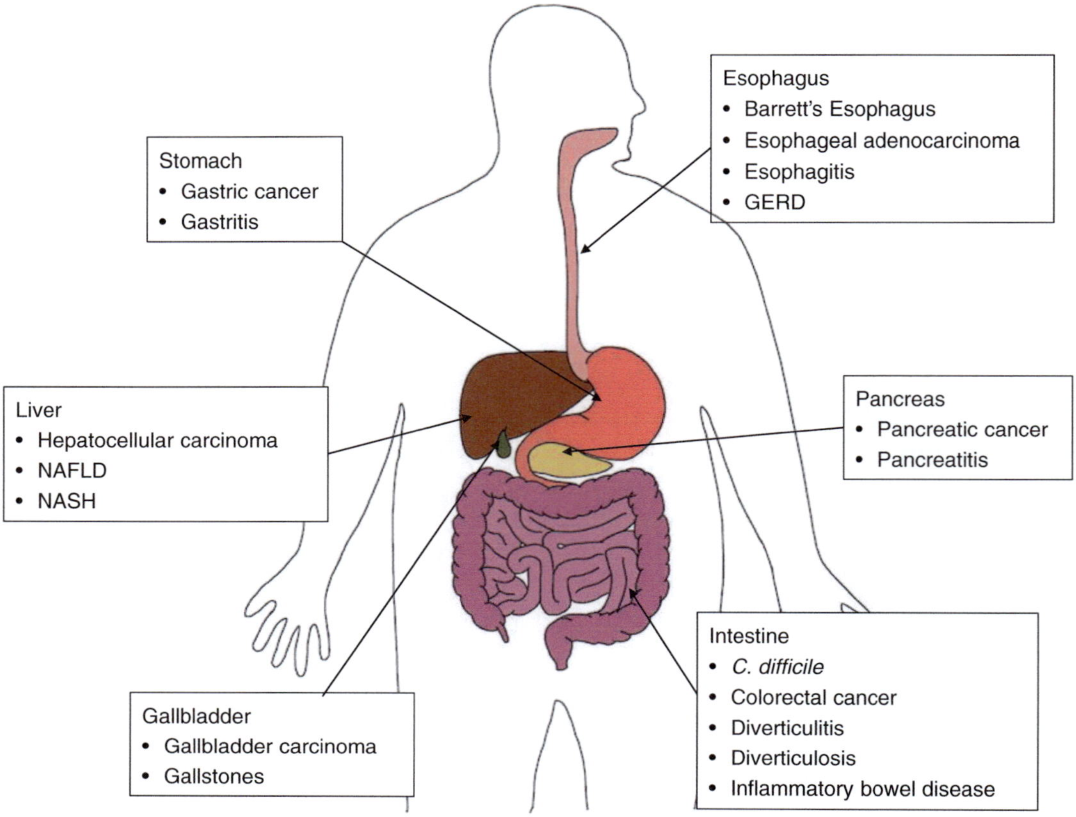

Fig. 13.1 Gastrointestinal disorders associated with obesity. (Author: Dr. Elissa Lin)

As a result, the integrity of the gastroesophageal junction is impaired.

As obesity increases the risk of GERD, studies have sought to answer whether there is resolution with weight loss. Multiple randomized controlled trials show that weight loss by lifestyle modification reduces esophageal acid exposure [8]. Successful weight loss by lifestyle modification also correlates with a decreased prevalence of reflux symptoms [8]. In the bariatric surgery population, the effect of bariatric surgery on gastroesophageal reflux is complicated by a number of factors including procedure type, presence or repair of hiatal hernia during surgery, post-bariatric diet, and the degree of lifestyle modification. Forty percent of patients with obesity have hiatal hernias prior to bariatric surgery [9]. Roux-en-Y gastric bypass is considered the most effective at alleviating symptoms of GERD and is sometimes performed in cases of failed fundoplication [7].

The relationship between sleeve gastrectomy and GERD is complex. Sleeve gastrectomy may worsen reflux symptoms or incite esophagitis in patients with preexisting GERD due to alterations in stomach anatomy that decrease the basal pressure of the LES while increasing intragastric pressure [7, 10]. However, some studies demonstrate an improvement in GERD symptoms following surgery possibly due to the resultant weight loss as well as decreased acid production and accelerated gastric emptying [10, 11]. Regardless, a retained fundus has been shown to increase the risk of GERD, and as such, complete resection of the fundus during sleeve gastrectomy is recommended [10].

Erosive Esophagitis

Erosive esophagitis is defined by esophageal mucosal erosive changes that occur with or without reflux. Obesity is associated with an increased risk of GERD and thereby erosive esophagitis. Additionally, visceral adiposity is metabolically active and creates a pro-inflammatory state that contributes to inflammation in esophageal tissue [12]. A cohort study of metabolically healthy adults who underwent upper endoscopy found that those with overweight and obesity had an increased risk of developing erosive esophagitis compared to normal-weight adults, even after adjustment for metabolic risk factors. Interestingly, a retrospective cross-sectional study with over 10,000 subjects showed that in the absence of obesity, metabolic comorbidities, specifically hypertension, hyperlipidemia, and diabetes, did not increase the risk for erosive esophagitis [13]. This suggests that metabolic health alone does not play a critical role in the development of erosive esophagitis. Thus, obesity even without metabolic comorbidities remains a risk factor for erosive esophagitis [14].

Barrett's Esophagus and Esophageal Adenocarcinoma

Barrett's esophagus (BE) is a pathologic state in which the stratified squamous epithelium of the distal esophagus is replaced by metaplastic columnar epithelium with goblet cells. BE predisposes patients to esophageal adenocarcinoma (EAC). Obesity is a known risk factor for both Barrett's esophagus and esophageal adenocarcinoma [15]. A systematic analysis of 46 studies demonstrated that abdominal obesity, defined as a waist-to-hip ratio >0.90 for men and >0.85 for women, increased the risk of BE by 30% (OR 1.30, 95% CI 1.11–1.52) [16]. With regard to esophageal malignancies, it is important to distinguish the risk of esophageal adenocarcinoma from the risk of squamous cell carcinoma. A meta-analysis on studies prior to 2010 revealed a relative risk (RR) of developing all esophageal cancers (both adenocarcinoma and squamous cell carcinoma) to be 1.21 (0.97–1.52) and 1.20 (0.95–1.53) in men and women with obesity, respectively, compared to normal-weight counterparts [17]. While these results were not statistically significant, more recent studies on the effect of obesity on exclusively EAC found that those with obesity were at least four times as likely to develop EAC [15, 18, 19]. The mechanisms of the association of obesity with BE and EAC are thought to be both mechanical and non-mechanical, similar to GERD. Abdominal fat can decrease lower esophageal sphincter pressure resulting in increased reflux events while also potentiating reflux-mediated inflammation [18]. A 2019 population-based case-control study demonstrated that metabolic syndrome is associated with the risk of BE in males but not in females, which may explain the higher prevalence of BE in males [20]. Additionally, some bariatric procedures, specifically sleeve gastrectomy, are associated with an increased risk of developing BE [21]. A 2019 meta-analysis revealed an incidence of BE following sleeve gastrectomy of 13.6% when patients were followed for longer than 5 years after the surgery in studies that performed endoscopies on all patients before and after laparoscopic sleeve gastrectomy irrespective of reflux symptoms [21]. This study also demonstrated higher rates of GERD, hiatal hernia, and erosive esophagitis in the same cohort, which can mediate the association between sleeve gastrectomy and BE. Increased reflux may be related to anatomic changes after sleeve gastrectomy such as reduced gastric compliance with preserved pylorus leading to a high-pressure system. Additionally, sleeve gastrectomy can be associated with disruption of intrinsic anti-reflux mechanisms related to alteration of the angle of His and resection of gastric sling fibers, thus affecting lower esophageal sphincter integrity [10, 22–25].

Gastric Disorders

The complex interplay of gastric physiology contributes to appetite, satiety, and thereby obesity. Among the many orexigenic and anorexigenic peptides, ghrelin is the only orexigenic hormone that is secreted by the stomach, with a significant role in hunger [26]. Gastric motility also appears to play a role in obesity as gastric emptying may be faster, thereby delaying satiation in those with obesity [26]. In addition to the baseline physiologic roles of the stomach in weight regulation, obesity appears to be associated with several gastric-related disease states.

Gastritis

Obesity has been shown to be associated with not only endoscopic erosive gastritis but also histologic inflammation of the gastric mucosa [27]. Studies assessing the relationship between obesity and histologic gastritis have mostly been performed in patients undergoing bariatric surgery [28, 29]. These studies show that patients with morbid obesity have a significantly increased prevalence of histologically confirmed gastritis compared to age- and sex-matched control subjects with normal BMI [28]. There was no difference in *Helicobacter pylori* infection between patients with morbid obesity versus nonobese cohorts. It is unclear if an increased risk of gastritis is seen in those with less severe degrees of obesity. The mechanisms of the development of gastritis in obesity are not well understood beyond the pro-inflammatory nature of adipose tissue. However, there is evidence that adiponectin, an adipokine known to increase insulin sensitivity, may play a role. It has been shown that lower serum levels of adiponectin, as seen in obesity, are significantly associated with endoscopic erosive gastritis [30]. This is consistent with the anti-inflammatory nature of adiponectin in which it has been noted to promote ulcer healing and reduces leukocyte infiltration in the submucosa [31].

Gastric Cancer

Gastric cancer is one of the leading causes of cancer-related mortality worldwide [32]. The etiology of gastric cancer is both environmental and genetic and includes modifiable risk factors such as *H. pylori* and GERD. Given that obesity is a known risk factor for GERD [1], it is reasonably also a risk factor for gastric cancer. Interestingly, risk factors for cancer development differ depending on the region of the stomach. In the setting of obesity, there is a two- to threefold increased risk of cancer of the esophagogastric junction including the cardia [19]. However, increased BMI may not be associated with gastric non-cardia cancer [33]. Instead, risk factors associated with gastric non-cardia cancer include *H. pylori* infection, low socioeconomic status, and high intake of salty and smoked food [32].

Hepatobiliary Disorders

A variety of disorders of the liver and biliary tract are affected by obesity. The liver plays an important role in metabolism as it receives and stores nutrients from the intestines and peripheral tissues. Due to its metabolic activity, the liver is susceptible to changes in nutritional status including excessive calorie intake in the setting of obesity. In the biliary system, gallstone disease is defined by symptoms or complications caused by gallstones in the gallbladder or bile ducts. Gallstone disease, also exacerbated by obesity, is a chronic condition that increases with age and can greatly affect quality of life. As obesity increases the risk of metabolic abnormalities, the development of these comorbidities in turn predisposes one to an increased risk of gallbladder malignancy [34].

Gallstone Disease

Cholelithiasis, the formation of gallstones, is a known complication of obesity [35]. Multiple epidemiological studies have demonstrated an increased risk of gallstones in those with obesity, though the association of BMI with the development of gallstones is more frequently seen in women than in men [35]. A meta-analysis by Goh et al. [17] found obesity to increase the risk of gallstone disease 43% and 132% in men and women, respectively. It is hypothesized that differences in hormone secretion may explain the difference between the risk of gallstones in men and women [36]. One study found that women with a BMI greater than 30 kg/mg^2 had a 1% yearly incidence of gallstones [37]. The true prevalence of gallstones in those with obesity might be underestimated due to decreased sensitivity of ultrasound in detecting gallstones with increasing adipose tissue.

Cholesterol stones are the most common types of gallstones in those with obesity [35]. Cholesterol stone formation is primarily promoted by the supersaturation of bile with cholesterol such that the cholesterol to bile acid ratio is disproportionately increased [35]. In those with obesity, bile is significantly more saturated with cholesterol due to a greater degree of cholesterol secretion [35].

Though obesity is associated with cholelithiasis, weight loss may not always reduce the incidence of gallstones [35]. In fact, higher rates of weight loss and long periods of fasting are associated with the formation of gallstones regardless of sex [35]. An increased saturation of bile with cholesterol may occur during weight loss as caloric restriction leads to decreased secretion of biliary lipids and subsequent smaller bile acid pool. This may explain an increased incidence of gallstones during weight loss, and subsequently an increased risk of choledocholithiasis and cholecystitis. Of those with gallstones, approximately 1–4% of patients will develop symptoms of gallstone disease annually [38].

Gallbladder Cancer

Gallbladder cancer (GBC) is an uncommon malignancy that only arises in 1 in 200 cases of gallstone disease [39]. The association between obesity and GBC has been demonstrated in a number of studies worldwide [40, 41]. Women compared to men have a higher risk of developing GBC [41]. For each 5-point increase in BMI, there is a 59% and 9% increased risk of developing gallbladder cancer in women and men, respectively [34]. Other factors increasing the risk for GBC include abdominal obesity specifically and obesity in early adulthood [42]. Not only is obesity a risk factor for gallstones, obesity can also lead to an increased risk of GBC in the absence of gallstones [41]. The mechanisms of obesity in GBC development are primarily fatty infiltration of the gallbladder along with obesity-induced insulin resistance and resultant increased production of insulin-like growth factors (IGF) [41]. Increased fatty infiltration in the gallbladder enhances local chronic inflammation which is hypothesized to favor epithelial cell transformation [41]. A systematic analysis of the expression of IGF in gallbladder carcinomas showed that IGFs are involved in the early stage of carcinogenesis and are expressed in lymph nodes and hepatic metastases [43].

NAFLD/NASH

The incidence and severity of nonalcoholic fatty liver disease (NAFLD) has rapidly increased in parallel with the obesity epidemic. Obesity is an independent risk factor NAFLD, with a 3.5-fold higher relative risk (RR) of developing NAFLD and a dose-dependent RR of 1.20 for each 1-point increase in BMI [44]. The global burden of NAFLD is estimated to be 25%, with the highest prevalence in the Middle East and South America and lowest prevalence in Sub-Saharan Africa [45]. NAFLD is a major cause of liver disease and may progress to nonalcoholic steatohepatitis (NASH), liver fibrosis, cirrhosis, and hepatocellular carcinoma (HCC) [46]. Out of 100 patients with NAFLD, approximately 5 will go on to develop cirrhosis and 1–2 will ultimately die from a liver-related etiology [45]. Patients with NAFLD also have higher rates of hypertension, dyslipidemia, and increased insulin resistance or type 2 diabetes which are major risk factors for cardiovascular disease, a leading cause of death among patients with NAFLD and NASH [47].

Clinically, NAFLD is generally asymptomatic but may cause mild liver test abnormalities.

Diagnosis of NAFLD is typically confirmed by ultrasound, which is the most common screening test. In North America, prevalence of NAFLD with ultrasound was 24% but only 13% with serum measurement of AST and ALT [45], suggesting that blood tests alone are insufficient to diagnosis NAFLD. Several clinical calculators have been developed to predict NAFLD severity and risk of progression to NASH, but these tools are imperfect [48]. The gold standard for diagnosis of NASH is liver biopsy and is reserved for cases where the diagnosis is uncertain or there is high suspicion for advanced NAFLD-related liver disease. A noninvasive method to detect NASH is through ultrasound or magnetic resonance liver elastography, a measurement of liver stiffness, and is commonly used to monitor patients with NASH for progression to cirrhosis [48].

Treatment of NAFLD and NASH primarily consists of lifestyle changes with the goal of weight loss. Even a modest 5% weight loss lead to improvement of NAFLD in 65% of patients and NASH-resolution in 26% of patients [49]. A more impressive 10% weight loss leads to improvement NAFLD in 100% of patients and NASH-resolution in 90% of patients [49]. A Mediterranean diet is recommended as the most effective diet for weight loss with beneficial reductions in cardiometabolic risk factors [49]. Evidence for pharmacologic therapy for NAFLD and NASH is limited; patients with non-diabetic, biopsy-proven NASH may benefit from vitamin E and pioglitazone [48]. Many other pharmacologic agents are in trial. Bariatric surgery is a highly effective treatment for NASH but is reserved only for cases who have failed lifestyle and pharmacologic therapy and meet a separate criterion for weight loss surgery [50].

Cirrhosis

In patients with obesity and NASH, an estimated 3–15% progress to cirrhosis [51, 52]. In addition, obesity is considered an independent risk factor for the development of cirrhosis [51]. Obesity is a poor prognostic indicator in those who have existing liver disease. For example, obesity increases the risk of portal vein thrombosis by way of pro-inflammatory and prothrombotic mechanisms [51]. In addition to the negative effects of excess adipose tissue, the coexistence of sarcopenia and obesity magnifies the risk of cirrhosis complications such as sepsis and hepatic encephalopathy [51]. In liver transplantation, obesity is associated with increased perioperative complications, length of stay, and risk of infection [51].

Bariatric surgery is the most effective currently available therapy to treat obesity and can be considered in patients with Child-Pugh class A cirrhosis, though more severe forms of liver disease are often a contraindication. In a systematic review of bariatric surgery outcomes in patients with cirrhosis [53], bariatric surgery was found to potentially halt or reverse liver damage with corresponding improvements in metabolic parameters. Furthermore, bariatric surgery with resultant weight loss could improve the likelihood of liver transplant in patients with obesity as a BMI $\geq$40 kg/m^2 is often a contraindication to transplantation.

Hepatocellular Carcinoma

Hepatocellular carcinoma (HCC) is the most common primary liver malignancy [54]. The increasing incidence of obesity and development of NASH is largely responsible for the increase in HCC cases across the United States [55]. For every 5-point BMI increase, the relative risk of developing liver cancer increased 24% [56]. When comparing NASH and NAFLD, the risk of HCC is more associated with NASH-cirrhosis than with NAFLD [55]. Nevertheless, obesity remains a well-known risk factor for HCC development in patients with other types of liver disease as well, such as viral hepatitis [57]. Additionally, the risk of dying from liver cancer is 4.5 times higher in men with a BMI of $\geq$35 kg/m^2 compared to normal-weight counterparts [57]. Obesity-related metabolic inflammation has been implicated in HCC progression through mechanisms that include neural regulation, innate immune responses, and endocrinal regulation [54, 58]. Previously labeled as cryptogenic HCC, the metabolic syndrome is now acknowledged as a cause of liver cancer. Insulin resistance and hepatic steatosis both promote tissue-derived inflammation which predisposes hepatocytes to carcinogenesis [57]. In addition, pro-inflammatory adipocytokines in obesity are associated with a worse prognosis of HCC [54]. NAFLD and NASH can be prevented by maintaining a healthy lifestyle and avoiding the development of hypertension, diabetes, and hyperlipidemia. Doing so decreases fatty liver-related disease, which then reduces both cirrhosis and HCC cases.

Pancreatic Disorders

Increased pancreatic volume and fatty infiltration of pancreatic tissue is seen more commonly in patients who are overweight or obese [59, 60]. Presently, it remains unclear how closely BMI and pancreatic steatosis correlate. Pancreatic steatosis is associated with multiple diseases ranging from cystic fibrosis to diabetes [59, 61]. Although there is no consensus as to whether increased pancreatic fat is clinically relevant, obesity appears to be an independent risk factor for the development and severity of pancreatic diseases, notably acute pancreatitis (AP) and pancreatic cancer (PC) [61].

Acute Pancreatitis

In the last several decades, the incidence of acute pancreatitis (AP) has risen in parallel to the prevalence of obesity [62]. Patients with obesity have a higher incidence of pancreatitis. Obesity has several known mechanisms that contribute to the risk of acute pancreatitis. First, obesity is a known risk factor for biliary disease, specifically gallstones which cause acute pancreatitis by obstruction of biliopancreatic ducts [35]. Second, hypertriglyceridemia is a common lipid abnormality in patients with visceral obesity [63]. Elevated lipid triglycerides can form microthrombi in the pancreatic vasculature and subsequent ischemia [63]. Third, obesity and diabetes mellitus type 2 (DM2) are highly associated. DM2 increases the risk of AP by various mechanisms including islet cell hypertrophy which can result in duct obstruction [64]. Other mechanisms include hypertriglyceridemia and medications for diabetes such as glucagon-like peptide-1 agonists which have been implicated in drug-associated pancreatitis. Obesity is also an independent risk factor for the severity of AP as well as mortality from AP [65]. Increased intra- and peri-pancreatic fat is associated with a worse degree of pancreatic necrosis and systemic unsaturated fatty acid toxicity, respectively [64].

The association between obesity and the development of chronic pancreatitis (CP) is not well understood. One study found that patients with CP were more likely to have higher degrees of pancreatic fat [60]. However, BMI was not found to be significantly associated with CP [60]. The data on the association between pancreatic steatosis and CP is insufficient to conclude that pancreatic steatosis or obesity is an etiological factor for CP.

Pancreatic Cancer

Pancreatic cancer (PC) is one of the most lethal malignancies with a 5-year survival rate of less than 10% [66]. Multiple cohort studies and meta-analyses have demonstrated a positive association between BMI and risk of PC [67]. Geography and ethnicity appear to play a role in PC risk. A 2016 meta-analysis found a relative risk of PC to be 1.07 and 1.18 for every 5 kg/m^2 increase in BMI in North American and European-Australian populations, respectively, but no association with BMI in the Asia-Pacific group [68]. Some studies show a positive association between BMI and risk of PC in men but not in women [67]. Childhood obesity is an independent risk factor for PC [69]. With regard to the mechanism of PC in those with obesity, obesity is known to cause a pro-inflammatory state, and this chronic low-grade inflammation is thought to play a primary role in PC development. PC is promoted by the carcinogenic effects of adipokines, insulin resistance, and IGF-1 [67]. Both prevention and treatment of obesity may help to prevent the development of PC. A meta-analysis involving over 10,000 PC patients showed physical activity to be weakly associated with a reduced PC risk;

this association was stronger for consistent physical activity over time [70]. The role of bariatric surgery in PC risk has not yet been clearly elucidated.

Bowel Disorders

In the past two decades, new studies have emerged that redefine the relationship between the gastrointestinal tract and obesity. In addition to the gastrointestinal tract's function in nutrient and calorie absorption, the gut microbiome also appears to be involved in the regulation of body weight [71]. Changes in the gut microbiome have been linked to pro-inflammatory states as seen in metabolic syndrome [71]. While there is still much more to be understood in the underlying mechanisms of the microbiome as a causal factor for obesity, it is also important to understand the impact obesity has on the gut itself. Here we discuss the complex relationships between obesity and four major diseases: colorectal cancer, diverticular disease, inflammatory bowel disease (IBD), and *Clostridium difficile* infection (CDI).

Colorectal Cancer

Multiple meta-analyses assessing obesity and CRC risk have consistently shown a significant increased risk of CRC in both men and women [72]. Relative risks of CRC in the setting of obesity vary from 1.19 to 1.95 [72, 73]. In a meta-analysis of more than 4.7 million subjects, early-life obesity (obesity before the age of 25) was associated with a 39% increased risk of CRC in adult men ($p < 0.0001$) and a 19% increased risk of CRC in adult women ($p = 0.004$) [74]. Obesity-related CRC has been linked to low physical activity and dietary habits such as higher consumption of red and processed meats [73]. Multiple hormones related to obesity have been implicated in the development of CRC, in particular insulin, adiponectin, leptin, ghrelin, and resistin [75]. When considering mechanisms of risk reduction, there is little evidence from randomized clinical trials showing the effects of weight loss interventions on colorectal cancer incidence. A large prospective cohort study using data from the Women's Health Initiative evaluated the association between intentional weight change by lifestyle modification and obesity-related cancer incidence [76]. Compared to women with stable weight, women with intentional weight loss had a lower risk of colorectal cancer (HR = 0.79, 95% CI = 0.63–0.99) [76]. However, there is a discordance on whether bariatric surgery may affect incident CRC risk [77, 78]. A potential mechanism of CRC risk reduction via bariatric surgery includes hormonal changes due to both structural and functional changes in the gastrointestinal tract. For example, IGF-I receptors are overexpressed in CRC suggesting their involvement in the pathogenesis of CRC. Bariatric surgery may reduce levels of free IGF-1. Conversely, bariatric surgery may also cause increased gut-specific inflammation and dietary changes which contribute to an increased risk of CRC. Additionally, certain gut bacteria directly promote colon carcinogenesis by immune regulation and toxin production [79]. Thus, modulation of the gut microbiota due to surgical manipulation may also contribute to CRC risk.

Diverticular Disease

Diverticular disease of the colon is a complex disorder arising from multiple risk factors, though the exact pathogenesis is not known [80]. Diverticulosis refers to the presence of colonic diverticula, while diverticulitis refers to the presence of inflammation of diverticula. Genetics and lifestyle factors have both been implicated in the development of diverticular disease. A diet high in red meat and refined grains increases the risk of diverticular disease while a plant-based diet decreases risk [80]. Obesity, in particular central obesity, is associated with an increased risk of diverticular disease [81]. Diverticulosis has been shown to be independently associated with increasing visceral adipose tissue and subcutaneous adipose tissue [82, 83]. The odds of colonic diverticulosis in subjects with obesity is 40%

greater than those without obesity [83]. The mechanism by which obesity increases the risk of diverticulosis is unclear. However, the microbiome in the setting of obesity has been hypothesized to play an important role. Another theory is that increasing cytokines produced by adipocytes leads to delayed colonic motility and a subsequent increase in intraluminal pressure. Similar to diverticulosis, a large prospective cohort study of over 45,000 men demonstrated that BMI, waist circumference, and waist-to-hip ratio significantly increased the risks of diverticulitis and diverticular bleeding [81].

Inflammatory Bowel Disease

Approximately 15–40% of patients with IBD are also diagnosed with obesity [84]. Given that most studies evaluating the IBD population with obesity are retrospective in nature, it is unclear if obesity is a manifestation or a significant predictor of disease severity. Since obesity is associated with a pro-inflammatory state, it has been postulated that this inflammation may be involved in the etiology of IBD. While one prospective cohort study demonstrated no increased risk of incident ulcerative colitis (UC) or Crohn's disease (CD) cases in participants with obesity [85], others have demonstrated an increased risk of CD among individuals with obesity, but no increased risk of UC [86]. Obesity has multiple implications on diagnostic imaging, severity of IBD, and treatment of patients with IBD. For instance, inflammatory markers may be elevated in patients with obesity irrespective of inflammation related to IBD disease [87]. Imaging access and quality may be compromised in patients with obesity. Not only do patients with obesity face challenges related to equipment weight limits, but layers of adipose tissue can result in poor image quality. Obesity may also result in a suboptimal response to therapies for IBD due to excess adipose tissue promoting rapid clearance of biologic agents [86, 88]. Cross-sectional and cohort studies have shown a statistically significant higher risk of IBD surgery-related complications and hospitalizations in patients with obesity versus controls with IBD without obesity [89, 90].

Clostridium Difficile Infection

Clostridium difficile causes a diarrheal infection that manifests from asymptomatic, mild diarrhea, to fulminant disease. Commonly acknowledged risk factors include advanced age and alterations in the intestinal microbiome (e.g., antibiotic use) [91]. Obesity is often found to be a risk factor for hospital infections, although it is not a well-defined risk factor for *Clostridium difficile* infection (CDI). Previous studies have shown obesity to be associated with an increased risk of CDI [92]. One retrospective cohort study involving nearly 200 patients found that a BMI >35 kg/m^2 was 1.7-fold more likely to be associated with severe CDI compared to normal-weight or overweight counterparts ($p < 0.005$) [93]. The pathogenesis of CDI in the setting of obesity has been thought to be related to disruption of the gut microbiome, persistent low-grade inflammation, and alterations in leptin signaling that affect immunity [92]. More recent studies challenge this notion. Based on a nationwide retrospective cohort study with 1.43 million patients, obesity was independently associated with a decreased risk of postoperative CDI [94]. In this study, the incidence of postoperative CDI was 0.36% in those with class III obesity compared to 0.56% in the normal-weight group (p for the trend from lowest to highest BMI group <0.001) [94]. A case-control study examining obesity as an exposure risk for CDI found no statistically significant difference in the odds of acquiring CDI when those with obesity were compared to age and gender-matched controls [95]. Overall, the relationship and mechanism of obesity-mediated effects on CDI are both complex and likely to be mediated by additional factors that alter immunity.

Conclusion

The relationship between obesity and diseases of the gastrointestinal tract is multifaceted and bidirectional. While the gastrointestinal tract is itself a conduit for excess calorie absorption, obesity also contributes to gastrointestinal complications.

Obesity is characterized by a chronic low-grade inflammatory state of adipose tissue [88]. Of the several compartments of body fat, visceral deposits have been found to be the most metabolically active and predictive of intestinal inflammation [96]. There is also growing interest in distinguishing "metabolically healthy obese (MHO)" individuals from those with obesity and metabolic syndrome in order to more accurately assess the relationship between obesity and disease. A chronic pro-inflammatory state is thought to contribute to the development of multiple gastrointestinal diseases in the setting of obesity. Furthermore, excess adipose tissue can lead to anatomical changes that alter organ function. It is important to note that evidence for the role of obesity in the development of gastrointestinal illnesses is often based on observational studies which carry several limitations. In addition to the presence of confounding variables, BMI does not describe the composition of fat versus lean tissues. Furthermore, dietary variables may have a significant effect on health but dietary composition is often not detailed in studies. Future studies are needed to better elucidate the mechanisms by which obesity influences diseases of the gut in order to better manage obesity and its related comorbidities.

References

1. Chang P, Friedenberg F. Obesity and GERD. Gastroenterol Clin N Am. 2014;43(1):161–73.
2. El-Serag H. The association between obesity and GERD: a review of the epidemiological evidence. Dig Dis Sci. 2008;53(9):2307–12.
3. Eslami O, Shahraki M, Bahari A, Shahraki T. Dietary habits and obesity indices in patients with gastro-esophageal reflux disease: a comparative cross-sectional study. BMC Gastroenterol. 2017;17(1):132.
4. Wu JC, Mui LM, Cheung CM, Chan Y, Sung JJ. Obesity is associated with increased transient lower esophageal sphincter relaxation. Gastroenterology. 2007;132(3):883–9.
5. Kouklakis G, Moschos J, Kountouras J, Mpoumponaris A, Molyvas E, Minopoulos G. Relationship between obesity and gastroesophageal reflux disease as recorded by 3-hour esophageal pH monitoring. Rom J Gastroenterol. 2005;14(2):117–21.
6. Varela JE, Hinojosa M, Nguyen N. Correlations between intra-abdominal pressure and obesity-related co-morbidities. Surg Obes Relat Dis. 2009;5(5):524–8.
7. Schlottmann F, Herbella FAM, Patti MG. Bariatric surgery and gastroesophageal reflux. J Laparoendosc Adv Surg Tech A. 2018;28(8):953–5.
8. Ness-Jensen E, Hveem K, El-Serag H, Lagergren J. Lifestyle intervention in gastroesophageal reflux disease. Clin Gastroenterol Hepatol. 2016;14(2):175–82.e1–3.
9. Hutopila I, Copaescu C. Hiatal hernia is more frequent than expected in bariatric patients. Intraoperative findings during laparoscopic sleeve gastrectomy. Chirurgia (Bucur). 2019;114(6):779–89.
10. Oor JE, Roks DJ, Ünlü Ç, Hazebroek EJ. Laparoscopic sleeve gastrectomy and gastroesophageal reflux disease: a systematic review and meta-analysis. Am J Surg. 2016;211(1):250–67.
11. Rebecchi F, Allaix ME, Giaccone C, Ugliono E, Scozzari G, Morino M. Gastroesophageal reflux disease and laparoscopic sleeve gastrectomy: a physiopathologic evaluation. Ann Surg. 2014;260(5):909–14. discussion 14–5.
12. Anggiansah R, Sweis R, Anggiansah A, Wong T, Cooper D, Fox M. The effects of obesity on oesophageal function, acid exposure and the symptoms of gastro-oesophageal reflux disease. Aliment Pharmacol Ther. 2013;37(5):555–63.
13. Baeg MK, Ko SH, Ko SY, Jung HS, Choi MG. Obesity increases the risk of erosive esophagitis but metabolic unhealthiness alone does not: a large-scale cross-sectional study. BMC Gastroenterol. 2018;18(1):82.
14. Kim TJ, Lee H, Baek SY, et al. Metabolically healthy obesity and the risk of erosive esophagitis: a cohort study. Clin Transl Gastroenterol. 2019;10(9):e00077.
15. Monardo A, McCullough J. Incidence of dysplasia in obese vs nonobese patients with nondysplastic Barrett esophagus. Ochsner J. 2019;19(4):347–52.
16. Di J, Cheng Y, Chang D, Liu Y. A meta-analysis of the impact of obesity, metabolic syndrome, insulin resistance, and microbiome on the diagnosis of Barrett's esophagus. Dig Dis. 2020;38(3):165–77.
17. Goh GB, Schauer PR, McCullough AJ. Considerations for bariatric surgery in patients with cirrhosis. World J Gastroenterol. 2018;24(28):3112–9.
18. Chandar AK, Iyer PG. Role of obesity in the pathogenesis and progression of Barrett's esophagus. Gastroenterol Clin N Am. 2015;44(2):249–64.
19. Hoyo C, Cook MB, Kamangar F, et al. Body mass index in relation to oesophageal and oesophagogastric junction adenocarcinomas: a pooled analysis from the International BEACON Consortium. Int J Epidemiol. 2012;41(6):1706–18.
20. Kendall BJ, Macdonald GA, Prins JB, O'Brien S, Thrift AP, Whiteman DC. Sex differences in the risk of Barrett's esophagus associated with the metabolic effects of obesity. J Clin Gastroenterol. 2020;54(9):795–800.
21. Hoerter N, Smukalla S, Pitman M, Popov V. Barrett's esophagus is a long-term complication of sleeve gastrectomy: a systematic review and meta-analysis. The

Society for Surgery of the Alimentary Tract 2019; 60th Annual Meeting. 18–21 May 2019. San Diego, CA.
22. Stenard F, Iannelli A. Laparoscopic sleeve gastrectomy and gastroesophageal reflux. World J Gastroenterol. 2015;21:10348–57.
23. Ali M, El Chaar M, Ghiassi S, et al. American Society for Metabolic and Bariatric Surgery updated position statement on sleeve gastrectomy as a bariatric procedure. Surg Obes Relat Dis. 2017;13:1652–7.
24. Felsenreich DM, Kefurt R, Schermann M, et al. Reflux, sleeve dilation, and Barrett's esophagus after laparoscopic sleeve gastrectomy: long-term follow-up. Obes Surg. 2017;27:3092–101.
25. Sebastianelli L, Benois M, Vanbiervliet G, et al. Systematic endoscopy 5 years after sleeve gastrectomy results in a high rate of Barrett's esophagus: results of a multicenter study. Obes Surg. 2019;29(5):1462–9.
26. Hunt RH, Camilleri M, Crowe SE, et al. The stomach in health and disease. Gut. 2015;64(10):1650–68.
27. Yamamoto S, Watabe K, Takehara T. Is obesity a new risk factor for gastritis? Digestion. 2012;85(2):108–10.
28. Dutta SK, Arora M, Kireet A, Bashandy H, Gandsas A. Upper gastrointestinal symptoms and associated disorders in morbidly obese patients: a prospective study. Dig Dis Sci. 2009;54(6):1243–6.
29. Csendes A, Burgos AM, Smok G, Beltran M. Endoscopic and histologic findings of the foregut in 426 patients with morbid obesity. Obes Surg. 2007;17(1):28–34.
30. Yamamoto S, Watabe K, Tsutsui S, et al. Lower serum level of adiponectin is associated with increased risk of endoscopic erosive gastritis. Dig Dis Sci. 2011;56(8):2354–60.
31. Fard AA, Hajrezaie M, Kadir FA, et al. The effects of combined adiponectin-metformin on glucose and lipids levels in mice and acute toxicity and anti-ulcerogenic activity of adiponectin against ethanol-induced gastric mucosal injuries in rat. Molecules. 2011;16(11):9534–52.
32. Karimi P, Islami F, Anandasabapathy S, Freedman ND, Kamangar F. Gastric cancer: descriptive epidemiology, risk factors, screening, and prevention. Cancer Epidemiol Biomark Prev. 2014;23(5):700–13.
33. Chen Y, Liu L, Wang X, et al. Body mass index and risk of gastric cancer: a meta-analysis of a population with more than ten million from 24 prospective studies. Cancer Epidemiol Biomark Prev. 2013;22(8):1395–408.
34. Wolin KY, Carson K, Colditz GA. Obesity and cancer. Oncologist. 2010;15(6):556–65.
35. Erlinger S. Gallstones in obesity and weight loss. Eur J Gastroenterol Hepatol. 2000;12(12):1347–52.
36. Lammert F, Gurusamy K, Ko CW, et al. Gallstones. Nat Rev Dis Primers. 2016;2(1):16024.
37. Maclure KM, Hayes KC, Colditz GA, Stampfer MJ, Speizer FE, Willett WC. Weight, diet, and the risk of symptomatic gallstones in middle-aged women. N Engl J Med. 1989;321(9):563–9.
38. Lee JY, Keane MG, Pereira S. Diagnosis and treatment of gallstone disease. Practitioner. 2015;259(1783):15–9. 2
39. Baiu I, Visser B. Gallbladder cancer. JAMA. 2018;320(12):1294.
40. Jeong SU, Lee SK. Obesity and gallbladder diseases. Korean J Gastroenterol. 2012;59(1):27–34.
41. Wang F, Wang B, Qiao L. Association between obesity and gallbladder cancer. Front Biosci (Landmark Ed). 2012;17:2550–8.
42. Hsing AW, Sakoda LC, Rashid A, et al. Body size and the risk of biliary tract cancer: a population-based study in China. Br J Cancer. 2008;99(5):811–5.
43. Kornprat P, Rehak P, Rüschoff J, Langner C. Expression of IGF-I, IGF-II, and IGF-IR in gallbladder carcinoma. A systematic analysis including primary and corresponding metastatic tumours. J Clin Pathol. 2006;59(2):202–6.
44. Li L, Liu DW, Yan HY, Wang ZY, Zhao SH, Wang B. Obesity is an independent risk factor for non-alcoholic fatty liver disease: evidence from a meta-analysis of 21 cohort studies. Obes Rev. 2016;17(6):510–9.
45. Younossi ZM, Koenig AB, Abdelatif D, Fazel Y, Henry L, Wymer M. Global epidemiology of nonalcoholic fatty liver disease-meta-analytic assessment of prevalence, incidence, and outcomes. Hepatology. 2016;64(1):73–84.
46. De Minicis S, Day C, Svegliati-Baroni G. From NAFLD to NASH and HCC: pathogenetic mechanisms and therapeutic insights. Curr Pharm Des. 2013;19(29):5239–49.
47. Vernon G, Baranova A, Younossi ZM. Systematic review: the epidemiology and natural history of non-alcoholic fatty liver disease and non-alcoholic steatohepatitis in adults. Aliment Pharmacol Ther. 2011;34(3):274–85.
48. Leoni S, Tovoli F, Napoli L, Serio I, Ferri S, Bolondi L. Current guidelines for the management of non-alcoholic fatty liver disease: a systematic review with comparative analysis. World J Gastroenterol. 2018;24(30):3361–73.
49. Romero-Gomez M, Zelber-Sagi S, Trenell M. Treatment of NAFLD with diet, physical activity and exercise. J Hepatol. 2017;67(4):829–46.
50. Lassailly G, Caiazzo R, Buob D, et al. Bariatric surgery reduces features of nonalcoholic steatohepatitis in morbidly obese patients. Gastroenterology. 2015;149(2):379–88; quiz e15–6.
51. Schiavo L, Busetto L, Cesaretti M, Zelber-Sagi S, Deutsch L, Iannelli A. Nutritional issues in patients with obesity and cirrhosis. World J Gastroenterol. 2018;24(30):3330–46.
52. Dhamija E, Paul SB, Kedia S. Non-alcoholic fatty liver disease associated with hepatocellular carci-

noma: an increasing concern. Indian J Med Res. 2019;149(1):9–17.
53. Jan A, Narwaria M, Mahawar KK. A systematic review of bariatric surgery in patients with liver cirrhosis. Obes Surg. 2015;25(8):1518–26.
54. Gan L, Liu Z, Sun C. Obesity linking to hepatocellular carcinoma: a global view. Biochim Biophys Acta Rev Cancer. 2018;1869(2):97–102.
55. Mittal S, El-Serag HB. Epidemiology of hepatocellular carcinoma: consider the population. J Clin Gastroenterol. 2013;47 Suppl(0):S2–6.
56. Larsson SC, Wolk A. Overweight, obesity and risk of liver cancer: a meta-analysis of cohort studies. Br J Cancer. 2007;97(7):1005–8.
57. Marengo A, Rosso C, Bugianesi E. Liver cancer: connections with obesity, fatty liver, and cirrhosis. Annu Rev Med. 2016;67:103–17.
58. Kew MC. Obesity as a cause of hepatocellular carcinoma. Ann Hepatol. 2015;14(3):299–303.
59. DeSouza SV, Singh RG, Yoon HD, Murphy R, Plank LD, Petrov MS. Pancreas volume in health and disease: a systematic review and meta-analysis. Expert Rev Gastroenterol Hepatol. 2018;12(8):757–66.
60. Tirkes T, Jeon CY, Li L, et al. Association of pancreatic steatosis with chronic pancreatitis, obesity, and type 2 diabetes mellitus. Pancreas. 2019;48(3):420–6.
61. Majumder S, Philip NA, Takahashi N, Levy MJ, Singh VP, Chari ST. Fatty pancreas: should we be concerned? Pancreas. 2017;46(10):1251–8.
62. Lowenfels AB, Maisonneuve P, Sullivan T. The changing character of acute pancreatitis: epidemiology, etiology, and prognosis. Curr Gastroenterol Rep. 2009;11(2):97–103.
63. Kushner PA, Cobble ME. Hypertriglyceridemia: the importance of identifying patients at risk. Postgrad Med. 2016;128(8):848–58.
64. Khatua B, El-Kurdi B, Singh VP. Obesity and pancreatitis. Curr Opin Gastroenterol. 2017;33(5):374–82.
65. Dobszai D, Mátrai P, Gyöngyi Z, et al. Body-mass index correlates with severity and mortality in acute pancreatitis: a meta-analysis. World J Gastroenterol. 2019;25(6):729–43.
66. Rawla P, Sunkara T, Gaduputi V. Epidemiology of pancreatic cancer: global trends, etiology and risk factors. World J Oncol. 2019;10(1):10–27.
67. Zhou B, Wu D, Liu H, et al. Obesity and pancreatic cancer: an update of epidemiological evidence and molecular mechanisms. Pancreatology. 2019;19(7):941–50.
68. Wang J, Yang DL, Chen ZZ, Gou BF. Associations of body mass index with cancer incidence among populations, genders, and menopausal status: a systematic review and meta-analysis. Cancer Epidemiol. 2016;42:1–8.
69. Nogueira L, Stolzenberg-Solomon R, Gamborg M, Sørensen TIA, Baker JL. Childhood body mass index and risk of adult pancreatic cancer. Curr Dev Nutr. 2017;1(10):cdn.117.001362.
70. Behrens G, Jochem C, Schmid D, Keimling M, Ricci C, Leitzmann MF. Physical activity and risk of pancreatic cancer: a systematic review and meta-analysis. Eur J Epidemiol. 2015;30(4):279–98.
71. Chen X, Devaraj S. Gut microbiome in obesity, metabolic syndrome, and diabetes. Curr Diab Rep. 2018;18(12):129.
72. Bardou M, Barkun AN, Martel M. Obesity and colorectal cancer. Gut. 2013;62(6):933–47.
73. Baena R, Salinas P. Diet and colorectal cancer. Maturitas. 2015;80(3):258–64.
74. Garcia H, Song M. Early-life obesity and adulthood colorectal cancer risk: a meta-analysis. Rev Panam Salud Publica. 2019;43:e3.
75. Uyar GO, Sanlier N. Association of adipokines and insulin, which have a role in obesity, with colorectal cancer. Eurasian J Med. 2019;51(2):191–5.
76. Luo J, Hendryx M, Manson JE, et al. Intentional weight loss and obesity-related cancer risk. JNCI Cancer Spectr. 2019;3(4):pkz054.
77. Tao W, Artama M, von Euler-Chelpin M, et al. Colon and rectal cancer risk after bariatric surgery in a multicountry Nordic cohort study. Int J Cancer. 2019; https://doi.org/10.1002/ijc.32770.
78. Bailly L, Fabre R, Pradier C, Iannelli A. Colorectal cancer risk following bariatric surgery in a nationwide study of French individuals with obesity. JAMA Surg. 2020;155(5):395–402.
79. Wong SH, Yu J. Gut microbiota in colorectal cancer: mechanisms of action and clinical applications. Nat Rev Gastroenterol Hepatol. 2019;16(11):690–704.
80. Kupcinskas J, Strate LL, Bassotti G, et al. Pathogenesis of diverticulosis and diverticular disease. J Gastrointestin Liver Dis. 2019;28(suppl. 4):7–10.
81. Strate LL, Liu YL, Aldoori WH, Syngal S, Giovannucci EL. Obesity increases the risks of diverticulitis and diverticular bleeding. Gastroenterology. 2009;136(1):115–22.e1.
82. Nagata N, Sakamoto K, Arai T, et al. Visceral abdominal obesity measured by computed tomography is associated with increased risk of colonic diverticulosis. J Clin Gastroenterol. 2015;49(10):816–22.
83. Wijarnpreecha K, Ahuja W, Chesdachai S, et al. Obesity and the risk of colonic diverticulosis: a meta-analysis. Dis Colon Rectum. 2018;61(4):476–83.
84. Singh S, Dulai PS, Zarrinpar A, Ramamoorthy S, Sandborn WJ. Obesity in IBD: epidemiology, pathogenesis, disease course and treatment outcomes. Nat Rev Gastroenterol Hepatol. 2017;14(2):110–21.
85. Chan SS, Luben R, Olsen A, et al. Body mass index and the risk for Crohn's disease and ulcerative colitis: data from a European Prospective Cohort Study (The IBD in EPIC Study). Am J Gastroenterol. 2013;108(4):575–82.
86. Harper JW, Zisman TL. Interaction of obesity and inflammatory bowel disease. World J Gastroenterol. 2016;22(35):7868–81.
87. Swanson SM, Harper J, Zisman TL. Obesity and inflammatory bowel disease: diagnostic and therapeutic implications. Curr Opin Gastroenterol. 2018;34(2):112–9.

88. Smit C, De Hoogd S, Bruggemann RJM, Knibbe CAJ. Obesity and drug pharmacology: a review of the influence of obesity on pharmacokinetic and pharmacodynamic parameters. Expert Opin Drug Metab Toxicol. 2018;14(3):275–85.
89. Seminerio JL, Koutroubakis IE, Ramos-Rivers C, et al. Impact of obesity on the management and clinical course of patients with inflammatory bowel disease. Inflamm Bowel Dis. 2015;21(12):2857–63.
90. Singh S, Khera R, Sandborn WJ. Obesity is associated with worse outcomes in hospitalized patients with inflammatory bowel diseases: a Nationwide analysis: 591. Am J Gastroenterol. 2016;111:S271.
91. Czepiel J, Dróżdż M, Pituch H, et al. Clostridium difficile infection: review. Eur J Clin Microbiol Infect Dis. 2019;38(7):1211–21.
92. Madan R, Petri WA Jr. Role of obesity and adipose tissue-derived cytokine leptin during Clostridium difficile infection. Anaerobe. 2015;34:182–6.
93. Mulki R, Baumann AJ, Alnabelsi T, et al. Body mass index greater than 35 is associated with severe Clostridium difficile infection. Aliment Pharmacol Ther. 2017;45(1):75–81.
94. Meier K, Nordestgaard AT, Eid AI, et al. Obesity as protective against, rather than a risk factor for, postoperative Clostridium difficile infection: a nationwide retrospective analysis of 1,426,807 surgical patients. J Trauma Acute Care Surg. 2019;86(6):1001–9.
95. Punni E, Pula JL, Asslo F, Baddoura W, DeBari VA. Is obesity a risk factor for Clostridium difficile infection? Obes Res Clin Pract. 2015;9(1):50–4.
96. Kredel LI, Siegmund B. Adipose-tissue and intestinal inflammation – visceral obesity and creeping fat. Front Immunol. 2014;5:462.

14 Clinical Evaluation, Lifestyle, and Pharmacological Management of Obesity

Sindhura Kolli, Beverly G. Tchang, Ilana P. Redmond, Sarah Barenbaum, and Katherine H. Saunders

Section 1: Clinical Evaluation of Obesity

Introduction

The prevalence of adults aged ≥18 years delineated into overweight or obesity based on body mass index (BMI) has steadily increased on a global scale. In the United States, in particular, as prevalence of obesity increases annually, predictive models suggest 1 in 2 adults will have obesity by the year 2030 [1, 2].

Obesity's influence on the pathophysiology of multiple comorbidities, such as type 2 diabetes mellitus (DM2), non-alcoholic fatty liver disease (NAFLD), metabolic syndrome, hyperlipidemia, hypertension (HTN), and obstructive sleep apnea (OSA), has been well established [3]. Its deleterious effects on lifespan and quality of life, compounded by its associated healthcare costs, warrant a recalibration of preventative, primary, and subspecialty fields of medicine to focus on identifying, evaluating, and treating this multifactorial, multisystemic, chronic medical condition [3, 4].

Approaching the Patient with Obesity

Reducing Stigma

Weight bias is highly prevalent within the healthcare system. Preconceived notions about patients with obesity result in shorter clinic visits, dismissal of illness-related symptoms, and/or attributing them to weight, potentially creating a distrustful relationship between healthcare providers and patients [5–9]. Weight bias can be reduced by following these strategies:

- Acknowledging the complex, multifactorial causes of obesity, rather than attributing obesity to poor personal choices [8]
- Using people-first language (i.e., addressing "people *with* obesity" rather than "obese people")
- Furnishing waiting rooms with wide-berth seating and medical examinationrooms with scales and beds that accommodate weights ≥400 lbs. (181 kg)

S. Kolli (✉)
Department of Internal Medicine, NYU Langone Comprehensive Program on Obesity, NYU School of Medicine, New York, NY, USA
e-mail: sree.kolli@nyulangone.org

B. G. Tchang · I. P. Redmond · S. Barenbaum
Department of Internal Medicine, Division of Endocrinology, Comprehensive Weight Control Center, NewYork-Presbyterian Hospital, Weill Cornell Medicine, New York, NY, USA
e-mail: bgt9001@med.cornell.edu; imp9005@med.cornell.edu; srb9023@med.cornell.edu

K. H. Saunders
Division of Endocrinology, Diabetes and Metabolism, New York-Presbyterian Hospital and Weill Cornell Medical Center, New York, NY, USA
e-mail: kph2001@med.cornell.edu

C. Newberry et al. (eds.), *Nutrition, Weight, and Digestive Health*,
https://doi.org/10.1007/978-3-030-94953-2_14

Table 14.1 Vitals and measurements collected at each patient visit

Height (in. or cm)
Weight (lb or kg)
Heart rate
Blood pressure
Waist circumference
Hip circumference

$$\text{BMI} = \frac{\text{Weight (kg) x 703}}{\text{Height (m)}^2}$$

Fig. 14.1 BMI calculation

- Providing appropriately sized blood pressure cuffs and gowns [9]

Clinical Evaluation of Obesity

Vital Signs

Obtaining baseline and follow-up measurements of the following allows for a thorough assessment of patients' metabolic progress (Table 14.1):

Waist Circumference (WC)

A WC of ≥35 in in women and ≥40 in in men functions as an independent risk factor in the development of DM2, metabolic syndrome, and cardiovascular disease (CVD), as well as decrease in life expectancy of 3 years for men and 5 years for women on average [10, 11]. The WC is an inexpensive and fast way to assess central and visceral fat and can be measured at the halfway point between the iliac crest and the last rib [12, 13].

Waist-to-Hip Ratio (WHR)

A WHR is calculated by waist circumference (cm) divided by hip circumference (measured across the widest part of the buttocks) (cm). Abdominal obesity is defined as a ratio of >0.85 in women and >0.90 in men. The WHR serves as a risk factor for the development of CVD and DM2 [14, 15].

Body Mass Index

BMI correlates with body fat percentage in certain groups of patients. While it cannot discriminate between body fat and lean mass, it serves as a widely used diagnostic, classification, and risk assessment tool (Fig. 14.1) [16].

To garner a better assessment of an individual's metabolic health [17], BMI is best used in conjunction with other tools that evaluate body composition, such as the following:

- Waist circumference
- Bioelectric impedance, which runs an electric current throughout the body in order to classify body mass into fat, muscle, fat free mass, visceral fat, and resting metabolic rate
- Dual-energy X-ray absorption (DEXA) scan
- Computed tomography (CT)
- Magnetic resonance imaging (MRI)

Laboratory Evaluation

Recommended baseline screening laboratory tests include a complete blood count (CBC), comprehensive metabolic panel (CMP), hemoglobin A1c (HbA1c), lipid panel, and thyroid-stimulating hormone (TSH). Additional testing is dependent upon underlying comorbidities. Cancer screening tests based on current standard guidelines are recommended.

Physical Exam

Physical exam findings aid in identifying possible underlying causes of obesity, obesity-related comorbidities, patterns of fat distribution (Fig. 14.2), and mechanical consequences of obesity.

History

The initial assessment should include *medical/psychiatric history* to determine underlying diseases caused by or contributing to obesity, *surgical history*, and *family history* of obesity to evaluate for genetic causes. In addition, *weight history* and *social history* are important to obtain.

Weight History

- Onset of obesity (e.g., childhood, life events, pregnancy)
- Highest nonpregnant weight
- Rate of weight gain
- Frequency of weight cycling (i.e., dieting resulting in losing and regaining weight repeatedly)

Clinical Tip **Physical Exam: Fat Distribution and Lipodystrophies**

Lipodystrophies are a collection of diseases encompassing abnormal distribution of adipose tissue. They are important to identify as they are resistant to traditional weight loss strategies including diet and exercise. Treatment options are very limited and liposuction might show some promise.

One of the most common pathologies within the group is known as lipedema, which is a chronic, progressive, painful, and symmetrical abnormal accumulation of fat in the arms or legs, most commonly in females. It is often disproportionate to the size of the patient's trunk, hands, and feet.

Signs of lipedema include:

- Shouldering sign (right): an abnormal "cut off" at the ankle as lipedema spares the feet while affecting the calf
- Stemmer's sign: Pinch and lift the skin of the second toe; if it is not feasible (positive), it suggests lymphedema. If it does lift (negative), it supports the diagnosis of lipedema.

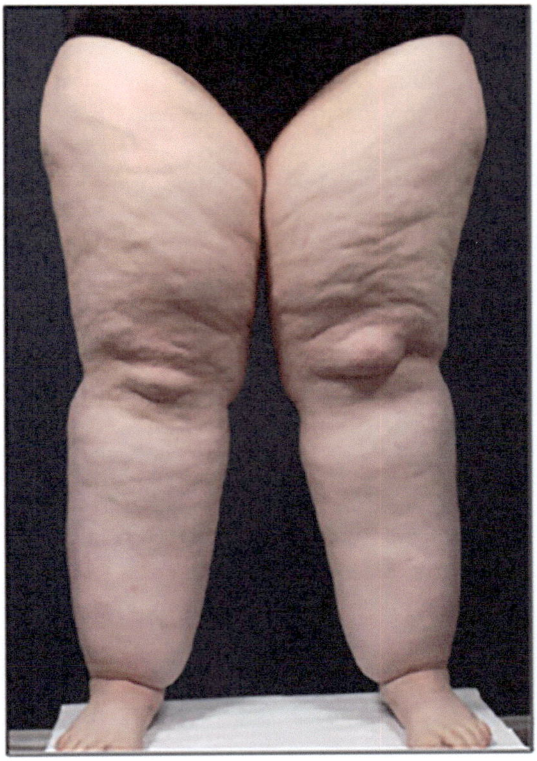

Other diseases include Dercum's disease, which are painful lipomas located on the extremities, and Madelung Disease, which is fat accumulation either around the neck, upper arms and shoulder or pelvis occurring in men with alcohol-induced liver damage.

Fig. 14.2 Clinical tip: physical exam – fat distribution and lipodystrophies (Image reprinted without changes from Wiedner et al., Differential diagnoses and treatment of lipedema, *Plastic and Aesthetic Research* (2020), under open access license Creative Commons Attribution 4.0 International License (https://creativecommons.org/licenses/by/4.0/) [18, 19])

- Current or history of eating disorders: anorexia, bulimia, binge eating, night eating syndrome, sleep-related eating disorder
- Methods used in previous weight loss attempts and sustained weight loss (e.g., weight loss medications, types of diets, bariatric surgery)
- Effect of weight on quality of life
- Nutrition (e.g., 24-hour food recall)
- Activity level, including both sedentary time and physical activity [20]

- Medications that cause weight gain and whether they can be replaced with weight-neutral medications or medications associated with weight loss (Table 14.2) [17, 21, 22]

NSAIDs nonsteroidal anti-inflammatory drugs, *GLP-1* glucagon-like peptide-1, *SGLT2* sodium-glucose co-transporter 2, *DPP-4* dipeptidyl peptidase-4, *ACE* angiotensin-converting enzyme, *ARB* angiotensin II receptor blocker, *CCB* calcium channel blocker, *NNRTI* non-nucleoside reverse transcriptase inhibitors, *PI* protease inhibitors, *IM* intramuscular, *IUD* intrauterine device [17, 21–23].

Social History

- Socioeconomic status
- Stresses related to occupation, relationships, etc.
- Life events contributing to weight such as recent death, family illness, upcoming weddings, change of domicile, job transitions, divorce, etc.
- Mental health status, illicit substance use, smoking, and alcohol intake
- Disrupted circadian rhythms or sleep deprivation [24–26]

Section 2: Lifestyle Management of Obesity

Introduction

The management of overweight and obesity begins with the identification of goals and the understanding that greater weight loss confers greater benefit [27, 28]:

• Overweight without metabolic risk factors	Avoid weight gain
• Overweight with metabolic risk factors	5–10% weight loss over 6 months
• Obesity	5–10% weight loss over 6 months

Lifestyle Modification

The foundation of obesity management is lifestyle modification. More frequent patient contact with providers has been shown to result in greater weight loss. Intensive lifestyle interventions (ILIs) are structured as 14 individual or group sessions over 6 months that provide patients with the knowledge and tools to address their weight [27, 29]. Nutrition, physical activity, and behav-

Table 14.2 Examples of medications associated with weight gain and their alternatives

Medications associated with weight gain and alternatives		
Drug category	Medications associated with weight gain	Medications not associated with weight gain
Antipsychotics	Thioridazine, olanzapine, quetiapine, risperidone, clozapine, lithium	Ziprasidone, lurasidone
Antidepressants	Amitriptyline, nortriptyline, imipramine, doxepin, phenelzine, paroxetine, mirtazapine, lithium	Bupropion, fluoxetine, sertraline
Anti-inflammatories	Glucocorticoids	NSAIDs, inhaled or topical steroids
Antiepileptics	Valproate, carbamazepine, gabapentin, pregabalin	Topiramate, lamotrigine, zonisamide, phenytoin, levetiracetam
Antidiabetics	Insulin, sulfonylureas, thiazolidinediones, meglitinides	Metformin, acarbose, GLP-1 analogues, SGLT2 inhibitors, DPP-4 inhibitors
Migraines	Pizotifen	
Antihistamines	Cyproheptadine, diphenhydramine	Loratadine, decongestants
Antihypertensives	Metoprolol, atenolol, propranolol, terazosin, nadolol	ACE inhibitors, ARBs, CCBs, carvedilol, nebivolol, diuretics
Antiretrovirals	Integrase inhibitors, NNRTIs, PIs	Not applicable
Contraception	Medroxyprogesterone (IM), levonorgestrel (IUD)	Nonhormonal IUD

Changes in medication regimens should always be performed in consultation with the prescriber

ior change are the three tenets of lifestyle modification.

Nutrition

The best diet for weight loss is difficult to identify because of the different pathophysiologies that cause each individual's obesity (i.e., variation in basal metabolic rates (BMR), different homeostatic and hedonic stimuli of food intake). Historically, the "calories-in vs. calories-out" model was widely touted, but there is increasing emphasis on the importance of both quantity and quality of calories. As far as quantity, a caloric deficit is required to achieve weight loss. Expert guidelines recommend a hypocaloric diet (e.g., 1200–1500 kcal for women and 1500–1800 kcal for men) that achieves a deficit of 500–750 kcal/day [27, 28]. Very-low-calorie diets (VLCD), which are typically ≤800 kcal/day and often utilize meal replacements, are effective short-term options that should be performed only under medical supervision [27]. However, the type of calories consumed (i.e., carbohydrate, fat, or protein) may affect the quantity consumed, with some macronutrients resulting in greater satiety than others, thereby making a caloric deficit potentially more attainable.

The macronutrient composition of the "ideal" diet has long been debated. Historically, low-fat diets (<20–30% of total daily calories) [27] were recommended because of the positive association between limiting dietary fat and improvement in plasma cholesterol and cardiovascular risk [30]. Gold standard randomized controlled trials (RCTs) of long duration, such as Look Action for Health in Diabetes (Look AHEAD) and Diabetes Prevention Program (DPP), showed that sustained low-fat diets resulted in weight loss and metabolic benefits, including improvements in blood pressure, lipid profile, and risk for diabetes [31–33]. In the landmark Look AHEAD study, 50.3% of individuals randomized to ILI lost ≥5% of baseline weight at 8 years, as compared to 35.7% in the control group [32].

However, a low-carbohydrate diet (≤150 g/day or <40% of total daily calories) has become increasingly popular because of research suggesting that not all calories are equal. For example, calories obtained from carbohydrates, more so than fat or protein, stimulate insulin secretion, and insulin increases lipogenesis and suppresses lipolysis resulting in an accumulation of fat storage. As such, a low-carbohydrate diet may provide a metabolic advantage to weight loss by reducing insulin levels [36, 37]. Meta-analyses comparing low-carbohydrate to low-fat diets have had conflicting conclusions depending on the protocols of the RCTs included [38, 39], which can vary from <20 g/day to ≤150 g/day of carbohydrate intake. However, the adoption of a very-low-carbohydrate diet (<20-50 g/day), such as the Atkins diet or ketogenic diet, has demonstrated more weight loss than low-fat diets [40] but is limited by poor long-term adherence [41].

Within low-carbohydrate and low-fat diets, the relative contribution of protein varies. Studies have found that high protein intake (>1.0 g/kg/day) is more effective than moderate protein intake (0.8–1.0 g/kg/day) for fat mass loss during weight loss and for fat-free mass preservation during weight maintenance [42].

Diets that avoid macronutrient restrictions, such as the Mediterranean, Dietary Approaches to Stop Hypertension (DASH), vegetarian, or vegan, demonstrate evidence-based benefits in obesity or obesity-related comorbidities [27, 43]. For example, the Mediterranean diet is associated with a roughly 30% reduction in CVD [34]. The DASH diet is a widely recommended intervention for HTN, reducing systolic blood pressure by 5.5 mmHg and diastolic blood pressure by 3.0 mmHg, independent of weight loss [35]. The United States Department of Agriculture (USDA) currently recommends the "MyPlate" strategy for general health [44]. With MyPlate, 50% of each meal comprises fruits and vegetables, 25% carbohydrates, and 25% protein.

Significant public interest has developed in the timing of food consumption, broadly known as intermittent fasting. Intermittent fasting utilizes a variety of eating patterns to achieve a hypocaloric diet (Table 14.3). In alternate-day fasting, individuals adopt a hypocaloric diet every other day and eat a normal or higher caloric diet on the interceding days. With the 5:2 diet, two consecutive or nonconsecutive days of the

Table 14.3 Types of intermittent fasting

	Pattern of eating
Alternate-day fast [47, 48]	Alternating days of very low caloric intake (−75% of baseline) with normal or increased caloric intake (+125% of baseline)
5:2 [49, 50]	2 days per week of hypocaloric intake (500–800 kcal/day) with 5 days per week of normal caloric intake; hypocaloric days can be consecutive or nonconsecutive
Fast-mimicking [51, 52]	Hypocaloric intake (classically 600 kcal/day) for 5–14 days at a time, repeated monthly or "as needed"
Time-restricting feeding [53, 54]	Limiting daily caloric intake to designated hours of the day, most commonly 8 hours of food intake followed by 16 hours of fasting; total caloric intake is not specified

week are dedicated to low calorie intakes. The fast-mimicking diet is defined by an extended period (5–15 consecutive days) of a very-low-calorie diet, which may be repeated at regular intervals. Time-restricted feeding limits daily caloric intake to a specified window of food intake, commonly 8 hours, allowing the individual to fast for the remaining hours of the day. Greater caloric intake earlier in the day (e.g., larger breakfast and smaller dinner; early instead of late time-restricted feeding) results in more weight loss (about 2.5-fold over 12 weeks) and lower 24-hour glucose levels (about 20%) [45, 46].

Overall, because RCTs have demonstrated little clinical difference in long-term weight loss among different macronutrient diet patterns when accompanied by a caloric deficit [43, 55, 56], multiple guidelines recommend any diet that provides the best adherence [27, 28]. Identifying the most effective diet requires individualized counseling and regular feedback.

Physical Activity

Increasing energy expenditure aids in the achievement and maintenance of a caloric deficit required for weight loss. Total energy expenditure (TEE) is partitioned into basal metabolic rate, diet-induced thermogenesis (DIT), non-exercise activity thermogenesis (NEAT), and exercise

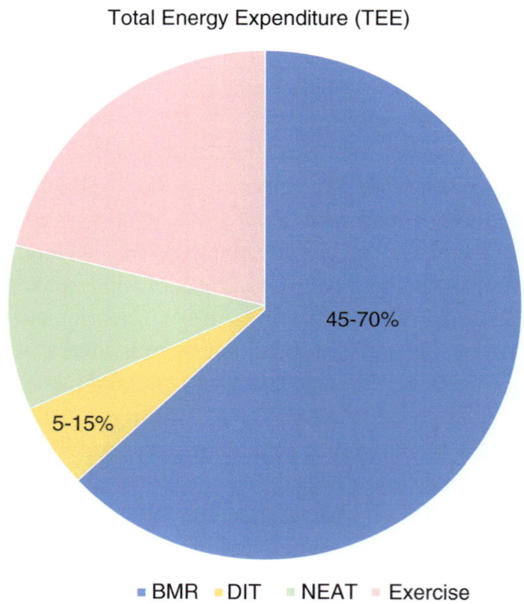

Fig. 14.3 BMR comprises 45–70% of TEE [58]. DIT on a mixed diet contributes 5–15% to TEE [59]. NEAT and exercise, components of physical activity, are targets of interventions to increase TEE. BMR, basal metabolic rate; DIT, diet-induced thermogenesis; NEAT, non-exercise activity thermogenesis

(Fig. 14.3). BMR is the minimum amount of energy required to maintain necessary physiologic functions at rest and is mostly determined by the amount of lean muscle mass. DIT is the energy utilized for the catabolism of food (5–15% of TEE). NEAT encompasses physical activities outside of exercise bouts (e.g., walking to the bus stop, fidgeting, housework) and can vary significantly among individuals. While BMR is the largest contributor to energy expenditure at rest (45–70%), only exercise is significantly modifiable by lifestyle [57].

Cardiovascular Exercise

Physical activity as exercise is categorized as cardiovascular exercise or resistance/strength training. Cardiovascular exercise is often described with three levels of intensity—light, moderate, or vigorous—that are expressed in terms of metabolic equivalent of task (MET) (Table 14.4) [60]. The MET of a particular activity is its rate of energy expenditure compared to the rate of energy expenditure at rest. Light-intensity activ-

Table 14.4 Defined intensity levels of physical activity

	Light intensity	Moderate intensity	Vigorous intensity
MET	<3.0	3.0–5.9	≥6.0
Patient exertion	Easily holds a conversation	Can talk but not sing	Unable to talk secondary to shortness of breath
Examples	Leisurely walking, basic household chores	Brisk walking, dancing, bike riding	Running, climbing stairs

Abbreviations: *MET* metabolic equivalent of task

ity is defined as MET <3.0, moderate-intensity activity is defined by MET 3.0–5.9, and vigorous-intensity activity occurs when MET is at least 6.0. When counseling patients, light-intensity activity may be better described as "able to hold a conversation," moderate-intensity activity as "able to talk but not sing," and vigorous-intensity activity as "too out of breath to talk."

The Department of Health and Human Services (DOHHS) Physical Activity Guidelines Advisory Committee provides evidence-based recommendations to prevent weight gain, achieve weight loss, maintain weight loss, and/or improve overall health with cardiovascular exercise [60].

The DOHHS recommends at least 150 minutes/week of moderate-intensity activity or 75 minutes/week of vigorous-intensity activity to prevent weight gain (Table 14.4). At least 150 minutes/week of moderate-intensity exercise is required to achieve weight loss and maintain weight loss, with many individuals requiring at least 300 minutes/week; these goals may also be attained with >75 minutes/week of vigorous-intensity exercise. Similar to patients' responses to dietary changes and anti-obesity medication, individual response to exercise is heterogeneous. In the landmark Midwest Exercise Trial-1, for example, most men lost weight, but 50% of women gained weight with 225 minutes/week of moderate-intensity cardiovascular exercise [61]. Weight loss is also dose responsive in relation to exercise; more exercise results in greater weight loss [57]. When combined with modest hypocaloric diets, cardiovascular exercise is effective at stimulating more weight loss than diet alone [57, 62].

While the DOHHS provides specific ranges for physical activity targets, data supports health benefits at all levels of activity regardless of weight loss [60]. For example, reducing sedentary time by walking for 2 minutes every hour is associated with a 33% reduction in all-cause mortality [63]. High-intensity interval training (HIIT) of 4-minute bouts is equally effective as moderate-intensity continuous exercise in reducing abdominal fat mass [64]. At least 150 minutes/week of moderate-intensity exercise consistently demonstrates benefits in all-cause mortality, CVD and CVD mortality, HTN, DM2, dyslipidemia, cancers (e.g., colon, breast, endometrium, bladder, kidney, lung, stomach, esophagus), cognition, dementia, anxiety, depression, sleep, bone health, physical function, and fall prevention [60].

Resistance Training (RT)

RT alone has demonstrated varied results in its effects on weight, body fat, and lean muscle mass [57]. RT without caloric restriction reduces body fat but not weight. When added to a hypocaloric diet, it does not provide additional weight or fat loss, but when added to a hypocaloric diet plus aerobic exercise, it does provide more weight loss than either modality alone.

Because weight loss is accompanied by a reduction in BMR [65] and BMR increases with more lean mass, RT may help in preventing weight regain. RT has been shown to increase lean muscle mass in isocaloric diets and mitigate lean muscle loss in hypocaloric diets, and a few studies have demonstrated its effect on increasing metabolism [66, 67].

Behavior

In addition to nutrition and physical activity modifications, behavioral changes also assist in weight loss success. The tenets of behavioral treatment for obesity are goal setting, self-monitoring, and stimulus control [68]. Setting goals for behavior changes should be specific and feasible, with clear delineation of how, when, and where these goals will be achieved. Self-monitoring of food intake, activity, and weight is strongly associated with weight loss and weight maintenance success, with greater success rates correlated to more frequent monitoring [68, 69]. The National Weight Control Registry (NWCR), a database of individuals who have lost ≥30 kg and maintained ≥13.6 kg lost for 5 years or more, found that 75% of participants weighed themselves at least once a week [70]. Stimulus control teaches patients to modify external cues in order to create an environment that is more conducive to behavior change. The classic example has patients identify highly palatable foods and avoid bringing them into the household. Other components of behavior modification include problem solving therapy, cognitive restructuring, coping strategies, stress management, and sleep hygiene and may also provide benefit especially in weight loss maintenance [71].

Section 3: Pharmacological Management of Obesity

Introduction

In 2013, the American Heart Association (AHA), American College of Cardiology (ACC), and The Obesity Society (TOS) released a joint practice guideline on the management of overweight/obesity in adults [27]. As described above, the initial intervention for all patients with overweight or obesity should be a comprehensive lifestyle program, including behavioral and dietary modifications, as well as regular physical activity. However, given the adaptive physiological changes that occur with weight loss, such as decreased metabolic rate and upregulation of orexigenic hormones, lifestyle modifications alone may result in insufficient or unsustainable weight loss [72–74]. For these individuals, anti-obesity medications should be considered to counteract metabolic adaptations, improve adherence to behavioral modifications, and help achieve clinically significant weight loss, defined as ≥5% total body weight loss (TBWL) [22].

Anti-obesity medications should be considered in individuals with a BMI ≥30 kg/m^2 or ≥ 27 kg/m^2 with cardiovascular risk factors (e.g., HTN, insulin resistance, dyslipidemia, elevated WC) or obesity-associated comorbidities (e.g., OSA, NAFLD) if a comprehensive lifestyle regimen fails to result in ≥5% weight loss and improvement in health targets. Despite proven efficacy for anti-obesity medications, they are underused clinically [75]. Identifiable barriers include physician and patient reluctance to discuss obesity, lack of insurance reimbursement, medical contraindications, and adverse effects of the medications [76]. Joint guidelines released in 2016 by the Endocrine Society, the European Society of Endocrinology, and The Obesity Society provide detailed clinical practice guidelines for the pharmacologic management of obesity [22].

Tailoring the Regimen to the Patient

The decision of which pharmacotherapy to initiate is based on the patient's unique challenges with weight loss, the presence of coexisting comorbidities or social habits, potential drug-drug interactions, and medication contraindications. Obesity is considered a chronic disease, and therefore a majority of agents have been approved for long-term use.

Once pharmacotherapy for weight management is initiated, the following general prescribing guidelines should be followed:

- Reassess patients at regular intervals (preferably at least once monthly during the first 3 months of treatment) to assess efficacy (typically defined as ≥5% TBWL over 3 months) and tolerability of the medication.
- If ineffective, intolerable, or unsafe, the medication should be discontinued, and another agent may be considered.
- There can be significant individual variability in response to medications for weight management. Lack of response to one medication should not preclude consideration of other medications.
- When a patient reaches a weight loss plateau (i.e., no weight loss over 1–3 months) or expe-

riences weight regain, abrupt discontinuation of a medication may lead to increased weight. Instead, it is appropriate to consider dose escalation or the addition of another pharmacotherapy to target multiple pathways simultaneously.
- Once a desired weight has been achieved, the provider may consider reducing the dose of one or more medications or the number of overall medications the patient is on, though with great caution and careful attention to weight fluctuation and hunger/fullness.
- Given that obesity is a chronic disease, patients will require long-term treatment and follow-up to maintain weight loss and prevent or treat relapse.

Medications

This topic is divided into two parts. Part A discusses medications that are approved by the Food and Drug Administration (FDA) for weight loss. Part B highlights medications used for the treatment of DM2 that are associated with weight loss as many patients with obesity also have insulin resistance and/or DM2 (Tables 14.5 and 14.6).

Table 14.5 Categorization of available weight loss medications

Part	Medications
A. FDA-approved pharmacotherapy	Phentermine Phentermine/topiramate Orlistat Naltrexone/bupropion Liraglutide 3.0 mg
B. DM2 medications associated with weight loss	Metformin SGLT2 inhibitors (canagliflozin, dapagliflozin, empagliflozin, and ertugliflozin) Pramlintide GLP-1 receptor agonists other than liraglutide 3.0 mg (liraglutide 1.8 mg, semaglutide, dulaglutide, exenatide, lixisenatide)

FDA Food and Drug Administration, *DM2* type 2 diabetes mellitus, *GLP-1* glucagon-like peptide-1, *SGLT2* sodium-glucose transporter 2

FDA-Approved Pharmacotherapy for Weight Management

Phentermine

Phentermine received FDA approval for weight management in 1959. It is approved for short-term use (3 months) in adolescents over the age of 16 and adults, as longer-term safety trials have not been performed. However, it is approved for chronic weight management in combination with topiramate and used long term in an off-label fashion with close monitoring. Phentermine is a sympathomimetic agent that results in hypothalamic release of norepinephrine causing appetite suppression [87]. A number of structurally similar adrenergic agonists, including diethylpropion and phendimetrazine, are also available in the United States and global markets.

Efficacy

A meta-analysis of 9 studies from 1975 to1999 found an average weight loss of 3.6 kg with phentermine 15–30 mg/day for 2–24 weeks of treatment [88]. A more recent, 28-week RCT comparing the efficacy of phentermine and/or topiramate monotherapy with phentermine/topiramate combination therapy versus placebo found a weight loss of 5.45% with phentermine 7.5 mg/day and 6.06% with phentermine 15 mg/day, versus 1.71% with placebo [78].

Dosing and Precautions

Phentermine is available in capsule/tablet formulation with recommended dosing of 15–37.5 mg daily. A low-dose 8 mg tablet is available for use up to 3 times daily. The lowest effective dose should be used with dose escalation based on managing hunger and weight plateaus. Phentermine should be avoided 6–8 hours prior to bedtime due to risk of insomnia. It is a Schedule IV controlled substance due to pharmacologic similarity to amphetamines. However, phentermine at higher-than recommended doses and for prolonged duration (up to 21 years) has not been

Table 14.6 FDA-approved pharmacotherapy for weight loss

	Mechanism of action	Clinical effects	Estimated % TBWL	Adverse events (most common)	Contraindications	Discontinuation criteria
Phentermine [77]	Norepinephrine-releasing agent	Appetite suppression	5.45% at 28 weeks with 7.5 mg daily, 6.06% with 15 mg daily, versus 1.71% with placebo [78]	Dizziness Dry mouth Insomnia Irritability HTN Tachycardia	Hx of CVD (arrhythmia, HF, CAD, stroke, uncontrolled HTN) Hyperthyroidism Angle closure glaucoma Agitated states Hx of drug abuse Concurrent MAOI use (during or 14 days after) Pregnancy or breastfeeding	Not specified
Phentermine/ topiramate [79]	Norepinephrine-releasing agent /blocks voltage-gated Na channels and Ca channels and inhibits carbonic anhydrase	Appetite suppression, enhanced satiety	7.8% at 1 year with 7.5/46 mg daily, 9.8% with 15/92 mg daily, versus 1.2% with placebo [80]	Paresthesia Dizziness Dysgeusia Insomnia Constipation Dry mouth	Hyperthyroidism Angle closure glaucoma Concurrent MAOI use (during or 14 days after) Pregnancy or breastfeeding[a]	<3% weight loss at 12 weeks on 7.5/46 mg daily (or increase dose) <5% weight loss at 12 weeks on 15/92 mg daily
Orlistat [81]	Lipase inhibitor	Caloric deficit via unabsorbed triglycerides	8.8% at 1 year with 120 mg TID versus 5.8% with placebo [82]	Steatorrhea Oily spotting Fatty stool Fecal urgency Flatus with discharge Fecal incontinence	Chronic malabsorption syndrome Cholestasis Pregnancy or breastfeeding	Not specified
Bupropion/ naltrexone [83]	Norepinephrine and dopamine reuptake inhibitor/opioid receptor antagonist	Appetite suppression via effects on the brain's appetite regulatory center and reward system	5.0% at 56 weeks with 160/16 mg BID versus 1.3% with placebo [84]	Nausea/vomiting Diarrhea Constipation Headache Dizziness Insomnia Dry mouth	Hx of suicidal behavior[b] Concurrent MAOI use (during or 14 days after) Opioid agonist or partial agonist use Abrupt discontinuation of benzodiazepines, alcohol, barbiturates, or antiepileptic medications Uncontrolled HTN Seizure disorder or hx of seizure Anorexia nervosa or bulimia Pregnancy or breastfeeding	<5% weight loss at 12 weeks

Liraglutide 3.0 mg [85]	GLP-1 receptor agonist	Appetite suppression via effects on the brain's regulatory center	8.0% at 56 weeks with 3 mg daily versus 2.6% with placebo [86]	Hypoglycemia (especially if used in combination with insulin) Diarrhea Constipation Abdominal pain Dyspepsia Increased lipase Headache Fatigue Dizziness Acute pancreatitis Cholelithiasis	Personal or family hx of medullary thyroid cancer or MEN2[c] Pregnancy or breastfeeding	<4% weight loss at 16 weeks

Abbreviations: BID twice daily, *CAD* coronary artery disease, *CVD* cardiovascular disease, *eGFR* estimated glomerular filtration rate, *GLP-1* glucagon-like peptide-1, *HF* heart failure, *HTN* hypertension, *hx* history, *MAOI* monoamine oxidase inhibitor, *MEN2* multiple endocrine neoplasia syndrome type 2, *TBWL* total body weight loss, *TID* three times daily

[a]The FDA requires a Risk Evaluation and Mitigation Strategy (REMS) given the increased risk of orofacial clefts with topiramate when taken during the first trimester of pregnancy [79]

[b]Black box warning: increased risk of suicidal thoughts and behaviors in children, adolescents, and young adults taking antidepressants for major depressive disorder and other psychiatric disorders. However, no evidence of suicidality was found in phase 3 studies

[c]Black box warning: risk of thyroid C-cell tumors in rodents. However, no evidence was found of comparable malignancy in humans

shown to result in addiction, intoxication, withdrawal, or medication abuse [89].

Phentermine/Topiramate Extended Release

Phentermine/topiramate combination therapy was approved by the FDA in 2012 for chronic weight management. The phentermine/topiramate capsule is designed such that the phentermine component peaks in the morning, while the topiramate component peaks in the afternoon [90]. Topiramate is FDA approved for the treatment of epilepsy and for migraine prophylaxis. Although topiramate monotherapy has not been approved for weight management, topiramate can be successfully used without phentermine for weight loss. It can be particularly helpful in the off-label treatment of night-eating syndrome and binge-eating disorder [91, 92]. Topiramate is thought to cause weight loss via increased satiety and appetite suppression through a combination of enhanced GABA activity, glutamate receptor antagonism, blockage of neuronal voltage-dependent sodium channels, lipogenesis suppression, increased insulin sensitization and adiponectin secretion, and weak carbonic anhydrase inhibition [93].

Efficacy

The efficacy of phentermine/topiramate was evaluated in three RCTs:

- *EQUIP*: At 56 weeks, significantly more weight loss was seen with phentermine/topiramate 3.75/23 mg/day and 15/92 mg/day versus placebo (5.1% and 10.9% of baseline body weight, versus 1.6% with placebo). Several markers of cardiometabolic function (WC, systolic and diastolic blood pressure, fasting glucose, and cholesterol) significantly improved with phentermine/topiramate 15/92 mg/day versus placebo [94].
- *CONQUER*: At 56 weeks, significantly more weight loss was seen with phentermine/topiramate 7.5/46 mg/day and 15/92 mg/day versus placebo (7.8% and 9.8% of baseline body weight, versus 1.2% with placebo). Significantly more study participants achieved ≥5% and ≥10% TBWL with respective phentermine/topiramate doses versus placebo [80].
- *SEQUEL*: A 2-year extension study of the CONQUER trial. Weight loss of 9.3%, 10.5%, and 1.8% was seen with phentermine/topiramate 7.5/46 mg/day, 15/92 mg/day, and placebo. Significantly more patients in the treatment group achieved ≥5%, 10%, 15%, and 20% weight loss. The treatment group required fewer antihypertensive agents than the placebo group, despite having similar blood pressure readings at the study's conclusion. A decreased rate of incident DM2 was noted in the treatment group, with a reduction in progression to diabetes compared to placebo by 54% and 76% for phentermine/topiramate 7.5/46 mg/day and 15/92 mg/day. There was also a significant reduction in HbA1c in the treatment group versus placebo group for those with preexisting diabetes [95].

Dosing and Precautions

Phentermine/topiramate is available in a fixed-dose capsule. Dosing is initiated at 3.75/23 mg for 14 days, increasing to 7.5/46 mg for 12 weeks, with subsequent escalation as needed to 11.25/69 mg and 15/92 mg. The 3.75/23 and 11.25/69 doses are intended for titration purposes. When discontinuing phentermine/topiramate 15/92 mg, the dose should be tapered to one dose every other day for 1 week before stopping in order to reduce the risk of precipitating a seizure. Due to the phentermine component, it is a Schedule IV controlled substance in the United States [79].

Orlistat

Orlistat received FDA approval for the management of obesity in adults 18 years and older in 1999, and in adolescents age 12 and older in 2003. Orlistat reversibly inhibits pancreatic and gastric lipases, preventing 30% of triglycerides from being digested and absorbed within the gastrointestinal tract.

Efficacy

In the XENDOS study, significantly greater weight loss with orlistat 120 mg TID than placebo was seen at 1 year (10.6 kg versus 6.2 kg) [96]. This weight change remained statistically significant at the end of the four-year trial. Orlistat treatment was associated with a 37.3% risk reduction in the incidence of DM2. A meta-analysis of pharmacotherapeutic options for obesity found that orlistat treatment was associated with a reduced incidence of DM2 and improved glycemic control, as well as improved cholesterol (total and LDL) and blood pressure [97].

Dosing and Precautions

Orlistat is available in capsule form at a recommended dose of 120 mg TID, to be taken during or up to 1 hour after a meal containing fat. An over-the-counter half-dose formulation (60 mg TID) is also available that results in 25% TBWL with those with a BMI of 25 and above and 18 years and older. Use is limited by gastrointestinal side effects given its mechanism of action. It requires a 2- or 4-hour gap to prevent interference with the absorption of a number of medications, including levothyroxine, antiretroviral medications, antiepileptic agents, cyclosporine, and fat-soluble vitamins.

Naltrexone Sustained Release (SR)/ Bupropion SR

Bupropion, a norepinephrine and dopamine reuptake inhibitor, was approved by the FDA for the treatment of depression in the 1980s, and for smoking cessation in 1997. Naltrexone, an opioid receptor antagonist, was approved by the FDA for the treatment of opiate dependency in 1984, and for the treatment of alcohol addiction in 1994. The combination of naltrexone SR/bupropion SR (N/B) was approved by the FDA for the treatment of obesity in 2014. Bupropion stimulates hypothalamic proopiomelanocortin (POMC) neurons in the arcuate nucleus, which leads to release of alpha-melanocyte-stimulating hormone (α-MSH; a potent anorectic neuropeptide). Release of α-MSH has downstream effects of increasing energy expenditure and decreasing food intake. Naltrexone antagonizes an inhibitory feedback loop that limits bupropion's anorectic properties [98, 99]. Combined, bupropion and naltrexone have a synergistic effect [98].

Efficacy

The combination of N/B was found to lead to significant weight loss through four 56-week, phase 3, multicenter, double-blind, placebo-controlled trials: Contrave Obesity Research (COR)-I, COR-II, and COR-Behavior Modification (COR-BMOD) and COR-Diabetes. COR-I, COR-II, and COR-BMOD evaluated patients with a BMI of 30 kg/m^2 or greater or a BMI of 27 kg/m^2 or greater and at least one weight-related comorbidity. COR-Diabetes enrolled patients with a BMI of 27 kg/m^2 or greater with DM2 and with or without dyslipidemia and HTN.

- *COR-I*: At 56 weeks, greater weight loss was seen with naltrexone SR 32 mg plus bupropion SR 360 mg (N/B32) versus placebo (6.1% versus 1.3%, respectively). Significantly more subjects on N/B32 lost ≥5% body weight compared with placebo (48% versus 15%) [84].
- *COR-II*: At 56 weeks, subjects on N/B32 had superior outcomes in mean changes in body weight versus placebo (6.4% versus 1.2%, respectively). A greater percentage of those on N/B 32 mg also achieved ≥5% weight loss versus placebo (50.5% versus 12.1%) [100].
- *COR-BMOD*: This study compared patients who received intensive group behavioral modifications in addition to medication or placebo. At 56 weeks, patients on N/B had superior outcomes (9.3% versus 5.1% weight loss; 66.4% versus 42.5% lost ≥5% body weight on N/B versus placebo) [101].
- *COR-Diabetes*: Subjects on N/B lost more weight than subjects receiving placebo (5.0% versus 1.8%) and more subjects achieved ≥5% weight loss on N/B versus placebo (44.5% versus 18.9%,). Subjects on N/B also had a greater reduction in HbA1c (0.6%) compared to placebo (0.1%) [102].

Of note, all subjects on treatment in the COR trials achieved significant improvements in triglycerides and high-density lipoproteins, and all trials except for COR-Diabetes found significant improvements in waist circumference, insulin resistance index (HOMA-IR), and fasting insulin.

Dosing and Precautions

Each N/B tablet contains naltrexone 8 mg and bupropion 90 mg. Dosing is started at 1 tablet daily and increased by 1 tablet per week as needed up to a maximum dose of two tablets twice daily (naltrexone 32 mg and bupropion 360 mg daily). It should not be prescribed if the patient is on or is planning to be on an opiate, opiate agonist, or partial agonist, as naltrexone can antagonize the effect leading to inadequate pain relief.

Although neither naltrexone nor bupropion is FDA approved as monotherapy for the treatment of obesity, off-label use of bupropion monotherapy is used effectively as part of a tailored regimen based on a patient's individual presentation.

Liraglutide 3.0 mg

Liraglutide is a glucagon-like peptide-1 (GLP-1) receptor agonist that was approved in 2010 by the FDA for the treatment of DM2 (liraglutide 1.8 mg). In 2017, an additional indication was approved by the FDA for the use of liraglutide 1.8 mg to reduce the risk of major adverse cardiovascular events in patients with DM2 and established CVD. Liraglutide 3.0 mg was approved by the FDA in 2014 for the treatment of obesity.

Human GLP-1 is an incretin hormone secreted in the gut in response to nutrients with a half-life of 1–2 minutes. It binds to GLP-1 receptors which are expressed in various tissues throughout the body. GLP-1 slows gastric emptying at 1 hour and reduces food intake. GLP-1 regulates appetite centers within the brain [103]. Peripherally, it stimulates insulin secretion and decreases glucagon secretion decreasing energy storage. Liraglutide has 97% homology to human GLP-1, but with a half-life of approximately 13 hours.

Efficacy

The efficacy of liraglutide was demonstrated in the Satiety and Clinical Adiposity – Liraglutide Evidence (SCALE) trials which were RCTs conducted over 56 weeks.

- *SCALE Obesity and Prediabetes*: This trial evaluated liraglutide 3.0 mg in patients with overweight or obesity and prediabetes; it found significantly greater weight loss with liraglutide 3.0 mg than with placebo (8.0% versus 2.6%) [86].
- *SCALE Diabetes*: This trial evaluated liraglutide 3.0 mg in patients with overweight or obesity and DM2; it found significantly greater weight in the liraglutide 3.0 mg than with placebo (5.9% versus 2.0%) [104].
- *SCALE Maintenance*: This trial enrolled participants with obesity or overweight and had dyslipidemia or HTN who lost at least 5% of initial weight during a run-in period of 4–12 weeks (mean weight loss was 6%). After successful completion of the run-in period, participants were randomized to liraglutide 3.0 mg or placebo for 56 weeks. Participants randomized to liraglutide 3.0 mg were more successful at maintaining weight loss versus those on placebo (81.4% versus 48.9%, respectively). In addition, participants receiving liraglutide 3.0 mg were more likely to lose an additional 5% or more of their body weight versus placebo (50.5% versus 21.8%) [105].

Dosing and Precautions

Liraglutide is administered once daily as a subcutaneous injection into the abdomen, thigh, or upper arm. It is initiated at 0.6 mg daily for 1 week and then increased as needed by 0.6 mg weekly until a maximum dose of 3.0 mg daily is achieved. Titration can be slowed if the patient exhibits a response at a lower dose or if the patient experiences side effects.

Diabetes Medications Associated with Weight Loss

In addition to GLP-1 receptor agonists, a number of medications that are approved for the treatment of DM2, while not FDA approved for weight management, have been shown to be associated with weight loss. These medications can be considered as part of a weight-centric approach to treating diabetes [22].

Metformin

Metformin, available in Europe since the 1950s, received FDA approval for the treatment of DM2 in adults in 1994, and for children over age 10 in 2000. Numerous possible mechanisms by which metformin causes weight loss have been proposed. Metformin decreases hepatic gluconeogenesis, decreases intestinal absorption of glucose, and increases insulin sensitivity via increased peripheral glucose uptake and utilization [106]. By improving glycemic control and decreasing circulating glucose levels, there is less glucose available for storage, and this may lead to subsequent weight loss [107]. By decreasing circulating insulin levels, metformin prevents postprandial hypoglycemia and associated hypoglycemia-induced hunger [108]. It has been shown to induce a catabolic state by increasing AMP-activated protein kinase [109]. Metformin also has hormonal effects that can influence hunger, satiety, and weight setpoints. It has been shown to increase leptin sensitivity in rats and increase GLP-1 activity in humans [110, 111]. Most recently, rodent models have shown metformin to increase circulating levels of GDF15, a peptide hormone which acts in the hindbrain to suppress appetite and increase energy expenditure [112].

Metformin's role in improving glycemic control is well established. Multiple studies have additionally found that metformin promotes modest weight loss and can confer a cardiometabolic benefit in populations both with and without diabetes. Metformin can be useful in mitigating medication-induced weight gain, including weight gain secondary to antipsychotic medications [113]. A meta-analysis of 13 studies in patients with overweight/obesity without an obesity-related comorbidity found that metformin use was associated with a significant reduction in body weight (weighted mean difference 2.33 kg) and BMI (weighted mean difference 0.57 kg/m^2) [114]. In the DPP, patients with overweight/obesity and prediabetes were randomized to receive standard lifestyle modification with placebo, standard lifestyle modification with metformin 850 mg twice daily, or intensive lifestyle modification [115]. Total body weight was significantly reduced in the metformin group versus standard lifestyle at both 1 and 2 years (2.7% versus 0.43%, and 2.1% versus 0.02%, respectively), albeit less than in the intensive lifestyle group. However, recently published long-term follow-up data found that the metformin group maintained a weight loss of 6.2% of baseline weight between years 6 and 15, compared to 3.7% in the intensive lifestyle group and 2.8% in the placebo group [116].

Canagliflozin, Dapagliflozin, Empagliflozin, and Ertugliflozin

Canagliflozin, dapagliflozin, empagliflozin, and ertugliflozin are sodium glucose co-transporter 2 (SGLT2) inhibitors. SGLT2 is expressed in the proximal tubule of the kidney and mediates reabsorption of the majority of the filtered glucose load. SGLT2 inhibitors promote renal excretion of glucose, which leads to modest weight loss and moderate decreases in blood pressure [117, 118]. SGLT2 inhibitors are FDA approved for the treatment of DM2. These medications are not FDA approved for weight loss, but they have been associated with weight loss of 1–3 kg. Therefore, some providers prescribe these medications as part of a weight-centric approach to diabetes [119].

Pramlintide

Pramlintide is an amylin analogue that is FDA approved for the treatment of type 1 diabetes and insulin-treated DM2. Amylin is an amino acid peptide that is stored in pancreatic beta cells and is co-secreted with insulin. Amylin complements insulin in glucose regulation and leads to slowing of postprandial rise of glucagon, slowed gastric emptying, and reduction in food intake [120]. It also binds to receptors in the area postrema, which may contribute to satiety [121]. With amylin, endogenous and exogenous sources of glucose are better regulated, and insulin can match physiologic needs more closely. The effects of amylin are glucose dependent, so it is administered with meals. Pramlintide is not FDA approved for weight loss but is associated with weight loss and therefore is used by providers as part of a weight-centric approach to the treatment of diabetes.

Liraglutide 1.8 mg Daily, Semaglutide (Subcutaneous and Oral), Dulaglutide, Exenatide (Immediate Release and Extended Release), and Lixisenatide

GLP-1 receptor agonists are discussed in detail above under liraglutide 3.0 mg daily. While liraglutide 3.0 mg daily is a GLP-1 receptor agonist that is FDA approved specifically for weight loss, there are other GLP-1 receptor agonists that are FDA approved for DM2, which are associated with weight loss and may be prescribed as a weight-centric approach to the treatment of type 2 diabetes. These medications include liraglutide 1.8 mg daily, semaglutide (subcutaneous and oral), dulaglutide, exenatide (immediate release and extended release), and lixisenatide.

Conclusion

The evaluation of individuals with obesity should include a detailed weight history and exam with special attention to signs or symptoms of obesity-related comorbidities. The cornerstones of weight management are lifestyle modifications guided by nutrition, physical activity, and behavioral counseling. As weight loss achieved by lifestyle modifications alone is often limited and difficult to maintain, anti-obesity medication is an additional tool to support patients in achieving and maintaining clinically significant weight loss in order to improve health.

References

1. Ward ZJ, Bleich SN, Cradock AL, Barrett JL, Giles CM, Flax C, et al. Projected U.S. state-level prevalence of adult obesity and severe obesity. N Engl J Med. 2019;381(25):2440–50.
2. Centers for Disease Control and Prevention. Prevalence of self-reported obesity among U.S. adults by state and territory. Behavioral Risk Factor Surveillance System 2018.
3. Pi-Sunyer FX. Comorbidities of overweight and obesity: current evidence and research issues. Med Sci Sports Exerc. 1999;31(11 SUPPL): S602–8.
4. Bean M. Weighing the cost of care: how hospitals accommodate obese patients. 2016.
5. Rubino F, Puhl RM, Cummings DE, Eckel RH, Ryan DH, Mechanick JI, et al. Joint international consensus statement for ending stigma of obesity. Nat Med. 2020;26(4):485–97.
6. Phelan SM, Burgess DJ, Yeazel MW, Hellerstedt WL, Griffin JM, van Ryn M. Impact of weight bias and stigma on quality of care and outcomes for patients with obesity. Obes Rev. 2015;16(4):319–26.
7. Albury C, Strain WD, Brocq SL, Logue J, Lloyd C, Tahrani A. The importance of language in engagement between health-care professionals and people living with obesity: a joint consensus statement. Lancet Diabetes Endocrinol. 2020;8(5):447–55.
8. Teachman BA, Gapinski KD, Brownell KD, Rawlins M, Jeyaram S. Demonstrations of implicit anti-fat bias: the impact of providing causal information and evoking empathy. Health Psychol. 2003;22(1):68–78.
9. Fujioka K, Crockett T. In: Bray GA, Bouchard C, editors. Obesity and the primary care physician. 4th ed. Taylor & Francis; 2014.
10. Cerhan JR, Moore SC, Jacobs EJ, Kitahara CM, Rosenberg PS, Adami HO, et al. A pooled analysis of waist circumference and mortality in 650,000 adults. Mayo Clin Proc. 2014;89(3):335–45.
11. Jacobs EJ, Newton CC, Wang Y, Patel AV, McCullough ML, Campbell PT, et al. Waist circumference and all-cause mortality in a large US cohort. Arch Intern Med. 2010;170(15):1293–301.
12. World Health Organization (WHO) Expert Consultation. Waist circumference and waist-hip ratio. World Health Organization; 2008.
13. Ma WY, Yang CY, Shih SR, Hsieh HJ, Hung CS, Chiu FC, et al. Measurement of waist circumference: midabdominal or iliac crest? Diabetes Care. 2013;36(6):1660–6.
14. Pouliot MC, Després JP, Lemieux S, Moorjani S, Bouchard C, Tremblay A, et al. Waist circumference and abdominal sagittal diameter: best simple anthropometric indexes of abdominal visceral adipose tissue accumulation and related cardiovascular risk in men and women. Am J Cardiol. 1994;73(7):460–8.
15. Vazquez G, Duval S, Jacobs DR, Silventoinen K. Comparison of body mass index, waist circumference, and waist/hip ratio in predicting incident diabetes: a meta-analysis. Epidemiol Rev. 2007;29:115–28.
16. Romero-Corral A, Somers VK, Sierra-Johnson J, Thomas RJ, Collazo-Clavell ML, Korinek J, et al. Accuracy of body mass index in diagnosing obesity in the adult general population. Int J Obes. 2008;32(6):959–66.
17. Kushner RF, Bray GA. Classification and evaluation of the overweight patient. 2014.
18. Wiedner M, Aghajanzadeh D, Richter DF. Differential diagnoses and treatment of lipedema. Plast Aesthetic Res. 2020;7(10):1–10.

19. Rapprich S, Baum S, Kaak I, Kottmann T, Podda M. Treatment of lipoedema using liposuction: results of our own surveys. Phlebologie. 2015;44:121–32.
20. Kushner RF, Batsis JA, Butsch WS, Davis N, Golden A, Halperin F, et al. Weight history in clinical practice: the state of the science and future directions. Obesity (Silver Spring). 2020;28(1):9–17.
21. Igel LI, Kumar RB, Saunders KH, Aronne LJ. Practical use of pharmacotherapy for obesity. Gastroenterology. 2017;152(7):1765–79.
22. Apovian CM, Aronne LJ, Bessesen DH, McDonnell ME, Murad MH, Pagotto U, et al. Pharmacological management of obesity: an endocrine society clinical practice guideline. J Clin Endocrinol Metab. 2015;100(2):342–62.
23. Sax PE, Erlandson KM, Lake JE, McComsey GA, Orkin C, Esser S, et al. Weight gain following initiation of antiretroviral therapy: risk factors in randomized comparative clinical trials. Clin Infect Dis. 2020;71(6):1379–89.
24. Obayashi K, Saeki K, Iwamoto J, Okamoto N, Tomioka K, Nezu S, et al. Exposure to light at night, nocturnal urinary melatonin excretion, and obesity/dyslipidemia in the elderly: a cross-sectional analysis of the HEIJO-KYO study. J Clin Endocrinol Metab. 2013;98(1):337–44.
25. Fonken LK, Lieberman RA, Weil ZM, Nelson RJ. Dim light at night exaggerates weight gain and inflammation associated with a high-fat diet in male mice. Endocrinology. 2013;154(10):3817–25.
26. Engin A. Circadian rhythms in diet-induced obesity, vol. 960. New York: Springer New York LLC; 2017. p. 19–52.
27. Jensen MD, Ryan DH, Apovian CM, Ard JD, Comuzzie AG, Donato KA, et al. 2013 AHA/ACC/TOS guideline for the management of overweight and obesity in adults: a report of the American College of Cardiology/American Heart Association Task Force on Practice Guidelines and The Obesity Society. Circulation. 2014;129(25 SUPPL. 1):102–38.
28. Garvey WT, Mechanick JI, Brett EM, Garber AJ, Hurley DL, Jastreboff AM, et al. American Association of Clinical Endocrinologists (AACE) and American College of Endocrinology (ACE) comprehensive clinical practice guidelines for medical care of patients with obesity. Endocr Pract. 2016;22(Suppl 3):1–203.
29. Wadden TA, Tronieri JS, Butryn ML. Lifestyle modification approaches for the treatment of obesity in adults. Am Psychol. 2020;75(2):235–51.
30. McGandy RB, Hegsted DM, Stare FJ. Dietary fats, carbohydrates and atherosclerotic vascular disease. N Engl J Med. 1967;277(4):186–92. contd.
31. Knowler WC, Barrett-Connor E, Fowler SE, Hamman RF, Lachin JM, Walker EA, et al. Reduction in the incidence of type 2 diabetes with lifestyle intervention or metformin. N Engl J Med. 2002;346(6):393–403.
32. Pi-Sunyer X. The look AHEAD trial: a review and discussion of its outcomes. Curr Nutr Rep. 2014;3(4):387–91.
33. Diabetes Prevention Program Research Group. The Diabetes Prevention Program (DPP): description of lifestyle intervention. Diabetes Care. 2002;25(12):2165–71.
34. Estruch R, Ros E, Salas-Salvadó J, Covas MI, Corella D, Arós F, et al. Primary prevention of cardiovascular disease with a mediterranean diet supplemented with extra-virgin olive oil or nuts. N Engl J Med. 2018;378(25):1–14.
35. Harsha DW, Lin PH, Obarzanek E, Karanja NM, Moore TJ, Caballero B. Dietary approaches to stop hypertension: a summary of study results. DASH Collaborative Research Group. J Am Diet Assoc. 1999;99(8 Suppl):S35–9.
36. Ludwig DS, Ebbeling CB. The carbohydrate-insulin model of obesity: beyond "calories in, calories out". JAMA Intern Med. 2018;178(8):1098–103.
37. Westman EC, Feinman RD, Mavropoulos JC, Vernon MC, Volek JS, Wortman JA, et al. Low-carbohydrate nutrition and metabolism. Am J Clin Nutr. 2007;86(2):276–84.
38. Hu T, Mills KT, Yao L, Demanelis K, Eloustaz M, Yancy WS Jr, et al. Effects of low-carbohydrate diets versus low-fat diets on metabolic risk factors: a meta-analysis of randomized controlled clinical trials. Am J Epidemiol. 2012;176(Suppl):S44–54.
39. Tobias DK, Chen M, Manson JE, Ludwig DS, Willett W, Hu FB. Effect of low-fat diet interventions versus other diet interventions on long-term weight change in adults: a systematic review and meta-analysis. Lancet Diabetes Endocrinol. 2015;3(12):968–79.
40. Bueno NB, de Melo IS, de Oliveira SL, da Rocha AT. Very-low-carbohydrate ketogenic diet v. low-fat diet for long-term weight loss: a meta-analysis of randomised controlled trials. Br J Nutr. 2013;110(7):1178–87.
41. Athinarayanan SJ, Adams RN, Hallberg SJ, McKenzie AL, Bhanpuri NH, Campbell WW, et al. Long-term effects of a novel continuous remote care intervention including nutritional ketosis for the management of Type 2 diabetes: a 2-year non-randomized clinical trial. Front Endocrinol (Lausanne). 2019;10:348.
42. Westerterp-Plantenga MS, Lemmens SG, Westerterp KR. Dietary protein - its role in satiety, energetics, weight loss and health. Br J Nutr. 2012;108(Suppl 2):S105–12.
43. Shai I, Schwarzfuch D, Yaakov H, Shaha DR, Witkow S, Greenberg I. Weight loss with a low-carbohydrate, mediterranean, or low-fat diet. N Engl J Med. 2009;362(15):1329–38.
44. United States Department of Agriculture. ChooseMyPlate Alexandria, VA: United States Department of Agriculture (USDA) Center for

Nutrition Policy & Promotion; 1994. Available from: www.choosemyplate.gov.
45. Jakubowicz D, Barnea M, Wainstein J, Froy O. High caloric intake at breakfast vs. dinner differentially influences weight loss of overweight and obese women. Obesity (Silver Spring). 2013;21(12):2504–12.
46. Hutchison AT, Regmi P, Manoogian ENC, Fleischer JG, Wittert GA, Panda S, et al. Time-restricted feeding improves glucose tolerance in men at risk for Type 2 diabetes: a randomized crossover trial. Obesity (Silver Spring). 2019;27(5):724–32.
47. Varady KA, Bhutani S, Klempel MC, Lamarche B. Improvements in LDL particle size and distribution by short-term alternate day modified fasting in obese adults. Br J Nutr. 2011;105(4):580–3.
48. Trepanowski JF, Kroeger CM, Barnosky A, Klempel MC, Bhutani S, Hoddy KK, et al. Effect of alternate-day fasting on weight loss, weight maintenance, and cardioprotection among metabolically healthy obese adults: a randomized clinical trial. JAMA Intern Med. 2017;177(7):930–8.
49. Harvie M, Wright C, Pegington M, McMullan D, Mitchell E, Martin B, et al. The effect of intermittent energy and carbohydrate restriction v. daily energy restriction on weight loss and metabolic disease risk markers in overweight women. Br J Nutr. 2013;110(8):1534–47.
50. Harvie MN, Pegington M, Mattson MP, Frystyk J, Dillon B, Evans G, et al. The effects of intermittent or continuous energy restriction on weight loss and metabolic disease risk markers: a randomized trial in young overweight women. Int J Obes. 2011;35(5):714–27.
51. Brandhorst S, Choi IY, Wei M, Cheng CW, Sedrakyan S, Navarrete G, et al. A periodic diet that mimics fasting promotes multi-system regeneration, enhanced cognitive performance, and healthspan. Cell Metab. 2015;22(1):86–99.
52. Longo VD, Panda S. Fasting, circadian rhythms, and time-restricted feeding in healthy lifespan. Cell Metab. 2016;23(6):1048–59.
53. Gabel K, Hoddy KK, Haggerty N, Song J, Kroeger CM, Trepanowski JF, et al. Effects of 8-hour time restricted feeding on body weight and metabolic disease risk factors in obese adults: a pilot study. Nutr Healthy Aging. 2018;4(4):345–53.
54. Sutton EF, Beyl R, Early KS, Cefalu WT, Ravussin E, Peterson CM. Early time-restricted feeding improves insulin sensitivity, blood pressure, and oxidative stress even without weight loss in men with prediabetes. Cell Metab. 2018;27(6):1212–21.e3.
55. Dansinger ML, Gleason JA, Griffith JL, Selker HP, Schaefer EJ. Comparison of the Atkins, Ornish, Weight Watchers, and Zone diets for weight loss and heart disease risk reduction: a randomized trial. JAMA. 2005;293(1):43–53.
56. Sacks FM, Bray GA, Carey VJ, Smith SR, Ryan DH, Anton SD, et al. Comparison of weight-loss diets with different compositions of fat, protein, and carbohydrates. N Engl J Med. 2009;360(9): 859–73.
57. Donnelly JE, Blair SN, Jakicic JM, Manore MM, Rankin JW, Smith BK. American College of Sports Medicine position stand: appropriate physical activity intervention strategies for weight loss and prevention of weight regain for adults. Med Sci Sports Exerc. 2009;41(2):459–71.
58. Food and Agriculture Organization (FAO)/World Health Organization (WHO)/United Nations University (UNU). Human energy requirements. Food Nutr Tech Rep Ser. 2001;1(1):1–103.
59. Westerterp KR. Diet induced thermogenesis. Nutr Metab 2004;1(1):1–5.
60. Department of Health and Human Services. Physical activity guidelines for Americans, 2nd edition [Internet]. United States Department of Health and Human Services. 2018.
61. Donnelly JE, Hill JO, Jacobsen DJ, Potteiger J, Sullivan DK, Johnson SL, et al. Effects of a 16-month randomized controlled exercise trial on body weight and composition in young, overweight men and women: the Midwest Exercise Trial. Arch Intern Med. 2003;163(11):1343–50.
62. Shaw K, Gennat H, O'Rourke P, Del Mar C. Exercise for overweight or obesity. Cochrane Database Syst Rev. 2006;(4):CD003817.
63. Beddhu S, Wei G, Marcus RL, Chonchol M, Greene T. Light-intensity physical activities and mortality in the United States general population and CKD subpopulation. Clin J Am Soc Nephrol. 2015;10(7):1145–53.
64. Zhang H, Tong TK, Qiu W, Zhang X, Zhou S, Liu Y, et al. Comparable effects of high-intensity interval training and prolonged continuous exercise training on abdominal visceral fat reduction in obese young women. J Diabetes Res. 2017;2017(5071740): 13–23.
65. Fothergill E, Guo J, Howard L, Kerns JC, Knuth ND, Brychta R, et al. Persistent metabolic adaptation 6 years after "The Biggest Loser" competition. Obesity (Silver Spring). 2016;24(8):1612–9.
66. Aristizabal JC, Freidenreich DJ, Volk BM, Kupchak BR, Saenz C, Maresh CM, et al. Effect of resistance training on resting metabolic rate and its estimation by a dual-energy X-ray absorptiometry metabolic map. Eur J Clin Nutr. 2015;69(7):831–6.
67. Pratley R, Nicklas B, Rubin M, Miller J, Smith A, Smith M, et al. Strength training increases resting metabolic rate and norepinephrine levels in healthy 50- to 65-yr-old men. J Appl Physiol (1985). 1994;76(1):133–7.
68. Butryn ML, Webb V, Wadden TA. Behavioral treatment of obesity. Psychiatr Clin North Am. 2011;34(4):841–59.
69. Zheng Y, Klem ML, Sereika SM, Danford CA, Ewing LJ, Burke LE. Self-weighing in weight management: a systematic literature review. Obesity (Silver Spring). 2015;23(2):256–65.

70. Klem ML, Wing RR, McGuire MT, Seagle HM, Hill JO. A descriptive study of individuals successful at long-term maintenance of substantial weight loss. Am J Clin Nutr. 1997;66(2):239–46.
71. Perri MG, Nezu AM, McKelvey WF, Shermer RL, Renjilian DA, Viegener BJ. Relapse prevention training and problem-solving therapy in the long-term management of obesity. J Consult Clin Psychol. 2001;69(4):722–6.
72. Hinkle W, Cordell M, Leibel R, Rosenbaum M, Hirsch J. Effects of reduced weight maintenance and leptin repletion on functional connectivity of the hypothalamus in obese humans. PLoS One. 2013;8(3):e59114-e.
73. Rosenbaum M, Goldsmith R, Bloomfield D, Magnano A, Weimer L, Heymsfield S, et al. Low-dose leptin reverses skeletal muscle, autonomic, and neuroendocrine adaptations to maintenance of reduced weight. J Clin Invest. 2005;115(12):3579–86.
74. Rosenbaum M, Hirsch J, Gallagher DA, Leibel RL. Long-term persistence of adaptive thermogenesis in subjects who have maintained a reduced body weight. Am J Clin Nutr. 2008;88(4):906–12.
75. Thomas CE, Mauer EA, Shukla AP, Rathi S, Aronne LJ. Low adoption of weight loss medications: a comparison of prescribing patterns of antiobesity pharmacotherapies and SGLT2s. Obesity (Silver Spring). 2016;24(9):1955–61.
76. Kanj A, Levine D. Overcoming obesity: weight-loss drugs are underused. Cleve Clin J Med. 2020;87(10):602–4.
77. Adipex-p (phentermine) [package insert]. Sellersville: Teva Pharmaceuticals; 2012.
78. Aronne LJ, Wadden TA, Peterson C, Winslow D, Odeh S, Gadde KM. Evaluation of phentermine and topiramate versus phentermine/topiramate extended-release in obese adults (EQUATE). Obesity (Silver Spring). 2013;21(11):2163–71.
79. Qsymia (phentermine and topiramate extended-release) [package insert]. Winchester: VIVUS Inc.; 2012.
80. Gadde KM, Allison DB, Ryan DH, Peterson CA, Troupin B, Schwiers ML, et al. Effects of low-dose, controlled-release, phentermine plus topiramate combination on weight and associated comorbidities in overweight and obese adults (CONQUER): a randomised, placebo-controlled, phase 3 trial. Lancet. 2011;377(9774):1341–52.
81. Xenical (orlistat) [package insert]. San Francisco: Genentech USA, Inc.; 1999.
82. Davidson MH, Hauptman J, DiGirolamo M, Foreyt JP, Halsted CH, Heber D, et al. Weight control and risk factor reduction in obese subjects treated for 2 years with orlistat: a randomized controlled trial. JAMA. 1999;281(3):235–42.
83. Contrave (naltrexone HCl and bupropion HCl) [package insert]. San Diego: Nalpropion Pharmaceuticals, Inc.; 2014.
84. Greenway FL, Fujioka K, Plodkowski RA, Mudaliar S, Guttadauria M, Erickson J, et al. Effect of naltrexone plus bupropion on weight loss in overweight and obese adults (COR-I): a multicentre, randomised, double-blind, placebo-controlled, phase 3 trial. Lancet. 2010;376(9741):595–605.
85. Saxenda (liraglutide) [package insert]. Plainsboro: Novo Nordisk; 2014.
86. Pi-Sunyer X, Astrup A, Fujioka K, Greenway F, Halpern A, Krempf M, et al. A randomized, controlled trial of 3.0 mg of liraglutide in weight management. N Engl J Med. 2015;373(1):11–22.
87. Rothman RB, Baumann MH, Dersch CM, Romero DV, Rice KC, Carroll FI, et al. Amphetamine-type central nervous system stimulants release norepinephrine more potently than they release dopamine and serotonin. Synapse. 2001;39(1):32–41.
88. Li Z, Maglione M, Tu W, Mojica W, Arterburn D, Shugarman LR, et al. Meta-analysis: pharmacologic treatment of obesity. Ann Intern Med. 2005;142(7):532–46.
89. Hendricks EJ, Srisurapanont M, Schmidt SL, Haggard M, Souter S, Mitchell CL, et al. Addiction potential of phentermine prescribed during long-term treatment of obesity. Int J Obes. 2014;38(2):292–8.
90. Endocrinologic Metabolic Drugs Advisory Committee. VI-0521 (QNEXA) briefing document NDA 022580. Food and Drug Administration 2012:1–166.
91. McElroy SL, Hudson JI, Capece JA, Beyers K, Fisher AC, Rosenthal NR. Topiramate for the treatment of binge eating disorder associated with obesity: a placebo-controlled study. Biol Psychiatry. 2007;61(9):1039–48.
92. Milano W, De Rosa M, Milano L, Capasso A. Night eating syndrome: an overview. J Pharm Pharmacol. 2011;64(1):2–10.
93. Kushner RF. Weight loss strategies for treatment of obesity. Prog Cardiovasc Dis. 2014;61(2): 246–52.
94. Allison DB, Gadde KM, Garvey WT, Peterson CA, Schwiers ML, Najarian T, et al. Controlled-release phentermine/topiramate in severely obese adults: a randomized controlled trial (EQUIP). Obesity (Silver Spring). 2012;20(2):330–42.
95. Garvey WT, Ryan DH, Look M, Gadde KM, Allison DB, Peterson CA, et al. Two-year sustained weight loss and metabolic benefits with controlled-release phentermine/topiramate in obese and overweight adults (SEQUEL): a randomized, placebo-controlled, phase 3 extension study. Am J Clin Nutr. 2012;95(2):297–308.
96. Torgerson JS, Hauptman J, Boldrin MN, Sjostrom L. XENical in the prevention of diabetes in obese subjects (XENDOS) study: a randomized study of orlistat as an adjunct to lifestyle changes for the prevention of type 2 diabetes in obese patients. Diabetes Care. 2004;27(1):155–61.
97. Rucker D, Padwal R, Li SK, Curioni C, Lau DCW. Long term pharmacotherapy for obesity and overweight: updated meta-analysis. Br Med J. 2007;335(7631):1194–9.

98. Greenway FL, Whitehouse MJ, Guttadauria M, Anderson JW, Atkinson RL, Fujioka K, et al. Rational design of a combination medication for the treatment of obesity. Obesity (Silver Spring). 2009;17(1):30–9.
99. Apovian CM, Aronne L, Powell AG. Clinical management of obesity. 1st ed. West Islip: Professional Communications, Inc.; 2015.
100. Apovian CM, Aronne L, Rubino D, Still C, Wyatt H, Burns C, et al. A randomized, phase 3 trial of naltrexone SR/bupropion SR on weight and obesity-related risk factors (COR-II). Obesity (Silver Spring). 2013;21(5):935–43.
101. Wadden TA, Foreyt JP, Foster GD, Hill JO, Klein S, O'Neil PM, et al. Weight loss with naltrexone SR/bupropion SR combination therapy as an adjunct to behavior modification: the COR-BMOD trial. Obesity (Silver Spring). 2011;19(1):110–20.
102. Hollander P, Gupta AK, Plodkowski R, Greenway F, Bays H, Burns C, et al. Effects of naltrexone sustained-release/bupropion sustained-release combination therapy on body weight and glycemic parameters in overweight and obese patients with type 2 diabetes (COR-diabetes). Diabetes Care. 2013;36(12):4022–9.
103. van Can J, Sloth B, Jensen CB, Flint A, Blaak EE, Saris WHM. Effects of the once-daily GLP-1 analog liraglutide on gastric emptying, glycemic parameters, appetite and energy metabolism in obese, non-diabetic adults. Int J Obes. 2014;38(6):784–93.
104. Davies MJ, Bergenstal R, Bode B, Kushner RF, Lewin A, Skjøth TV, et al. Efficacy of liraglutide for weight loss among patients with type 2 diabetes: the SCALE diabetes randomized clinical trial. JAMA J Am Med Assoc. 2015;314(7):687–99.
105. Wadden TA, Hollander P, Klein S, Niswender K, Woo V, Hale PM, et al. Weight maintenance and additional weight loss with liraglutide after low-calorie-diet-induced weight loss: the SCALE maintenance randomized study. Int J Obes. 2013;37(11):1443–51.
106. Glucophage (metformin hydrochloride) [package insert]. Princeton: Bristol-Myers Squibb Company; 1995.
107. Seifarth C, Schehler B, Schneider HJ. Effectiveness of metformin on weight loss in non-diabetic individuals with obesity. Exp Clin Endocrinol Diabetes. 2013;121(1):27–31.
108. Schultes B, Oltmanns KM, Kern W, Fehm HL, Born J, Peters A. Modulation of hunger by plasma glucose and metformin. J Clin Endocrinol Metab. 2003;88(3):1133–41.
109. Hawley SA, Gadalla AE, Olsen GS, Grahame HD. The antidiabetic drug metformin activates the AMP-activated protein kinase cascade via an adenine nucleotide-independent mechanism. Diabetes. 2002;51(8):2420–5.
110. Kim YW, Kim JY, Park YH, Park SY, Won KC, Choi KH, et al. Metformin restores leptin sensitivity in high-fat-fed obese rats with leptin resistance. Diabetes. 2006;55(3):716–24.
111. Hostalek U, Gwilt M, Hildemann S. Therapeutic use of metformin in prediabetes and diabetes prevention. Drugs. 2015;75(10):1071–94.
112. Coll AP, Chen M, Taskar P, Rimmington D, Patel S, Tadross JA, et al. GDF15 mediates the effects of metformin on body weight and energy balance. Nature. 2020;578(2295):444–8.
113. Igel LI, Sinha A, Saunders KH, Apovian CM, Vojta D, Aronne LJ. Metformin: an old therapy that deserves a new indication for the treatment of obesity. Curr Atheroscler Rep. 2016;18(4):16. –.
114. Ning HH, Le J, Wang Q, Young CA, Deng B, Gao PX, et al. The effects of metformin on simple obesity: a meta-analysis. Endocrine. 2018;62(3):528–34.
115. Diabetes Prevention Program Research Group. 10-year follow-up of diabetes incidence and weight loss in the Diabetes Prevention Program Outcomes Study (DPPOS). Lancet. 2009;374(9702):1677–86.
116. Apolzan JW, Venditti EM, Edelstein SL, Knowler WC, Dabelea D, Boyko EJ, et al. Long-term weight loss with metformin or lifestyle intervention in the diabetes prevention program (DPP) outcomes study (DPPOS). Ann Intern Med. 2019;170(10):682–90.
117. Ribola FA, Cançado FB, Schoueri JHM, De Toni VF, Medeiros VHR, Feder D. Effects of SGLT2 inhibitors on weight loss in patients with type 2 diabetes mellitus. Eur Rev Med Pharmacol Sci. 2017;21(1):199–211.
118. Abdul-Ghani MA, Defronzo RA. Lowering plasma glucose concentration by inhibiting renal sodium-glucose cotransport. J Intern Med. 2014;276(4):352–63.
119. Lee PC, Ganguly S, Goh SY. Weight loss associated with sodium-glucose cotransporter-2 inhibition: a review of evidence and underlying mechanisms. 2018.
120. Riddle M, Frias J, Zhang B, Maier H, Brown C, Lutz K, et al. Pramlintide improved glycemic control and reduced weight in patients with type 2 diabetes using basal insulin. Diabetes Care. 2007;30(11):2794–9.
121. Ratner RE, Want LL, Fineman MS, Velte MJ, Ruggles JA, Gottlieb A, et al. Adjunctive therapy with the amylin analogue pramlintide leads to a combined improvement in glycemic and weight control in insulin-treated subjects with type 2 diabetes. Diabetes Technol Therap. 2002;4(1):51–61.

15 Endoscopic Management of Obesity

Russ Dolan, Pichamol Jirapinyo, and Janese Laster

Introduction

Endoscopic bariatric and metabolic therapies (EBMT) provide an alternative weight loss strategy to bariatric surgery when conservative measures such as diet and exercise have been unsuccessful or in the case of surgical ineligibility. These innovative techniques have gained popularity among physicians and patients alike due to reduced procedural and recovery times and lower risk of associated complications. The primary objectives of EBMT include (1) achieving meaningful weight loss and thereby (2) improving obesity-related comorbid conditions (i.e., hypertension, type 2 diabetes mellitus, nonalcoholic fatty liver disease). This group of therapies typically requires endoscopic delivery and removal. The two most common gastrointestinal targets for therapeutic intervention are the stomach and small bowel, with the majority of experience with gastric therapies. Although there are no currently FDA-approved small bowel interventions, this is expected to change in the coming years as new techniques are refined. The following is a review of endoscopic management of obesity highlighting currently approved devices and investigational products.

FDA-Approved Gastric Therapies

Intragastric Balloons (IGBs)

Intragastric balloons (IGBs) reached the market over 30 years ago and have evolved greatly since their inception. Despite years of use, the American Gastroenterological Association (AGA) recently published guidelines for their use in the management of obesity [1]. They are indicated for short-term use (6–12 months) when traditional methods of exercise and dietary lifestyle modifications have been unsuccessful. Currently, in the United States, patients with a BMI between 30 and 40 kg/m^2 are eligible for IGB placement. Patients in Europe are eligible with BMI >27 kg/m^2. Weight loss with IGB is primarily achieved through device space occupation within the stomach as well as delayed gastric emptying, thereby generating early satiety, prolonged satiation, and subsequent reduced caloric intake [2, 3]. IGB use is recommended in conjunction with supervised dietary and behavioral modifications for sus-

The original version of this chapter was revised. The erratum to this chapter can be found at https://doi.org/10.1007/978-3-030-94953-2_19

R. Dolan · P. Jirapinyo
Brigham and Women's Hospital and Harvard Medical School, Boston, MA, USA
e-mail: rddolan@bwh.harvard.edu; pjirapinyo@bwh.harvard.edu

J. Laster (✉)
Gastroenterology, Obesity Medicine, Nutrition and Bariatric Endoscopist, Gut Theory Total Digestive Care, George Washington University Hospital, 1712 N St NW, Suite 101, Washington, DC, USA
e-mail: jlaster@guttheoryhealth.com

C. Newberry et al. (eds.), *Nutrition, Weight, and Digestive Health*,
https://doi.org/10.1007/978-3-030-94953-2_15

tained weight loss with new habit formation. Although they are often used as primary therapy, IGBs are also utilized as a bridge to gastric bypass surgery, more definitive EBMT procedures, or to achieve weight loss prior to other elective surgeries or organ transplantation [1].

IGB placement requires careful patient selection to assure tolerability and achievement of defined weight loss goals. IGB contraindications include the presence of additional IGB; prior gastrointestinal surgery or bariatric surgery; the presence of gastric mass; large (>5 cm) hiatal hernia; active gastrointestinal inflammation (i.e., esophagitis, gastric ulceration, Crohn's disease, etc.); motility disorders such as achalasia, cirrhosis, or severe coagulopathy; alcoholism or drug addiction; patients unwilling to take concomitant proton pump inhibitor therapy or pursue concomitant counseling and follow-up; and those who are pregnant or breastfeeding [4]. There are several choices of IGB on the market, which include both fluid-filled and gas-filled options.

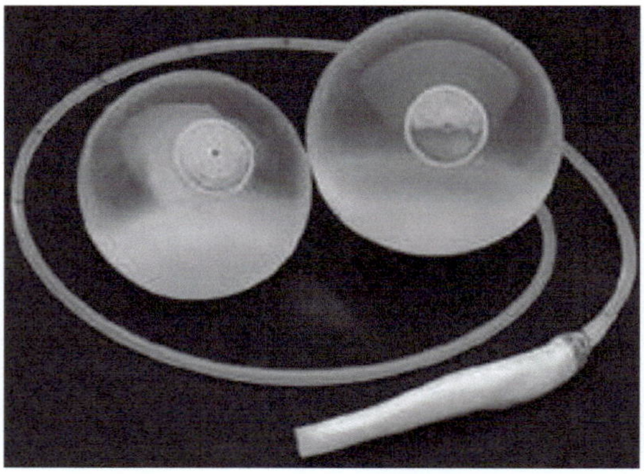

Fig. 15.1 Orbera single balloon device. (Image used with permission from Apollo Endosurgery)

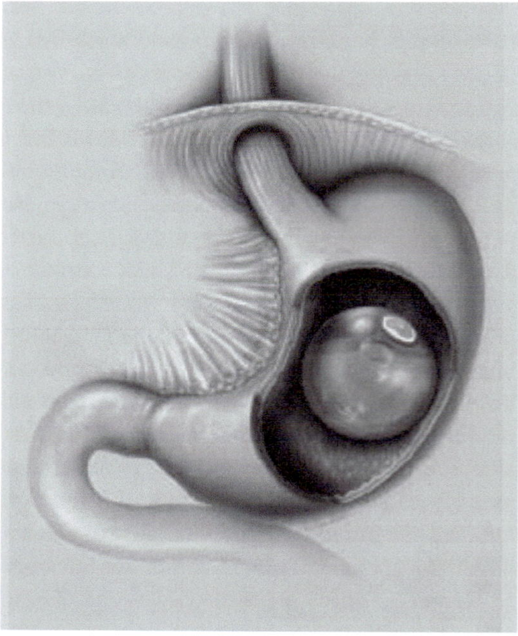

Fig. 15.2 Orbera single balloon device in situ. (Image used with permission from Apollo Endosurgery)

Orbera Balloon

The Orbera balloon (Apollo Endosurgery, Austin, TX) was first FDA approved in 2015, initially named the Bioenteric intragastric balloon (BIB), and later renamed Orbera. It deploys as a single spherical fluid-filled (volume ranges 400–700 mL) balloon with free movement in the stomach and has a self-sealing external valve following catheter removal (Figs. 15.1 and 15.2). Following initial placement, the balloon is no longer adjustable. Both deployment and removal require endoscopy.

The Orbera balloon is intended to be used in combination with long-term behavioral and dietary modification to sustain durable weight loss. The maximum placement period recommended is 6 months; however, there are Orbera balloons in the European market that can be placed for up to 1 year. The Orbera balloon achieved FDA approval shortly following the IB-005 pivotal study in 2015. This was a multicenter, prospective, unblinded, randomized control trial consisting of 1:1 randomization comparing a 12-month behavioral modification program alone with the Orbera balloon (6 months with balloon in place; 6 months following balloon removal) [4]. A total of 448 participants were enrolled in the trial. The study failed to meet the 95% confidence interval primary endpoint of mean percent excess weight loss (EWL) of at least 25% at 9 months in the Orbera group (mean EWL of 26.5% in Orbera vs 9.7% in control group at 9 months; $p < 0.001$). However, the Orbera group achieved significantly greater total body weight loss (TBWL) in comparison to the control group (mean TBWL 9.1% vs 3.4% at 9 months; $p < 0.001$). Although there was significant improvement in TBWL, the study did report a 15.1% early device removal rate predominantly due to device intolerance (5%) and the presence of adverse events including aspiration pneumonia (0.63%), gastric outlet obstruction (0.63%), gastric perforation and sepsis (0.63%), abdominal infection with fluid positive for *Candida* (0.63%), and dehydration (1.3%).

Following FDA approval, the balloon has been trialed in several real-world studies, including a retrospective safety and efficacy study in 2018 with 321 patients across 18 centers [5] which reported a reduction in mean TBWL of 11.8% at 6 months (EWL not reported), which was minimally improved from the pivotal study. The device removal rate at 6 months remained high at 16.7%, similar to the clinical trial. The American Society for Gastrointestinal Endoscopy Bariatric Endoscopy Task Force meta-analysis demonstrated the Orbera balloon surpassed preservation and incorporation of valuable endoscopic intervention thresholds by achieving >5% TBWL at 12 months as a nonprimary (bridge) therapy [6]. Specifically, the Orbera was shown to achieve 25.44% EWL and 11.27% TBWL at 12 months.

ReShape Dual Intragastric Balloon

The ReShape dual intragastric balloon (ReShape Medical Inc., San Clemente, CA) was initially FDA approved on July 28, 2015, as the first approved dual-balloon system filled with sterile saline and methylene blue solution (maximum 450 mL per balloon). Following removal of the ReShape Delivery Catheter, a mineral-oil based valve sealant prevents further adjustment. Endoscopic placement and removal are required. Eventual approval was primarily based on the REDUCE Pivotal Trial in 2015, a double-blinded, prospective, sham-controlled multicenter study of 330 subjects randomized in 1:1 fashion [7]. Reshape balloon retrieval occurred at 6 months, with an additional 6 months of dietary and exercise counseling post-removal. The mean intent-to-treat EWL at 6 months was 25.1% in the treatment group versus 11.3% with the sham control group (13.9% mean difference; $p = 0.0041$). The mean intent-to-treat TBWL at 6 months was 6.8% versus 3.3% for the treatment and control groups, respectively.

Although the serious adverse event or non-accommodative device event rate was low (3.0%), 35% of participants experienced gastric ulcerations, almost entirely located at gastric incisura, which was suspected to be device related. This prompted alteration to a smaller, smoother, and softer distal device tip. This adjustment led to a 74% reduction in ulceration rate. A real-world safety and efficacy study in 2018 subsequently demonstrated mean TBWL of 11.1% and mean EWL of 29.9% at 6 months [8]. This retrospective study included 202 adults that received treatment with the dual intragastric balloon. Serious adverse events were uncommon; however, there was a single case of balloon migration that precipitated small bowel obstruction. Despite efficacy and tolerance, the manufacturer removed the device from the market in 2019, focusing instead on single balloon liquid-filled options.

Obalon Balloon

The Obalon balloon (Obalon Therapeutics, Carlsbad, CA) was FDA approved on September 8, 2016. Like the Orbera, it is a spherical balloon with free movement in the stomach following placement (Fig. 15.3). However, the Obalon offers an alternative deployment option. Instead of endoscopic placement, the patient swallows a

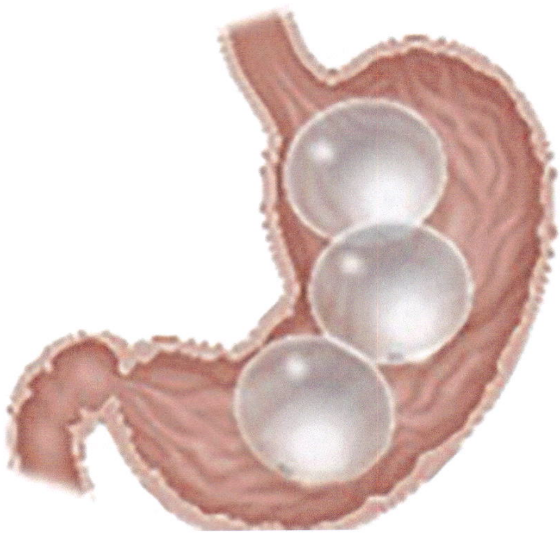

Fig. 15.3 Obalon balloons in situ. (Image use with permission of Wolters Kluwer Health, Inc. and American Journal of Gastroenterology)

thin capsule attached to an inflation catheter. Following dissolution of the gelatin capsule and radiologic confirmation of placement, the balloon is insufflated with 250 mL of a gas mixture. Up to 3 balloons may be inserted simultaneously within the stomach. Despite a non-procedural option for deployment, the Obalon balloon requires endoscopic removal following the treatment period.

The Obalon balloon maximum dwell period recommendation is 6 months. The balloon was first analyzed in a 12-week single-arm pilot feasibility study of 17 patients who achieved significant EWL at 4, 8, and 12 weeks and reported minimal side effects [9]. The Six-Month Adjunctive Weight Reduction (SMART) Trial in 2018, a multicenter, prospective, sham-controlled, randomized trial, later amplified these results after enrolling 430 subjects who were randomized to treatment (6 months Obalon balloon) versus sham (swallowed capsule without balloon). Overall, 387 patients completed the study (198 Obalon, 189 sham) over 24 weeks, after which participants were unblinded, and the Obalon balloons were retrieved [10]. Continued diet and exercise counseling was performed between 24 and 48 weeks at the conclusion of study. The co-primary effectiveness endpoint was TBWL, with 6.6% for treatment subjects and 3.4% for control subjects reported at 24 weeks (mean difference TBWL being 3.2%; $p = 0.0354$). The mean EWL was 24.1% for the treatment group versus 12.2% for the sham group.

Effect on Obesity-Related Comorbidities

IGBs have been shown to induce weight loss and improve obesity-related comorbid metabolic conditions such as insulin resistance and hypertension. This was demonstrated in a recent meta-analysis including 10 RCTs and 30 observational studies that reported a reduction in fasting hyperglycemia by 12.7 mg/dL and diastolic blood pressure by 2.9 mmHg [11].

Balloon Selection

In an analysis by Bazerbachi et al., 4 IGBs were evaluated (2 fluid and 2 gas filled) across 15 trials (seen in Table 15.1). Fluid-filled balloons demonstrated significant results (Orbera mean TBWL of 6.72% and ReShape mean TBWL of 4% at 6 months) in comparison to one of the gas-filled options (Obalon mean TBWL of 3.3% at 6 months) [12]. The other gas-filled balloon, the investigational heliosphere, demonstrated a mean TBWL of 6.7% at 6 months; however, this was not significant. Notably, this meta-analysis demonstrated improved tolerance of the gas-filled Obalon balloon in comparison to fluid-filled balloons, with fewer adverse events and early device removals. Based on this study, providers are encouraged to discuss data on weight loss, tolerance, and baseline gastrointestinal complaints including bloating, nausea, and vomiting with patients prior to selecting saline-filled vs gas-filled balloons.

Plication and Suturing

A more permanent endoscopic alternative to IGB therapy includes both plication and suturing techniques, which achieve tissue apposition. The primary objective of these EBMTs is reduction in gastric volume, effectively providing a less invasive alternative to the traditional surgical gastric sleeve. Additionally, there may be neurohormonal alterations that augment weight loss including changes in satiety hormones and insulin sensitivity [13]. The most commonly

Table 15.1 Comparison of FDA-approved intragastric balloons

Balloon	Subtype	Shape, volume	Balloon versus control at 6 months (TBWL %, confidence interval)[12]
Orbera	Fluid-filled	Single spherical, 400–700 cc	6.72 (5.55, 7.89)
ReShape	Fluid-filled	Dual spherical, 900 cc (450 cc × 2)	4.00 (2.69, 5.31)
Obalon	Gas-filled	Single spherical, 250 cc (up to 3)	3.30 (2.30, 4.30)

performed procedures are the endoscopic sleeve gastroplasty (ESG), utilizing the Overstitch device (Apollo Endosurgery, Austin, TX), and Primary Obesity Surgery, Endoluminal (POSE), utilizing the Incisionless Operative Platform (IOP; USGI medical, San Clemente, CA). These techniques are indicated in patients with a BMI 30–40 kg/m^2 who desire a less invasive procedural approach or who do not qualify for surgical interventions due to lower BMI class or significant comorbidities. A recent study has revealed that endoscopic plication and suturing can also be used in patients with BMI >40 kg/m^2 (achieving 20.5% TBWL at 1 year) as a bridge therapy to surgical approach or as primary treatment of obesity [14]. Contraindications to these procedures are similar to those of IGBs and include prior gastric surgery, active gastritis, coagulation disorders, pregnancy, and inability to maintain appropriate post-procedural care including medications and follow-up appointments [11].

Endoscopic Sleeve Gastroplasty (ESG)

Endoscopic sleeve gastroplasty (ESG) utilizes the Overstitch device (Apollo Endosurgery, Austin, TX) for tissue apposition, which obtained initial FDA approval in 2017 for general use rather than specifically for primary ESG. The ESG technique has been demonstrated to induce early satiety and delay gastric emptying, thereby reducing caloric intake [15] and producing subsequent weight loss. There are now two versions of the Overstitch device, one requiring a double-channel endoscope (Fig. 15.4), occupying the large channel, and permitting use of the second instrument channel, and another that is suitable for a single-channel endoscope. The device has an attached curved needle driver that permits full-thickness suturing in an interrupted or running fashion (Fig. 15.5b). ESG serves as a reasonable option for those who prefer a less invasive procedure or who are not surgical candidates. Additionally, this procedure may be more

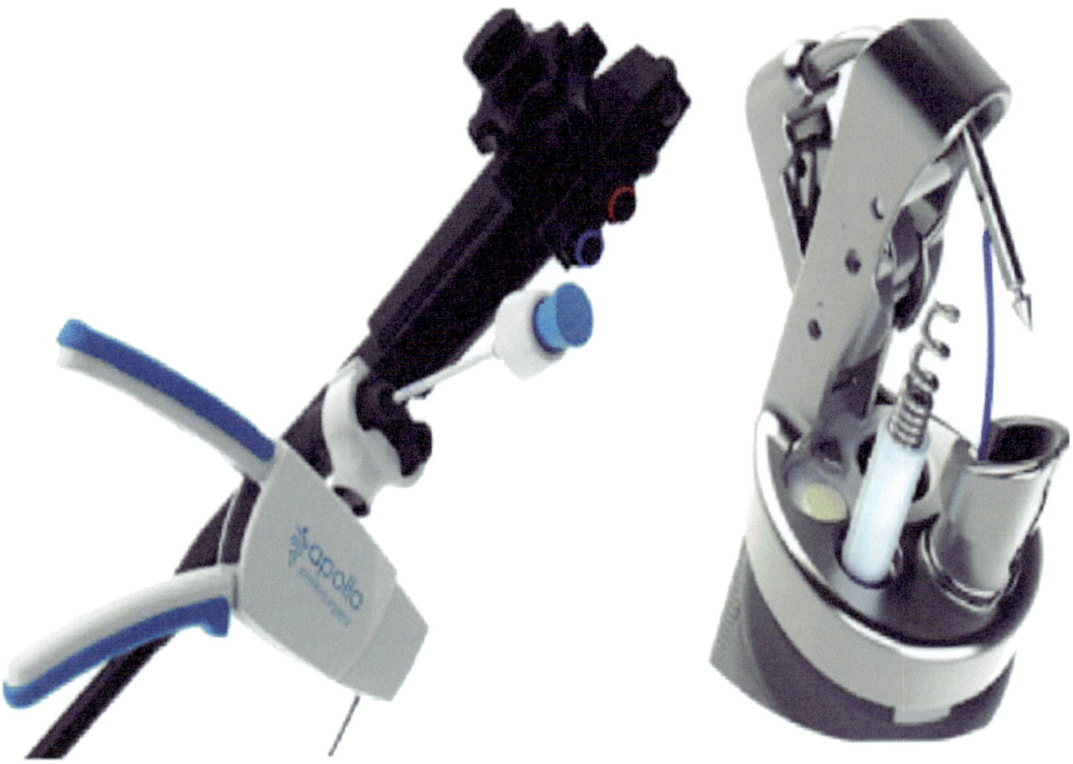

Fig. 15.4 Apollo overstitch device . (Images used with permission of Apollo Endosurgery)

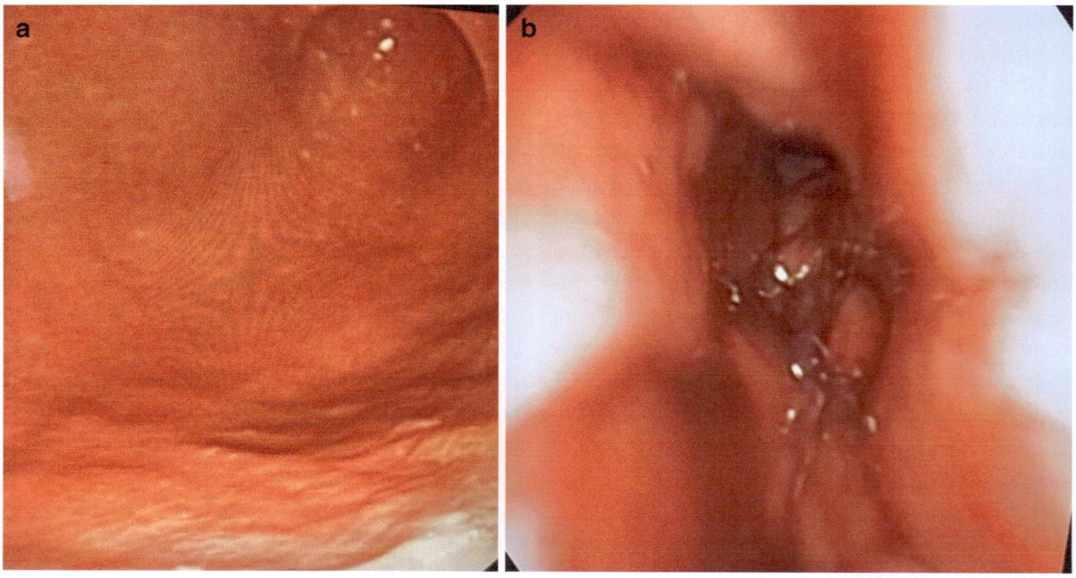

Fig. 15.5 (**a**) Endoscopic view of native stomach. (**b**) Endoscopic view after endoscopic sleeve gastroplasty with tubular configuration. (Image courtesy of Janese Laster, MD, Gut Theory Total Digestive Care, Washington, DC)

efficacious, more durable, and better tolerated than other endoscopic options such as IGBs.

The initial human safety and efficacy study evaluating ESG was published in 2018, consisting of three phases [15]. Phase I established safety and efficacy with reported short-term weight loss. Phase II trialed varying stitch patterns for technique refinement. Phase III established technique conformity and weight loss outcomes. A total of 77 patients were included with demonstrated mean %TBWL of 16.2% and 17.4% at 6 and 12 months, respectively. Although nausea and epigastric pain were common following ESG, there were no significant adverse events during the procedure or in the months following the procedure.

Shortly after these initial analyses, a large international multicenter retrospective trial with 112 patients demonstrated ESG to be a safe, effective, and reproducible for weight loss therapy [16]. At 6 months, mean TBWL was 14.9% and EWL was 50.3%, which eclipsed the magnitude of weight loss seen with IGBs. Furthermore, there were far less gastrointestinal complaints of GERD, nausea, and abdominal discomfort [17, 18] when compared to IGBs. Three (2.7%) significant adverse events were reported during the follow-up period in this ESG study (two gastrointestinal hemorrhage cases, one 3 cm peri-gastric fluid collection formation).

The efficacy of ESG has now been reproduced across several studies, with meta-analyses demonstrating 6-month TBWL of 15.1%. Relative EWL was 57.7% in one study [19] and TBWL of 14.47% and EWL 53.14% in another [20]. A low rate of serious adverse events was consistent across analyses, ranging from 1% to 2.2% [19, 20].

Primary Obesity Surgery Endoluminal (POSE)

Primary obesity surgery endoluminal (POSE) utilizes the incisionless operating platform (IOP; USGI medical, San Clemente, CA) for tissue apposition, which is currently undergoing clinical trial for FDA approval in the United States and is widely utilized abroad. The IOP device is similar to an endoscope with a control handle to maneuver the flexible tube tip in both vertical and horizontal directions; however, this is much larger (54 Fr) owing to its four working channels that accommodate an ultra-slim endoscope for visualization and dedicated instruments required for tissue plication (Fig. 15.6). The physiologic

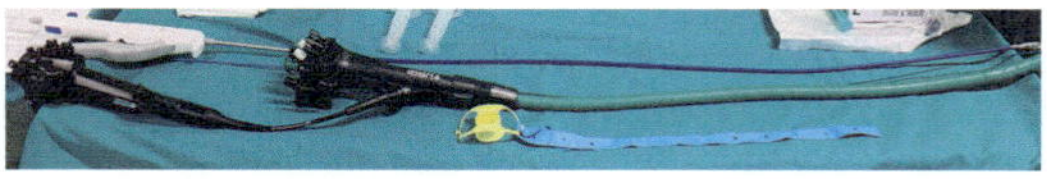

Fig. 15.6 Incisionless operative platform. (Image courtesy of Janese Laster, MD from HM Sanchinarro University Hospital, Madrid, Spain)

alterations following the POSE procedure have been proposed to be predominantly neuroendocrine driven, as gastric emptying (although initially delayed at 2 months post-procedure) was not significantly reduced at 6 months. A significant reduction in ghrelin secretion and postprandial increase in peptide YY has also been demonstrated [21], although it remains unclear whether these changes are directly due to the procedure or a product of weight loss itself.

The initial experience of POSE was published in 2013 as a single-center, prospective observational study that reported 6-month outcomes on safety and efficacy [22]. This study demonstrated a mean TBWL of 15.5% and mean EWL of 49.4% at 6 months among 45 patients. There were no serious adverse events reported. This was followed by the MILEPOST trial in 2016, which was designed as a multicenter, prospective, unblinded trial randomized in 3:1 fashion between POSE and control (diet and exercise only) groups [23]. At 12 months, POSE demonstrated a mean TBWL of 13.0%, compared to the control group with mean TBWL of 5.3%. Similarly, there was a significant increase in EWL (45.0%) compared with the control group (18.1%). Furthermore, this study demonstrated significant reductions in three satiety parameters (satiety volume, caloric intake, and satiety time) for individuals that underwent the POSE procedure compared to control. A larger study of 147 patients that underwent the POSE procedure were prospectively followed for 1 year at a single center. This study demonstrated similar results, with a TBWL of 15.1% and EWL 44.9% at 12 months [24]. There were no serious short- or long-term adverse events, strengthening data regarding overall safety of the procedure. POSE also appears to be durable, with sustainable weight loss reported after 12 months [25].

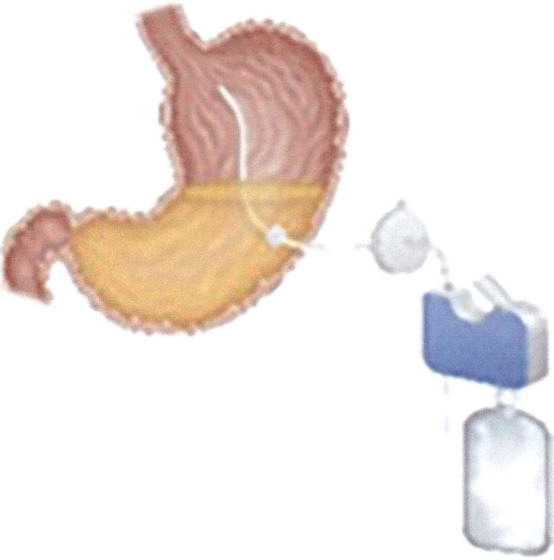

Fig. 15.7 Aspiration assist therapy device. (Image use with permission of Wolters Kluwer Health, Inc. and American Journal of Gastroenterology)

AspireAssist (AT)

The AspireAssist (AT) device (Aspire Bariatrics Inc., Exton, PA) obtained FDA approval on June 24, 2014. This device assists in draining a portion of gastric contents through a gastrostomy tube following meals (Fig. 15.7). The "A-tube" is connected to a gravity flow director system (via skin port) and is accessed 20–30 minutes postprandially with a goal to remove ~30% of meal contents, which are then directly disposed of into a toilet bowl. The predominant weight loss mechanisms include direct removal of ingested calories following a meal (through gastrostomy tube aspiration) as well as behavioral modifications such as increased mastication, which prevents tube clogging, promotes slower consumption, and increases satiety thereby reducing caloric intake. The device is intended for long-term use along with adjunctive weight loss measures with exercise and dietary modifications.

The AT device is indicated for adults >22 years of age with a BMI between 35 and 55 kg/m^2 who have previously failed nonsurgical weight loss. Contraindications for AT include the presence of prior abdominal surgery that complicates gastrostomy tube placement, history of refractory gastric ulcers, uncontrolled hypertension (blood pressure >160/110 mmHg), presence of esophageal narrowing or stricture, gastric masses, presence of anemia or coagulopathy, or presence of bulimia/binge-eating disorders.

An initial single-center pilot study of 18 patients, randomized in 2:1 fashion with AT device vs control group undergoing lifestyle therapy only, was published in 2013 [26]. At 1 year after placement, patients in the AT treatment arm experienced a mean TBWL of 18.6% and EWL of 49% compared to TBWL of 5.9% and EWL of 14.9% in the control group. There were no reported serious adverse events or altered eating behaviors such as binge eating. Later, the PATHWAY Pivotal trial, a large, controlled, multicenter, open-label, prospective trial randomized in a 2:1 fashion between device and 1 year of lifestyle management confirmed similarly positive results [27]. After 52 weeks, the AT group achieved a mean EWL of 31.5% compared to the control group, which reported a mean EWL of 9.8%. The AT group achieved 12.1% TBWL compared to the control group of 3.5%. Serious adverse events were reported in 3.6% of the AT group. Adverse events noted included peristomal granulation tissue formation, peristomal bleeding/irritation and infection, pain, nausea/vomiting, abdominal discomfort, and change in bowel habits.

A post-marketing study evaluating long-term (4 years) safety and efficacy results involving the AT device was published in 2018 [28]. This 201-participant study was multicentered and prospective in nature. After 4 years of follow-up, the mean TBWL was 19.2% (EWL not reported). There were 8 total serious adverse events reported including 7 participants who developed buried bumper syndrome which resolved with removal/replacement of A-tube and 1 participant who developed peritonitis that resolved with a 2-day course of intravenous antibiotics.

Comparison of Plication and Suturing Devices

A large meta-analysis involving the Overstitch ESG and POSE procedures was published in 2019 and included 22 cohort studies involving 7 different devices [29]. Comparative weight loss metrics favored ESG following 6- and 12-month outcomes, with an EWL at 6 months of 57.9% versus 44.4% (p = 0.02) and at 12 months of 68.3% versus 44.9% (p = 0.04) for ESG and POSE, respectively. Another large meta-analysis that included 12 studies (1149 patients) that evaluated both ESG and POSE procedures was also published in 2019 [30] and found similar results, with ESG producing more overall weight loss. Following 6- and 12-month intervals, ESG produced mean EWL 49.67% and 52.75% (TBWL 16.01% and 17.41%), respectively, compared to POSE, which resulted in mean EWL 43.79% and 44.91% (TBWL 13.82% and 10.98%). Notably given nonuniformity of reporting adverse events across studies, this was not included in the meta-analysis.

Transpyloric Shuttle (TPS)

The Transpyloric Shuttle (TPS; BAROnova Inc., San Carlos, CA), FDA approved on April 16, 2019, is designed as a removable gastric implant (Fig. 15.8). Following endoscopic deployment, it

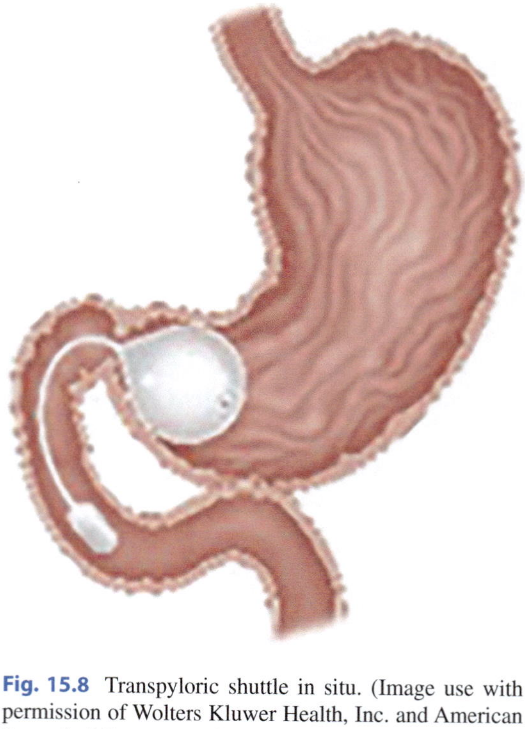

Fig. 15.8 Transpyloric shuttle in situ. (Image use with permission of Wolters Kluwer Health, Inc. and American Journal of Gastroenterology)

facilitates weight loss by positioning across the pylorus and inducing intermittent pyloric obstruction with subsequent delay in gastric emptying. This is accomplished by the presence of a flexible silicone catheter connected to both a small and large bulb, with the larger bulb remaining in the stomach. The size of the large bulb prevents device migration into the small intestine. Recommended duration of use is 12 months, followed by endoscopic retrieval.

The TPS is indicated for adults with a BMI between 35 and 40 kg/m^2 or between 30 and 35 kg/m^2 with one or more obesity-related comorbidities. It is intended to be used as an adjunctive measure to dietary and exercise lifestyle modifications. Contraindications to device use include prior surgery or endoscopic intervention that has altered esophageal, gastric or duodenal anatomy, structural abnormality in the esophagus or pharynx (i.e., diverticulum or stricture), esophageal abnormality (i.e., erosive esophagitis, varices, eosinophilic esophagitis, telangiectasias), structural or functional disorders of the stomach (i.e., gastritis, gastric varices, hiatal hernia >4 cm, pyloric stricture, gastric mass, ulcers), untreated *Helicobacter pylori* infection, coagulopathy, continuous use with ulcerogenic medication (i.e., aspirin, NSAIDs), pregnancy or planned pregnancy or history of bulimia nervosa, binge-eating behavior, or other severe psychiatric disorders.

The TPS was initially studied in 2014, with the outcomes of 22 patients evaluated at 3- and 6-months post-procedurally [31]. The achieved EWL was 41.0% and TBWL 14.5% at 6 months. Two patients required early device removal due to symptomatic gastric ulcerations that resolved following device removal.

The pivotal Endobesity II study in 2019 was a multicenter, double-blinded, prospective [32] study that enrolled 302 individuals (32 open-label following 270 randomized) in randomized, 2:1 fashion favoring treatment with TPS vs control (sham endoscopic procedure in addition to exercise/diet modifications). Following 12 months, the TPS group achieved a mean TBWL of 9.5% compared to 2.8% in the control group. Mean EWL was 30.9% in the TPS group compared to 9.8% in the control group. There was a total of 9 serious adverse events, including 1 esophageal rupture causing pneumothorax during unsuccessful deployment and 4 gastric impactions that resolved following device removal.

Hydrogel

Plenity (Gelesis, Boston, MA) is a novel orally administered three-dimensional hydrogel that uses two naturally occurring components, cellulose and citric acid, to modify gastric contents following ingestion. As compared to natural fibers, which are typically linear in structure, Plenity absorbs larger fluid volumes, thereby operating as a space-occupying material that promotes early satiety.

The Gelesis Loss of Weight (GLOW) pivotal study, published in 2019, was a 24-week prospective, multicenter, double-blinded, placebo-controlled, randomized trial involving 436 patients (223 Gelesis, 213 placebo). At the end of the study period, Gelesis patients experienced greater %EWL (29.0% vs 21.0%) and %TBWL (6.41% vs 4.39%) compared to controls [33]. There were no serious adverse events reported. The results of this study helped Plenity achieve FDA clearance for individuals with BMI between 25 kg/m^2 and 40 kg/m^2 on April 12, 2019, and was subsequently approved.

Investigational Therapies: Gastric

New EBMT technologies targeting gastric anatomy and physiology are emerging rapidly, with a number of devices in the investigational phase of study. These include alternative IGB options along with devices for gastric tissue apposition and suturing.

Intragastric Balloons (IGBs)

In addition to the FDA-approved IGBs previously discussed, other iterations of these space-occupying devices are being studied. These newer IGBs have innovative designs that allow

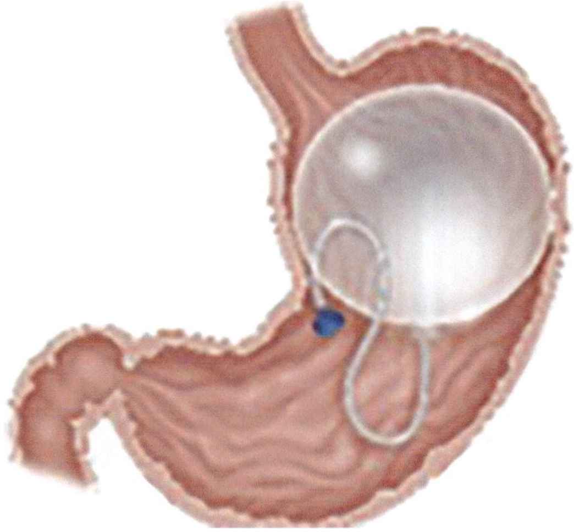

Fig. 15.9 Spatz3 adjustable balloon in situ. (Images use with permission of Wolters Kluwer Health, Inc. and American Journal of Gastroenterology)

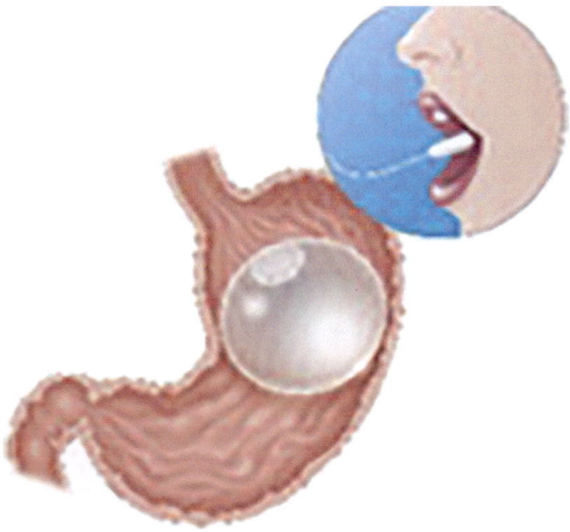

Fig. 15.10 Elipse balloon in situ. (Images use with permission of Wolters Kluwer Health, Inc. and American Journal of Gastroenterology)

for post-procedure adjustment (Spatz adjustable balloon, Fig. 15.9) and alternative deployment and removal options (Elipse balloon, which can be swallowed and then degrades over time, Fig. 15.10). Additional options are also under investigation with a goal to alleviate adverse effects, improve tolerability, and reduce premature removal [34–38].

Endosleeves

Endomina

The Endomina device (Endo Tools Therapeutics, Gosselies, Belgium) has been developed as a novel endoscopic suturing platform utilizing a triangulation system that allows for operation within close proximity to the endoscope tip. It was evaluated as a suturing platform initially in the setting of gastric volume reduction [39] and later as an instrument for ESG in 51 patients in 2018. The outcomes at 1-year revealed weight loss metrics of 29.0% EWL and 7.4% TBWL without severe adverse events reported.

Endozip

An additional endosleeve device currently under investigation is the Endozip (Nitinotes Ltd, Caesarea, Israel), which serves as an automated endoscopic device that forms wall-to-wall longitudinal attachments in the stomach and allows for reduced gastric volume. It was developed to provide ease of device operation (when compared to other suturing and plication devices) in creating a smaller gastric volume (Fig. 15.11) and subsequent weight loss, with a goal of increasing universal use among physicians trained in endoscopy. The device has been investigated in a single-center pilot study in 2020, which analyzed 11 patients with BMI between 30 kg/m^2 and 40 kg/m^2 and demonstrated 100% technical success and 54.3% EWL and 16.2% TBWL at 6 months [40].

Investigational Therapies: Small Bowel

In addition to a large spectrum of gastric devices developed for weight loss, there are also a number of small bowel devices under investigation. As the main gastrointestinal site for absorption of nutrients and glucoregulatory measures, the small bowel provides an opportunity for innovative weight loss technologies. Although no small bowel devices are currently FDA approved, they are currently under investigation.

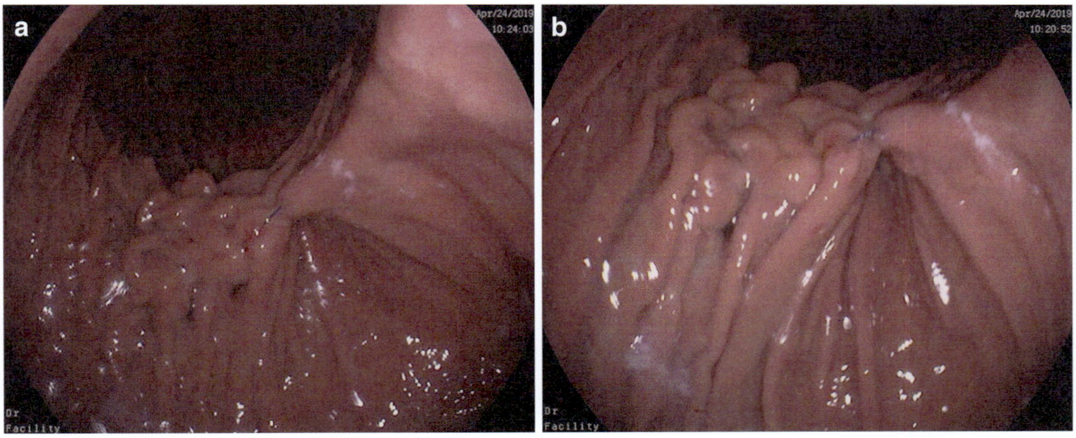

Fig. 15.11 Endoscopic view of gastric mucosa after Endozip plication. (Image courtesy of Ravishankar Asokkumar, MBBS from HM Sanchinarro University Hospital, Madrid, Spain and Singapore General Hospital, Singapore)

Endoluminal Bypass Techniques

Endobarrier

The Endobarrier (GI Dynamics, Boston, MA) has been developed as a duodenal-jejunal bypass liner composed of an ultra-slim Teflon sleeve anchored into the muscularis propria at the level of the duodenal bulb and extending 60 cm distally to bypass the duodenum and proximal jejunum (Fig. 15.12). It requires endoscopic placement and is intended for endoscopic removal at 12 months. The device was designed to mimic the excluded biliopancreatic limb of a Roux-en-Y gastric bypass surgery, and the mechanism for weight loss is proposed to be malabsorptive and neurohormonal. There have been a number of small randomized controlled trials investigating the Endobarrier for weight loss [41], and a large multicenter trial is currently enrolling participants to investigate the device's role in refractory type 2 diabetes.

Although moderately efficacious in the short term with reported reductions in BMI of 3–5 kg/m^2 and hemoglobin A1C (HbA1C) of 1–2% over the course of 6–12 months, long-term durability of response remains unclear. A multicenter randomized controlled trial with median duration of 42 months in 2019 which included 29 patients demonstrated no significant weight loss (TBWL of 2.2%), suggesting diminished effect with longer duration [42]. This study was followed by an investigation of a longer device dwell time of 24 months in 24 patients who were previously enrolled in the shorter study [43]. Although the weight loss achieved after 12 months remained stable through the 24 months, the rate of adverse

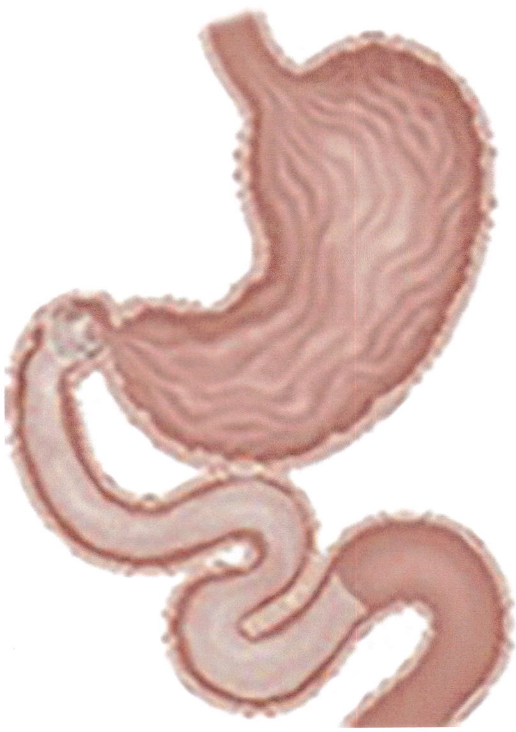

Fig. 15.12 Endobarrier (duodenal-jejunal bypass liner). (Image use with permission of Wolters Kluwer Health, Inc. and American Journal of Gastroenterology)

events (including 2 patients with hepatic abscesses requiring hospitalization) increased during the second year of implantation and necessitated a 45% early explanation in this cohort. Additional adverse events encountered during this study included partial migration [11], migration >5 cm [8], and abdominal pain, nausea, or vomiting.

Several meta-analyses have been performed, including one in 2016 of 5 RCTs (235 patients) and 10 observational studies (211 patients). An analysis of 4 RCTs demonstrated EWL of 12.6% compared to controls (diet alone) [44]. A large early explantation rate was also observed, with a total of 66 devices explanted early due to device migration, gastrointestinal bleeding, obstruction, abdominal pain, or investigator request.

Endosleeve

The Endosleeve (Metamodix, Plymouth, MN) provides a similar mechanism to the aforementioned Endobarrier, in which a sleeve is anchored at the level of the pyloric sphincter and prohibits contact of food contents within the proximal small bowel. The device is currently undergoing preliminary investigation outside of the United States, and there is no data available on safety or efficacy at this time.

ValenTx

ValenTx (ValenTx Inc., Maple Grove, MN) is a novel form of endoluminal bypass therapy designed to mimic the Roux-en-Y surgical bypass surgery. The device, implanted via endoscopy, is a 120 cm adjustable and removable sleeve anchored at the level of the gastroesophageal junction and designed to create an endoluminal gastro-duodena-jejunal bypass. After placement, food contents bypass the gastric lumen and proximal small bowel, emptying into the jejunum. A prospective, single-center, 1-year trial involving 13 patients with mean BMI of 42 kg/m^2 reported a EWL of 54%; however, 3 patients required early device removal secondary to intolerance, and an additional 4 patients had premature detachment [45]. No additional studies have been performed on the device, and to date, the device is not FDA approved and is undergoing initial investigation.

Duodenal Mucosal Resurfacing (DMR)

Revita DMR (Fractyl, Lexington, MA) serves as a novel single-use balloon catheter designed to deliver hydrothermal therapy across the duodenal barrier with the intent to remove the excessive layer of mucosa that develops in the setting of a high-fat diet (Fig. 15.13). The procedure was developed in response to previous animal studies reporting proximal small bowel hypertrophy in the setting of diabetes highlighting the importance of the small bowel in glucoregulation [46].

To date, DMR has been studied predominantly in the diabetes setting, where it has been shown to be technically feasible and safe with an estimated reduction in HbA1C values of 0.9–1.2% after 6–24 months [47, 48]. Investigation into

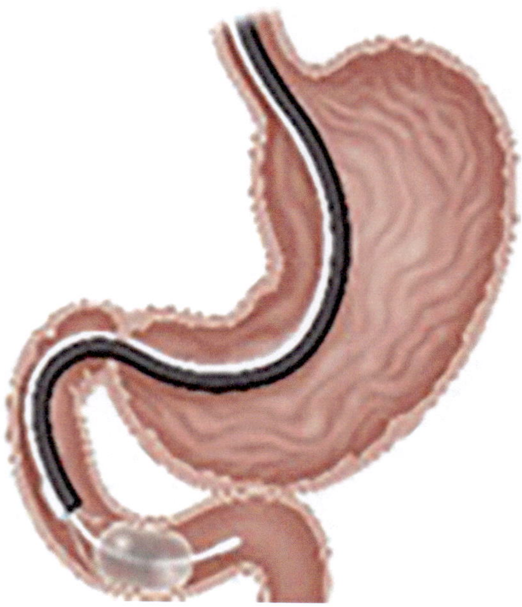

Fig. 15.13 Duodenal mucosal resurfacing in situ. (Image use with permission of Wolters Kluwer Health, Inc. and American Journal of Gastroenterology)

utility as a weight loss procedure will require future studies.

Incisionless Magnetic Anastomosis System

The Incisionless Magnetic Anastomosis System (IMAS; GI Windows, West Bridgewater, MA) was developed as a self-assembling magnetic system that forms an octagonal shape following deployment. The system is designed to be delivered endoscopically via both upper endoscopy and colonoscopy. The two deployed linear "smart" magnets develop a self-forming octagonal ring and approximate one another, forming a partial jejunal diversion (PJD). This diversion maintains patency of the native path and allows food contents through the small bowel in addition to a partial diversion of contents into the ileum at an earlier phase, subsequently inducing secretion of peptide YY and glucagon-1 peptide, among other hormones.

The feasibility study in humans was published in 2017 and included 14 patients evaluated over a 12-month period [49]. At 12 months, there were no serious adverse events reported, all PJD sites remained patent, and patients experienced an average TBWL of 14.6% and an average HbA1c reduction of 1.9%. The IMAS provides promise; however, it requires further investigation prior to FDA approval.

Conclusion

Although diet and exercise lifestyle modifications remain the foundation of sustained weight management, many patients may benefit from procedural options, including both surgical and endoscopic techniques. The latter is an area of increasing interest, due to reproducibility, safety, efficacy, noninvasiveness, and decreased complication rates when compared to surgical alternatives. Current FDA-approved EBMT modalities include intragastric balloons, endoscopic plication and suturing procedures, transpyloric bypass devices, and Plenity, with additional options undergoing active investigation.

References

1. Muniraj T, Day LW, Teigen LM, Ho EY, Sultan S, Davitkov P, et al. AGA clinical practice guidelines on intragastric balloons in the management of obesity. Gastroenterology. 2021;160(5):1799–808. https://doi.org/10.1053/j.gastro.2021.03.003.
2. Lopez-Nava G, Bautista-Castaño I, Acosta A, Bazerbachi F, Vargas EJ, Rizk M, et al. Utility of the office-based gastric emptying breath test (GEBT) in lieu of gastric scintigraphy to measure physiological response to the single fluid-filled intragastric balloon. Gastroenterolgy. 2018;154(6):S-1053. https://doi.org/10.1016/S0016-5085(18)33524-8.
3. Gomez V, Woodman G, Abu Dayyeh BK. Delayed gastric emptying as a proposed mechanism of action during intragastric balloon therapy: results of a prospective study. Obesity (Silver Spring). 2016;24(9):1849–53. https://doi.org/10.1002/oby.21555. Epub 2016/07/29. PubMed PMID: 27465076.
4. Abu Dayyeh BK, Eaton LL, Woodman G, Fusco M, Shayani V, Billy HT, et al. 444 A randomized, multi-center study to evaluate the safety and effectiveness of an intragastric balloon as an adjunct to a behavioral modification program, in comparison with a behavioral modification program alone in the weight management of obese subjects. Gastrointest Endosc. 2015;81(5, Supplement):AB147. https://doi.org/10.1016/j.gie.2015.03.1235.
5. Vargas EJ, Pesta CM, Bali A, Ibegbu E, Bazerbachi F, Moore RL, et al. Single fluid-filled intragastric balloon safe and effective for inducing weight loss in a real-world population. Clin Gastroenterol Hepatol. 2018;16(7):1073–80.e1. Epub 2018/02/10. https://doi.org/10.1016/j.cgh.2018.01.046.
6. Abu Dayyeh BK, Kumar N, Edmundowicz SA, Jonnalagadda S, Larsen M, Sullivan S, et al. ASGE Bariatric Endoscopy Task Force systematic review and meta-analysis assessing the ASGE PIVI thresholds for adopting endoscopic bariatric therapies. Gastrointest Endosc. 2015;82(3):425–38.e5. Epub 2015/08/02. https://doi.org/10.1016/j.gie.2015.03.1964.
7. Ponce J, Woodman G, Swain J, Wilson E, English W, Ikramuddin S, et al. The REDUCE pivotal trial: a prospective, randomized controlled pivotal trial of a dual intragastric balloon for the treatment of obesity. Surg Obes Relat Dis. 2015;11(4):874–81. https://doi.org/10.1016/j.soard.2014.12.006. Epub 2015/04/15. PubMed PMID: 25868829.
8. Agnihotri A, Xie A, Bartalos C, Kushnir V, Sullivan S, Islam S, et al. Real-world safety and efficacy of fluid-filled dual intragastric balloon for weight loss. Clin Gastroenterol Hepatol. 2018;16(7):1081–8.

e1. https://doi.org/10.1016/j.cgh.2018.02.026. Epub 2018/02/27. PubMed PMID: 29481969.
9. Mion F, Ibrahim M, Marjoux S, Ponchon T, Dugardeyn S, Roman S, et al. Swallowable Obalon gastric balloons as an aid for weight loss: a pilot feasibility study. Obes Surg. 2013;23(5):730–3. https://doi.org/10.1007/s11695-013-0927-x.
10. Sullivan S, Swain J, Woodman G, Edmundowicz S, Hassanein T, Shayani V, et al. Randomized sham-controlled trial of the 6-month swallowable gas-filled intragastric balloon system for weight loss. Surg Obes Relat Dis. 2018;14(12):1876–89. https://doi.org/10.1016/j.soard.2018.09.486.
11. Popov VB, Ou A, Schulman AR, Thompson CC. The impact of intragastric balloons on obesity-related co-morbidities: a systematic review and meta-analysis. Am J Gastroenterol. 2017;112(3):429–39. Epub 2017/01/25. https://doi.org/10.1038/ajg.2016.530.
12. Bazerbachi F, Haffar S, Sawas T, Vargas EJ, Kaur RJ, Wang Z, et al. Fluid-filled versus gas-filled intragastric balloons as obesity interventions: a network meta-analysis of randomized trials. Obes Surg. 2018;28(9):2617–25. Epub 2018/04/18. https://doi.org/10.1007/s11695-018-3227-7.
13. Abu Dayyeh BK, Acosta A, Camilleri M, Mundi MS, Rajan E, Topazian MD, et al. Endoscopic sleeve gastroplasty alters gastric physiology and induces loss of body weight in obese individuals. Clin Gastroenterol Hepatol. 2017;15(1):37–43.e1. Epub 2016/01/10. https://doi.org/10.1016/j.cgh.2015.12.030.
14. Lopez-Nava G, Laster J, Anuradha N, Fook-Chong S, Bautista-Castano I, Asokkumar R. Endoscopic Sleeve Gastroplasty (ESG) for morbid obesity: how effective is it? Surg Endosc. Epub 2021/1/25. https://doi.org/10.1007/s00464-021-08289-1.
15. Kumar N, Abu Dayyeh BK, Lopez-Nava Breviere G, Galvao Neto MP, Sahdala NP, Shaikh SN, et al. Endoscopic sutured gastroplasty: procedure evolution from first-in-man cases through current technique. Surg Endosc. 2018;32(4):2159–64. Epub 2017/10/28. https://doi.org/10.1007/s00464-017-5869-2.
16. Sartoretto A, Sui Z, Hill C, Dunlap M, Rivera AR, Khashab MA, et al. Endoscopic sleeve gastroplasty (ESG) is a reproducible and effective endoscopic bariatric therapy suitable for widespread clinical adoption: a large, international multicenter study. Obes Surg. 2018;28(7):1812–21. Epub 2018/02/17. https://doi.org/10.1007/s11695-018-3135-x.
17. Kim SH, Chun HJ, Choi HS, Kim ES, Keum B, Jeen YT. Current status of intragastric balloon for obesity treatment. World J Gastroenterol. 2016;22(24):5495–504. Epub 2016/06/29. https://doi.org/10.3748/wjg.v22.i24.5495.
18. Gaur S, Levy S, Mathus-Vliegen L, Chuttani R. Balancing risk and reward: a critical review of the intragastric balloon for weight loss. Gastrointest Endosc. 2015;81(6):1330–6. Epub 2015/04/19. https://doi.org/10.1016/j.gie.2015.01.054.
19. Hedjoudje A, Dayyeh BA, Cheskin LJ, Adam A, Neto MG, Badurdeen D, et al. Efficacy and safety of endoscopic sleeve gastroplasty: a systematic review and meta-analysis. Clin Gastroenterol Hepatol. 2019. Epub 2019/08/24; https://doi.org/10.1016/j.cgh.2019.08.022.
20. Li P, Ma B, Gong S, Zhang X, Li W. Efficacy and safety of endoscopic sleeve gastroplasty for obesity patients: a meta-analysis. Surg Endosc. 2019. Epub 2019/06/27; https://doi.org/10.1007/s00464-019-06889-6.
21. Espinos JC, Turro R, Moragas G, Bronstone A, Buchwald JN, Mearin F, et al. Gastrointestinal physiological changes and their relationship to weight loss following the POSE procedure. Obes Surg. 2016;26(5):1081–9. Epub 2015/09/05. https://doi.org/10.1007/s11695-015-1863-8.
22. Espinos JC, Turro R, Mata A, Cruz M, da Costa M, Villa V, et al. Early experience with the incisionless operating platform (IOP) for the treatment of obesity : the primary obesity surgery endolumenal (POSE) procedure. Obes Surg. 2013;23(9):1375–83. Epub 2013/04/18. https://doi.org/10.1007/s11695-013-0937-8.
23. Miller K, Turro R, Greve JW, Bakker CM, Buchwald JN, Espinos JC. MILEPOST multicenter randomized controlled trial: 12-month weight loss and satiety outcomes after pose (SM) vs. medical therapy. Obes Surg. 2017;27(2):310–22. Epub 2016/07/30. https://doi.org/10.1007/s11695-016-2295-9.
24. Lopez-Nava G, Bautista-Castano I, Jimenez A, de Grado T, Fernandez-Corbelle JP. The primary obesity surgery endolumenal (POSE) procedure: one-year patient weight loss and safety outcomes. Surg Obes Relat Dis. 2015;11(4):861–5. Epub 2015/02/24. https://doi.org/10.1016/j.soard.2014.09.026.
25. Singh S, Bazarbashi AN, Khan A, Chowdhry M, et al. Primary obesity surgery endoluminal (POSE) for the treatment of obesity: a systematic review and meta-analysis. Surg Endo. 2021; https://doi.org/10.1007/s00464-020-08267-z.
26. Sullivan S, Stein R, Jonnalagadda S, Mullady D, Edmundowicz S. Aspiration therapy leads to weight loss in obese subjects: a pilot study. Gastroenterology. 2013;145(6):1245–52.e1–5. Epub 2013/09/10. https://doi.org/10.1053/j.gastro.2013.08.056.
27. Thompson CC, Abu Dayyeh BK, Kushner R, Sullivan S, Schorr AB, Amaro A, et al. Percutaneous gastrostomy device for the treatment of class II and class III obesity: results of a randomized controlled trial. Am J Gastroenterol. 2017;112(3):447–57. Epub 2016/12/07. https://doi.org/10.1038/ajg.2016.500.
28. Nystrom M, Machytka E, Noren E, Testoni PA, Janssen I, Turro Homedes J, et al. Aspiration therapy as a tool to treat obesity: 1- to 4-year results in a 201-patient multi-center post-market European registry study. Obes Surg. 2018;28(7):1860–8. Epub 2018/02/02. https://doi.org/10.1007/s11695-017-3096-5.
29. Gys B, Plaeke P, Lamme B, Lafullarde T, Komen N, Beunis A, et al. Endoscopic gastric plication for morbid obesity: a systematic review and meta-analysis of published data over time. Obes Surg.

2019;29(9):3021–9. Epub 2019/06/24. https://doi.org/10.1007/s11695-019-04010-3.

30. Khan Z, Khan MA, Hajifathalian K, Shah S, Abdul M, Saumoy M, et al. Efficacy of endoscopic interventions for the management of obesity: a meta-analysis to compare endoscopic sleeve gastroplasty, aspire assist, and primary obesity surgery endolumenal. Obes Surg. 2019;29(7):2287–98. Epub 2019/04/15. https://doi.org/10.1007/s11695-019-03865-w.
31. Marinos G, Eliades C, Raman Muthusamy V, Greenway F. Weight loss and improved quality of life with a nonsurgical endoscopic treatment for obesity: clinical results from a 3- and 6-month study. Surg Obes Relat Dis. 2014;10(5):929–34. Epub 2014/07/30. https://doi.org/10.1016/j.soard.2014.03.005.
32. Rothstein RI, Woodman G, Swain J, de La Cruz N, Kushnir V, Pryor AD, et al. Transpyloric shuttle treatment improves cardiometabolic risk factors and quality of life in patients with obesity: results from a randomized, double-blind, sham-controlled trial. Gastroenterology. 2019;156(6):S-237. https://doi.org/10.1016/S0016-5085(19)37393-7.
33. Greenway FL, Aronne LJ, Raben A, Astrup A, et al. A randomized, double-blind, placebo-controlled study of Gelesis100: a novel nonsystemic oral hydrogel for weight loss. Obesity. 2018 Nov;27(2):205–16. https://doi.org/10.1002/oby.22347.
34. Machytka E, Klvana P, Kornbluth A, Peikin S, Mathus-Vliegen LE, Gostout C, et al. Adjustable intragastric balloons: a 12-month pilot trial in endoscopic weight loss management. Obes Surg. 2011;21(10):1499–507. Epub 2011/05/10. https://doi.org/10.1007/s11695-011-0424-z.
35. Brooks J, Srivastava ED, Mathus-Vliegen EM. One-year adjustable intragastric balloons: results in 73 consecutive patients in the U.K. Obes Surg. 2014;24(5):813–9. Epub 2014/01/21. https://doi.org/10.1007/s11695-014-1176-3.
36. Machytka E, Gaur S, Chuttani R, Bojkova M, Kupka T, Buzga M, et al. Elipse, the first procedureless gastric balloon for weight loss: a prospective, observational, open-label, multicenter study. Endoscopy. 2017;49(2):154–60. Epub 2016/12/13. https://doi.org/10.1055/s-0042-119296.
37. Alsabah S, Al Haddad E, Ekrouf S, Almulla A, Al-Subaie S, Al Kendari M. The safety and efficacy of the procedureless intragastric balloon. Surg Obes Relat Dis. 2018;14(3):311–7. Epub 2018/01/07. https://doi.org/10.1016/j.soard.2017.12.001.
38. Choi SJ, Choi HS. Various intragastric balloons under clinical investigation. Clin Endosc. 2018;51(5):407–15. Epub 2018/09/28. https://doi.org/10.5946/ce.2018.140.
39. Huberty V, Ibrahim M, Hiernaux M, Chau A, Dugardeyn S, Deviere J. Safety and feasibility of an endoluminal-suturing device for endoscopic gastric reduction (with video). Gastrointest Endosc. 2017;85(4):833–7. Epub 2016/08/27. https://doi.org/10.1016/j.gie.2016.08.007.
40. Lopez-Nava G, Asokkumar R, Rull A, Fernandez C, Bautista I, Dayyeh BA. Safety and feasibility of a novel endoscopic suturing device (EndoZip TM) for treatment of obesity: first-in-human study. Obes Surg. 2020; https://doi.org/10.1007/s11695-019-04370-w.
41. Ruban A, Teare. The EndoBarrier: duodenal-jejunal bypass liner for diabetes and weight loss. Gastroenterol Res Pract. 2018;2018:7823182–9. https://doi.org/10.1155/2018/7823182.
42. van Rijn S, Roebroek YGM, de Jonge C, Greve JWM, Bouvy ND. Effect of the EndoBarrier device: a 4-year follow-up of a multicenter randomized clinical trial. Obes Surg. 2019;29(4):1117–21. Epub 2019/01/11. https://doi.org/10.1007/s11695-018-03659-6.
43. Betzel B, Cooiman MI, Aarts EO, Janssen IMC, Wahab PJ, Groenen MJM, et al. Clinical follow-up on weight loss, glycemic control, and safety aspects of 24 months of duodenal-jejunal bypass liner implantation. Surg Endosc. 2020;34(1):209–15. Epub 2019/03/17. https://doi.org/10.1007/s00464-019-06752-8.
44. Rohde U, Hedback N, Gluud LL, Vilsboll T, Knop FK. Effect of the EndoBarrier gastrointestinal liner on obesity and type 2 diabetes: a systematic review and meta-analysis. Diabetes Obes Metab. 2016;18(3):300–5. Epub 2015/11/06. https://doi.org/10.1111/dom.12603.
45. Sandler BJ, Rumbaut R, Swain CP, Torres G, Morales L, Gonzales L, et al. One-year human experience with a novel endoluminal, endoscopic gastric bypass sleeve for morbid obesity. Surg Endosc. 2015 Nov;29(11):3298–303. https://doi.org/10.1007/s00464-015-4081-5.
46. Gniuli D, Calcagno A, Dalla Libera L, Calvani R, Leccesi L, Caristo ME, et al. High-fat feeding stimulates endocrine, glucose-dependent insulinotropic polypeptide (GIP)-expressing cell hyperplasia in the duodenum of Wistar rats. Diabetologia. 2010;53(10):2233–40. https://doi.org/10.1007/s00125-010-1830-9. Epub 2010/06/30. PubMed PMID: 20585935.
47. van Baar ACG, Holleman F, Crenier L, Haidry R, Magee C, Hopkins D, et al. Endoscopic duodenal mucosal resurfacing for the treatment of type 2 diabetes mellitus: one-year results from the first international, open-label, prospective, multicenter study. Gut. 2020;69(2):295–303. Epub 2019/07/25. https://doi.org/10.1136/gutjnl-2019-318349.
48. Rajagopalan H, Cherrington AD, Thompson CC, Kaplan LM, Rubino F, Mingrone G, et al. Endoscopic duodenal mucosal resurfacing for the treatment of type 2 diabetes: 6-month interim analysis from the first-in-human proof-of-concept study. Diabetes Care. 2016;39(12):2254–61. Epub 2016/08/16. https://doi.org/10.2337/dc16-0383.
49. Machytka E, Buzga M, Zonca P, Lautz DB, Ryou M, Simonson DC, et al. Partial jejunal diversion using an incisionless magnetic anastomosis system: 1-year interim results in patients with obesity and diabetes. Gastrointest Endosc. 2017;86(5):904–12. Epub 2017/07/19. https://doi.org/10.1016/j.gie.2017.07.009.

Surgical Management of Obesity

16

Danny Mou and Ali Tavakkoli

Bariatric Surgery Is the Most Effective Treatment for Obesity

Obesity is a chronic disease that results from neurobehavioral, genetic, and environmental factors [1]. Obesity has become a global pandemic and contributes to increased mortality, morbidity, and healthcare costs [2–4]. The majority of the world's population inhabit countries in which the consequences of obesity outweigh those of malnutrition. Half a billion adults suffer from obesity globally, while one billion adults have a diagnosis of overweight [5]. In the USA, 93 million adults suffered from obesity in 2016 [6]. US medical costs associated with obesity is now over $100 billion annually, driven by obesity-associated comorbidities [7, 8]. Obesity is also a major risk factor for many medical comorbidities including type 2 diabetes (T2D), hypertension, Nonalcoholic Steateohepatitis (NASH), cardiovascular disease, and malignancy. Every 5 unit increase in BMI is estimated to increase mortality rate by 22% [9, 10].

Many studies have shown that bariatric surgery is an effective treatment option for patients with morbid obesity who have failed medical management. Bariatric surgery outcomes have been shown to confer durable weight loss, induce remission of obesity-related comorbidities, improve quality of life (QOL), and prolong life expectancy [11]. Bariatric surgery volume has steadily increased in the USA from 158,000 cases in 2011 to 252,000 cases in 2018 [12]. Global bariatric surgery volumes have also increased. Among the International Federation for the Surgery of Obesity and Metabolic Disorder (IFSO) national members, there were an estimated 685,000 annual operations in 2016 [13]. The majority of bariatric surgeries are now performed laparoscopically, which has minimized surgical complications, reduced surgical morbidity and mortality, and decreased length of hospital stay to 1–2 postoperative days [14, 15].

Current indications of bariatric surgery as established by the American National Institute of Health dictate that bariatric surgery should be offered to patients with a body mass index (BMI) of 35 kg/m^2 who also have an obesity-related comorbidity including T2D, hypertension, or obstructive sleep apnea [16, 17]. For those with BMI of 40 kg/m^2 or greater, bariatric surgery should be offered regardless of the presence of obesity-related comorbidities. As more bariatric surgery-related long-term data accumulate, these guidelines are being reconsidered with a joint statement by several international diabetic societies, recommending bariatric surgery in T2D

D. Mou (✉)
Department of Surgery, Brigham and Women's Hospital, Boston, MA, USA
e-mail: dmou2@partners.org

A. Tavakkoli
Division of General and GI Surgery, Brigham and Women's Hospital, Boston, MA, USA
e-mail: atavakkoli@bwh.harvard.edu

C. Newberry et al. (eds.), *Nutrition, Weight, and Digestive Health*,
https://doi.org/10.1007/978-3-030-94953-2_16

patients with BMI >30, and further reduced to 27.5 for Asians who experience adverse metabolic effect of obesity at a lower BMI.

History of Bariatric Surgery

Since its inception, bariatric surgery has evolved significantly. Bariatric surgeons have refined surgical techniques, developed novel procedures and devices, and standardized quality of care by establishing a nationalized accreditations system known as the Metabolic and Bariatric Surgery Accreditation and Quality Improvement Program (MBSAQIP) [15, 18, 19].

The first bariatric surgeries were performed in the 1950s. The concept of weight loss surgery emerged from patients who lost significant weight after undergoing bowel resections and other food restricting surgeries. These procedures were generally regarded as "restrictive" if there was a reduction in the gastric pouch size or "malabsorptive" if a portion of the intestine is bypassed. However, our current understanding of these mechanisms in the induction of weight loss has challenged this oversimplification; the classification continues to be used by many.

Dr. Kremen was credited for performing the first malabsorptive procedure, the jejunoileal bypass, in 1954 [16]. This procedure bypasses 50–70% of small bowel while creating a long loop of bowel with a blind end. Though this procedure conferred significant weight loss, it also resulted in diarrhea and cirrhosis, which led to its eventual abandonment [20].

Dr. Mason was accredited for performing the first gastric bypass surgery in 1966 [21]. By horizontally transecting the stomach and creating a bowel loop anastomosis to the proximal portion of the stomach, he achieved weight loss through both malabsorptive and restrictive methods. However, this anatomic configuration was prone to the development of bile reflux. This was addressed with the Roux-en-Y configuration, which promoted anterograde flow of bile and minimized its reflux into the stomach.

Several weight loss surgery variations were developed in the following years, including the biliopancreatic diversion in 1979 and the duodenal switch in 1993 [22]. Today, these procedures are infrequently performed and are usually indicated for patients with BMIs over 50.

Restrictive surgical techniques include the horizontal gastroplasty and the vertical banded gastroplasty. These purely restrictive procedures were considered less invasive and more physiologic, as they avoided bowel manipulation. Another purely restrictive surgical approach for weight loss was known as the gastric band [15, 18, 19, 23]. Started in 1978 in Europe, the gastric band gained significant popularity in the mid- to late 2000s when it accounted for about 40% of all bariatric operations in the USA [24]. This intervention has since become less popular due to inadequate long-term weight loss and complications such as band slippage and erosion.

Laparoscopy has made a markedly significant impact in bariatric surgery. Laparoscopic techniques enabled elective bariatric surgeries to have fewer complications, faster recovery, and decreased length of hospital stay. This has significantly contributed to the popularity of bariatric surgery [14, 15]. The first laparoscopic gastric bypass took place in 1994, and by 2004, laparoscopic bariatric surgeries exceeded open bariatric surgeries [15, 18]. Today, over 95% of all bariatric surgeries are performed laparoscopically [12, 25].

Contemporary Bariatric Surgeries

The most common bariatric surgeries performed today include the Roux-en-Y gastric bypass (RYGB), laparoscopic sleeve gastrectomy (LSG), and laparoscopic adjustable gastric banding (LAGB) [12].

Roux-En-Y Gastric Bypass (RYGB)

RYGB is considered one of the most effective and durable bariatric surgeries to date. This procedure confers roughly 30% total body weight loss (TBWL) at 2 years. Significant technical refinements have been made to the RYGB over the years. Though variations still exist, the size of the gastric pouch is 20–30 mL, often compared to the size of an egg to aid in patient understanding. The jejunum is transected 40–80 cm distal to the ligament of Treitz (Fig. 16.1). The distal end of the transected jejunum is anastomosed to the gastric pouch. The proximal end of the transected jejunum is anastomosed to the distal jejunum (i.e., creating the jejuno-jejunostomy) to create a 100–150 cm alimentary limb, or Roux limb.

The average reported weight loss after RYGB is 31% TBWL at 2 years and 26% TBWL at 5 years. The mechanism through which RYGB induces weight loss was originally described as a combination of physical restriction of food intake and caloric malabsorption from the bypassed bowel. However, there is increasing evidence describing the significant neurohormonal impact of bariatric surgery on weight loss success. The changes in gut hormones contribute to profound alterations in metabolism, appetite, and satiety. Ghrelin, known as the hunger hormone, has been shown to be notably decreased in patients after RYGB [26, 27]. Changes in other incretin hormones, such as glucagon-like peptide-1 (GLP-1) and peptide YY (PYY), alter satiety and glucose homeostasis [26–29]. Changes in bile salt levels and the intestinal microbiome have also been posited as potential contributors to weight loss.

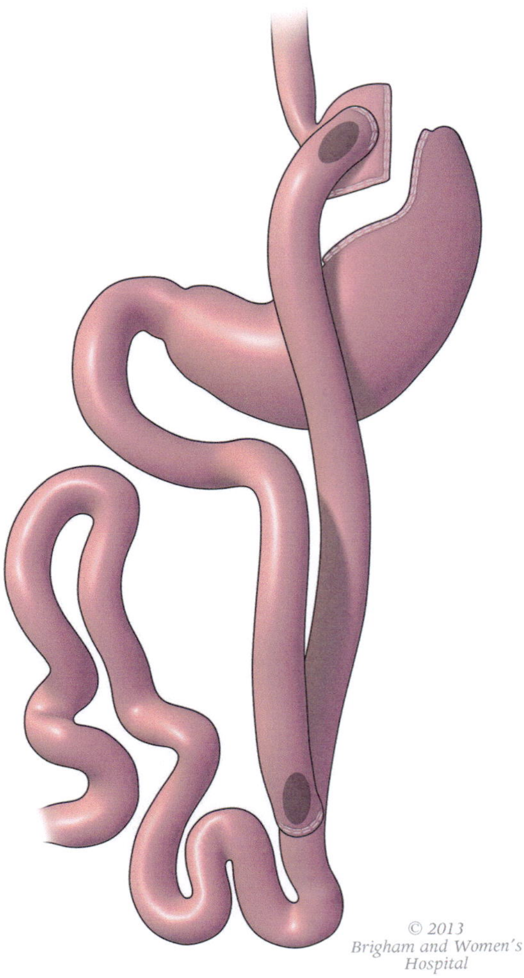

Fig. 16.1 Depiction of a Roux-en-Y gastric bypass (RYGB)

Over the years, RYGB has become a much safer surgery, with current mortality rates at 0.2%, similar to many common operations such as an appendectomy or knee arthroplasty. Complications early in the postoperative period include anastomotic leak, surgical site infections, bowel obstruction, thromboembolic events, and bleeding. The 30-day complication rate is approximately 3.4% for serious complications and 8.3% for all complications [30]. Anastomotic leaks, which were a major complication after this surgery, are now reduced with leak rates at <1%. Most bariatric procedures are performed with venous thromboembolism (VTE) prophylaxis. Therefore, the risk for VTE has decreased to 0.04% [31, 32]. Length of hospital stay after surgery is reduced to 1–2 days, with many patients able to discharge on postoperative day 1 and to return to work within 2–4 weeks.

Longer-term complications include marginal ulcers, internal hernias, vitamin and mineral deficiencies, and dumping syndrome. Development of marginal ulcers at the gastrojejunal anastomosis ranges from 0.6% to 7.6%. Risk factors include smoking, NSAID use, steroid use, large pouch size, and tension at the gastrojejunal anastomosis [33, 34]. Marginal ulcers can be treated with avoidance of risk factors, proton pump inhibitors, and sucralfate. Rarely, marginal ulcers can lead to bleeding and intestinal perforation, which will require operative intervention.

Internal hernias, bowel herniation through a mesenteric defect, can lead to obstruction and possible ischemia. This complication typically arises 2–3 years after RYGB in patients who have lost significant weight [35]. Presentation can be nonspecific abdominal pain. Given the potential for evolving ischemic bowel, a high index of suspicion is warranted [35, 36]. Abdominal CT scan with oral and intravenous contrast is helpful in the diagnosis of internal hernias. Urgent operative exploration is warranted for patients with internal hernia.

RYGB patients require long-term monitoring to ensure compliance with multivitamins. Postoperative patients are at risk for deficiencies in vitamin B12, iron, vitamin D, folate, zinc, copper, and selenium which can be minimized by regular use of supplementation and lifelong annual bariatric follow-up [37–42]. Finally, dumping syndrome refers to a constellation of symptoms due to the rapid transit of chyme through the small bowel. Symptoms include nausea, emesis, dizziness, light-headedness, abdominal pain, diarrhea, flushing, and palpitations. Early dumping takes place within 30 minutes of food ingestion and is secondary to rapid osmotic fluid shifts. Late dumping takes place 2–3 hours postprandially and is secondary to reactive hypoglycemia [43]. Of the RYGB patients, 10–20% experience early dumping syndrome, while 5–10% experience late dumping syndrome [44, 45]. Dumping syndrome can often be addressed with dietary adjustments such as increasing protein and fiber intake and initiation of small, frequent meals. Should the symptoms be refractory to dietary changes, medical management can be initiated often using acarbose as the initial agent.

Laparoscopic Sleeve Gastrectomy (LSG)

LSG was originally intended to be the first step of the biliopancreatic diversion. However, it was observed that patients lost a significant amount of weight with only this procedure, and it was thus adopted as a standalone procedure approximately 10 years ago. The LSG is currently the most popular bariatric surgery performed in the USA.

This procedure confers a 20–25% TBWL at 2 years with 5-year average weight loss of 18% TBWL. In this procedure, 80% of the stomach is vertically resected, resulting in a narrow gastric tube, often described as banana shaped (Fig. 16.2). No small bowel manipulation or resection is performed, and as a result, the surgery is accomplished quicker than a RYGB. The mechanisms that yield weight loss continue to be investigated but include decreasing the secretion of hunger-related hormones such as ghrelin. Ghrelin is produced in the oxyntic glands of cells in the gastric fundus, much of which is removed during LSG.

Early surgical complications include bleeding from the staple line, gastric leak, as well as dysphagia due to sleeve strictures. Both staple line bleeding and gastric leaks occur in 1–3% of LSG patients [46–49]. Postoperative strictures can often be managed by endoscopic dilations. Long-term complications include vitamin deficiencies and exacerbation of reflux symptoms. Persistent abdominal pain, nausea, and emesis can also occur due to sleeve stenosis. Such stenosis typically occurs at the incisura area of the sleeve and can often be addressed with endoscopic dilation [50].

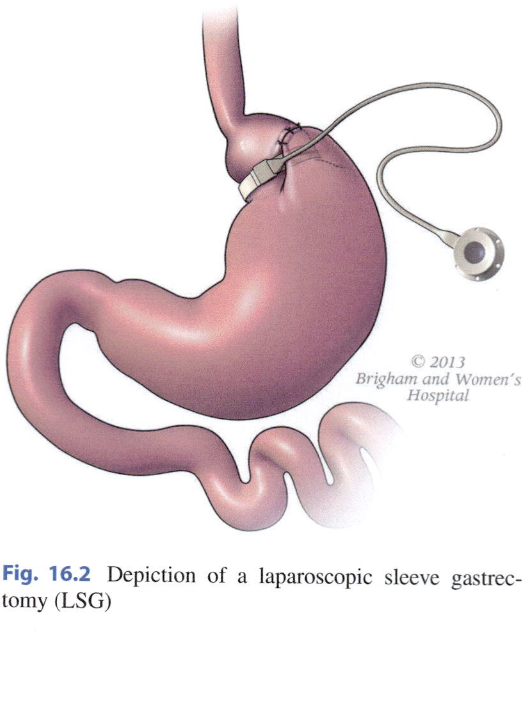

Fig. 16.2 Depiction of a laparoscopic sleeve gastrectomy (LSG)

Similar to RYGB patients, LSG patients are at risk for deficiencies in vitamin D, iron, folate, and vitamin B12 [39, 41, 51]. There is evidence that 32% of patients suffering from mild gastroesophageal reflux disease (GERD) may have worsened symptoms after LSG [52]. But there is also evidence that after LSG, reflux symptoms can improve as well, presumably due to overall weight loss. Due to these mixed results, surgeons are often cautious when recommending a LSG in patients with severe preoperative reflux symptoms and often perform a careful intraoperative assessment at the time of a LSG with the goal of repairing a hiatal hernia if identified. In a position piece, the ASMBS did not state a strong opinion on whether GERD should be deemed a relative contraindication to LSG [53].

Given its lower technical complexity relative to the RYGB, LSG has become the most common bariatric surgery performed in the USA. Of all bariatric surgeries performed, LSG increased from 33% in 2012 to over 60% in 2018 [12].

Laparoscopic Adjustable Gastric Banding (LAGB)

LAGB uses a silicone ring with an inflatable balloon that is placed 1–2 cm below the gastroesophageal junction to create a small superior gastric compartment (Fig. 16.3). This reservoir is approximately 30 mL in volume. Constriction of the band can be modified by injecting or aspirating saline from a port placed in the subcutaneous tissue. The port is attached to the inflatable balloon around the ring, which can be inflated or deflated to achieve the desired level of constriction. This procedure can result in early satiety, which leads to weight loss. However, long-term data have revealed that weight loss from LAGB is less than alternative surgical procedures and may not be as durable. LAGB results in 15% TBWL at 2 years and 10% at 5 years. The poor long-term weight loss outcomes and need for frequent band adjustments have contributed to the decline in popularity of LAGB.

Furthermore, LAGB outcomes have shown late postoperative complications, including band slippage and erosion. These complications often result in band removal and possibly conversions to other weight loss surgeries. In a retrospective study of 19,000 LAGB operations, 34% required surgical revision in 7 years [54]. The combination of suboptimal efficacy and concern for complications has decreased the popularity of LAGB. Of all bariatric surgeries performed in the USA, the percentage of LAGB placements has decreased drastically, from 35% of all bariatric operations in 2011 to 1.1% in 2018 [12].

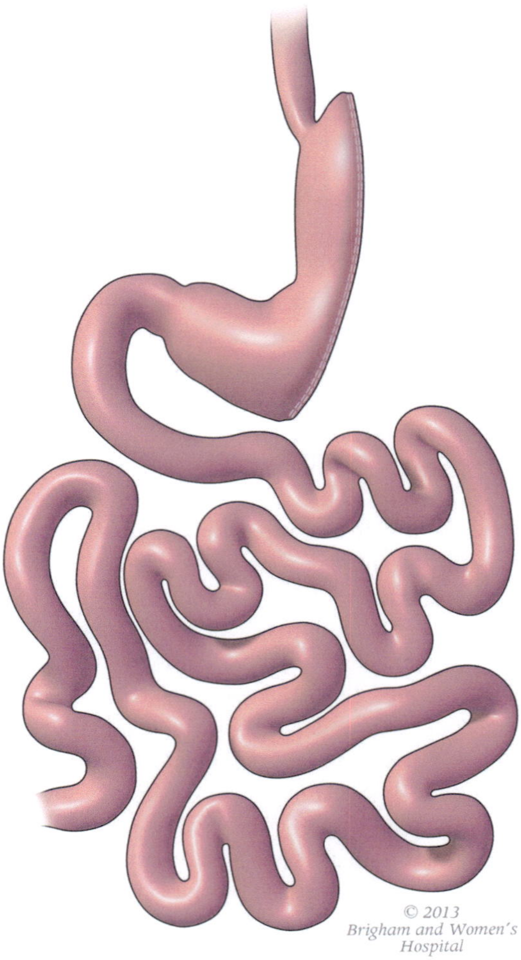

Fig. 16.3 Depiction of a laparoscopic adjustable gastric band (LAGB)

The Patient-Centered Outcomes Research Institute (PCORI) recently funded the national Patient-Centered Clinical Research Network

(PCORnet) Bariatric Study to compare the outcomes of RYGB, LSG, and LAGB. This longitudinal study of 40,000 patients demonstrated that at 5 years after surgery, RYGB conferred the most weight loss (26% TBWL), with LSG (19% TBWL) and LAGB (12% TBWL) trailing in effectiveness. However, RYGB also resulted in the highest 30-day major adverse event (5.0%) compared to LSG (2.6%) and LAGB (2.9%) [55]. Thoughtful assessment of risks and benefits should be undertaken to determine the most appropriate bariatric surgery for each individual patient [55]. Table 16.1 summarizes some of the important considerations when reviewing surgical options with patients.

Revisional Operations for Weight Gain

Bariatric surgery patients who experience complications, weight regain, or insufficient weight loss are considered treatment nonresponders and may be considered for revisional procedures and reintervention [56]. Despite this general recommendation, there is not a well-defined guideline of the degree of weight regain that warrants reintervention [57]. Although post-bariatric surgery weight regain is often attributed to patient eating habits and diet, it is most likely multifactorial, including procedure type as well as patient genotypes and baseline hormonal levels. In a study of 100 RYGB, our group has shown that preoperative hormones such as glucagon can predict the risk of postoperative weight regain highlighting the role of biological drivers of weight regain [58].

All modifiable risk factors should be optimized prior to pursuing reoperation [56, 59]. Specifically, for RYGB, weight regain has been attributed to gastric pouch dilatation, dilated gastrojejunal anastomosis, and gastro-gastric fistula. Although data supporting these hypotheses are mixed, endoscopic interventions to reduce gastric pouch size or a dilated anastomosis have gained popularity. These endoscopic approaches are typically the preferred approach for intervention due to high surgical complication rates. For gastro-gastric fistulas, endoscopic approaches have not been successful and surgical take down of the fistulas remains the gold standard [60, 61]. Though revisional bariatric surgeries certainly have a role in obesity management, they are associated with increased risk of complications. Therefore, thoughtful discussions with patients are necessary to clarify their goals, risks, and benefits, prior to committing to additional surgical intervention [62, 63].

Impact on Metabolism

Data has shown that bariatric surgery also significantly impacts the various metabolic syndrome-related comorbidities [64, 65] in addition to weight loss. The Longitudinal Assessment of Bariatric Surgery (LABS) showed that at 7 years following RYGB surgery, patients maintained remission of multiple comorbidities including 60% for T2D, 63% for hyperlipidemia, and 32% for hypertension [66]. A meta-analysis of ran-

Table 16.1 Relevant information to consider when selecting bariatric surgery for patients

	Laparoscopic adjustable gastric band (LAGB)	Laparoscopic sleeve gastrectomy (LSG)	Laparoscopic Roux-en-Y gastric bypass (RYGB)
Length of surgery	<1 hour	1 hour	1.5–2 hours
Time in hospital	0–1 day	1–2 days	1–2 days
%TBWL at 1 year	Around 15%	Around 25%	Around 31%
Risk of major adverse events	2.9%	2.6%	5%
Risk of death	<0.05%	0.1–0.3%	0.2–0.5%
Long-term rates of T2D remission[a]	65%	84%	86%
Postoperative adverse events	Slipped band Band erosion	Can cause reflux Strictures/twists Leaks	Dumping syndrome Ulcers Internal hernias

[a]T2D remission at some point in 5 years after surgery

domized control trials reveal that LSG patients achieve 46% remission in T2D 5 years after surgery [67].

The impact of bariatric surgery on T2D is well described. The procedure improves insulin sensitivity and often induces T2D remission [20, 23, 34, 35]. The precise mechanism of this process is poorly understood. It was initially thought that the weight loss itself was the primary contributor to T2D remission, but it has been observed that bariatric surgery confers immediate improvement in T2D that appears to be independent of weight. This is likely due to the neurohormonal impact of the surgery [23–26, 36]. The remarkable T2D remission rates reported have been confirmed in several randomized studies when comparing T2D patients who received intensive medical therapy, to patients who underwent RYGB and LSG who achieved significantly higher rates of remission, and for those not in remission, they required less T2D-related medications and achieved superior glycemic control [68–70]. Furthermore, the Longitudinal Assessment of Bariatric Surgery (LABS) study evaluated weight loss and changes in co-morbid conditions in 2348 patients 7 years after RYGB and LAGB. Of the RYGB patients, 60% achieved T2D remission, though this was not observed in LAGB patients [66].

Other Benefits of Bariatric Surgery

Beyond weight loss and improvement of various obesity-related comorbidities, bariatric surgery also confers longer life expectancy. In a longitudinal study that followed over 2000 patients with obesity compared with case-matched controls over 11 years, it was found that patients who underwent bariatric surgery had a decreased mortality (hazard ratio = 0.76) [71]. Another observational cohort study of 1000 patients with 5 years follow-up revealed an 89% decrease in the relative risk of mortality [72]. Additionally, in a large retrospective study with 8000 patients per arm comparing RYGB patients with nonsurgical controls matched for age, sex, and BMI, it was found that all-cause mortality was reduced by 40% in the RYGB group. With this mortality decline, there was a 56% reduction of mortality related to coronary artery disease (CAD), 92% reduction of mortality related to T2D, and 60% reduction of mortality related to cancer [73].

Bariatric surgery has also been shown to decrease systemic inflammation and reduce obesity-related cancer incidence [74, 75]. A meta-analysis of over 105,000 patients followed over 12 years revealed that bariatric surgery led to a 27% reduction of colorectal cancer [75]. Similar benefits have been described in the reduced rates of breast cancer, endometrial cancer, and pancreatic cancer [76, 77].

Expanded Indications for Bariatric Surgery

Childhood obesity has increased drastically in the past 40 years [3]. In the USA, nearly 1 in 5 adolescents have obesity [78]. The ASMBS has published revised guidelines for bariatric surgery in the pediatric population [79]. Current guidelines recommend that bariatric surgery should be considered for adolescents with similar guidelines to those of adults: BMI >35 with comorbidity or BMI >40. Extensive multidisciplinary team involvement is strongly recommended. There is a growing consensus that obesity is a disease that often requires intervention beyond healthy eating habits. There is accumulating evidence of the effectiveness of bariatric surgery in the adolescent population [80–82].

Utilization of Bariatric Surgery

Despite the benefits of bariatric surgery, only 1% of medically indicated individuals ultimately undergo this intervention. Barriers to bariatric surgery include lack of patient education, lack of experience with this intervention from referring providers, insurance barriers, limited access for care, and a perception that bariatric surgery often leads to severe complications [83–85]. Further studies are needed to understand the barriers to obtaining this therapy [86, 87].

Though bariatric surgery may not be cost saving, it has been shown to be cost effective [88]. Unfortunately, health insurance companies are inconsistent in their coverage for bariatric surgery [86]. Patients with public insurance and patients who belong to racial and ethnic minority groups are less likely to receive bariatric surgery compared to Caucasians [89]. These findings may be confounded by geographic variations [90, 91]. Further studies are needed to assess disparities in access to bariatric surgery.

Conclusion

Over the past few decades, bariatric surgery has proven to be effective, safe, life saving, and life improving. Further research is needed to understand the mechanisms behind its various metabolic benefits. Importantly, bariatric surgery is severely underutilized and education for patients and providers should be prioritized.

References

1. Bray GA, Kim KK, Wilding JPH, World Obesity Federation. Obesity: a chronic relapsing progressive disease process. A position statement of the World Obesity Federation. Obes Rev. 2017;18(7):715–23. PubMed PMID: 28489290.
2. Biener A, Cawley J, Meyerhoefer C. The high and rising costs of obesity to the US health care system. J Gen Intern Med. 2017;32(Suppl 1):6–8. PubMed PMID: 28271429. Pubmed Central PMCID: 5359159.
3. Katz DA, McHorney CA, Atkinson RL. Impact of obesity on health-related quality of life in patients with chronic illness. J Gen Intern Med. 2000;15(11):789–96. PubMed PMID: 11119171. Pubmed Central PMCID: 1495614.
4. Hedley AA, Ogden CL, Johnson CL, Carroll MD, Curtin LR, Flegal KM. Prevalence of overweight and obesity among US children, adolescents, and adults, 1999-2002. JAMA. 2004;291(23):2847–50. PubMed PMID: 15199035.
5. Stevens G, Mascarenhas M, Mathers C. WHO: global health risks. 2009 [cited 2020 5/11]. Available from: https://doi.org/10.2471/BLT.09.070565.
6. National health and Nutrition Examination Survey (NHANES) 2017 [cited 2020 5/11]. Available from: https://www.cdc.gov/nchs/data/factsheets/factsheet_nhanes.pdf.
7. Kim AR, Lee SM, An S. Estimating the economic value of counselling services using the contingent valuation method. Psychother Res. 2018;28(5):820–8. PubMed PMID: 28134035.
8. Tsai AG, Williamson DF, Glick HA. Direct medical cost of overweight and obesity in the USA: a quantitative systematic review. Obes Rev. 2011;12(1):50–61. PubMed PMID: 20059703. Pubmed Central PMCID: 2891924.
9. Prospective Studies C, Whitlock G, Lewington S, Sherliker P, Clarke R, Emberson J, et al. Body-mass index and cause-specific mortality in 900 000 adults: collaborative analyses of 57 prospective studies. Lancet. 2009;373(9669):1083–96. PubMed PMID: 19299006. Pubmed Central PMCID: 2662372.
10. Xu H, Cupples LA, Stokes A, Liu CT. Association of obesity with mortality over 24 years of weight history: findings from the Framingham heart study. JAMA Netw Open. 2018;1(7):e184587. PubMed PMID: 30646366. Pubmed Central PMCID: 6324399.
11. Aguilar-Olivos NE, Almeda-Valdes P, Aguilar-Salinas CA, Uribe M, Mendez-Sanchez N. The role of bariatric surgery in the management of nonalcoholic fatty liver disease and metabolic syndrome. Metab Clin Exp. 2016;65(8):1196–207. PubMed PMID: 26435078.
12. American Society for Metabolic and Bariatric Surgery: Estimate of Bariatric Surgery Numbers - American Society for Metabolic and Bariatric Surgery. www.asmbs.org 2014 [cited 2019]. Available from: https://asmbs.org/resources/estimate-of-bariatric-surgery-numbers.
13. Aangrisani L, Santonicola A, Iovino P, et al. IFSO worldwide survey 2016: primary, endoluminal, and revisional procedures. Obes Surg. 2018;28:3783–94.
14. Reoch J, Mottillo S, Shimony A, Filion KB, Christou NV, Joseph L, et al. Safety of laparoscopic vs open bariatric surgery: a systematic review and meta-analysis. Arch Surg. 2011;146(11):1314–22. PubMed PMID: 22106325.
15. Sundbom M. Laparoscopic revolution in bariatric surgery. World J Gastroenterol. 2014;20(41):15135–43. PubMed PMID: 25386062. Pubmed Central PMCID: 4223247.
16. NICE. Surgery for obese adults. In: Excellence NIfHaC, editor. NICE Pathways 2019.
17. Courcoulas A, Pories WJ. Potential candidates for bariatric surgery NIDDK. Natl Inst Health 2016 [cited 2020 5/12]. Available from: https://www.niddk.nih.gov/health-information/weight-management/bariatric-surgery/potential-candidates.
18. Phillips BT, Shikora SA. The history of metabolic and bariatric surgery: development of standards for patient safety and efficacy. Metab Clin Exp. 2018;79:97–107. PubMed PMID: 29307519.
19. Buchwald H. The evolution of metabolic/bariatric surgery. Obes Surg. 2014;24(8):1126–35. PubMed PMID: 25008469.
20. Singh D, Laya AS, Clarkston WK, Allen MJ. Jejunoileal bypass: a surgery of the past and a review of its complications. World J Gastroenterol. 2009;15(18):2277–9. PubMed PMID: 19437570. Pubmed Central PMCID: 2682245.

21. Mason EE, Ito C. Gastric bypass in obesity. 1967. Obes Res. 1996;4(3):316–9. PubMed PMID: 8732969.
22. Marceau P, Biron S, Hould FS, Lebel S, Marceau S, Lescelleur O, et al. Duodenal switch: long-term results. Obes Surg. 2007;17(11):1421–30. PubMed PMID: 18219767.
23. Gass M, Beglinger C, Peterli R. Metabolic surgery-principles and current concepts. Langenbeck's Arch Surg. 2011;396(7):949–72. PubMed PMID: 21870176.
24. Steffen R. The history and role of gastric banding. Surg Obes Relat Dis. 2008;4(3 Suppl):S7–13. PubMed PMID: 18501318.
25. Welbourn R, Pournaras DJ, Dixon J, Higa K, Kinsman R, Ottosson J, et al. Bariatric surgery worldwide: baseline demographic description and one-year outcomes from the second IFSO global registry report 2013-2015. Obes Surg. 2018;28(2):313–22. PubMed PMID: 28822052.
26. Peterli R, Wolnerhanssen B, Peters T, Devaux N, Kern B, Christoffel-Courtin C, et al. Improvement in glucose metabolism after bariatric surgery: comparison of laparoscopic Roux-en-Y gastric bypass and laparoscopic sleeve gastrectomy: a prospective randomized trial. Ann Surg. 2009;250(2):234–41. PubMed PMID: 19638921.
27. le Roux CW, Aylwin SJ, Batterham RL, Borg CM, Coyle F, Prasad V, et al. Gut hormone profiles following bariatric surgery favor an anorectic state, facilitate weight loss, and improve metabolic parameters. Ann Surg. 2006;243(1):108–14. PubMed PMID: 16371744. Pubmed Central PMCID: 1449984.
28. Hutch CR, Sandoval D. The role of GLP-1 in the metabolic success of bariatric surgery. Endocrinology. 2017;158(12):4139–51. PubMed PMID: 29040429. Pubmed Central PMCID: 5711387.
29. Magouliotis DE, Tasiopoulou VS, Sioka E, Chatedaki C, Zacharoulis D. Impact of bariatric surgery on metabolic and gut microbiota profile: a systematic review and meta-analysis. Obes Surg. 2017;27(5):1345–57. PubMed PMID: 28265960.
30. Stenberg E, Szabo E, Agren G, Naslund E, Boman L, Bylund A, et al. Early complications after laparoscopic gastric bypass surgery: results from the Scandinavian Obesity Surgery Registry. Ann Surg. 2014;260(6):1040–7. PubMed PMID: 24374541.
31. Dang JT, Switzer N, Delisle M, Laffin M, Gill R, Birch DW, et al. Predicting venous thromboembolism following laparoscopic bariatric surgery: development of the BariClot tool using the MBSAQIP database. Surg Endosc. 2019;33(3):821–31. PubMed PMID: 30003351.
32. American Society for Metabolic and Bariatric Surgery Clinical Issues Committee. ASMBS updated position statement on prophylactic measures to reduce the risk of venous thromboembolism in bariatric surgery patients. Surg Obes Relat Dis. 2013;9(4):493–7. PubMed PMID: 23769113.
33. Coblijn UK, Goucham AB, Lagarde SM, Kuiken SD, van Wagensveld BA. Development of ulcer disease after Roux-en-Y gastric bypass, incidence, risk factors, and patient presentation: a systematic review. Obes Surg. 2014;24(2):299–309. PubMed PMID: 24234733.
34. Coblijn UK, Lagarde SM, de Castro SM, Kuiken SD, van Wagensveld BA. Symptomatic marginal ulcer disease after Roux-en-Y gastric bypass: incidence, risk factors and management. Obes Surg. 2015;25(5):805–11. PubMed PMID: 25381115.
35. Greenstein AJ, O'Rourke RW. Abdominal pain after gastric bypass: suspects and solutions. Am J Surg. 2011;201(6):819–27. PubMed PMID: 21333269. Pubmed Central PMCID: 3123682.
36. Al-Mansour MR, Mundy R, Canoy JM, Dulaimy K, Kuhn JN, Romanelli J. Internal hernia after laparoscopic antecolic Roux-en-Y gastric bypass. Obes Surg. 2015;25(11):2106–11. PubMed PMID: 26037306.
37. Bal BS, Finelli FC, Shope TR, Koch TR. Nutritional deficiencies after bariatric surgery. Nat Rev Endocrinol. 2012;8(9):544–56. PubMed PMID: 22525731.
38. Weng TC, Chang CH, Dong YH, Chang YC, Chuang LM. Anaemia and related nutrient deficiencies after Roux-en-Y gastric bypass surgery: a systematic review and meta-analysis. BMJ Open. 2015;5(7):e006964. PubMed PMID: 26185175. Pubmed Central PMCID: 4513480.
39. Maghrabi AH, Wolski K, Abood B, Licata A, Pothier C, Bhatt DL, et al. Two-year outcomes on bone density and fracture incidence in patients with T2DM randomized to bariatric surgery versus intensive medical therapy. Obesity. 2015;23(12):2344–8. PubMed PMID: 26193177. Pubmed Central PMCID: 4701611.
40. Rodriguez-Carmona Y, Lopez-Alavez FJ, Gonzalez-Garay AG, Solis-Galicia C, Melendez G, Serralde-Zuniga AE. Bone mineral density after bariatric surgery. A systematic review. Int J Surg. 2014;12(9):976–82. PubMed PMID: 25110331.
41. Chakhtoura MT, Nakhoul NN, Shawwa K, Mantzoros C, El Hajj Fuleihan GA. Hypovitaminosis D in bariatric surgery: a systematic review of observational studies. Metab Clin Exp. 2016;65(4):574–85. PubMed PMID: 26805016. Pubmed Central PMCID: 4792683.
42. Zhang Q, Chen Y, Li J, Chen D, Cheng Z, Xu S, et al. A meta-analysis of the effects of bariatric surgery on fracture risk. Obes Rev. 2018;19(5):728–36. PubMed PMID: 29334691.
43. Berg P, McCallum R. Dumping syndrome: a review of the current concepts of pathophysiology, diagnosis, and treatment. Dig Dis Sci. 2016;61(1):11–8. PubMed PMID: 26396002.
44. Emous M, Wolffenbuttel BHR, van Dijk G, Totte E, van Beek AP. Long-term self-reported symptom prevalence of early and late dumping in a patient population after sleeve gastrectomy, primary, and revisional gastric bypass surgery. Surg Obes Relat Dis. 2018;14(8):1173–81. PubMed PMID: 29858129.

45. Nielsen JB, Pedersen AM, Gribsholt SB, Svensson E, Richelsen B. Prevalence, severity, and predictors of symptoms of dumping and hypoglycemia after Roux-en-Y gastric bypass. Surg Obes Relat Dis. 2016;12(8):1562–8. PubMed PMID: 27425831.
46. Berger ER, Clements RH, Morton JM, Huffman KM, Wolfe BM, Nguyen NT, et al. The impact of different surgical techniques on outcomes in laparoscopic sleeve gastrectomies: the first report from the metabolic and bariatric surgery accreditation and quality improvement program (MBSAQIP). Ann Surg. 2016;264(3):464–73. PubMed PMID: 27433904.
47. Dhar VK, Hanseman DJ, Watkins BM, Paquette IM, Shah SA, Thompson JR. What matters after sleeve gastrectomy: patient characteristics or surgical technique? Surgery. 2018;163(3):571–7. PubMed PMID: 29398036.
48. Aurora AR, Khaitan L, Saber AA. Sleeve gastrectomy and the risk of leak: a systematic analysis of 4,888 patients. Surg Endosc. 2012;26(6):1509–15. PubMed PMID: 22179470.
49. Gagner M, Kemmeter P. Comparison of laparoscopic sleeve gastrectomy leak rates in five staple-line reinforcement options: a systematic review. Surg Endosc. 2020;34(1):396–407. PubMed PMID: 30993513. Pubmed Central PMCID: 6946737.
50. Schulman AR, Thompson CC. Complications of bariatric surgery: what you can expect to see in your GI practice. Am J Gastroenterol. 2017;112(11):1640–55. PubMed PMID: 28809386.
51. Ben-Porat T, Elazary R, Goldenshluger A, Sherf Dagan S, Mintz Y, Weiss R. Nutritional deficiencies four years after laparoscopic sleeve gastrectomy-are supplements required for a lifetime? Surg Obes Relat Dis. 2017;13(7):1138–44. PubMed PMID: 28416186.
52. Peterli R, Wolnerhanssen BK, Peters T, Vetter D, Kroll D, Borbely Y, et al. Effect of laparoscopic sleeve gastrectomy vs laparoscopic Roux-en-Y gastric bypass on weight loss in patients with morbid obesity: the SM-BOSS randomized clinical trial. JAMA. 2018;319(3):255–65. PubMed PMID: 29340679. Pubmed Central PMCID: 5833546.
53. Ali M, El Chaar M, Ghiassi S, Rogers AM, American Society for Metabolic and Bariatric Surgery Clinical Issues Committee. American Society for Metabolic and Bariatric Surgery updated position statement on sleeve gastrectomy as a bariatric procedure. Surg Obes Relat Dis. 2017;13(10):1652–7. PubMed PMID: 29054173.
54. Altieri MS, Yang J, Telem DA, Meng Z, Frenkel C, Halbert C, et al. Lap band outcomes from 19,221 patients across centers and over a decade within the state of New York. Surg Endosc. 2016;30(5):1725–32. PubMed PMID: 26201412.
55. Arterburn D, Wellman R, Emiliano A, Smith SR, Odegaard AO, Murali S, et al. Comparative effectiveness and safety of bariatric procedures for weight loss: a PCORnet cohort study. Ann Intern Med. 2018;169(11):741–50. PubMed PMID: 30383139. Pubmed Central PMCID: 6652193.
56. Brethauer SA, Kothari S, Sudan R, Williams B, English WJ, Brengman M, et al. Systematic review on reoperative bariatric surgery: American Society for Metabolic and Bariatric Surgery Revision Task Force. Surg Obes Relat Dis. 2014;10(5):952–72. PubMed PMID: 24776071.
57. Mann JP, Jakes AD, Hayden JD, Barth JH. Systematic review of definitions of failure in revisional bariatric surgery. Obes Surg. 2015;25(3):571–4. PubMed PMID: 25515500.
58. Aliakbarian H, Bhutta HY, Heshmati K, Unes Kunju S, Sheu EG, Tavakkoli A. Pre-operative predictors of weight loss and weight regain following Roux-en-Y gastric bypass surgery: a prospective human study. Obes Surg. 2020;30(12):4852–9. PubMed PMID: 32748203.
59. Osland E, Yunus RM, Khan S, Memon B, Memon MA. Weight loss outcomes in laparoscopic vertical sleeve gastrectomy (LVSG) versus laparoscopic Roux-en-Y gastric bypass (LRYGB) procedures: a meta-analysis and systematic review of randomized controlled trials. Surg Laparosc Endosc Percutan Tech. 2017;27(1):8–18. PubMed PMID: 28145963.
60. Abu Dayyeh BK. Endoscopic revision of bariatric surgery: expanding the toolbox. Endoscopy. 2020;52(3):166–7. PubMed PMID: 32097962.
61. Keith JN. Endoscopic management of common bariatric surgical complications. Gastrointest Endosc Clin N Am. 2011;21(2):275–85. PubMed PMID: 21569979.
62. Nedelcu M, Khwaja HA, Rogula TG. Weight regain after bariatric surgery-how should it be defined? Surg Obes Relat Dis. 2016;12(5):1129–30. PubMed PMID: 27350180.
63. Mahawar KK, Nimeri A, Adamo M, Borg CM, Singhal R, Khan O, et al. Practices concerning revisional bariatric surgery: a survey of 460 surgeons. Obes Surg. 2018;28(9):2650–60. PubMed PMID: 29616464.
64. Knop FK, Taylor R. Mechanism of metabolic advantages after bariatric surgery: it's all gastrointestinal factors versus it's all food restriction. Diabetes Care. 2013;36(Suppl 2):S287–91. PubMed PMID: 23882061. Pubmed Central PMCID: 3920787.
65. Yu J, Zhou X, Li L, Li S, Tan J, Li Y, et al. The long-term effects of bariatric surgery for type 2 diabetes: systematic review and meta-analysis of randomized and non-randomized evidence. Obes Surg. 2015;25(1):143–58. PubMed PMID: 25355456.
66. Courcoulas AP, King WC, Belle SH, Berk P, Flum DR, Garcia L, et al. Seven-year weight trajectories and health outcomes in the longitudinal assessment of bariatric surgery (LABS) study. JAMA Surg. 2018;153(5):427–34. PubMed PMID: 29214306. Pubmed Central PMCID: 6584318.
67. Borgeraas H, Hofso D, Hertel JK, Hjelmesaeth J. Comparison of the effect of Roux-en-Y gastric bypass and sleeve gastrectomy on remission of type 2 diabetes: a systematic review and meta-analysis of randomized controlled trials. Obes Rev.

2020;21(6):e13011. PubMed PMID: 32162437. Pubmed Central PMCID: 7317556.
68. Schauer PR, Bhatt DL, Kirwan JP, Wolski K, Aminian A, Brethauer SA, et al. Bariatric surgery versus intensive medical therapy for diabetes – 5-year outcomes. N Engl J Med. 2017;376(7):641–51. PubMed PMID: 28199805. Pubmed Central PMCID: 5451258.
69. Rubino F, Nathan DM, Eckel RH, Schauer PR, Alberti KG, Zimmet PZ, et al. Metabolic surgery in the treatment algorithm for type 2 diabetes: a joint statement by international diabetes organizations. Surg Obes Relat Dis. 2016;12(6):1144–62. PubMed PMID: 27568469.
70. Khorgami Z, Shoar S, Saber AA, Howard CA, Danaei G, Sclabas GM. Outcomes of bariatric surgery versus medical management for Type 2 diabetes mellitus: a meta-analysis of randomized controlled trials. Obes Surg. 2019;29(3):964–74. PubMed PMID: 30402804.
71. Sjostrom L, Gummesson A, Sjostrom CD, Narbro K, Peltonen M, Wedel H, et al. Effects of bariatric surgery on cancer incidence in obese patients in Sweden (Swedish Obese Subjects Study): a prospective, controlled intervention trial. Lancet Oncol. 2009;10(7):653–62. PubMed PMID: 19556163.
72. Christou NV, Sampalis JS, Liberman M, Look D, Auger S, McLean AP, et al. Surgery decreases long-term mortality, morbidity, and health care use in morbidly obese patients. Ann Surg. 2004;240(3):416–23; discussion 23–4. PubMed PMID: 15319713. Pubmed Central PMCID: 1356432.
73. Adams TD, Hunt SC. Cancer and obesity: effect of bariatric surgery. World J Surg. 2009;33(10):2028–33. PubMed PMID: 19672652.
74. Adams TD, Gress RE, Smith SC, Halverson RC, Simper SC, Rosamond WD, et al. Long-term mortality after gastric bypass surgery. N Engl J Med. 2007;357(8):753–61. PubMed PMID: 17715409.
75. Afshar S, Kelly SB, Seymour K, Lara J, Woodcock S, Mathers JC. The effects of bariatric surgery on colorectal cancer risk: systematic review and meta-analysis. Obes Surg. 2014;24(10):1793–9. PubMed PMID: 25015708.
76. Heshmati K, Harris DA, Rosner B, Pranckevicius E, Ardestani A, Cho N, et al. Association of bariatric surgery status with reduced HER2+ breast cancers: a retrospective cohort study. Obes Surg. 2019;29(4):1092–8. PubMed PMID: 30659466.
77. Schauer DP, Feigelson HS, Koebnick C, Caan B, Weinmann S, Leonard AC, et al. Bariatric surgery and the risk of cancer in a large multisite cohort. Ann Surg. 2019;269(1):95–101. PubMed PMID: 28938270. Pubmed Central PMCID: 6201282.
78. Ogden CL, Carroll MD, Kit BK, Flegal KM. Prevalence of childhood and adult obesity in the United States, 2011-2012. JAMA. 2014;311(8):806–14. PubMed PMID: 24570244. Pubmed Central PMCID: 4770258.
79. Pratt JSA, Browne A, Browne NT, Bruzoni M, Cohen M, Desai A, et al. ASMBS pediatric metabolic and bariatric surgery guidelines, 2018. Surg Obes Relat Dis. 2018;14(7):882–901. PubMed PMID: 30077361. Pubmed Central PMCID: 6097871.
80. Inge TH, Jenkins TM, Xanthakos SA, Dixon JB, Daniels SR, Zeller MH, et al. Long-term outcomes of bariatric surgery in adolescents with severe obesity (FABS-5+): a prospective follow-up analysis. Lancet Diabetes Endocrinol. 2017;5(3):165–73. PubMed PMID: 28065736.
81. Beamish AJ, Johansson SE, Olbers T. Bariatric surgery in adolescents: what do we know so far? Scand J Surg. 2015;104(1):24–32. PubMed PMID: 25388886.
82. Qi L, Guo Y, Liu CQ, Huang ZP, Sheng Y, Zou DJ. Effects of bariatric surgery on glycemic and lipid metabolism, surgical complication and quality of life in adolescents with obesity: a systematic review and meta-analysis. Surg Obes Relat Dis. 2017;13(12):2037–55. PubMed PMID: 29079384.
83. Funk LM, Jolles SA, Greenberg CC, Schwarze ML, Safdar N, McVay MA, et al. Primary care physician decision making regarding severe obesity treatment and bariatric surgery: a qualitative study. Surg Obes Relat Dis. 2016;12(4):893–901. PubMed PMID: 26948943.
84. Funk LM, Jolles S, Fischer LE, Voils CI. Patient and referring practitioner characteristics associated with the likelihood of undergoing bariatric surgery: a systematic review. JAMA Surg. 2015;150(10):999–1005. PubMed PMID: 26222655. Pubmed Central PMCID: 4992360.
85. Simon R, Lahiri SW. Provider practice habits and barriers to care in obesity management in a large multicenter health system. Endocr Pract. 2018;24(4):321–8. PubMed PMID: 29561192.
86. Kim DD, Arterburn DE, Sullivan SD, Basu A. Economic value of greater access to bariatric procedures for patients with severe obesity and diabetes. Med Care. 2018;56(7):583–8. PubMed PMID: 29762271.
87. Kim DD, Arterburn DE, Sullivan SD, Basu A. Association between the publication of clinical evidence and the use of bariatric surgery. Obes Surg. 2018;28(5):1321–8. PubMed PMID: 29086183.
88. Alsumali A, Eguale T, Bairdain S, Samnaliev M. Cost-effectiveness analysis of bariatric surgery for morbid obesity. Obes Surg. 2018;28(8):2203–14. PubMed PMID: 29335933.
89. Hennings DL, Baimas-George M, Al-Quarayshi Z, Moore R, Kandil E, DuCoin CG. The inequity of bariatric surgery: publicly insured patients undergo lower rates of bariatric surgery with worse outcomes. Obes Surg. 2018;28(1):44–51. PubMed PMID: 28667512.
90. Birkmeyer NJ, Gu N. Race, socioeconomic status, and the use of bariatric surgery in Michigan. Obes Surg. 2012;22(2):259–65. PubMed PMID: 20559894.
91. Stanford FC, Jones DB, Schneider BE, Blackburn GL, Apovian CM, Hess DT, et al. Patient race and the likelihood of undergoing bariatric surgery among patients seeking surgery. Surg Endosc. 2015;29(9):2794–9. PubMed PMID: 25492453. Pubmed Central PMCID: 4597304.

Part IV

Nutrition Support

Parenteral Nutrition

17

Ennaliza Salazar, Nicha Somlaw, Sara Bonnes, and Ryan T. Hurt

Introduction

In the late 1960s, Dudrick et al. successfully infused total parenteral nutrition (PN) in a 1-month-old infant with small bowel atresia for at least 5 months [1]. Since its initial inception, PN has now evolved to include three major components, namely, macronutrient, micronutrient, and fluid. The macronutrient component consists of carbohydrate, lipid, and protein, the micronutrient component is made up of multivitamins and trace elements, and the volume comprises sterile water with or without electrolytes.

Since the proven clinical application of PN in malnourished postoperative patients, its use has evolved from a supplement in patients whose oral or enteral intake is less than 60% requirement to total nutrition support in patients who have nonfunctioning gastrointestinal tract (GIT) [2, 3]. Previous attempts of PN infusion were complicated by erroneous mixtures of macronutrients causing phlebitis or embolic event [1]. Establishing adequate venous access proved to be an additional challenge to provide PN therapy for hypertonic nutrient administration. This was eventually resolved by subclavian vein catherization to minimize thrombotic complication associated with peripheral PN infusion.

Routes of Infusion

Parenteral nutrition can be infused peripherally or centrally. The route of administration is determined by its osmolarity. Peripheral PN has a similar composition to that of central PN but has a lower caloric concentration and higher volume to allow for peripheral administration. As a general rule, the osmolarity of peripheral PN should be between 600 and 900 mOSM to avoid the risk of thrombophlebitis [4]. Therefore, adequate peripheral venous access is required to avoid complications and to maintain patient tolerance of large volumes of PN. Due to the lower caloric concentration of PN, it is utilized for short periods (up to 2 weeks) as a supplement to oral or enteral intake or as a bridge to central PN. Central PN is higher in caloric concentration and is used to provide all nutritional needs, often referred to as total PN. Central PN is hyperosmolar (greater than 1000 mOsm) and requires infusion via a large-diameter vessel, such as the superior vein

E. Salazar
Department of Gastroenterology and Hepatology, Singapore General Hospital, Singapore, Singapore
e-mail: ennaliza.salazar@sgh.com.sg

N. Somlaw
Department of Medicine, King Chulalongkorn Memorial Hospital and Chulalongkorn University, Bangkok, Thailand

S. Bonnes (✉) · R. T. Hurt
Department of General Internal Medicine, Mayo Clinic, Rochester, MN, USA
e-mail: bonnes.sara@mayo.edu; hurt.ryan@mayo.edu

C. Newberry et al. (eds.), *Nutrition, Weight, and Digestive Health*,
https://doi.org/10.1007/978-3-030-94953-2_17

cava (SVC) or small peripherally inserted central venous catheters (PICC). Infusion of central PN into large-diameter vein allows higher rate of infusion and is the preferred route of administration for patients who require PN support for greater than 7 days.

Types of Parenteral Nutrition

There are both ready-to-use PN and compound PN formulations available for use. Ready-to-use PN has a fixed number of calories with or without electrolytes and is available for central or peripheral PN use. The macronutrients are separated into chambers by an internal membrane that is broken just before its administration to mix the components. The mixing is done prior to administration to prevent metabolic instability that may occur after 24 hours of mixing micronutrition and micronutrients [5]. Compounded PN is customizable to meet individual patient requirements. This PN requires a sterile central compounding facility for daily composition. Potential advantages of ready-to-use PN include reduced cost, fewer ordering and compounding errors, and fewer bloodstream infections [6]. However, ready-to-use PN may not meet each patient's total calorie or electrolyte requirement, in addition to the added inconvenience of adding multivitamins just prior to administration.

Indication of Parenteral Nutrition

PN is indicated in patients who are malnourished or at risk of malnutrition when enteral feeding is not possible to meet nutritional needs. Screening for malnutrition can be performed by using a quick and easy screening tool such as malnutrition screening tool (MST), Malnutrition Universal Screening tool (MUST), or Nutritional Risk Screening (NRS) which usually involves three questionnaires. Types of screening tool vary among institutions. Typical screening questions include body mass index, percentage of weight loss, presence of loss of appetite, or presence of illness. A score is then calculated, and patients are categorized as low, moderate, or high risk of malnutrition [7]. Patients who have moderate- to high-risk malnutrition should receive formal dietician assessment such as Subjective Global Assessment (SGA, see perioperative malnutrition section) and dietary counselling.

Despite the innovation provided by PN, it remains a costly intervention and is not without complication. Prior to initiation of PN, a consideration of enteral feeding with utilizing the gastrointestinal tract (GIT) is always preferred. In a functional GIT, oral or enteral feeding are a less expensive option and aid in maintaining the mucosal barrier, preventing bacterial translocation, or additional risks discussed in the following section (Table 17.1) [8].

Critical Illness

The prevalence of malnutrition ranges from 38 to 78% in critically ill patients in the intensive care unit (ICU) and is associated with increased morbidity, mortality, and healthcare cost [10]. To determine risks in this population, nutrition screening should take place within 48 hours of admission using the nutritional risk screening (NRS 2002) and NUTRIC scores [11]. Patients who are at high nutrition risk, defined by NRS 2002 ≥ 5 or NUTRIC score ≥ 5, are more likely to benefit from early nutrition intervention within 48 hours with improved outcomes vs those at low nutrition risk. Enteral nutrition is the preferred route of nutrition therapy. However, if enteral

Table 17.1 Indication of parenteral nutrition

Malnourished or at risk of malnutrition patients who are not able to meet nutrition requirement with enteral nutrition
Impaired GIT function as a result of underlying disease or treatment
Paralytic ileus
GIT obstruction
GIT fistula when enteral feeding past fistula is not possible
Prolonged diarrhea
Short bowel syndrome

Source: Adapted from ASPEN [8, 9]
GIT gastrointestinal tract

nutrition is not feasible, PN should be started as soon as possible following ICU admission [11]. Alternatively, in patients with a low nutrition risk (NRS 2002 ≤3 or NUTRIC score ≤5), exclusive PN can be withheld for 7 days following ICU admission if the patient cannot maintain oral or enteral feeding [11].

Perioperative Malnutrition

Perioperative malnutrition is identified by utilizing the validated subjective global assessment (SGA), which was developed to quickly and accurately assess physiological symptoms of malnutrition and functional capacity. Patients with SGA B and C should receive dietetic counselling to rectify malnutrition issues (scoring with A as normal, B as mild to moderate, and C as severe malnutrition). These measures are paramount due to known pro-inflammatory mediators that are elicited during surgical intervention [12]. This cascade of inflammatory mediators induce protein catabolism resulting in loss of muscle tissue which can impede overall functional recovery. The post-surgical Enhanced Recovery After Surgery (ERAS) protocol is a widely adopted multidisciplinary approach for patients who undergo elective surgery [12]. The protocol starts before, during, and after surgery involving surgeons, anesthetists, dieticians, nurses, and physiotherapists. The multispecialty approach has shown to reduce hospital stay, surgical complication, and overall cost [13]. From a metabolic and nutritional aspect, perioperative care includes nutritional counselling for patients with a high risk of malnutrition prior to surgery, avoidance of long periods of preoperative fasting (2 hours of liquid and 6 hours of solid is allowed), resumption of oral feeding as early as possible after surgery, blood sugar control, minimizing paralytic agents for ventilator management in the postoperative period, and early mobilization to facilitate protein synthesis and muscle function [12]. While enteral nutrition is the preferred form of nutrition therapy, PN is usually reserved when enteral nutrition is not feasible and maximal benefit is derived in severely malnourished patient who receive PN for more than 7–10 days preoperatively [14].

Home Parenteral Nutrition

The indication for home PN mirrors those of hospitalized patients, however, with an expected prolonged duration of need after discharge [15]. Patients who have chronic intestinal failure, which is defined a as chronic condition where there is reduction of gut function below the minimum necessary for the absorption of macronutrition and/or water and electrolytes such that intravenous supplementation is required to maintain health and/or growth. These patients are usually metabolically stable with a condition that may or may not be reversible [16]. Patients who have chronic intestinal failure may require home PN indefinitely as reversibility of chronic intestinal failure is only reported approximately 20–50% [17]. Careful consideration must be given to the capabilities of patients and caregivers as well as social circumstances. Outcomes of home PN patients depend on the underlying disease process with cancer patients having more frequent PN complications and a poorer prognosis [15]. Patients who receive home PN should be managed by trained physicians, dieticians, nurses, and pharmacists for careful monitoring to avoid both short- and long-term complications.

Parenteral Nutrition Formulation

Carbohydrate

Carbohydrates are the main sources of energy in PN. It makes up 50–60% of total calories or 70–85% of non-protein calories [18, 19]. The most commonly used carbohydrate substrate in PN is dextrose monohydrate that provides 3.4 kcal/g. Higher concentrations of dextrose (>10%) are reserved for central venous administration to avoid thrombophlebitis in peripheral veins.

Minimum glucose intake of at least 100–120 g/day is widely suggested in order to suppress both gluconeogenesis and protein catabolism in healthy individuals [18, 20]. During catabolic stress, maximum oxidation rate of glucose is theoretically about 4–7 mg/kg/min. Thus, it is recommended that glucose infusion rate (GIR) should not exceed 5 mg/kg/day in critically ill patients; otherwise, it can lead to hyperglycemia, hypertriglyceridemia, and lipogenesis. In stable non-acutely ill patients, glucose oxidation rate of 5–7 mg/kg/day is tolerated [3, 20].

Protein

Crystalline amino acids (AAs) provide protein source in PN formulation and yield 4 kcal/g. Standard amino acid products offer varying mixtures of essential and non-essential AAs in concentrations ranging from 3.5% to 20%. Some amino acid formulations also contain a combination of electrolytes [9].

Specialized amino acid products are available for use in specific conditions such as hepatic or renal disease. However, its efficacy in clinical outcome has not been proven in either patient population [21, 22].

Fat

Intravenous lipid emulsions (ILEs) are included in PN regimens to provide a dense source of non-protein energy and essential fatty acids (EFAs; *n-6* linoleic acid and *n-3* alpha-linolenic acid). ILEs are mainly composed of long-chain triglycerides from a variety of oils. ILES also contain egg yolk phospholipid and glycerol, which provide additional energy yielding 10–11 kcal/g.

The first-generation ILEs are soybean oil (SO)-based formulations, 100% SO, and a combination of SO and safflower oil, which offer a great amount of both EFAs. However, the high content of n-6 linoleic acid in these products has been associated with pro-inflammatory and immunosuppressive effects. Moreover, the conventional ILEs have been associated with hypertriglyceridemia. Newer alternative ILEs with lower *n*-6 content have been introduced and gradually replaced SO-based ILE. These reduced *n*-6 ILEs are the second generation ILEs; medium chain triglycerides (MCTs) mixed with SO, third generation; olive oil (OO) and SO, and the fourth generation; fish oil (FO) based ILEs. MCTs accumulate less in adipose tissue and the liver, are metabolized faster, and do not produce pro-inflammatory mediators. OO is high in oleic acid and mono-unsaturated fatty acid (MUFA), which produce less oxidative stress than SO and is not metabolized to mediators of inflammation. FO is high in n-3 fatty acids with anti-inflammatory properties and may potentially reverse intestinal failure associated liver disease in children receiving long-term PN. One of the FO-based ILEs, Smoflipid (Fresenius Kabi), is a mixture of four oils (SO, MCTs, OO, and FO), with lower ratios of *n*-6 to *n*-3 fatty acid and has been recommended in the critically ill and surgical patient populations [22].

The recommended dose for ILE infusion is 1–2 g/kg/kg/day. Many clinicians limit the use of SO-based ILE to 1 g/kg/day due to its pro-inflammatory effect. The dose of lipid infusion and infusion rate should not exceed 2.5 g/kg/day and 0.11 g/kg/hour, respectively. Higher doses or infusion rates are associated with increased risks of hypertriglyceridemia, infection, and fat overload syndrome, characterized by headache, fever, jaundice, hepatosplenomegaly, respiratory distress, spontaneous bleeding, pancytopenia, and shock [23].

Propofol is a lipid-soluble, short-acting intravenous anesthetic available in an emulsion similar to an ILE 10% yielding 1.1 kcal/ml. Therefore, when propofol is administered, the daily dose of ILE in the PN regimen should be adjusted accordingly.

Electrolytes

Electrolytes are added to PN formulations as a maintenance or therapeutic measure according to individual patient requirements. Suggested doses of electrolyte additions in adult PN formulation and commonly used forms are listed in Table 17.2. Maximum limits of electrolyte additives are based on both clinical and PN compounding

Table 17.2 Electrolyte PN additions in adult [9, 19]

Electrolyte	Suggested maintenance ranges	Salt forms that commonly used
Sodium	1–2 mEq/kg	Acetate, chloride, phosphate
Potassium	1–2 mEq/kg	Acetate, chloride, phosphate
Calcium	10–15 mEq/day	Gluconate
Magnesium	8–20 mEq/day	Sulfate
Phosphorus	20–40 mmol/day	Sodium, potassium
Chloride	As needed to maintain acid-base balance	Sodium, potassium
Acetate	As needed to maintain acid-base balance	Sodium, potassium

Based on generally healthy adults with normal losses

parameters. Particular attention should be paid to calcium and phosphate amounts due to the potential risk of precipitate formation in the PN solution when excessive amounts are added [24]. Electrolytes are available in various parenteral salt forms; however, not all electrolyte forms can be used in PN formulations due to their physiochemical incompatibilities. For example, sodium bicarbonate should not be added to PN solutions because it can interact with calcium to form insoluble calcium carbonate.

Vitamins

Commercially available vitamins for PN addition include multivitamin products with both water-soluble and fat-soluble vitamins with or without vitamin K, water-soluble vitamin admixtures, fat-soluble vitamin admixtures, and some single-entity products. Multivitamin products are designed to meet the requirements outlined by the American Medical Association (AMA) and the US Food and Drug administration (FDA). Compositions of adult multivitamin preparation are listed in Table 17.3.

Trace Elements

Trace elements (TEs) are minerals present at very low concentrations in the human body but essential for metabolic activities. PN solution contains several TEs from direct supplementation and contamination with PN components. TEs for PN addition are commercially available as single-entity products and in various multi-TE combinations which usually include zinc, copper, manganese, chromium, and selenium. Most multi-TE products provide trace element amounts to meet the requirement outlined by AMA. In 2012 the American Society of Parenteral and Enteral Nutrition (ASPEN) recommended significant changes in commercially available adult multi-TE products [25]. The recommendations included reducing doses of copper, manganese, and chromium, limiting trace elements, while increasing selenium. The recommendations were made after several findings of organ accumulations of copper, manganese, and chromium. The discrepancies between adult parenteral TE requirement and the dose provided from multi-TE products are shown in Table 17.4.

Iron is not routinely added to PN formulation in the USA because of the risk of anaphylaxis and the concern of incompatibilities. Thus, long-

Table 17.3 Contents of adult parenteral multivitamin preparations [9, 18, 25]

Components	Daily parenteral dose
Fat-soluble vitamins	
Vitamin A	1 mg or 3300 IU[a]
Vitamin D	5 mcg or 200 IU[b]
Vitamin E	10 mg or 10 IU[c]
Vitamin K	0–150 mcg[d]
Water-soluble vitamins	
Vitamin B1 (thiamine)	6 mg
Vitamin B2 (riboflavin)	3.6 mg
Vitamin B3 (niacin)	40 mg
Vitamin B5 (pantothenic acid)	15 mg
Vitamin B6 (pyridoxine)	6 mg
Vitamin B12 (cyanocobalamin)	5 mcg
Vitamin C (ascorbic acid)	200 mg
Folate	600 mcg
Biotin	60 mcg

[a]1 mcg retinol = 1 mcg retinol-activity equivalent (RAE) = 3.33 IU retinol.

[b]1 mcg cholecalciferol = 40 IU.

[c]1 mg = 1 IU = 1 United States Pharmacopeia (USP) unit is used in IV multivitamin preparation.

[d]Products without vitamin K are designed for patients receiving warfarin.

Table 17.4 Current recommended adult daily trace element requirements and ranges provided by multi-TE products

Trace elements	Daily dose provided from multi-TE products	Current recommended daily dose[a]
Copper (mg)	0.4–1.3	0.3–0.5
Chromium (mcg)	10–12	1–1.5
Manganese (mcg)	100–800	55
Selenium (mcg)	0–60	60–100
Zinc (mg)	1–6.5	2.5–5
Iron (mg)	1.1	None[b]

[a]Parenteral supplementations with PN therapy [25, 28]
[b]Iron, iodine, molybdenum, and fluoride are not routinely added to PN products in the USA but in Europe.

term PN patients are susceptible to iron deficiency [26]. Among multiple intravenous iron products available, only low-molecular-weight iron dextran can be added to non-lipid containing (2-in-1) PN formulation [27]. However, intravenous iron supplementation outside of the PN regimen is often more practical.

Copper and manganese are excreted via the biliary system; as a result to prevent accumulations of excess copper (in liver, kidney, brain) and manganese (in brain), a reduction of both TE supplementations in patients with hepatobiliary disease should be considered. Supplementation of zinc above the standard recommendation is required by patients with excessive gastrointestinal (GI) loss such as severe diarrhea, high-output ostomy, or fistula. Supplementation of selenium with higher dose should be considered in patients with malnutrition, critical illness, and burn injuries as selenium needs are increased [25, 28].

Use of Filter

Use of in-line filters are recommended for PN administration to reduce the potential for harm due to particulates (e.g., plastic fragments from the bag), microprecipitates (e.g., calcium phosphate), microorganisms, and air emboli. Use of a 0.22 micron filter for 2-in-1 admixture and a 1.2 micron filter for TNA and separately infused ILE is recommended [29, 30].

Complication of Parenteral Nutrition

Introduction of Complication of Parenteral Nutrition

There are a number of complications that must be considered when delivering PN to patients in the hospital and home settings. Central venous catheter (CVC) infections are the most serious complications which can result in increased morbidity and mortality and require immediate treatment. Repeated catheter-related bloodstream infections (CRBSI) can eventually lead to loss of access in short-term and long-term PN patients. Metabolic complications are commonly encountered, such as metabolic bone disease, intestinal failure associated liver disease (IFALD), and essential fatty acid deficiency (EFAD), after weeks to months of PN administration. Other metabolic complications such as hypo- or hyperglycemia and hypertriglyceridemia can occur after only a few hours of PN. The following section will review common metabolic and CVC infections including CRBSI in PN patients.

Catheter-Related Infection

Catheter-related infection can occur anywhere from the insertion site (exit site, tunnel, pocket where the device is implanted) to bloodstream [31]. Infection at the exit, tunnel, or pocket sites is usually visibly red and tender and occurs in the absence of concomitant bloodstream infection (BSI) [31]. In pocket site infections, purulent fluid and discharge may occur and removal of device is necessary.

Catheter-related bloodstream infection (CRBSI) and central line–associated bloodstream infection (CLABSI) are often used interchangeably for catheter-related infection, although they differ [31]. CRBSI is a clinical definition that requires quantitative blood cultures of differential time positivity to identify the catheter as the source of BSI [31]. CRBSI is often difficult to diagnose due to the inability to perform appropriate cultures due to time sensitivity and specimen source labeling and the inability to remove catheters [31], while CLABSI is both a clinical and surveillance term used for diagnosis of BSI in a patient with a central line placed within a period of 48 hours of developing a BSI that is not due to an infection of another etiology [31]. Three criteria for CLABSI include clinical signs and symptoms of infection, no alternate source for BSI, and blood culture positivity [31].

There are four possible routes of transmission in CLABSI: endogenous skin flora at the site of insertion, contamination of catheter hub by hand or device, hematogenous seeding from distant infection, and infusion contamination [32]. The most common routes of contamination are skin insertion site and the hub [32].

In patients receiving parenteral nutrition and are suspected to have CLABSI, paired blood samples should be taken from the catheter and peripheral vein before initiation of antimicrobial therapy [33]. The bottles should be labeled appropriately to reflect the site from which the samples were obtained. It is recommended that at least two blood samples should be drawn through different catheter lumens if blood sample cannot be drawn from a peripheral vein [33].
Coagulase-negative staphylococci and gram-positive microorganisms are two common pathogens associated with CLABSI. Coagulase-negative staphylococci have the tendency to produce biofilm composed of exopolysaccharide which allow the staphylococcal cells to cling to the surface of the catheter. The biofilm can form on the catheter surfaces within 24 hours of device insertion. The emergence of drug-resistant microorganism such as methicillin-resistant *Staphylococcus aureus* and vancomycin-resistant *Enterococcus* continues to pose challenges in CLABSI management. Early consultation with an infection disease physician is warranted to guide antibiotic choice and duration. In addition to intravenous antibiotic, early removal of catheter is recommended in confirmed or suspected CLABSI in a hemodynamic unstable patient for source control [33]. In patients requiring long-term venous catheter or patients with limited vascular access, catheter salvage in uncomplicated coagulase-negative staphylococci with intravenous antibiotic and antimicrobial lock solution has been shown to be feasible in retrospective study [34]. However, gram-negative and fungemia CLABSI have lower rates of treatment success in salvaging catheter and require removal [33, 34]. Antimicrobial lock therapy should not be used as a sole therapy in CLABSI.

Prevention of Catheter-Related Infection

Prevention is the key to reduce catheter-related infection. The implementation of the central line bundle has resulted in significant reduction of CRBSI [35]. It includes hand hygiene, maximal barrier precaution during central venous catheter insertion, skin antisepsis with chlorhexidine, optimal catheter site selection by avoiding femoral site, and daily review of line necessity with prompt removal of unnecessary lines [35]. Due to concern for promoting antibiotic-resistant microorganisms, antimicrobial catheter lock solutions are restricted to treatment of infections. In patients requiring long-term catheters, there are various non-antimicrobial catheter lock solutions being studied to explore their potential role for CLABSI prophylaxis. Ethanol catheter lock solution in various concentrations has been successfully used to prevent CLABSI in home PN patients but its use is limited due to higher rates of mechanical complication such as occlusion and disruption of the integrity of the catheter requiring catheter replacement [36–38]. Taurolidine, a derivative of taurine, an amino acid is a bactericidal agent that is effective against gram-positive, gram-negative, and fungi. Its use in HPN as primary and secondary prevention of CLABSI in HPN patients appear promising [39–41]. Another potential non-antimicrobial solution anticoagulant that may reduce biofilm formation, bacterial colonization, and intraluminal thrombosis is tetrasodium ethylenediaminetetraacetic acid (EDTA) [42, 43]. Its use has been safely used in hemodialysis catheters [42].

However, there are no published studies of tetrasodium EDTA catheter lock solutions in home PN patients.

Noninfectious Catheter-Related Complication

Catheter occlusion can occur in up to 50% of central venous catheters [44]. Occlusion may be due to thrombotic or non-thrombotic causes. Catheter insertion potentially disrupts one of the Virchow's triad resulting in venous thrombosis. With the catheter tip against the vessel wall, an activated cascade of fibrin, platelet, coagulation factors, and erythrocytes interlink to form venous thrombi. This activation process is exacerbated by altered blood flow due to the presence of a catheter in the blood vessel. The types of catheter thrombosis include intraluminal clot, a fibrin sheath formation, and thrombosis of the vessel.

Intraluminal clotting is usually due to inadequate flushing, blood reflux, and drug or lipid precipitate resulting in sluggish catheter function or thrombosis [45]. The caregiver may find difficulty in infusing or aspirating from the catheter. The volume of flush solution is recommended to be at least twice the volume of catheter (typically 10 ml of normal saline) to prevent this complication [45]. Fibrin sheath formation at the distal catheter tip acts as a one-way valve, which usually allows infusion, but prevents aspiration of the blood sample. Catheter-related venous thrombosis with clinical signs of vascular obstruction, such as neck vein distension, swelling, and pain of ipsilateral arm and neck, will require anticoagulants for treatment [46]. Low-dose anticoagulant therapy has not been proven to be effective as primary prophylaxis in catheter-related thrombosis [47]. Catheter tip position has been identified as underlying etiology for thrombosis and should be positioned in the lower vena cava rather than proximal vena cava [48].

Lastly catheter pinch-off syndrome represents an intermittent mechanical obstruction caused by the catheter compression between the clavicle and the first rib [48]. This is due to the narrow anatomical triangle that exists at the junction of the axillary vein and the subclavian vein. Changing the patient's position by raising ipsilateral arm will open this angle and relieves the occlusion. Chest X-ray is sufficient to demonstrate the luminal narrowing of the catheter [48]. Removal is recommended as it may lead to catheter transection and embolus. Other noninfectious catheter-related complications include air embolism, catheter migration, pulmonary embolism, cardiac tamponade, and nerve injury [49].

Metabolic Complications

Given the mechanism of nutrient and electrolyte administration in PN, one must be cautious to monitor for metabolic complications. Metabolic complications can occur acutely or manifest over weeks, months, or years. These metabolic complications can often occur in patients without a diagnosis of a metabolic disorder prior to PN. PN-associated complications include hyper-/hypoglycemia, essential fatty acid deficiency (EFAD), hypertriglyceridemia, and hepatobiliary complications.

With the parenteral administration of dextrose, patients can develop complications from hyper- or hypoglycemia. Hyperglycemia is one of the most common complications associated with PN and can occur acutely in ICU patients or in long-term home parenteral nutrition (HPN) [9, 50]. Recommendations for target blood glucose and frequency of monitoring vary depending on institutional protocol and societal guidelines. The American Society of Parenteral and Enteral Nutrition (ASPEN) recommends for those high-risk adults receiving PN in acute hospital/ICU situations a target blood glucose between 140 and 180 mg/dL [51]. The Society of Critical Care Medicine (SCCM) recommends a similar target range of 150–180 mg/dL [52]. Monitoring of these high-risk patients is typically performed every 6 hours until patients remain stable in the target range and at goal PN calories. For low-risk patients, monitoring can be as simple as periodically monitoring for glucose in the urine. With evidence of glucosuria, follow up with a finger-stick or venous blood glucose to confirm. In patients on long-term cyclical HPN (10–12 hours) and at high risk of hyperglycemia, particularly those with diabetes, it is recommended that these patients check their blood glucose 1 hour after the start of PN administration and 1 hour after the infusion is completed [1]. In high-risk ICU PN patients, insulin drips are often used to maintain the target glucose range (140–180 mg/dL) [51, 52]. In long-term HPN or stable non-ICU hospitalized patients, regular insulin can be added to the PN to cover the dextrose load of the infusion. We generally recommend adding insulin to the PN if the blood sugar is >200 mg/dL 1 hour into the PN infusion. Some patients, particularly those with oral intake in addition to the PN, may require additional insulin or other management of their blood sugars. To help prevent metabolic complications, dextrose administration should not be infused at a rate greater of 5 mg/kg/min in acutely ill patients [53, 54]. In patients who are routinely monitoring blood glucose levels, an acute change to previously normal levels should raise concern for a potential infection and should be discussed with their managing team as blood glucose may rise before other symptoms of infection manifest.

In pediatric patients, there is concern for rebound hypoglycemia after the PN infusion is completed [55, 56]. For prevention, the rate of PN infusion should be decreased to half the "normal" rate for the last hour of infusion. This allows time for the body to decrease insulin release and minimize risk of hypoglycemia. Some patients may benefit from a longer (generally 2 hours) taper prior to discontinuation.

If long-term or stable non-ICU hospitalized patients who require insulin in their PN have rebound hypoglycemia, it is generally due to overcompensation in the production of insulin and is recommend to optimize blood glucose control during PN infusion to avoid excess endogenous insulin secretion. Each patient's needs should be carefully considered in addition to close monitoring while appropriate insulin adjustments are made. Initial insulin regimens in the PN solution start at 0.05–0.1 units of insulin/g dextrose, and it is not advised to give over 0.2 units of insulin/g dextrose [50, 51]. While this recommendation is not based on clinical trials, it has been utilized historically and adjustments beyond this should be considered with caution.

In addition to the potential complications of acute hyperglycemia, elevated blood glucose can also contribute to hypertriglyceridemia. Given the risk of hypertriglyceridemia with infusion of glucose and lipids, periodic monitoring of triglyceride levels is recommended. This may reveal underlying familial hypertriglyceridemia requiring treatment, or metabolic complications attributable to the PN itself. In patients with triglyceride levels >400, it is important to consider the dextrose infusion rates and whether decreased infusion rates would provide improved physiologic compensation [57]. Alternatively, in patients with both hyperglycemia and hypertriglyceridemia, improving blood sugar control with insulin may also improve triglyceride levels. However, in some cases, there is a need to increase infusion times or adjust macronutrient compositions with the consideration of both glucose and lipid content to achieve an adequate triglyceride level that minimizes risk of complications.

Essential Fatty Acid Deficiency

Essential fatty acids, linoleic and alpha-linoleinic, are fatty acids that are unable to be synthesized by the human body and must be ingested. These fatty acids are present in significant amounts in soy-based intravenous lipid emulsions (ILE), in a lesser concentration in olive oil-based ILE, and even less in fish oil-based ILE. Without adequate ingestion, patients are at risk for developing essential fatty acid deficiency (EFAD). Symptomatically these patients may develop scaly skin, hair loss, and potentially liver enzyme abnormalities which can manifest after weeks to months without adequate fatty acid intake. EFAD is diagnosed by an elevated triene/tetraene ratio in the blood. Calculations can be performed to assess the minimal lipid concentration needed based on the composition of the lipid product being used; however, initial studies demonstrated that EFAD could be avoided if 0.2–0.3% of kilocalories were provided as alpha-linolenic acid

[58]. This recommendation has later been extrapolated to 1–4% of kilocalories from lipid emulsion [59, 60]. There are patients that are unable to tolerate ILE infusion due to allergies or other limitations. In rare cases, there are reports of topical administration of sunflower or safflower oil which allow sufficient absorption of essential fatty acids to prevent EFAD. However, the effectiveness of these topical preparations has not been well studied [59, 61].

Hepatobiliary Complication

While the prior metabolic complications tend to manifest acutely to subacutely, longer-term PN patients may develop intestinal failure associated liver disease (IFALD) previously known as parenteral nutrition associated liver disease (PNALD). Complications range from increased risk of cholelithiasis to cholestasis, steatosis, and rarely cirrhosis [62, 63]. Studies have reported significant variations in the rates of IFALD from 30 to 60% of children and 15 to 40% of adults requiring long-term hospital-based PN or HPN with soybean oil as the source of lipid [63]. The pathophysiology of IFALD remains unclear, but recent work has shown that changing to a mixed oil ILE or fish oil-based ILE can result in the reversal of hepatic steatosis [62–64]. Without treatment and reversal of hepatic steatosis, IFALD can progress to cirrhosis and end-stage liver disease. Soy-based ILEs have been associated with IFALD due to excess caloric intake, overfeeding, or high dextrose load. The IFALD associated with 100% soy-based ILE may be related to the pro-inflammatory lipids that are found in soybean oil [17]. Other research has shown that carnitine and choline deficiency may contribute to IFLAD, theoretically related to their role in lipid transport and metabolism [16]. Additionally, other studies have shown the potential impact of gut microbiota composition and change and potential benefit of antimicrobial therapy to help adjust bowel flora [62, 63]. However, this is an area that is still undergoing prospective investigation and does not have clear causality or treatment recommendations determined.

In patients requiring long-term PN therapy, it is advisable to routinely monitor liver enzymes, specifically alkaline phosphatase and bilirubin [62]. If there is an acute rise, the patient should be assessed for possible infection. If a slow rise, then consideration is given to development of early stages of IFALD and should be evaluated with hepatic structural assessment with an ultrasound, and laboratory evaluation to calculate of FIB-4 for fibrosis staging [62, 65]. It is important to assess other risk factors these patients may have for developing liver disease such as alcohol, viral or genetic etiologies, as well as PN formulation, and daily caloric infusion rate. Decreasing reliance on soybean-based ILEs has been shown to decrease risk of developing IFALD. For patients that have some oral or enteral intake, it may be beneficial to decrease their PN ILEs to minimize exposure. In patients that are not able to obtain essential fatty acids or enough calories with oral or enteral supplementation, it may be beneficial to change their ILE to a mixed oil or fish oil ILE [64, 66, 67]. Early work is showing the potential of regression of IFALD with fish oil-based ILE, but there is still much work to be done in this area [67]. Cyclic PN is an infusion run for <24 hrs per day which allows the body a period free from nutrient infusion and has been shown to decrease the risk of developing IFALD. This cyclical strategy is often used in long-term hospital-based PN or HPN patients. Other IFALD treatment strategies include pharmacologic therapies such as bile acid binding agents, or antimicrobial therapy. If IFALD persists despite exhaustion of all treatment modalities, a referral for a combined liver/small bowel transplant should be considered.

Metabolic Bone Disease

Metabolic bone disease (MBD) may present as osteomalacia, osteopenia, or osteoporosis. Prevalence of PN-associated MBD is unknown, but it is estimated that 40%–100% of adult patients receiving chronic PN may have some degree of bone demineralization [68]. However, it is unclear whether the PN solution is the direct

Table 17.5 PN factors related to MBD and suggested modification [9, 69]

PN factors	Effects on bone metabolism	Consideration
Amino acids	↑ urinary Ca excretion	Limit dose (1 g/kg/day) after nutrition repletion
Dextrose	↑ urinary Ca excretion	Avoid excessive dose
Sodium	↑ urinary Ca excretion	Provide enough to meet amounts loss in stool and urine
Metabolic acidosis	↑ urinary Ca excretion	Provide acetate to maintain normal bicarbonate
Calcium	↑ urinary Ca excretion	Calcium 10–15 mEq/day
Phosphate	↓ urinary Ca excretion	Phosphate 20–40 mmol/day
Magnesium	Low serum level inhibits PTH release	Provide enough to meet amounts loss meet amounts loss in stool/fistula
Copper	Low serum level correlated with low BMD	Maintain adequate intake
Aluminum	Defects in bone mineralization	Minimize contamination in PN components
Vitamin D	Variable	Maintain adequate intake and oral supplementation if patient has deficiency
Cyclic infusion	↑ urinary Ca excretion	–

Ca calcium, *PTH* parathyroid hormone, *BMD* bone mineral density

cause of MBD as all patients on long-term PN have at least one of numerous predisposing factors for bone loss such as undernutrition, endocrine diseases, gastrointestinal malabsorption, malignancies, concomitant medications, etc. [68, 69] Several factors related to PN formulation and administration can have negative effects on bone metabolism and are outlined in Table 17.5 with modification strategies to prevent BMD (ref: practical gastroenterology, curriculum).

All long-term PN patients should be screened for MBD, as most are asymptomatic at diagnosis. Recommended screening modalities include dual-energy X-ray absorptiometry scan (DEXA) at baseline and every 12–18 months and monitoring of serum electrolytes, minerals, and acid base balance [70]. To prevent or slow progression of MBD, all potential contributing factors should be discontinued or treated as soon as identified. Besides PN modification, lifestyle modifications, to include weight-bearing exercise, smoking cessation, reducing alcohol and caffeine intake, and fall prevention measures should be introduced. Endocrinology referral for pharmacological managements in osteoporosis may also be considered.

References

1. Vassilyadi F, Panteliadou AK, Panteliadis C. Hallmarks in the history of enteral and parenteral nutrition: from antiquity to the 20th century. Nutr Clin Pract. 2013;28(2):209–17.
2. Pironi L, Arends J, Baxter J, et al. ESPEN endorsed recommendations. Definition and classification of intestinal failure in adults. Clin Nutr. 2015;34(2):171–80.
3. Singer P, Blaser AR, Berger MM, et al. ESPEN guideline on clinical nutrition in the intensive care unit. Clin Nutr. 2019;38(1):48–79.
4. Culebras JM, Martin-Pena G, Garcia-de-Lorenzo A, Zarazaga A, Rodriguez-Montes JA. Practical aspects of peripheral parenteral nutrition. Curr Opin Clin Nutr Metab Care. 2004;7(3):303–7.
5. Barnett MI, Pertkiewicz M, Cosslett AG, Muhlebach S. Basics in clinical nutrition: parenteral nutrition admixtures, how to prepare parenteral nutrition (PN) admixtures. Clin Nutr ESPEN. 2009;4(3):114–6.
6. Yu J, Wu G, Tang Y, Ye Y, Zhang Z. Efficacy, safety, and preparation of standardized parenteral nutrition regimens: three-chamber bags vs compounded monobags – a prospective, multicenter, randomized, single-blind clinical trial. Nutr Clin Pract. 2017;32(4):545–51.
7. Kondrup J, Allison SP, Elia M, et al. ESPEN guidelines for nutrition screening 2002. Clin Nutr. 2003;22(4):415–21.
8. ASPEN Board of Directors and the Clinical Guidelines Task Force. Guidelines for the use of parenteral and enteral nutrition in adult and pediatric patients. JPEN J Parenter Enteral Nutr. 2002;26:1SA–138SA.
9. Mueller CM. The ASPEN adult nutrition support core curriculum. Silver Spring: American Society for Parenteral and Enteral Nutrition; 2017.
10. Lew CCH, Yandell R, Fraser RJL, Chua AP, Chong MFF, Miller M. Association between malnutrition and clinical outcomes in the intensive care unit: a systematic review. JPEN J Parenter Enteral Nutr. 2017;41(5):744–58.
11. McClave SA, Taylor BE, Martindale RG, et al. Guidelines for the provision and assessment of

nutrition support therapy in the adult critically ill patient: Society of Critical Care Medicine (SCCM) and American Society for Parenteral and Enteral Nutrition (A.S.P.E.N.). JPEN J Parenter Enteral Nutr. 2016;40(2):159–211.
12. Weimann A, Braga M, Carli F, et al. ESPEN guideline: clinical nutrition in surgery. Clin Nutr. 2017;36(3):623–50.
13. Ljungqvist O, Scott M, Fearon KC. Enhanced recovery after surgery: a review. JAMA Surg. 2017;152(3):292–8.
14. Kudsk KA, Tolley EA, DeWitt RC, et al. Preoperative albumin and surgical site identify surgical risk for major postoperative complications. JPEN J Parenter Enteral Nutr. 2003;27(1):1–9.
15. Pironi L, Boeykens K, Bozzetti F, et al. ESPEN guideline on home parenteral nutrition. Clin Nutr. 2020;39(6):1645–66.
16. Pironi L, Arends J, Bozzetti F, et al. ESPEN guidelines on chronic intestinal failure in adults. Clin Nutr. 2016;35(2):247–307.
17. Pironi L, Goulet O, Buchman A, et al. Outcome on home parenteral nutrition for benign intestinal failure: a review of the literature and benchmarking with the European prospective survey of ESPEN. Clin Nutr. 2012;31(6):831–45.
18. Derenski K, Catlin J, Allen L. Parenteral nutrition basics for the clinician caring for the adult patient. Nutr Clin Pract. 2016;31(5):578–95.
19. Mirtallo J, Canada T, Johnson D, et al. Safe practices for parenteral nutrition. JPEN J Parenter Enteral Nutr. 2004;28(6):S39–70.
20. Singer P, Berger MM, Van den Berghe G, et al. ESPEN guidelines on parenteral nutrition: intensive care. Clin Nutr. 2009;28(4):387–400.
21. Brown RO, Compher C, American Society for Parenteral and Enteral Nutrition (A.S.P.E.N.) Board of Directors. A.S.P.E.N. clinical guidelines: nutrition support in adult acute and chronic renal failure. JPEN J Parenter Enteral Nutr. 2010;34(4):366–77.
22. Mirtallo JM, Ayers P, Boullata J, et al. ASPEN lipid injectable emulsion safety recommendations, part 1: background and adult considerations. Nutr Clin Pract. 2020;35(5)769–82.
23. Mirtallo JM, Dasta JF, Kleinschmidt KC, Varon J. State of the art review: intravenous fat emulsions: current applications, safety profile, and clinical implications. Ann Pharmacother. 2010;44(4):688–700.
24. Boullata JI, Gilbert K, Sacks G, et al. A.S.P.E.N. clinical guidelines: parenteral nutrition ordering, order review, compounding, labeling, and dispensing. JPEN J Parenter Enteral Nutr. 2014;38(3):334–77.
25. Vanek VW, Borum P, Buchman A, et al. A.S.P.E.N. position paper: recommendations for changes in commercially available parenteral multivitamin and multi-trace element products. Nutr Clin Pract. 2012;27(4):440–91.
26. Hwa YL, Rashtak S, Kelly DG, Murray JA. Iron deficiency in long-term parenteral nutrition therapy. JPEN J Parenter Enteral Nutr. 2016;40(6):869–76.
27. Kumpf VJ. Update on parenteral iron therapy. Nutr Clin Pract. 2003;18(4):318–26.
28. Jin J, Mulesa L, Carrilero RM. Trace elements in parenteral nutrition: considerations for the prescribing clinician. Nutrients. 2017;9(5):440
29. Ayers P, Adams S, Boullata J, et al. A.S.P.E.N. parenteral nutrition safety consensus recommendations. JPEN J Parenter Enteral Nutr. 2014;38(3):296–333.
30. Gorski LA. The 2016 infusion therapy standards of practice. Home Healthc Now. 2017;35(1):10–8.
31. Centers for Disease Control and Prevention. Guidelines for the prevention of intravascular catheter-related infection. https://www.cdc.gov/hai/pdfs/bsi-guidelines-2011.pdf. Published 2011. Accessed June 24 2020.
32. O'Grady NP, Alexander M, Burns LA, et al. Guidelines for the prevention of intravascular catheter-related infections. Clin Infect Dis. 2011;52(9):e162–93.
33. Mermel LA, Allon M, Bouza E, et al. Clinical practice guidelines for the diagnosis and management of intravascular catheter-related infection: 2009 update by the Infectious Diseases Society of America. Clin Infect Dis. 2009;49(1):1–45.
34. Edakkanambeth Varayil J, Whitaker JA, Okano A, et al. Catheter salvage after catheter-related bloodstream infection during home parenteral nutrition. JPEN J Parenter Enteral Nutr. 2017;41(3):481–8.
35. Pronovost P, Needham D, Berenholtz S, et al. An intervention to decrease catheter-related bloodstream infections in the ICU. N Engl J Med. 2006;355(26):2725–32.
36. Abu-El-Haija M, Schultz J, Rahhal RM. Effects of 70% ethanol locks on rates of central line infection, thrombosis, breakage, and replacement in pediatric intestinal failure. J Pediatr Gastroenterol Nutr. 2014;58(6):703–8.
37. Davidson JB, Edakkanambeth Varayil J, Okano A, et al. Prevention of subsequent catheter-related bloodstream infection using catheter locks in high-risk patients receiving home parenteral nutrition. JPEN J Parenter Enteral Nutr. 2017;41(4):685–90.
38. Rahhal R, Abu-El-Haija MA, Fei L, et al. Systematic review and meta-analysis of the utilization of ethanol locks in pediatric patients with intestinal failure. JPEN J Parenter Enteral Nutr. 2018;42(4):690–701.
39. Wouters Y, Theilla M, Singer P, et al. Randomised clinical trial: 2% taurolidine versus 0.9% saline locking in patients on home parenteral nutrition. Aliment Pharmacol Ther. 2018;48(4):410–22.
40. Bisseling TM, Willems MC, Versleijen MW, Hendriks JC, Vissers RK, Wanten GJ. Taurolidine lock is highly effective in preventing catheter-related bloodstream infections in patients on home parenteral nutrition: a heparin-controlled prospective trial. Clin Nutr. 2010;29(4):464–8.
41. Saunders J, Naghibi M, Leach Z, et al. Taurolidine locks significantly reduce the incidence of catheter-related blood stream infections in high-risk patients on home parenteral nutrition. Eur J Clin Nutr. 2015;69(2):282–4.

42. Kanaa M, Wright MJ, Akbani H, Laboi P, Bhandari S, Sandoe JA. Cathasept line lock and microbial colonization of tunneled hemodialysis catheters: a multicenter randomized controlled trial. Am J Kidney Dis. 2015;66(6):1015–23.
43. Percival SL, Kite P, Eastwood K, et al. Tetrasodium EDTA as a novel central venous catheter lock solution against biofilm. Infect Control Hosp Epidemiol. 2005;26(6):515–9.
44. Moureau N, Poole S, Murdock MA, Gray SM, Semba CP. Central venous catheters in home infusion care: outcomes analysis in 50,470 patients. J Vasc Interv Radiol. 2002;13(10):1009–16.
45. Ryder M. Evidence-based practice in the management of vascular access devices for home parenteral nutrition therapy. JPEN J Parenter Enteral Nutr. 2006;30(1 Suppl):S82–93, S98-89.
46. Kucher N. Clinical practice. Deep-vein thrombosis of the upper extremities. N Engl J Med. 2011;364(9):861–9.
47. Akl EA, Vasireddi SR, Gunukula S, et al. Anticoagulation for patients with cancer and central venous catheters. Cochrane Database Syst Rev. 2011;4:CD006468.
48. Cadman A, Lawrance JA, Fitzsimmons L, Spencer-Shaw A, Swindell R. To clot or not to clot? That is the question in central venous catheters. Clin Radiol. 2004;59(4):349–55.
49. McGee DC, Gould MK. Preventing complications of central venous catheterization. N Engl J Med. 2003;348(12):1123–33.
50. Edakkanambeth Varayil J, Yadav S, Miles JM, et al. Hyperglycemia during home parenteral nutrition administration in patients without diabetes. JPEN J Parenter Enteral Nutr. 2017;41(4):672–7.
51. McMahon MM, Nystrom E, Braunschweig C, Miles J, Compher C, American Society for Parenteral and Enteral Nutrition (A.S.P.E.N.) Board of Directors, et al. A.S.P.E.N. clinical guidelines: nutrition support of adult patients with hyperglycemia. JPEN J Parenter Enteral Nutr. 2013;37:23–36.
52. Jacobi JBN, Krinsley J, Agus M, Braithwaite SS, Deutschman C, et al. Guidelines for the use of an insulin infusion for the management of hyperglycemia in critically ill patients. Crit Care Med. 2012;12(40):3251–76.
53. McMahon MM. Management of parenteral nutrition in acutely ill patients with hyperglycemia. Nutr Clin Pract. 2004;19(2):120–8.
54. McMahon MM, Nystrom E, Braunschweig C, et al. A.S.P.E.N. clinical guidelines: nutrition support of adult patients with hyperglycemia. JPEN J Parenter Enteral Nutr. 2013;37(1):23–36.
55. Bendorf K, Friesen CA, Roberts CC. Glucose response to discontinuation of parenteral nutrition in patients less than 3 years of age. JPEN J Parenter Enteral Nutr. 1996;20(2):120–2.
56. Nirula R, Yamada K, Waxman K. The effect of abrupt cessation of total parenteral nutrition on serum glucose: a randomized trial. Am Surg. 2000;66(9):866–9.
57. Kochevar Me, McMahon MM. Management of nutrition, vol. 2. 2nd ed. Informa Healthcare: Abingdon; 2006.
58. Bjerve KS, Fischer S, Alme K. Alpha-linolenic acid deficiency in man: effect of ethyl linolenate on plasma and erythrocyte fatty acid composition and biosynthesis of prostanoids. Am J Clin Nutr. 1987;46(4):570–6.
59. Mogensen KM. Essential fatty acid deficiency. Pract Gastroenterol 2017.
60. Innis SM. Essential fatty acids in growth and development. Prog Lipid Res. 1991;30(1):39–103.
61. Miller DG, Williams SK, Palombo JD, Griffin RE, Bistrian BR, Blackburn GL. Cutaneous application of safflower oil in preventing essential fatty acid deficiency in patients on home parenteral nutrition. Am J Clin Nutr. 1987;46(3):419–23.
62. Lal S, Pironi L, Wanten G, et al. Clinical approach to the management of Intestinal Failure Associated Liver Disease (IFALD) in adults: A position paper from the Home Artificial Nutrition and Chronic Intestinal Failure Special Interest Group of ESPEN. Clin Nutr. 2018;37(6 Pt A):1794–7.
63. Mundi MS, Salonen BR, Bonnes S. Home parenteral nutrition: fat emulsions and potential complications. Nutr Clin Pract. 2016;31(5):629–41.
64. Klek S, Szczepanek K, Scislo L, et al. Intravenous lipid emulsions and liver function in adult chronic intestinal failure patients: results from a randomized clinical trial. Nutrition. 2018;55–56:45–50.
65. Blüthner E PU-F, Stockmann M, Karber M, Maasberg S, Pevny S, et al. Assessing non-invasive liver function in patients with intestinal failure receiving total parenteral nutrition—results from the prospective PNLiver trial. Nutrients. https://www.ncbi.nlm.nih.gov/pmc/articles/PMC7282264/. Published 26 Apr 2020. Assessed on 17 July 2020.
66. Mundi MS, Kuchkuntla AR, Salonen BR, Bonnes S, Hurt RT. Long-term use of mixed-oil lipid emulsion in soybean oil-intolerant home parenteral nutrition patients. JPEN J Parenter Enteral Nutr. 2020;44(2):301–7.
67. Zhang T, Wang N, Yan W, et al. Effect of a fish oil-based lipid emulsion on intestinal failure-associated liver disease in children. Eur J Clin Nutr. 2018;72(10):1364–72.
68. Ferrone MGM. A review of the relationship between parenteral nutrition and metabolic bone disease. Nutr Clin Pract. 2007;22:329–39.
69. Hamilton C, Seidner DL. Metabolic bone disease in the patient on long-term parenteral nutrition. Pract Gastroenterol. 2008;6(4):335–41.
70. Staun M, Pironi L, Bozzetti F, et al. ESPEN guidelines on parenteral nutrition: home parenteral nutrition (HPN) in adult patients. Clin Nutr. 2009;28(4):467–79.

Enteral Nutrition

18

Konika Sharma and Robin Mendelsohn

Introduction

The alimentary canal or gastrointestinal (GI) tract is a one-way tube that measures 25 feet in length when in vivo and 35 feet when the smooth muscle tone is lost. The tube begins at the mouth and terminates at the anus. The GI tract includes the esophagus, stomach, and small and large intestines, all of which have different roles in absorption of macronutrients, micronutrients, and water. In healthy people, food enters the body orally and goes through a series of physiological processes to extract calories and nutrients to sustain bodily functions (see Chap. 1 for more details). In certain anatomical conditions and disease states, oral intake is not possible and alternative means of providing nutrition are necessary including enteral and parenteral supplementation. Enteral nutrition is always preferred when technically feasible and appropriate (i.e., in a functional gastrointestinal tract.)

Enteral Nutrition

Indication

Enteral nutrition is indicated in patients who cannot adequately meet their nutritional requirements through oral intake, despite having a functional GI tract. When feasible, enteral nutrition is always preferred over parenteral nutrition in order to maintain gut barrier functions [1] and attempt to mimic normal physiology. In addition, there is a lower degree of overall infections in patients receiving enteral nutrition vs parenteral including a lower risk of cholecystitis as the gallbladder can function under normal physiological conditions by stimulating the release of cholecystokinin. Enteral nutrition maintains the structural integrity of gut epithelium and releases IgA, which prevents bacterial adherence and translocation [2] via gut-associated lymphoid tissue (GALT) and enhances immunity by stimulating mucosal-associated lymphoid tissue at distant sites (MALT) as in lungs, liver, and kidney [3].

Oral feeding is not feasible in patients with proximal obstructions (i.e., head and neck cancer, esophageal cancer, gastric outlet obstruction) neurologic disorders (stroke, dementia, Parkinson's disease, cerebral palsy, multiple sclerosis, motor neuron disease), and in times of reduced level of consciousness (i.e., head injury, ICU patients, prolonged coma). Although gastric feeding is appropriate for many of these patients, small intestinal feeds are indicated when patients are at risk of aspiration of gastric contents (i.e., nausea/vomiting, gastroparesis) or when gastric feeding is not feasible secondary to anatomy or underlying pathology.

K. Sharma · R. Mendelsohn (✉)
Division of Gastroenterology, Memorial Sloan Kettering Cancer Center, New York, NY, USA
e-mail: sharmak1@mskcc.org; mendelsr@mskcc.org

C. Newberry et al. (eds.), *Nutrition, Weight, and Digestive Health*,
https://doi.org/10.1007/978-3-030-94953-2_18

Contraindications

Enteral nutrition is contraindicated when the GI tract is not functional and adequate calories/ nutrition cannot be derived from enteral support. Examples include conditions resulting in less than 100 cm of small bowel (i.e., short gut syndrome) (3), paralytic ileus, generalized dysmotility, small or large bowel obstructions which are too distal for enteral access, high output proximal fistulas, or severe shock. Although often offered, enteral nutrition has also not been shown to change survival or increase patients' quality of life in the setting of dementia; however, it may improve quality of life of family and caregivers. Cochrane reviews have shown no evidence of increased survival in patients with dementia receiving enteral nutrition [4]. In fact, one-quarter of patients will die during hospitalization when enteral nutrition is initiated due to patients' underlying conditions and not associated with complications from enteral nutrition access placement or initiation (4). In this context, both the European Society for Clinical Nutrition and Metabolism (ESPEN) and the National Institute for Clinical Excellence (NICE) recommend against the initiation of tube feeding in patients with severe dementia. In patients with early stages of dementia, there should be a multidisciplinary discussion with the ethics committee, physician, and family members focusing on the patient's known wishes to guide clinical decision-making. Ultimately patient selection should be performed on a case-by-case basis based on physician and dietitian assessment, patient and caregiver needs and preferences, diagnosis and life expectancy.

Timing

Enteral feeding should be considered in patients in whom oral intake is unsafe, insufficient, or impossible. The American Society for Parenteral and Enteral Nutrition (ASPEN) suggests that specialized nutrition support be initiated in all patients with inadequate oral intake for >7–14 days [5]. In critically ill patients, enteral feeding should be started early, ideally within the first 24–48 hours following critical care admission or as soon as hemodynamic stability has been achieved [5, 6]. ESPEN [12] and the Canadian Guidelines for Nutrition [7] recommend nutrition initiation within 24 hours of admission for critically ill patients. If enteral nutrition is not thought to be possible within 7 days of critical care admission due to absolute contraindications, parenteral nutrition should be initiated.

Nutritional Risk Assessment

Nutritional status should be assessed and supplemental enteral nutrition considered in patients who are malnourished or at risk of developing protein-calorie malnutrition who do not have contraindication to enteral feeding. Protein-calorie malnutrition is defined as recent weight loss of greater than 10–15% or actual body weight less than 90% of ideal body weight. Most institutions assess patient nutritional status upon hospital admission. There are various methods for nutritional status assessment (see Chap. 3). Subjective Global Assessment (SGA) and Mini-Nutritional Assessment (MNA) are the most commonly used ones by providers in hospitalized patients [8]. Although often used, lab markers such as albumin, pre-albumin, and transferrin are less reliable as these have low specificity [9] and often correlate with overall illness severity and inflammatory state.

Enteral Access

The appropriate type of access to deliver enteral nutrition is determined by various factors including (1) the duration of enteral support, (2) underlying disease, and (3) availability of resources. When nutrition support is required for short term (<4–6 weeks), nasogastric (NG), orogastric (OG), or nasojejunal (NJ) tubes are recommended. For longer term support (>4–6 weeks), gastrostomy, jejunostomy, or gastrojejunostomy tubes are preferred (Fig. 18.1) [10].

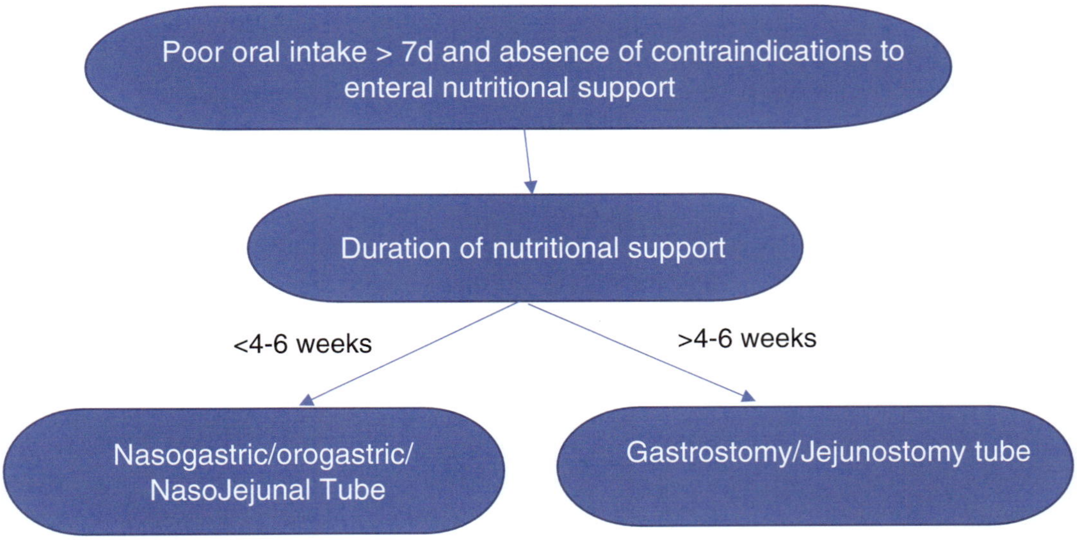

Fig. 18.1 Enteral access algorithm

Short-Term Access: Nasogastric and Orogastric Tubes

NG and OG tubes can be placed at the bedside. NJ tubes are usually placed under fluoroscopic or endoscopic assistance to ensure post-pyloric position. Tube position confirmation can avoid life-threatening respiratory complications of misplaced tubes into the respiratory tract [11]. The gold standard technique of tube position confirmation is radiographic visualization of the entire course of the tube [12, 13]. Other bedside techniques include checking the pH of the tube aspirate, though this is limited by acid-suppressant medications, and auscultatory confirmation after insufflation with air via an irrigating syringe.

The length of NG tube (NGT) to be inserted can be estimated by using an NGT placed externally and measuring from the tip of the patient's nose to the earlobe and then to the xiphoid process [14]. These tubes are very small in caliber, usually 8–14 French, and are at increased risk of clogging with tube feeds and medications. It is therefore important to flush these tubes with 30 mL of water before and after feeds or 10 mL of water after crushed medications are administered. These tubes can also become dislodged. Signs of dislodgement include a sharp increase in residual volume, sudden change in respiratory status, high negative pressure when attempting to withdraw the aspirate, and a change in the length of the tubing since the time of the confirmatory radiograph. Whenever there is a suspicion of dislodgement, feeds should be held and radiographic evaluation should be pursued [15].

Long-Term Access: Gastrotomy and Jejunostomy Tubes

Gastrostomy and jejunostomy tubes can be placed surgically, endoscopically, or fluoroscopically [16]. Studies comparing surgical gastrostomy with percutaneous endoscopic gastrotomy (PEG) have shown no difference in morbidity or mortality [17]. Endoscopic placement is less expensive and invasive. Surgical gastrostomy is usually reserved for patients who are already going to the operating room for another surgical indication. The difference in morbidity and mortality between endoscopic and radiologic gastrostomy tubes is not clear. Many studies indicate that PEG costs 44% more than percutaneous radiologic gastrostomy (PRG) initially, but in the end, the cost is usually similar given reinterventions and follow ups that are often requried [18]. Insertion approach may depend on local resources and expertise. In certain circumstances, such as oropharyngeal malignancies or anatomical limitations to endoscopic placement, radiologically placed tubes may be preferred [19].

For patients requiring long-term feeding tubes, gastrostomy and jejunostomy tubes can be replaced by low-profile options known as button tubes. This type of tube lies flat on the abdominal wall, is more aesthetically pleasing, and more easily hidden under clothing (Fig. 18.2). An adapter is required to administer feeds and medications through this type of tube.

Enteral Formulations

Enteral formulations are considered "medical foods" by the US Food and Drug Administration and are defined as foods which are formulated to be consumed or administered enterally under the supervision of a physician and intended for the specific dietary management of a disease or condition for which distinctive nutrition requirements based on recognized scientific principles are established [20]. The American Society for Parenteral and Enteral Nutrition (ASPEN) has published the "Enteral Nutrition Practice Recommendations" which include the following statements regarding formula selection [20]:

1. The accuracy and credibility of adult enteral formula labeling and product claims are dependent on formula vendors.
2. Nutrition support clinicians and consumers are responsible for determining the credibility of formulation.
3. It is important to interpret enteral formulation content/labeling and health claims with caution.

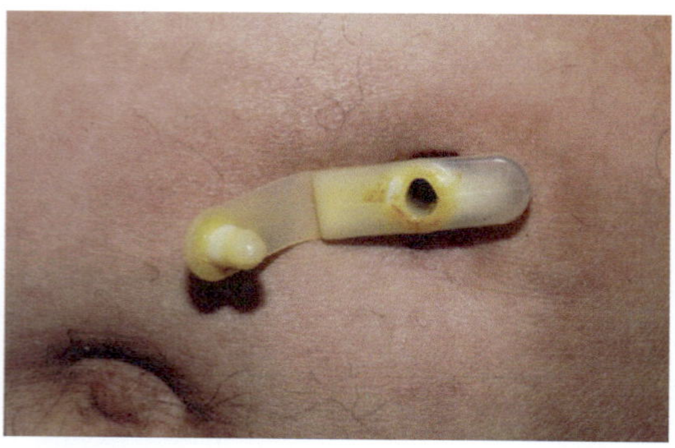

Fig. 18.2 Low-profile gastrotomy tube

Formula Classification

There are more than 200 different commercially prepared enteral formulations available on the market. Formulas are classified based on their composition as listed below. They all contain a unique combination of macronutrients and micronutrients including vitamins, minerals, and trace elements.

1. *Polymeric formulas:* These formulas contain intact protein, carbohydrates, and triglyceride polymers. These represent the most used formulas for enteral feeding and are the most cost-effective.
2. *Monomeric/hydrolyzed/elemental/semi-elemental formulas*: These formulas contain broken down products of macronutrients (i.e., amino acids/peptides instead of intact proteins, hydrolyzed starch, maltodextrin, or corn starch instead of complex carbohydrates, and medium- and long-chain fatty acids instead of intact fats). They are most used in patients with impaired digestion or absorption or intolerance of polymeric formulas.
3. *Modular formulas*: These formulas contain single nutritional components used for supplementation to create new formulas or enhance nutrient content of a preexisting formula.
4. *Disease-specific formulas*: There are formulas targeted for use in organ dysfunction or specific metabolic conditions.

Formula Composition

Carbohydrates

Carbohydrates are the main macronutrient and principal source of energy in most enteral formulations, accounting for 40–90% of calories [21]. The osmolarity of a formula is mainly influenced by the amount and source of carbohydrates in the form of monosaccharides (i.e., glucose) and disaccharides (i.e., sucrose).

Fat

The fat content of enteral formulas varies from less than 2 to 45% of total calories. A mixture of long-chain triglycerides (LCTs) and medium-chain triglycerides (MCTs) are often used. The most common sources of fat include corn oil, soybean oil, fish oil, and canola oil. MCTs are more easily hydrolyzed and absorbed via portal blood in comparison to LCTs, which require luminal transporters and lymphatics [22]. They do not, however, provide essential fatty acids, so a combination of MCTs and LCTs is usually recommended. Essential fatty acids like linolenic acid and linoleic acid are known to have some anti-inflammatory and anti-arrhythmic properties, slow platelet aggregation, and support metabolism [23].

Protein

Enteral formulas may contain intact proteins, hydrolyzed proteins, or free amino acids. Proteins are digested in the proximal intestinal tract and are absorbed in the form of dipeptides, tripeptides, or single amino acids. Intact proteins refer to whole proteins like casein and soy protein. These formulations require normal levels of pancreatic enzymes for digestion and absorption. Semi-elemental or elemental formulations contain hydrolyzed proteins and/or amino acids and are intended for patients with gastrointestinal dysfunction such as short bowel syndrome, malabsorption, or pancreatic exocrine insufficiency. Some enteral formulas add specific amino acids at pharmacological levels to help in wound and muscle repair (i.e., glutamine). Glutamine is a non-essential amino acid, synthesized mostly in muscles and serves as the primary energy source for the small intestine. In catabolic states, the release of glutamine from muscle and its utilization by the GI tract mucosa increase [24]. This process may result in loss of muscle tissue. Thus, glutamine has been proposed as an essential nutrient in catabolic processes and may be added to formulas designed for critical illness support [25].

Fiber

Fiber, both insoluble and soluble, is a polysaccharide found in plants that is not digestible by human enzymes. Soluble fermentable fiber is fermented by the gut microbiota in the distal intestine to produce short-chain fatty acids (SCFAs) which are a source of energy for colonocytes, supporting mucosal growth and promoting sodium and water absorption. Enteral formulas may contain a combination of both soluble and insoluble fiber or may be absent of fiber. Soluble fiber helps to control diarrhea by promoting sodium and water absorption. Insoluble fiber may treat constipation by decreasing colonic transit time through stool bulking [26, 27]. If a formula without fiber is used, fiber can be supplemented separately. The use of insoluble fiber–supplemented enteral formulas should be monitored closely, especially in critically ill patients, as cases of bowel obstruction have been reported. In such patients who have impaired gut motility or are at high risk of bowel ischemia, fiber-free formulas should be used [28].

Vitamins and Minerals

Most enteral formulas provide the recommended daily allowance of micronutrients including adequate trace elements such as iron, copper, zinc, and iodine. Studies have shown that people who are on enteral nutrition for more than 6 months have higher blood levels of various vitamins [29, 30]. Deficiencies can occur when the caloric intake from enteral feeding is low or when GI losses persistently exceed supplementation such as in patients with active inflammatory bowel disease or malabsorption secondary to other small intestinal or hepatobiliary pathology [31]. If vitamin or mineral deficiencies are identified, a different formula should be used and additional supplementation should be considered [32].

Water

Enteral formulas contain roughly 70–80% free water. The more calorically dense the formula, the less free water it contains [33]. Most patients receiving enteral nutrition will require an additional source of water to meet daily fluid needs, and this is often provided through the feeding tube as flushes.

Electrolytes

Mostly enteral formulas have adequate amounts of electrolytes to meet daily needs. Disease-specific formulations may have altered amounts as requirements of certain electrolytes may vary (i.e., renal disease formulations).

Osmolality

The osmolality of enteral formulas ranges from 270 to 700 mOSm/kg. The osmolality depends upon the concentration of free particles, molecules, and ions. The higher the concentration of such components, the higher the osmolality. Some patients may have intolerance of hyperosmolar/hypertonic formulas secondary to osmotic diarrhea.

Special Dietary Considerations

Many formulas are available which are lactose free, gluten free, and/or vegan to accommodate specific dietary needs and food intolerances.

Specific Disease States

Although most patients tolerate standard polymeric formulas, patients' current medical conditions and underlying medical history should be considered and may dictate specific formula selections and approaches to feeding.

Diabetes

Nutritional guidelines for patients with type II diabetes to reduce morbidity and mortality include appropriate blood glucose control (i.e., 80–130 mg/dL) and weight loss in the setting of overweight (BMI >25) or obese status (BMI >30) [5, 34]. The amount of carbohydrate in a formula is the main predictor of glycemic response and is important in maintaining blood sugar control. Enteral formulations designed to optimize glycemic control typically contain less monosaccharides and disaccharides, higher amounts of fat (usually in the form of monounsaturated fats), and higher fiber content. Although multiple formulations exist, the most widely studied is Glucerna©. For example, a randomized controlled trial of diabetic neurological patients with dysphagia who received either a diabetic formula or standard formula for up to 84 days showed that those on the diabetic formula had decreased insulin requirements, decreased fasting glucose, and decreased hypoglycemic episodes [35]. A follow-up meta-analysis of 23 other studies that compared diabetic to standard enteral formulas in patients with diabetes showed that diabetic formulas were associated with decreased post-prandial rise in blood glucose levels, decreased peak in blood glucose concentrations, and reduced overall HbA1c, though overall these findings lacked statistical power indicating that routine use is still controversial [36].

Renal Failure

Patients with acute renal failure tend to be hypermetabolic and hypercatabolic while those with chronic renal failure are at higher risk of sarcopenia and malnutrition [37]. Renal enteral formulations contain altered amounts of free water, proteins, electrolytes, vitamins, and minerals to accommodate kidney dysfunction. Protein content is the main variation among the various renal formulations. For example, formulas for patients who are not yet on dialysis have restricted protein content, whereas formulas for patients who are on dialysis have higher protein content as dialysis induces catabolism and protein wasting [38]. Studies that have looked at oral or tube feeding in patients with chronic kidney disease suggest that enteral nutrition support significantly increases serum albumin concentrations and improves total dietary intake. This may improve clinical outcomes, especially in malnourished patients, but insufficient published data exists to recommend these formulas routinely in patients with kidney disease [39]. In fact, current recommendations for critically ill patients with acute renal failure include nutritional support through standard formulations [5].

Pulmonary Disease/Critical Illness

There is decreased exhalation of carbon dioxide (CO_2) in patients with respiratory failure, which may lead to hypercarbia. In the 1980s, it was noted that high carbohydrate-containing nutritional support formulas were associated with enhanced CO_2 retention, and when carbohydrate substrate was decreased, respiratory rates also decreased [40–42]. During the acute and initial phases of critical illness, an exogenous energy supply in excess of 20–25 kcal/kg body weight (BW)/day should be avoided, whereas, during recovery, the aim should be to provide 25–30 total kcal/kg BW/day [43]. The enteral formulas that are designated specifically for respiratory failure patients are calorically dense, as these patients usually have fluid restrictions, and are lower in carbohydrates/higher in fats to improve respiratory quotients and reduce hypercarbia. Formulas for ambulatory and critically ill patients additionally differ in the type of lipid they contain, with alterations in ratios of omega-3 to omega-6 fatty acids. Non-critically ill formulas contain corn and safflower oils (which are higher in omega-6 fatty acids), while formulas for patients with acute respiratory distress syndrome (ARDS) or acute lung injury (ALI) contain marine oil and borage oil (which are higher in omega-3 fatty acids) [44]. Omega-3 fatty acids have been found to be more anti-inflammatory, reducing release of prostaglandins, thromboxanes, and leukotrienes. Use of formulas containing these types of fats in critical illness has been supported by meta-analysis, which associates a 60% reduction in 28 day in hospital all-cause mortality [45]. Another prospective, multicenter, randomized, double-blinded, controlled trial which evaluated an omega-3 rich ARDS/ALI formula in comparison to standard formula showed a benefit in the early stages of sepsis, preventing cardiovascular and respiratory deterioration [46]. Studies, however, have not routinely supported use of specialized critical care formulas as noted by a later randomized, placebo-controlled trial that failed to show mortality benefit with omega-3 fatty acid–supplemented options and a meta-analysis of six additional controlled trials which reported no improvement in all-cause mortality, 28-day ventilator-free days, or 28-day ICU-free days [47, 48]. There is no actual consensus on the use of supplementation of antioxidants in patients with ARDS/ALI; thus, the use is based on the prescriber's practice and an individual patient's risk profile.

Prone Positioning and Extracorporeal Membrane Oxygenation

During the SARS-CoV-2 pandemic, the use of lung-protective strategies such as prone positioning increased in frequency leading to safety analysis of enteral nutrition delivery in this position. Several retrospective and small prospective trials have shown that enteral nutrition during prone positioning is not associated with an increased risk of gastrointestinal or pulmonary complications and should still be used. Thus ASPEN recommends that patients requiring prone positioning also receive early enteral nutrition as is standardly recommended [49, 50]. When enteral nutrition is introduced during prone positioning, recommendations are to keep the head of the bed elevated (reverse Trendelenburg) to at least 10–25 degrees to decrease the risk of aspiration of gastric contents, facial edema, and intra-abdominal hypertension [51–53].

Another circumstance in critical illness that may affect nutritional needs is use of extracorporeal membrane oxygenation (ECMO), which can lead to delayed gastric emptying and bowel ischemia in the setting of enteral nutrition supplementation. Early observational data has reported bowel ischemia as high as 4.5% in patients on ECMO receiving enteral nutrition [54]; however, additional analysis has also reported much lower rates of complications and high tolerability of enteral nutrition during ECMO use [55]. Overall, recommendations include close monitoring for tolerance to enteral feeing and slow advancement to goal over the first week of critical illness, especially in the setting of ECMO use.

Inflammatory Bowel Disease

Adults with IBD are at increased risk of malnutrition, with deficits more common in patients with CD than UC [56]. Exclusive enteral nutrition (EEN) is one of the first-line therapies for pediatric CD, providing a complete nutritional feed while simultaneously inducing remission in up to

80% of cases. Although this approach can also be used in adults, evidence suggests higher efficacy in pediatric populations due to tolerance and mucosal inflammation patterns [57, 58]. Specific micronutrient deficiency states are relatively common in CD due to small bowel inflammation and should be trended closely. The most common deficiencies are iron and B12, especially in those with a history of ileal disease.

Standard EN (polymeric, moderate fat content, no specific supplements) is usually appropriate for primary and supportive nutritional therapy in active IBD [59, 60].

Liver Failure

Patients with hepatic encephalopathy have decreased levels of branched chain amino acids (BCAAs) and higher levels of aromatic amino acids (AAAs), both in blood and cerebrospinal fluid due to poor hepatic deamination [61, 62]. Liver failure formulations contain a lower total protein and AAA content, but a higher amount of BCAA to accommodate these metabolic changes. Formulas are more calorie dense and low in sodium to address underlying edema and ascites, and fat-soluble vitamins are given at lower doses to prevent accumulation. Although in theory these formulas have therapeutic benefit, studies have not consistently shown better outcomes, and standard polymeric regimens can often be trialed first.

Immune-Modulating Formulas

Specific nutrients can influence the immune system. As such, non-essential nutrients like arginine, glutamine, nucleotides, and omega- 3 fatty acids have been hypothesized to have beneficial effects on immune response, wound healing, inflammation, and defense against infection [23, 63, 64]. Arginine, a precursor of nitrous oxide, may not be adequately produced by critically ill patients. Many studies have been done in patients after major surgery, trauma, and burn injury addressing this question [65]. A recent study compared natural killer (NK) cell activity and related cytokine in patients receiving soybean oil-containing enteral nutrition (control group) versus a plant-derived *n*-3 fatty acid-enriched formulation. The study correlated plant-derived *n*-3 fatty acid supplementation with enhanced NK cell activity [66]. Based on this finding and additional literature, ASPEN now recommends consideration of "immune-modulating enteral formulations (supplemented with agents such as arginine, glutamine, nucleic acid, omega-3 fatty acids, and antioxidants)" in appropriate patient populations such as those post-major elective surgery, trauma, burns, head and neck cancer, and in critically ill patients on mechanical ventilation. These recommendations are classified as grade A for surgical ICU patients and grade B for medical ICU patients, recognizing that beneficial effects of immune-modulating formulas are more uniformly seen in patients undergoing major surgery than in critically ill mechanically ventilated patients [5]. There is no general indication for immune-modulating formula in patients with severe illness or sepsis and an APACHE II score > 15. Glutamine should be supplemented in patients suffering from burns or trauma [43].

Framework for Enteral Feeding Initiation

The society of Critical Care Medicine (SCCM), ASPEN, and the Canadian Clinical Practice Guidelines support the use of protocols and enteral order sets for safe delivery. These order sets contain (1) patient identifiers, (2) formula name, (3) enteral access device site, and (4) administration method [67].

Calculating Nutritional Needs

Determination of enteral nutrition prescription includes the following:

1. *Calorie Calculation*: Formula type dictates caloric density of the formula (i.e., standard polymeric formula is 1.0 kcal/milliliter (mL) of formula). Required kcal/day for a patient should be calculated using standard equations, indirect calorimetry, or approximation based on body weight (i.e., 25–35 kcal/kg of body weight/day). The amount of daily kcal needed is divided by a formula's caloric

density to determine the number of milliliters to be given per day (i.e., if 2000 kcal/day are needed and a standard polymeric formula is used which delivers 1.0 kcal/mL, the patient would need 2000 mL/day).

2. *Protein Calculation:* Total protein delivered/day is also important and is determined by calculating daily formula provision in mL by grams of protein/L found in the formula (i.e., if 2000 mL/day of formula is given and 1 L of formula provides 44 g of protein, 88 g of protein are delivered to the patient/day). Overall protein needs are calculated based on underlying condition and total body weight; on average, patients require 1–2 g protein/kg body weight/day (higher amounts in states of critical illness).
3. *Fluid Calculation*: To determine the total amount of fluid delivered by the formula in mL/day, the percent water of the formula is multiplied by the daily formula provision in mL. Additional fluid is often needed to meet overall daily fluid goal (i.e., if 2000 mL formula is delivered that is 84% water, 1680 mL of water is provided in the formula. If the patient requires 2200 mL of water/day, an additional 520 mL of water would need to be provided on top of the formula, often given as water boluses. Fluid needs of the average patient are also calculated as 25–25 mL/kg body weight/day).
4. *Flow Rate*: To determine the rate of feeding, the total number of mL of formula to be delivered is divided by the number of hours of delivery (i.e., 2000 mL formula/day over 24 hours would require 83.3 mL/hour of formula to be given) [20, 67].

Delivery Methods

Enteral formulas can be administered by bolus method, continuous feeds, or intermittent feeds. Which method to use is determined by the type and location of access device, patient tolerance to feeding, and clinical condition of the patient [68].

Bolus infusions are generally used when patients are being fed into the stomach. Bolus feeds cannot be used in the small intestine as the lumen is smaller in caliber than the stomach and it lacks a sphincter to control the outflow of contents. Bolus feeds are the most preferable method of enteral nutrition delivery as they are physiological and take the least amount of time. These types of feeds are achieved by administering a set volume of formula at specified time intervals over a short period of time through a syringe. Up to 500 mL/formula can be given at one time (usually over 5–10 minutes), though some patients may only tolerate lower total amounts (i.e., 200–300 mL) due to abdominal discomfort, pain, and nausea. If unable to tolerate true bolus feeds, delivery can be adjusted through a gravity bag and roller clamp [69].

Continuous infusion drips are used in patients who are being fed by jejunostomy tube, who are critically ill, and/or who are at high risk for refeeding syndrome [68]. Continuous feeds require a pump to control infusion rate. Typically feeds are started at 20–50 mL/hour and advanced as tolerated to achieve the goal rate, which can be as high as 120 mL/hour [70]. An intermittent infusion method uses gravity or pump delivery. This is popular for home enteral feeding. Approximately 1.5–2 liters of feeding can be delivered over an 8–16 hours period overnight [71]. A meta-analysis of 14 trials looking at continuous and intermittent feeding in critically ill patients showed that continuous feeding was associated with lower overall incidence of feeding intolerance, especially in high gastric volume and aspiration [72].

Complications

Enteral nutrition is a very safe modality. However, complications can occur due to the equipment used or conditions associated with feeding. These complications can be classified as minor or major [73]. Although there is low procedure-related mortality in most studies, the mortality rate may increase in patients with underlying comorbidities. A thorough evaluation of the patient must take place before starting on enteral nutrition, and frequent follows-ups are recommended to assess for complications [74].

Gastrointestinal

Nausea and vomiting occur in approximately 7–26% of patients who receive enteral nutrition [75]. Vomiting can increase risk of aspiration. Delayed gastric emptying is one of the most common causes of nausea and vomiting and is common in hospitalized patients. Infusing large-volume feeds in one setting may also be implicated. When delayed gastric emptying is suspected, switching to a low-fat and/or isotonic formula, administering at room temperature and at reduced rate of infusion, changing to infusion from bolus, and adding a prokinetic agent such as metoclopramide or erythromycin can be considered [76, 77].

Gastric residual volumes (GRVs) have been used to assess tolerance to enteral feeding. However, elevated GRVs do not always correlate with intolerance. Some studies in critically ill patients do report that high GRVs can be an early marker of upper digestive intolerance, which can lead to higher incidence of nosocomial pneumonia, longer ICU stays, and higher ICU mortality [78]. These studies, however, have been criticized as there are multiple confounders affecting GRV. First, there are no standardized methods for checking GRVs. Second, several factors can affect GRV measurement, such as the type and inner diameter of a feeding tube, the position of the feeding ports in the stomach, and the position of the patient's body. For example, if the end of an enteric tube is near the gastroesophageal junction, less fluid will be suctioned than a deeper positioned tube. Additionally, GRVs obtained from larger-diameter (14 and 18 Fr) sump tubes are noted to be approximately 1.2–1.7 times greater than those taken from smaller-diameter (10 Fr) tube. For these reasons, GRVs are often thought to have less clinical relevance than other indicators [79]. There is a Cochrane review currently under process to investigate the clinical efficacy and safety of monitoring GRV during enteral nutrition to continue to answer these questions [80]. As of now, ASPEN recommends against the use of GRV to assess enteral nutrition intolerance.

Alternative strategies to monitor critically ill patients receiving enteral nutrition include careful daily physical examinations, review of available abdominal radiologic films, and evaluation of clinical risk factors for aspiration. GRVs in the range of 200–500 mL may raise concern and lead to the implementation of measures to reduce risk of aspiration but should not be used alone for determining the need to stop enteral nutrition in the absence of other Enteral nutrition (EN) enteral feeding initiationgastrointestinal signs of intolerance [81, 82].

Abdominal distension and bloating are also common symptoms with enteral nutrition delivery. These symptoms can be due to many factors including presence of Ileus, ascites due to other medical comorbidities, constipation, or obstruction. Patients should be carefully assessed by overseeing clinician daily to identify these issues. Additionally, rapid formula administration, infusion of cold formula, or initial use of fiber supplemented formula may contribute to abdominal distension. Flat and upright abdominal X-rays are most often used to diagnose causes of distention. Injection of small amount of contrast material into the feeding tube, with observation of intestinal anatomy and motility under fluoroscopy or CT scan, can also provide a clear picture of the clinical situation. If no obstruction is seen, enteral nutrition may be continued with changes in delivery method as previously discussed.

Diarrhea

Diarrhea is one of the most common reported side effects of enteral nutrition. Normal water content of stools is about 100–200 mL/day. Diarrhea has been defined as >500 mL stool output every 24 hours, or more than three stools per day for at least 2 consecutive days [83]. Most formulas are of 1 kcal/mL strength, are lactose free, isotonic and not excessively high in fat so less likely to cause diarrhea, thus alternative causes of diarrhea should be identified before changing formula type. These include enteric infections and medications. Infusion of hypertonic enteral feeding products at a very high rate or by bolus in small bowel can induce diarrhea and should be considered in these select patients. In such cases, changing the formula to isotonic may be beneficial.

If the diarrhea is clinically significant and no other cause is identified, changing formula type can be considered [84]. Addition of supplemental soluble fiber or changing the formula to one with added fiber has been shown to help with diarrhea [85]. Addition of probiotics has also been investigated; however, studies are inconclusive and systemic review analysis questioned safety, so this approach is not currently recommended in guidelines [86–88].

Constipation

Common causes of constipation include dehydration and inadequate or fiber intake (as fiber reduced colonic transit time). Stool softeners, laxatives, and enemas can be used to alleviate constipation. Generally chronic use of stimulant laxatives is not recommend as this may result in tachyphylaxis.

A summary of enteral tube complications can be found in Table 18.1. One of the more common complications is buried bumper syndrome, which occurs when the internal gastric bumper migrates through the gastric wall. The tube should be adjusted and/or removed as soon as the diagnosis is made, as grave complications such as perforation of the stomach, peritonitis, and death may occur without appropriate management [89, 90]. The tube can be removed endoscopically, surgically, or at bedside by pulling it out directly if it was placed >30 days prior to the complication developing [91]. Buried bumper syndrome can be avoided by regular checking of the PEG tube position and leaving a small distance between the external bumper and the patient's skin.

Skin care is crucial for maintenance of enteral tubes and prevention of infection, both nasal and percutaneous. Patients with nasal tubes can have skin damage due to adhesives and tape products. To prevent pressure necrosis, repositioning nasal tubes is helpful. The skin around the percutaneous tubes should also be washed with mild soap and water and dried thoroughly. Routine hydrogen peroxide and antibiotic creams are not recommended. Zinc oxide ointment can be used locally for irritation from leakage of stomach acid. Dressings around the tube should be placed without excessive tension to prevent infection and buried bumper syndrome.

Table 18.1 Complications of enteral feeding tubes

Type of access	Tube-related complications
Short-term access	1. Nasal mucosal damage and ulceration 2. Discomfort 3. Gastritis, gastric bleeding 4. GI perforation 5. Pulmonary abscess 6. Pneumothorax 7. Aspiration pneumonia 8. Sinusitis 9. Clogging
Long-term access	1. Peritonitis 2. Necrotizing fasciitis 3. Buried bumper 4. Wound infection 5. Peristomal leakage 6. Bleeding 7. Gastric outlet obstruction 8. Inadvertent tube removal

Clogging of enteral tubes is common due to accumulation of formulas or pills. Flushing of tubes with water before and after feedings and medications is recommended to help prevent clogging. There are data on the use of pancreatic enzymes to prevent clogging, often in combination with other substrates [92]. For example, pancreatic enzymes with bicarbonate and 10 mL of warm water can help unclog tubes [93]. It is important to avoid using cytology brushes to clean out tubes, given the risk of perforation.

The development of hyper-granulation tissue around percutaneous enteral access is common. Factors such as friction from a poorly secured tube and excess moisture due to fluid leakage causing skin breakdown at the exit site can lead to granulation tissue development. Application of barrier creams may help with friction. Other treatment options include topical antimicrobials, low-dose steroid creams, cauterization via silver nitrate, and surgical removal with varying efficacy [94].

Metabolic

Electrolyte abnormalities can happen in patients receiving enteral feeding, most commonly due to dehydration or overhydration. Refeeding syndrome is one of the more serious metabolic complications and usually occurs in patients who were previously malnourished. With refeeding syndrome, decrements in electrolytes may occur in a matter of hours and may lead to arrythmias, respiratory and cardiac failure, aspiration, and even death. Clinicians should review the labs of malnourished patients before initiation of enteral feeding, looking for underlying electrolyte disturbances including hypophosphatemia, hypokalemia, or hypomagnesemia. Such patients should be well resuscitated prior to initiation of feeding and should be monitored with frequent electrolyte monitoring for first few days until stable. Furthermore, feeding should be advanced slowly and not exceed 15–20 kcal/kg of body weight/day in high-risk patients until clinically stable [95].

Aspiration

Aspiration of enteral feeding formula is a serious complication that can lead to pneumonitis, pneumonia, atelectasis, empyema, acute lung injury, acute respiratory distress syndrome, and even death. Studies have looked into aspiration events in critically ill patients using tracheal secretions tested either for pepsin (enzyme in gastric fluid) or yellow microscopic beads added to the enteral formula. These studies have reported a 22–31% presence of gastric contents in tracheal aspirates, a number that was highest in patients with low back rest elevation, gastric feeding, and gastroesophageal reflux disease [96]. The most significant independent risk factors for pneumonia were aspiration, use of paralytic agents, a high sedation level, and tube mispositioning including dislodgement when transporting within the hospital [97]. In terms of protective factors, head of bed elevation to 30°–45° has been found to reduce incidence of pneumonia from 23% to 5% [98]. Additionally, lower levels of sedation, which allows for a stronger cough/gag reflux, have also been found to be protective [97, 99].

Use of prokinetic agents such as erythromycin or metoclopramide has resulted in little change in clinical outcomes for ICU patients in terms of aspiration events. A total of 8 randomized controlled trials using metoclopramide and 1 trial combining erythromycin with metoclopramide were reviewed in a meta-analysis that reported no difference in terms of mortality or infection with the use of prokinetic agents [100–102]. Combination therapy with erythromycin and metoclopramide did demonstrate improved GRVs allowing for greater feeding success; however, neither hospital length of stay (LOS) nor mortality was improved. Both agents may have serious side effects including QTc prolongation that can lead to fatal arrhythmias. Additionally, metoclopramide has a black box warning for irreversible neurotoxicity (i.e., tardive dyskinesia), seen more frequently in the elderly. Such agents should therefore be used with caution [103]. Changing the level of infusion of enteral nutrition from the stomach to the small bowel has been shown to reduce the incidence of regurgitation, aspiration, and pneumonia [104, 105].

Head and Neck Tumor Seeding

A rare complication of enteral nutrition access placement in patients with head and neck cancers is tumor seeding. It is believed that seeding occurs during the "pull" or "push" method when the tube is in contact with the oropharyngeal cancer during insertion. The actual risk of this complication is unknown, with some studies suggesting this is related to hematogenous or lymphatic spread of cancer cells to a susceptible site and not from tube placement methods [106, 107].

Conclusion

If nutritional needs cannot be met through oral intake alone due to intolerance or contraindication, enteral nutrition support may be needed and is the preferred method of nutrition delivery in the presence of a functional gut. Access can be obtained for short- or long-term care, and recognizing appropriate patients, calculating needs, and managing complications are vital to success of enteral support.

References

1. Magnotti L, Deitch E. Mechanics and significance of gut barrier function and failure. Clin Nutr. 2005:23–31.
2. Kudsk KA. Current aspects of mucosal immunology and its influence by nutrition. Am J Surg. 2002;183(4):390–8.
3. Kang W, Kudsk KA. Is there evidence that the gut contributes to mucosal immunity in humans? JPEN J Parenter Enteral Nutr. 2007;31(3):246–58.

4. Sampson EL, Candy B, Jones L. Enteral tube feeding for older people with advanced dementia. Cochrane Database Syst Rev. 2009;2009(2):Cd007209.
5. McClave SA, et al. Guidelines for the provision and assessment of nutrition support therapy in the adult critically ill patient: Society of Critical Care Medicine (SCCM) and American Society for Parenteral and Enteral Nutrition (A.S.P.E.N.). JPEN J Parenter Enteral Nutr. 2016;40(2):159–211.
6. Artinian V, Krayem H, DiGiovine B. Effects of early enteral feeding on the outcome of critically ill mechanically ventilated medical patients. Chest. 2006;129(4):960–7.
7. Heyland DK, et al. Canadian clinical practice guidelines for nutrition support in mechanically ventilated, critically ill adult patients. JPEN J Parenter Enteral Nutr. 2003;27(5):355–73.
8. Young AM, et al. Malnutrition screening tools: comparison against two validated nutrition assessment methods in older medical inpatients. Nutrition. 2013;29(1):101–6.
9. Keller U. Nutritional laboratory markers in malnutrition. J Clin Med. 2019;8(6):775.
10. American Gastroenterological Association Medical Position Statement: guidelines for the use of enteral nutrition. Gastroenterology. 1995;108(4):1280–1.
11. Metheny N. Minimizing respiratory complications of nasoenteric tube feedings: state of the science. Heart Lung. 1993;22(3):213–23.
12. Baskin WN. Acute complications associated with bedside placement of feeding tubes. Nutr Clin Pract. 2006;21(1):40–55.
13. Metheny NA, Meert KL. Monitoring feeding tube placement. Nutr Clin Pract. 2004;19(5):487–95.
14. Meguid M, Eldar S, Wahba A. The delivery of nutritional support. A potpourri of new devices and methods. Cancer. 1985;55:279–89.
15. Metheny NA, Titler MG. Assessing placement of feeding tubes. Am J Nurs. 2001;101(5):36–45; quiz 45-6.
16. Given MF, Hanson JJ, Lee MJ. Interventional radiology techniques for provision of enteral feeding. Cardiovasc Intervent Radiol. 2005;28(6):692–703.
17. Stiegmann GV, et al. Endoscopic versus operative gastrostomy: final results of a prospective randomized trial. Gastrointest Endosc. 1990;36(1):1–5.
18. Wollman B, et al. Radiologic, endoscopic, and surgical gastrostomy: an institutional evaluation and meta-analysis of the literature. Radiology. 1995;197(3):699–704.
19. Cappell MS. Risk factors and risk reduction of malignant seeding of the percutaneous endoscopic gastrostomy track from pharyngoesophageal malignancy: a review of all 44 known reported cases. Am J Gastroenterol. 2007;102(6):1307–11.
20. Bankhead R, et al. Enteral nutrition practice recommendations. JPEN J Parenter Enteral Nutr. 2009;33(2):122–67.
21. Windsor AC, et al. Compared with parenteral nutrition, enteral feeding attenuates the acute phase response and improves disease severity in acute pancreatitis. Gut. 1998;42(3):431–5.
22. Bach AC, Babayan VK. Medium-chain triglycerides: an update. Am J Clin Nutr. 1982;36(5):950–62.
23. Worthington ML, Cresci G. Immune-modulating formulas: who wins the meta-analysis race? Nutr Clin Pract. 2011;26(6):650–5.
24. Souba WW, Herskowitz K, Plumley DA. Lung glutamine metabolism. JPEN J Parenter Enteral Nutr. 1990;14(4 Suppl):68s–70s.
25. Smith RJ, Wilmore DW. Glutamine nutrition and requirements. JPEN J Parenter Enteral Nutr. 1990;14(4 Suppl):94s–9s.
26. Spapen H, et al. Soluble fiber reduces the incidence of diarrhea in septic patients receiving total enteral nutrition: a prospective, double-blind, randomized, and controlled trial. Clin Nutr. 2001;20(4):301–5.
27. Slavin JL, et al. A review of the role of soluble fiber in health with specific reference to wheat dextrin. J Int Med Res. 2009;37(1):1–17.
28. Scaife CL, Saffle JR, Morris SE. Intestinal obstruction secondary to enteral feedings in burn trauma patients. J Trauma. 1999;47(5):859–63.
29. Berner Y, et al. Vitamin plasma levels in long-term enteral feeding patients. JPEN J Parenter Enteral Nutr. 1989;13(5):525–8.
30. Russell MK, Charney P. Is there a role for specialized enteral nutrition in the intensive care unit? Nutr Clin Pract. 2002;17(3):156–68.
31. Gîlcă-Blanariu G-E, et al. New insights into the role of trace elements in IBD. Biomed Res Int. 2018;2018:1813047.
32. Kang JH, Baik HW, Chung H-K. Trace element deficiencies in long-term tube fed patients. e-SPEN J. 2014;9(2):e63–8.
33. Lord LM, Lipp J, Stull S. Adult tube feeding formulas. Medsurg Nurs. 1996;5(6):407–19; quiz 420-1.
34. Marathe PH, Gao HX, Close KL. American Diabetes Association standards of medical care in diabetes 2017. J Diabetes. 2017;9(4):320–4.
35. Pohl M, et al. Glycaemic control in type II diabetic tube-fed patients with a new enteral formula low in carbohydrates and high in monounsaturated fatty acids: a randomised controlled trial. Eur J Clin Nutr. 2005;59(11):1221–32.
36. Elia M, et al. Enteral nutritional support and use of diabetes-specific formulas for patients with diabetes: a systematic review and meta-analysis. Diabetes Care. 2005;28(9):2267–79.
37. Gervasio JM, Garmon WP, Holowatyj M. Nutrition support in acute kidney injury. Nutr Clin Pract. 2011;26(4):374–81.
38. Zha Y, Qian Q. Protein nutrition and malnutrition in CKD and ESRD. Nutrients. 2017;9(3):208.
39. Stratton RJ, et al. Multinutrient oral supplements and tube feeding in maintenance dialysis: a systematic review and meta-analysis. Am J Kidney Dis. 2005;46(3):387–405.
40. Anker SD, et al. ESPEN guidelines on enteral nutrition: cardiology and pulmonology. Clin Nutr. 2006;25(2):311–8.

41. Kirvelä O, et al. Metabolism in the intensive care unit. Baillière's Clin Anaesthesiol. 1989;3(2):423–46.
42. Covelli HD, et al. Respiratory failure precipitated by high carbohydrate loads. Ann Intern Med. 1981;95(5):579–81.
43. Kreymann KG, et al. ESPEN guidelines on enteral nutrition: intensive care. Clin Nutr. 2006;25(2):210–23.
44. Hegazi RA, Wischmeyer PE. Clinical review: optimizing enteral nutrition for critically ill patients--a simple data-driven formula. Crit Care. 2011;15(6):234.
45. Pontes-Arruda A, et al. The use of an inflammation-modulating diet in patients with acute lung injury or acute respiratory distress syndrome: a meta-analysis of outcome data. JPEN J Parenter Enteral Nutr. 2008;32(6):596–605.
46. Pontes-Arruda A, et al. Enteral nutrition with eicosapentaenoic acid, γ-linolenic acid and antioxidants in the early treatment of sepsis: results from a multicenter, prospective, randomized, double-blinded, controlled study: the INTERSEPT study. Crit Care. 2011;15(3):R144.
47. Rice TW, et al. Enteral omega-3 fatty acid, gamma-linolenic acid, and antioxidant supplementation in acute lung injury. JAMA. 2011;306(14):1574–81.
48. Li C, et al. Enteral immunomodulatory diet (Omega-3 fatty acid, γ-linolenic acid and antioxidant supplementation) for acute lung injury and acute respiratory distress syndrome: an updated systematic review and meta-analysis. Nutrients. 2015;7(7):5572–85.
49. Saez de la Fuente I, et al. Enteral nutrition in patients receiving mechanical ventilation in a prone position. JPEN J Parenter Enteral Nutr. 2016;40(2):250–5.
50. Thibault R, et al. Nutrition of the COVID-19 patient in the intensive care unit (ICU): a practical guidance. Crit Care. 2020;24(1):447.
51. Kallet RH. The vexing problem of ventilator-associated pneumonia: observations on pathophysiology, public policy, and clinical science. Respir Care. 2015;60(10):1495–508.
52. Barazzoni R, et al. ESPEN expert statements and practical guidance for nutritional management of individuals with SARS-CoV-2 infection. Clin Nutr. 2020;39(6):1631–8.
53. Martindale R, et al. Nutrition therapy in critically ill patients with coronavirus disease 2019. JPEN J Parenter Enteral Nutr. 2020;44(7):1174–84.
54. Ridley EJ, et al. Nutrition therapy in adult patients receiving extracorporeal membrane oxygenation: a prospective, multicentre, observational study. Crit Care Resusc. 2015;17(3):183–9.
55. Bear DE, Smith E, Barrett NA. Nutrition support in adult patients receiving extracorporeal membrane oxygenation. Nutr Clin Pract. 2018;33(6):738–46.
56. Nguyen GC, Munsell M, Harris ML. Nationwide prevalence and prognostic significance of clinically diagnosable protein-calorie malnutrition in hospitalized inflammatory bowel disease patients. Inflamm Bowel Dis. 2008;14(8):1105–11.
57. Lochs H, et al. ESPEN guidelines on enteral nutrition: gastroenterology. Clin Nutr. 2006;25(2):260–74.
58. Matsui T, Sakurai T, Yao T. Nutritional therapy for Crohn's disease in Japan. J Gastroenterol. 2005;40 Suppl 16:25–31.
59. Akobeng AK, Thomas AG. Enteral nutrition for maintenance of remission in Crohn's disease. Cochrane Database Syst Rev. 2007;3:Cd005984.
60. Forbes A, et al. ESPEN guideline: clinical nutrition in inflammatory bowel disease. Clin Nutr. 2017;36(2):321–47.
61. Sanaka MR, Ong JP, Mullen KD. Challenges of designing hepatic encephalopathy treatment trials. Hepatology. 2003;38(2):527–8.
62. Bémeur C, Desjardins P, Butterworth RF. Role of nutrition in the management of hepatic encephalopathy in end-stage liver failure. J Nutr Metab. 2010;2010:489823.
63. Marik PE, Zaloga GP. Immunonutrition in critically ill patients: a systematic review and analysis of the literature. Intensive Care Med. 2008;34(11):1980–90.
64. Marik PE, Zaloga GP. Immunonutrition in high-risk surgical patients: a systematic review and analysis of the literature. JPEN J Parenter Enteral Nutr. 2010;34(4):378–86.
65. Drover JW, et al. Perioperative use of arginine-supplemented diets: a systematic review of the evidence. J Am Coll Surg. 2011;212(3):385–99, 399.e1.
66. Cho JM, et al. Effect of immune-enhancing enteral nutrition formula enriched with plant-derived n-3 fatty acids on natural killer cell activity in rehabilitation patients. Nutr Res Pract. 2019;13(5):384–92.
67. Boullata JI, et al. ASPEN safe practices for enteral nutrition therapy [formula: see text]. JPEN J Parenter Enteral Nutr. 2017;41(1):15–103.
68. Ichimaru S. Methods of enteral nutrition administration in critically ill patients: continuous, cyclic, intermittent, and bolus feeding. Nutr Clin Pract. 2018;33(6):790–5.
69. Bankhead R, et al. A.S.P.E.N. enteral nutrition practice recommendations. JPEN J Parenter Enteral Nutr. 2009;33:122–67.
70. White H, King L. Enteral feeding pumps: efficacy, safety, and patient acceptability. Med Devices (Auckland, NZ). 2014;7:291–8.
71. Adeyinka A, Rouster AS, Valentine M. Enteric feedings. In: StatPearls. 2020, StatPearls Publishing. Copyright © 2020, StatPearls Publishing LLC.: Treasure Island (FL).
72. Ma Y, et al. Intermittent versus continuous enteral nutrition on feeding intolerance in critically ill adults: a meta-analysis of randomized controlled trials. Int J Nurs Stud. 2021;113:103783.
73. Rahnemai-Azar AA, et al. Percutaneous endoscopic gastrostomy: indications, technique, complications and management. World J Gastroenterol. 2014;20(24):7739–51.
74. Zopf Y, et al. Predictive factors of mortality after PEG insertion. J Parenter Enteral Nutr. 2011;35(1):50–5.

75. Montejo JC, et al. Multicenter, prospective, randomized, single-blind study comparing the efficacy and gastrointestinal complications of early jejunal feeding with early gastric feeding in critically ill patients. Crit Care Med. 2002;30(4):796–800.
76. Ali T, et al. Gastroparesis. South Med J. 2007:281+.
77. Taylor SJ, Manara AR, Brown J. Treating delayed gastric emptying in critical illness. J Parenter Enteral Nutr. 2010;34(3):289–94.
78. Mentec H, et al. Upper digestive intolerance during enteral nutrition in critically ill patients: frequency, risk factors, and complications. Crit Care Med. 2001;29(10):1955–61.
79. Metheny NA, et al. Gastric residual volume and aspiration in critically ill patients receiving gastric feedings. Am J Crit Care. 2008;17(6):512–9; quiz 520.
80. Yasuda H, et al. Monitoring of gastric residual volume during enteral nutrition. Cochrane Database Syst Rev. 2019;(5).
81. Pinilla JC, et al. Comparison of gastrointestinal tolerance to two enteral feeding protocols in critically ill patients: a prospective, randomized controlled trial. JPEN J Parenter Enteral Nutr. 2001;25(2):81–6.
82. Montejo JC, et al. Gastric residual volume during enteral nutrition in ICU patients: the REGANE study. Intensive Care Med. 2010;36(8):1386–93.
83. Mobarhan S, DeMeo M. Diarrhea induced by enteral feeding. Nutr Rev. 1995;53(3):67–70.
84. Edes TE, Walk BE, Austin JL. Diarrhea in tube-fed patients: feeding formula not necessarily the cause. Am J Med. 1990;88(2):91–3.
85. McClave SA, et al. Guidelines for the provision and assessment of nutrition support therapy in the adult critically ill patient: Society of Critical Care Medicine (SCCM) and American Society for Parenteral and Enteral Nutrition (A.S.P.E.N.). JPEN J Parenter Enteral Nutr. 2009;33(3):277–316.
86. Kamarul Zaman M, et al. Fiber and prebiotic supplementation in enteral nutrition: a systematic review and meta-analysis. World J Gastroenterol. 2015;21(17):5372–81.
87. Zhao R, et al. Effects of fiber and probiotics on diarrhea associated with enteral nutrition in gastric cancer patients: A prospective randomized and controlled trial. Medicine. 2017;96(43):e8418.
88. Whelan K, Myers CE. Safety of probiotics in patients receiving nutritional support: a systematic review of case reports, randomized controlled trials, and nonrandomized trials. Am J Clin Nutr. 2010;91(3):687–703.
89. Anagnostopoulos GK, Kostopoulos P, Arvanitidis DM. Buried bumper syndrome with a fatal outcome, presenting early as gastrointestinal bleeding after percutaneous endoscopic gastrostomy placement. J Postgrad Med. 2003;49(4):325–7.
90. Ma MM, et al. The buried gastrostomy bumper syndrome: prevention and endoscopic approaches to removal. Gastrointest Endosc. 1995;41(5):505–8.
91. Erkan G, et al. The advantage of retrieval PEG tubes in patients with buried bumper syndrome - a case report. Turk J Gastroenterol. 2012;23(6):773–5.
92. Sriram K, et al. Prophylactic locking of enteral feeding tubes with pancreatic enzymes. JPEN J Parenter Enteral Nutr. 1997;21(6):353–6.
93. Marcuard SP, et al. Clearing obstructed feeding tubes. JPEN J Parenter Enteral Nutr. 1989;13(1): 81–3. https://doi.org/10.1177/014860718901300181.
94. Borkowski S. G tube care: managing hypergranulation tissue. Nursing. 2005;35(8):24.
95. da Silva JSV, et al. ASPEN consensus recommendations for refeeding syndrome. Nutr Clin Pract. 2020;35(2):178–95.
96. Metheny NA, et al. Tracheobronchial aspiration of gastric contents in critically ill tube-fed patients: frequency, outcomes, and risk factors. Crit Care Med. 2006;34(4):1007–15.
97. Kollef MH, et al. Patient transport from intensive care increases the risk of developing ventilator-associated pneumonia. Chest. 1997;112(3):765–73.
98. Drakulovic MB, et al. Supine body position as a risk factor for nosocomial pneumonia in mechanically ventilated patients: a randomised trial. Lancet. 1999;354(9193):1851–8.
99. McClave SA, et al. North American summit on aspiration in the critically ill patient: consensus statement. JPEN J Parenter Enteral Nutr. 2002;26(6 Suppl):S80–5.
100. Chapman MJ, et al. Erythromycin improves gastric emptying in critically ill patients intolerant of nasogastric feeding. Crit Care Med. 2000;28(7):2334–7.
101. Yavagal DR, Karnad DR, Oak JL. Metoclopramide for preventing pneumonia in critically ill patients receiving enteral tube feeding: a randomized controlled trial. Crit Care Med. 2000;28(5):1408–11.
102. MacLaren R, et al. Erythromycin vs metoclopramide for facilitating gastric emptying and tolerance to intragastric nutrition in critically ill patients. JPEN J Parenter Enteral Nutr. 2008;32(4):412–9.
103. Al-Khatib SM, et al. What clinicians should know about the QT interval. JAMA. 2003;289(16):2120–7.
104. Lien HC, Chang CS, Chen GH. Can percutaneous endoscopic jejunostomy prevent gastroesophageal reflux in patients with preexisting esophagitis? Am J Gastroenterol. 2000;95(12):3439–43.
105. Heyland DK, et al. Effect of postpyloric feeding on gastroesophageal regurgitation and pulmonary microaspiration: results of a randomized controlled trial. Crit Care Med. 2001;29(8):1495–501.
106. Brown MC. Cancer metastasis at percutaneous endoscopic gastrostomy stomata is related to the hematogenous or lymphatic spread of circulating tumor cells. Am J Gastroenterol. 2000;95(11):3288–91.
107. Strodel WE, Kenady DE, Zweng TN. Avoiding stoma seeding in head and neck cancer patients. Surg Endosc. 1995;9(10):1142–3.

Correction to: Endoscopic Management of Obesity

Carolyn Newberry, Janese Laster,
and Octavia Pickett-Blakely

Correction to:
Chapter 15 in: C. Newberry et al. (eds.), *Nutrition, Weight, and Digestive Health*, https://doi.org/10.1007/978-3-030-94953-2_15

The incorrect current affiliation of Dr. Janese Laster has been changed to:

Janese Laster, MD
Gastroenterology, Obesity Medicine, Nutrition & Bariatric Endoscopist
Gut Theory Total Digestive Care
George Washington University Hospital
1712 N St NW, Suite 101
Washington, DC 20036
jlaster@guttheoryhealth.com

The updated version of this chapter can be found at
https://doi.org/10.1007/978-3-030-94953-2_15
https://doi.org/10.1007/978-3-030-94953-2

C. Newberry et al. (eds.), *Nutrition, Weight, and Digestive Health*,
https://doi.org/10.1007/978-3-030-94953-2_19

Index

C. Newberry et al. (eds.), *Nutrition, Weight, and Digestive Health*,
https://doi.org/10.1007/978-3-030-94953-2

H

I

W

Z

MIX
Papier aus verantwortungsvollen Quellen
Paper from responsible sources
FSC® C105338

If you have any concerns about our products,
you can contact us on
ProductSafety@springernature.com

In case Publisher is established outside the EU,
the EU authorized representative is:
Springer Nature Customer Service Center GmbH
Europaplatz 3, 69115 Heidelberg, Germany

Printed by Libri Plureos GmbH
in Hamburg, Germany